BRIEF INTERVENTIONS FOR ADOLESCENT ALCOHOL AND SUBSTANCE ABUSE

Also Available

**The Tobacco Dependence Treatment Handbook:
A Guide to Best Practices**
*David B. Abrams, Raymond Niaura, Richard A. Brown,
Karen M. Emmons, Michael G. Goldstein, and Peter M. Monti*

Brief Interventions for Adolescent Alcohol and Substance Abuse

Edited by
PETER M. MONTI
SUZANNE M. COLBY
TRACY O'LEARY TEVYAW

THE GUILFORD PRESS
New York   London

The authors have checked with sources believed to be reliable in their efforts to provide
information that is complete and generally in accord with the standards of practice
that are accepted at the time of publication. However, in view of the possibility of
human error or changes in behavioral, mental health, or medical sciences, neither the
authors, nor the editors and publisher, nor any other party who has been involved in
the preparation or publication of this work warrants that the information contained
herein is in every respect accurate or complete, and they are not responsible for any
errors or omissions or the results obtained from the use of such information. Readers
are encouraged to confirm the information contained in this book with other sources.

Library of Congress Cataloging-in-Publication Data

Names: Monti, Peter M., editor. | Colby, Suzanne M., editor. | Tevyaw, Tracy
   O'Leary, editor.
Title: Brief interventions for adolescent alcohol and substance abuse /
   edited by Peter M. Monti, Suzanne M. Colby, Tracy O'Leary Tevyaw.
Description: New York : The Guilford Press, [2018] | Includes bibliographical
   references and index.
Identifiers: LCCN 2018003342 | ISBN 9781462535002 (hardback)
Subjects: LCSH: Teenagers—Substance use. | Teenagers—Alcohol use. |
   Substance abuse—Prevention. | Alcoholism—Prevention. | Brief
   psychotherapy for teenagers. | BISAC: PSYCHOLOGY / Psychopathology /
   Addiction. | MEDICAL / Psychiatry / Child & Adolescent. | SOCIAL
SCIENCE /
   Social Work. | PSYCHOLOGY / Psychotherapy / Child & Adolescent.
Classification: LCC RJ506.D78 B75 2018 | DDC 618.9286—dc23
LC record available at *https://lccn.loc.gov/2018003342*

About the Editors

Peter M. Monti, PhD, is Donald G. Millar Distinguished Professor of Alcohol and Addiction Studies and Director of the Center for Alcohol and Addiction Studies at Brown University, where he also serves as Professor of Behavioral and Social Sciences and of Psychiatry and Human Behavior. He is a past president of the Research Society on Alcoholism (RSA) and a recipient of the Marlatt Mentorship Award and Distinguished Researcher Award from the RSA, the Lifetime Achievement Award from the Addictive Behaviors Special Interest Group of the Association for Behavioral and Cognitive Therapies, and the Distinguished Career Contributions to Education and Training Award from Division 50 (Society of Addiction Psychology) of the American Psychological Association. Dr. Monti is a recognized leader in understanding the biobehavioral mechanisms that underlie addictive behavior and its prevention and treatment. He has published several books and approximately 400 papers and chapters.

Suzanne M. Colby, PhD, is Professor of Psychiatry and Human Behavior and Associate Director of the Center for Alcohol and Addiction Studies at Brown University. She is a senior editor of the journal *Addiction* and a Fellow of Divisions 28 (Psychopharmacology and Substance Abuse) and 50 (Society of Addiction Psychology) of the American Psychological Association. She is president-elect of the Society for Research on Nicotine & Tobacco (SRNT) and Chair of SRNT's Adolescent Research Network. Dr. Colby's research focuses on the development of innovative brief alcohol and other substance use interventions, particularly for underserved adolescents and young adults. She has conducted numerous randomized controlled trials of brief motivational interventions for adolescent smoking cessation, along with a series of laboratory-based studies of adolescent nicotine dependence and withdrawal.

Tracy O'Leary Tevyaw, PhD, is Clinical Associate Professor of Psychiatry and Human Behavior at Brown University and Chief Psychologist and Director of Psychology Training at Providence VA Medical Center. She leads the Providence VA's Primary Care Behavioral Health program and is a primary supervisor in the Brown University Clinical Psychology Training Consortium. Dr. Tevyaw has served as principal investigator/co-investigator of randomized clinical trials examining brief interventions for reducing substance use in adolescents and college students. Her research areas include brief interventions, substance use disorders, anxiety disorders, integrated primary care, and shared medical appointments.

Contributors

Sara J. Becker, PhD, Center for Alcohol and Addiction Studies, Brown University School of Public Health, Providence, Rhode Island

Brandon Bergman, PhD, Recovery Research Institute, Boston, Massachusetts

Andria M. Botzet, MA, Department of Psychiatry, University of Minnesota, Minneapolis, Minnesota

Jordan M. Braciszewski, PhD, Center for Health Policy and Health Services Research, Henry Ford Health System, Detroit, Michigan

Suzanne M. Colby, PhD, Center for Alcohol and Addiction Studies and Department of Psychiatry and Human Behavior, Brown University, Providence, Rhode Island

Julie Cristello, BS, Recovery Research Institute, Boston, Massachusetts

Elizabeth J. D'Amico, PhD, RAND, Santa Monica, California

Emily F. Dauria, PhD, MPH, Department of Psychiatry and Weill Institute for Neurosciences, University of California, San Francisco, San Francisco, California

Heather A. Davis, MS, Department of Psychology, University of Kentucky, Lexington, Kentucky

Christianne Esposito-Smythers, PhD, Department of Psychology, George Mason University, Fairfax, Virginia

Sarah W. Feldstein Ewing, PhD, Division of Child and Adolescent Psychiatry, and Adolescent Behavioral Health Clinic, Oregon Health and Science University, Portland, Oregon

Sarah Fischer, PhD, Department of Psychology, George Mason University, Fairfax, Virginia

Kristi E. Gamarel, PhD, EdM, Department of Health Behavior and Health Education, University of Michigan School of Public Health, Ann Arbor, Michigan

Staci A. Gruber, PhD, Cognitive and Clinical Neuroimaging Core and MIND Program, McLean Hospital, Belmont, Massachusetts

Judy Havlicek, PhD, MSW, School of Social Work, University of Illinois at Urbana–Champaign, Urbana, Illinois

Lynn Hernandez, PhD, Center for Alcohol and Addiction Studies and Department of Behavioral and Social Sciences, Brown University, Providence, Rhode Island

Ralph Hingson, ScD, MPH, Division of Epidemiology and Prevention Research, National Institute on Alcohol Abuse and Alcoholism, National Institutes of Health, Bethesda, Maryland

Aaron Hogue, PhD, The National Center on Addiction and Substance Abuse, New York, New York

John F. Kelly, PhD, Department of Psychiatry, Harvard Medical School, and Center for Addiction Medicine, Boston, Massachusetts

Susanne Lee, PhD, Department of Psychiatry, University of Minnesota, Minneapolis, Minnesota

Krista M. Lisdahl, PhD, Department of Psychology, University of Wisconsin–Milwaukee, Milwaukee, Wisconsin

Kyla Machell, PhD, Department of Psychiatry and Behavioral Sciences, Duke University, Durham, North Carolina

Jennifer L. Maggs, PhD, Department of Human Development and Family Studies, The Pennsylvania State University, University Park, Pennsylvania

Julie Maslowsky, PhD, Department of Kinesiology and Health Education, University of Texas at Austin, Austin, Texas

Nadine R. Mastroleo, PhD, College of Community and Public Affairs, Binghamton University, Binghamton, New York

Melissa A. McWilliams, MA, School of Education, University of North Carolina at Chapel Hill, Chapel Hill, North Carolina

Ethan H. Mereish, PhD, Department of Health Studies, American University, Washington, DC

Robert Miranda Jr., PhD, Center for Alcohol and Addiction Studies and Department of Psychiatry and Human Behavior, Brown University, Providence, Rhode Island

Peter M. Monti, PhD, Center for Alcohol and Addiction Studies and Departments of Behavioral and Social Sciences and Psychiatry and Human Behavior, Brown University, Providence, Rhode Island

Oswaldo Moreno, PhD, Counseling Psychology Program, VCU iCubed, Virginia Commonwealth University, Richmond, Virginia

Don Operario, PhD, Center for Alcohol and Addiction Studies, Brown University School of Public Health, Providence, Rhode Island

Timothy J. Ozechowski, PhD, Oregon Research Institute, Eugene, Oregon

Bethany Rallis, PhD, Department of Counseling and Psychological Services, The Pennsylvania State University, University Park, Pennsylvania

Elizabeth N. Riley, MS, Department of Psychology, University of Kentucky, Lexington, Kentucky

Kelly A. Sagar, MS, Department of Psychiatry, McLean Hospital, Belmont, Massachusetts

John Schulenberg, PhD, Institute for Social Research and Department of Psychology, University of Michigan, Ann Arbor, Michigan

Skyler Shollenbarger, PhD, Department of Neuropsychology, Henry Ford Health System, Detroit, Michigan

Gregory T. Smith, PhD, Department of Psychology, University of Kentucky, Lexington, Kentucky

Nichea S. Spillane, PhD, Department of Psychology, University of Rhode Island, Kingston, Rhode Island

Anthony Spirito, PhD, Center for Alcohol and Addiction Studies and Department of Psychiatry and Human Behavior, Brown University, Providence, Rhode Island

Tracy O'Leary Tevyaw, PhD, Center for Alcohol and Addiction Studies and Department of Psychiatry and Human Behavior, Brown University, and Providence Veterans Affairs Medical Center, Providence, Rhode Island

Marina Tolou-Shams, PhD, Department of Psychiatry and Weill Institute for Neurosciences, University of California, San Francisco, San Francisco, California

Hayley Treloar, PhD, Center for Alcohol and Addiction Studies and Department of Psychiatry and Human Behavior, Brown University, Providence, Rhode Island

Kamilla Venner, PhD, Department of Psychology, Center on Alcoholism, Substance Abuse, and Addictions, University of New Mexico, Albuquerque, New Mexico

Aaron White, PhD, Office of the Director, National Institute on Alcohol Abuse and Alcoholism, National Institutes of Health, Bethesda, Maryland

Caitlin Williams, MA, Department of Psychology, George Mason University, Fairfax, Virginia

Ken C. Winters, PhD, Oregon Research Institute, Eugene, Oregon

Robert A. Zucker, PhD, Department of Psychiatry and Addiction Research Center, University of Michigan, Ann Arbor, Michigan

Contents

PART II. CLINICAL GUIDE:
Application of Brief Interventions
in Diverse Settings and Populations

Introduction

Peter M. Monti, Suzanne M. Colby,
and Tracy O'Leary Tevyaw

Almost 20 years ago, as we embarked on *Adolescents, Alcohol, and Substance Abuse* (Monti, Colby, & O'Leary, 2001), we had two goals. The first was to make a compelling case that important developmental differences between adolescents and adults necessitate different approaches to treating substance misuse in each. The second was to rigorously support the legitimacy of embracing a harm reduction (HR) perspective when working with adolescents and young adults, and to examine the value of emerging brief motivational treatments while not negating the vital importance of intensive, long-term treatments for those with substance use disorders (SUDs).

In retrospect, that book struck an unanticipated chord in the broader community. We were humbled to learn that many of our initial readers were undergraduates and master's-level students preparing for careers as clinicians, as well as practitioners new to the field of addiction research and treatment.

In preparing this new book, we have taken to heart the feedback we received from those readers, and from other reviewers, including those who used the first book as a textbook. First, we have aimed to simplify language and avoid unnecessarily technical content, and have focused more closely on presenting a wide variety of practical applications in a much greater range of settings. We have encouraged our authors to carefully consider the special challenges involved in effectively engaging adolescents in interventions and treatment efforts. We also asked them to comment on the growing use of technology in support of interventions and encouraged them to share their personal insights gained by their experiences.

The basic structure of this new book is similar to that of the earlier work. We present a foundation of knowledge related to the etiology and developmental context of adolescent substance use in Part I, followed by a survey of clinical applications in Part II, and conclude with a summary that spells out current priorities and future directions. Throughout, we include completely revised and updated versions of chapters on some topics that were covered in the first book. Part I features two new chapters. One of these, by Lisdahl, Shollenbarger, Sagar, and Gruber, presents a comprehensive state-of-the-art review of the effects of alcohol and marijuana use on brain development. This is an area of research that has transformed the field in recent years. Part I culminates in a comprehensive description of an evidence-based approach to proactive brief interventions, adapted for adolescents, that provides a valuable foundation for the clinical application chapters that follow.

Part II features 10 completely new chapters that illustrate the promise of brief interventions in a variety of diverse contexts and populations, particularly when delivered at a teachable moment. Among the novel applications are chapters describing brief interventions with adolescents involved in the justice system (Dauria, McWilliams, & Tolou-Shams), in foster care (Braciszewski & Havlicek), in colleges (Mastroleo), using group motivational interviewing in school settings (D'Amico & Feldstein Ewing), and to facilitate participation in mutual help groups (Kelly, Cristello, & Bergman). We have also included chapters on cultural adaptions of motivational interviewing for Latino (Hernandez & Moreno), American Indian (Spillane & Venner), and LGBTQ youth (Mereish, Gamarel, & Operario). To be sure, even this broad range of chapters does not cover every population of interest. We hope the chapters provide insights into the *process* of treatment adaptation that will serve to inform similar efforts in new populations.

Part II also includes a comprehensive chapter (Miranda & Treloar) on the current consensus regarding use of pharmacotherapies for treating adolescent SUDs, along with an illustration of how brief interventions may be used to facilitate medication initiation and adherence. A complementary chapter by Esposito-Smythers, Rallis, Machell, Williams, and Fisher addresses the additional complexities inherent in treating adolescents with co-occurring substance use and psychiatric problems, including implications for assessment, diagnosis, and treatment.

Part III, prepared by adolescent substance use experts at the National Institutes of Health (Hingson & White), provides a summation and blueprint for future directions, including the potential for melding brief interventions with prevention approaches. In this introduction, we briefly discuss pertinent epidemiological trends and several overriding themes that include the stages of change model, the notion of HR, the emerging role of mechanisms of behavior change, and the elements of brief interventions.

PATTERNS AND TRENDS

Despite more than three decades of the "war on drugs," adolescent substance misuse remains a major public health problem. The nationwide survey conducted by the University of Michigan (Monitoring the Future; Miech, Johnston, O'Malley, Bachman, & Schulenberg, 2015) of the behaviors, attitudes, and values of secondary school students, college students, and young adults has been tracking alcohol and other substance use among youth for the past 40 years. That study indicates 66% of adolescents have consumed alcohol by their senior year in high school, with nearly half having done so by 10th grade (Miech et al., 2015). Clearly, alcohol remains the most popular drug for youth, with nearly one-third of 12th graders and 40% of young adults reporting recent binge drinking (five standard drinks for males and four standard drinks for females; Johnston, O'Malley, Miech, Bachman, & Schulenberg, 2015). Miech and colleagues (2015) report that the annual prevalence of any illicit drug was 15% for 8th graders, 30% for 10th graders, and 39% for 12th graders.

Findings from such national surveys have recently pointed to historical shifts toward overall decreasing levels of use (Johnston, O'Malley, Bachman, & Schulenberg, 2013). Indeed, data from Monitoring the Future (2012; Johnston, O'Malley, Miech, Bachman, & Schulenberg, 2013) indicated that prevalence of alcohol use in three grade levels (8th, 10th, and 12th) had reached historic lows. Interestingly, Miech and colleagues (2015) concluded that long-term data on alcohol use suggest that it moves much more with illicit drug use than counter to it. Nevertheless, as Wendel (2016) points out, alcohol remains the substance of choice among youth and is still used by a majority of them. He further points to the increase in use of new alcohol products, such as flavored alcohol beverages, by youth of all three grade levels, but particularly among early adolescents.

However, national trends mask high levels of heterogeneity within the adolescent population—some subgroups of youth are at greater risk for early initiation of alcohol and other substance use and negative consequences. The clinical intervention chapters constituting Part II focus on many of these groups and present prevalence data specific to each.

As Winters, Botzet, and Lee (Chapter 3, this volume) note, adolescence is a developmental period characterized by relatively high rates of SUDs. They note that in 2008, 7.6% of 12- to 17-year-olds met diagnostic criteria for one or more past-year SUD. Furthermore, the onset of drug use during adolescence increases the likelihood of developing an SUD later (Brown et al., 2008). Hingson, Heeren, and Winter (2006) found lifetime prevalence rates of alcohol use disorder to be 47% among those who started drinking at age 14 or younger versus 9% among those who started drinking at age 21 or older. As Lisdahl and colleagues (Chapter 2, this volume) discuss, earlier onset of marijuana use has also been associated with increased risk for developing a cannabis use disorder. They present converging evidence that adolescent onset of regular alcohol exposure is associated with increased risk for neurocognitive deficits, consistent with evidence presented by Volkow, Compton, and Weiss (2014), suggesting adolescent drug use not only affects cognition but may alter brain maturation.

It has long been known that the transition of students from high school to college is associated with substantial increases in alcohol use and heavy drinking (Baer, Kivlahan, & Marlatt, 1995; Borsari, Murphy, & Barnett, 2007). Excessive use extending into later adolescence and young adulthood is also a cause for concern (see Schulenberg, Maslowsky, Maggs, & Zucker, Chapter 1, this volume). College students report high rates of past-month alcohol consumption (68% consumed alcohol and 40% report having been drunk; Johnston, O'Malley, Bachman, et al., 2013). Mastroleo (Chapter 16, this volume) points out that even more concerning are rates of extremely heavy drinking within the past 2 weeks: according to Johnston, O'Malley, Bachman, et al. (2013), 37% of students had five or more drinks in a row, 13% had 10 or more, and 5% had 15 or more.

Young adult college students who binge drink are significantly more likely to experience a host of negative consequences, such as engaging in unplanned and unprotected sexual activity, sexual aggression and assault, transmission of sexual diseases, physical assaults and injuries, and motor vehicle crashes and fatalities (Hingson, Zha, & Weitzman, 2009). Furthermore, as Hingson and White (2014) point out, alcohol misuse and abuse among college-age individuals is a serious problem affecting not only those individuals but also their college campuses and social networks.

It is not uncommon to identify mental health problems in adolescents who use alcohol and/or other substances (see Esposito-Smythers et al., Chapter 7, this volume). Rates of co-occurring diagnoses range from an average of 60% among substance-using youth in community settings to 80% in inpatient psychiatric settings (Storr, Pacek, & Martins, 2012). Most often, onset of psychiatric disorders occurs prior to SUD onset (Hovens, Cantwell, & Kiriakos, 1994; Kessler et al., 1997), suggesting that adolescents who develop alcohol and other substance use problems may have a preexisting vulnerability to psychopathology, which in turn intensifies the risk of subsequent alcohol and other substance use problems (Esposito-Smythers et al., Chapter 7, this volume). However, such temporal order is not always the case, and establishing order of onset is important as it not only informs theory but frequently holds implications for treatment. As Esposito-Smythers and her colleagues illustrate, it is imperative to conduct a comprehensive assessment for comorbid psychiatric disorders when working with adolescents who have substance misuse or SUDs.

STAGES OF CHANGE

Because some of our authors refer to the stages of change model, also called the transtheoretical model (TTM) of behavior change (Prochaska, 2013), a brief introduction is warranted. Several decades ago, psychologists sought to understand how individuals successfully changed health risk behaviors on their own. What kinds of strategies did people use? What stages did they go through? What predicted success? The rationale was that if we could learn how people change their behavior, perhaps we could help others apply similar strategies and achieve success. Although early thinking on the TTM did not focus on adolescents, utility of the model for adolescents has since been widely documented and is apparent in this book.

Researchers gained early insights from studying successful self-changers. First, they realized that the dichotomous distinction between those engaging in a healthy versus an unhealthy behavior pattern (e.g., smoker vs. nonsmoker, binge vs. moderate drinker), on which we typically relied for evaluating treatment outcomes, masked some important differences within these two groups. Prospective research determined that individuals pass through a series of *stages of change* rather than shifting from user to nonuser and back again. The stages include *precontemplation*, when one does not identify a behavior as problematic and/or has no intention of changing; *contemplation*, when one begins to consider change but has no immediate plans; *preparation*, when one is ready to make a change and begins to take steps toward healthier behavior; *action*, when an individual has changed his or her behavior but is still in the early stages of maintaining that change; and *maintenance*, when one has successfully changed the behavior and maintained the change for a prolonged period of time (Prochaska & DiClemente, 1983). Progress toward successful behavior change occurs with each step forward along this continuum.

Second, researchers saw that individuals tend to use different strategies at different points. These strategies were termed *processes of change* (Prochaska, Velicer, DiClemente, & Fava, 1988), and they could be categorized into two higher-order groups: experiential processes (e.g., raising one's consciousness about the harmful effects of use), which are relied on more heavily in the earlier stages of change; and behavioral processes (e.g., rewarding oneself for not using, removing substances from one's home to avoid reminders of use), which are employed during later stages. This insight was important because it highlighted the fact that traditional treatments tended to be action oriented and therefore potentially inappropriate for those in the earliest stages. Thus, until individuals were committed to change, they were alienated from traditional interventions.

Third, researchers realized that change is a dynamic process and people undertaking change often relapse to unhealthy behaviors several times before succeeding. This knowledge enabled professionals to reframe the relapse concept from one of failure to one of progress. People can learn from relapse, using the experience to identify their high-risk situations, to discover current strategies for change that are not working, and to come up with new plans that might work better.

The TTM has been successfully applied to myriad health behaviors, including alcohol and other substance use reduction, smoking cessation, stress management, and exercise. In this book, we promote intervention approaches that appreciate the need to tailor intervention to one's readiness to change, and acknowledge that all progress toward change, even small steps, are steps in the right direction. A particular strength of these brief interventions is that the threshold for participation is low—that is, even adolescents not particularly interested in change may be willing to participate because an ultimate commitment to lifelong change is not required up front.

HARM REDUCTION

Prevention and treatment of adolescent substance use problems has been influenced by the concept of HR (Marlatt & Witkiewitz, 2002). HR is an orientation and belief system characterized by five basic principles (Marlatt, 1998). First, HR is an alternative to the moral, criminal, and disease models of substance abuse. It is more compatible with a public health perspective in that its proponents focus on reducing the harmful consequences of drug use and addiction rather than on drug use per se. Second, it accepts alternatives to total abstinence when abstinence is not a realistic goal. Marlatt (1998) described abstinence as an ideal end point along a continuum that ranges from excessively harmful to less harmful. Third, compared with a "top-down" approach promoted by drug policy makers, HR has emerged as a "bottom-up" approach (i.e., one that originates from consumers). This is consistent with motivational interviewing principles, which emphasize the personal responsibility of the individual for decisions about his or her own behavior change. Fourth, as an alternative to high-threshold approaches to services, HR promotes easier access to treatment by not requiring abstinence as a precondition. And, fifth, HR embraces compassionate pragmatism versus moralistic idealism. Psychoactive substance use occurs in all known societies, and heavy use is particularly common among young people; HR offers strategies to reduce potential harmful consequences of adolescent substance use, acknowledging that many adolescents will at least try substances (Toumbourou et al., 2007).

In adolescents, HR goals might include reducing the frequency and/or quantity of use, or delaying the age of initiation of substance use—for example, by increasing the minimum legal age requirements. Based on a systematic international review, evidence supports the use of HR strategies for saving young lives and reducing consequences of use among adolescent substance users, with effects measurable at the population level (Toumbourou et al., 2007). In contrast, zero-tolerance approaches essentially criminalize use and deny services to those unwilling or unable to abstain, potentially leading to an increase in overall harm. The brief intervention program outlined by us in Chapter 6 (Tevyaw, Spirito, Colby, & Monti) of this volume illustrates how offering a low-threshold strategy in the emergency room can help get teens to attend to their problematic drinking without turning them off. Similarly, nearly all the clinical approaches described in the following chapters are both brief and consistent with HR.

BRIEF INTERVENTIONS

In 2003, the Substance Abuse and Mental Health Services Administration (SAMHSA) inaugurated its Screening, Brief Intervention, and Referral to Treatment (SBIRT) initiative (Substance Abuse and Mental Health Services Administration, 2014). As Becker, Ozechowski, and Hogue discuss in depth (Chapter 5, this volume), SBIRT is a public health approach to early identification and intervention for at-risk alcohol and other substance use in targeted settings (see also Mitchell, Gryczynski, O'Grady, & Schwartz, 2013, for a review of SBIRT for adolescent substance use). The pillars of SBIRT include (1) using standardized assessment tools to quickly screen for risky use; (2) conducting brief interventions that include a discussion of risky use, along with feedback and advice on changing; and (3) providing referrals for brief therapy or services as warranted. The general consensus is that brief interventions consist of one to five sessions with a provider and are intended to increase motivation to change, alter, or avoid a target behavior. Most alcohol-specific brief interventions include at least one of the following: review and discussion of one's alcohol use, feedback on risks related to drinking, social norms comparisons, and coping strategies and goal setting for changing risky use (Tanner-Smith & Lipsey, 2015).

Since our first book was published in 2001, there has been a dramatic proliferation in the use of alcohol brief interventions for adolescents. For instance, in a recent meta-analysis (Tanner-Smith & Lipsey, 2015) of 185 adolescent and young adult brief intervention studies, published between 1980 and 2012, nearly 90% were published from 2000 to 2012. Results show that brief interventions result in significantly lower levels of use or alcohol-related problems with effects maintained for up to a year.

As the evidence mounts in support of brief interventions for adolescent use, and as they are increasingly disseminated and adopted in the larger community, the key question has now become not whether brief interventions work, but rather, *how* they work for different adolescents and *when* they work from a developmental perspective. We have arrived at the point where identifying mechanisms of change and active ingredients of treatment is the next step toward enhancing and refining adolescent-based brief interventions. Longabaugh and Magill (2011) have defined mechanisms of change as "behaviors or processes occurring within the patient, either during or outside treatment, that have a causal effect on subsequent changes in addictive behavior," and defined active ingredients as "those treatment elements or therapist behaviors empirically found to positively affect patient mechanisms of change or overall change in addictive behaviors" (p. 383). The field is moving away from comparing the effectiveness of one treatment against another and toward examining factors that account for the relationship between treatment and outcome—in other words, mediation. In the case of brief interventions that use motivational enhancement techniques, there has been great interest in the relationship between therapist behaviors and client change talk, and in turn, how those relationships impact outcomes (Apodaca et al., 2016; Gaume et al., 2016; see also D'Amico & Feldstein Ewing, Chapter 14, this volume).

Another likely mechanism of change in motivational interviewing and other brief interventions is ambivalence, or simultaneously wanting and not wanting to change a behavior (Feldstein Ewing, Apodaca, & Gaume, 2016). One of the major conceptual underpinnings of motivational interviewing is the exploration and resolution of ambivalence, such that the clinician assists the individual in resolving ambivalence and moving toward reasons for change. While many adults with alcohol problems report negative consequences due to their use, many adolescents do not view their use as a problem, and in fact, often report positive expectancies and experiences related to using alcohol and/ or other substances. Feldstein Ewing and colleagues (2016) suggest that for adolescents, ambivalence is not necessarily a prerequisite for positive behavior change, and that therapist behaviors, such as exploring the pros and the cons of substance use, may help spark ambivalence, which in turn could lead to teens being able to identify and embrace reasons for change.

Alternatively, from a developmental perspective, we (Monti & Monnig, 2016) propose that ambivalence may depend on other factors, such as the social learning context, one's neurocognitive development, and one's capacity for abstract thinking, self-reflection, and self-regulation. Compared with adults and children, adolescents may experience greater sensitivity to and reinforcement from certain types of feedback, such as positive peer feedback—this can be linked to increased brain activation in regions associated with action planning and reward learning (Jones et al., 2014). For researchers who use experimental paradigms to test innovations in treatment delivery, we recently suggested the potential for using translational imaging paradigms to identify in-session therapist behaviors that are the most socially and neurobiologically reinforcing to adolescents, as well as to develop laboratory methods to examine the construct of ambivalence.

The better we understand mechanisms of change, the more we can do to enhance and refine the interventions, treatments, and services we provide to teens. Similarly, by examining the active ingredients of brief interventions, we can better understand those within-session clinician behaviors, and their timing, that are more likely to lead to positive changes. Taking this perspective illustrates how potentially dynamic, fluid, and powerful brief interventions can be, and underscores how critically important clinical skills are in the moment.

REFERENCES

Apodaca, T. R., Jackson, K. M., Borsari, B., Magill, M., Longabaugh, R., Mastroleo, N. R., et al. (2016). Which individual therapist behaviors elicit client change talk and sustain talk in motivational interviewing? *Journal of Substance Abuse Treatment, 61*, 60–65.

Baer, J. S., Kivlahan, D. R., & Marlatt, G. A. (1995). High-risk drinking across the transition from high school to college. *Alcoholism: Clinical and Experimental Research, 19,* 54–61.

Borsari, B., Murphy, J. G., & Barnett, N. P. (2007). Predictors of alcohol use during the first year of college: Implications for prevention. *Addictive Behaviors, 32*(10), 2062–2086.

Brown, S. A., McGue, M., Maggs, J. L., Schulenberg, J. E., Hingson, R., Swartzwelder, S., et al. (2008). A developmental perspective on alcohol and youths 16 to 20 years of age. *Pediatrics, 121,* S290–S310.

Feldstein Ewing, S. W., Apodaca, T. R., & Gaume, J. (2016). Ambivalence: Prerequisite for success in motivational interviewing with adolescents? *Addiction, 111*(11), 1900–1907.

Gaume, J., Longabaugh, R., Magill, M., Bertholet, N., Gmel, G., & Daeppen, J. B. (2016). Under what conditions?: Therapist and client characteristics moderate the role of change talk in brief motivational intervention. *Journal of Consulting and Clinical Psychology, 84,* 211–220.

Hingson, R. W., Heeren, T., & Winter, M. R. (2006). Age at drinking onset and alcohol dependence: Age at onset, duration, and severity. *Archives of Pediatric Adolescent Medicine, 160,* 739–746.

Hingson, R. W., & White, A. (2014). New research findings since the 2007 Surgeon General's Call to Action to Prevent and Reduce Underage Drinking: A review. *Journal of Studies on Alcohol and Drugs, 75*(1), 158–169.

Hingson, R. W., Zha, W., & Weitzman, E. R. (2009). Magnitude of and trends in alcohol-related mortality and morbidity among U.S. college students ages 18–24, 1998–2005. *Journal of Studies on Alcohol and Drugs Supplement, 16,* 12–20. Retrieved from *www.ncbi.n/m.nih.gov/pubmed/19538908.*

Hovens, J. G., Cantwell, D. P., & Kiriakos, R. (1994). Psychiatric comorbidity in hospitalized adolescent substance abusers. *Journal of the American Academy of Child and Adolescent Psychiatry, 33,* 476–483.

Johnston, L. D., O'Malley, P. M., Bachman, J. G., & Schulenberg, J. E. (2013). *Monitoring the Future national survey results on drug use, 1975–2012.* Ann Arbor: Institute for Social Research, University of Michigan.

Johnston, L. D., O'Malley, P. M., Miech, R. A., Bachman, J. G., & Schulenberg, J. E. (2013). *Demographic subgroup trends among adolescents for fifty-one classes of licit and illicit drugs, 1975–2012* (Monitoring the Future Occasional Paper, No. 79). Ann Arbor: Institute for Social Research, University of Michigan. Retrieved from *www.monitoringthefuture.org/pubs/occpapers/mtf-occ79.pdf.*

Johnston, L. D., O'Malley, P. M., Miech, R. A., Bachman, J. G., & Schulenberg, J. E. (2015). *Monitoring the Future national results on drug use: Overview of key findings, 2014.* Ann Arbor: Institute for Social Research, University of Michigan.

Jones, R. M., Somerville, L. H., Li, J., Ruberry, E. J., Powers, A., Mehta, N., et al. (2014). Adolescent-specific patterns of behavior and neural activity during social reinforcement learning. *Cognitive, Affective, and Behavioral Neuroscience, 14,* 683–697.

Kessler, R. C., Crum, R. M., Warner, L. A., Nelson, C. B., Schulenberg, J., & Anthony, J. C. (1997). Lifetime co-occurrence of DSM-III-R alcohol abuse and dependence with other psychiatric disorders in the National Comorbidity Study. *Archives of General Psychiatry, 54,* 313–321.

Longabaugh, R., & Magill, M. (2011). Recent advances in behavioral addictions treatment: Focusing on mechanisms of change. *Current Psychiatry Reports, 13*(5), 382–389.

Marlatt, G. A. (1998). Basic principles and strategies of harm reduction. In G. A. Marlatt (Ed.), *Harm reduction: Pragmatic strategies for managing high-risk behaviors* (pp. 49–66). New York: Guilford Press.

Marlatt, G. A., & Witkiewitz, K. (2002). Harm reduction approaches to alcohol use: Health promotion, prevention, and treatment. *Addictive Behaviors, 27*(6), 867–886.

Miech, R. A., Johnston, L. D., O'Malley, P. M., Bachman, J. C., & Schulenberg, J. E. (2015). *Monitoring the Future national survey results on drug use, 1975–2014: Vol. I. Secondary school students.* Ann Arbor: Institute for Social Research, University of Michigan.

Mitchell, S. G., Gryczynski, J., O'Grady, K. I. E., & Schwartz, R. P. (2013). SBIRT for adolescent drug and alcohol use: Current status and future directions. *Journal of Substance Abuse Treatment, 44,* 463–472.

Monti, P. M., Colby, S. M., & O'Leary, T. A. (Eds.). (2001). *Adolescents, alcohol, and substance abuse: Reaching teens through brief interventions.* New York: Guilford Press.

Monti, P. M., & Monnig, M. (2016). Ambivalence and motivational interviewing with adolescents: Ensuring that the baby does not get thrown out with the bathwater. *Addiction, 111*(11), 1909–1910.

Prochaska, J. O. (2013). Transtheoretical model of behavior change. In M. Gellman & J. R. Turner (Eds.), *Encyclopedia of behavioral medicine* (pp. 1997–2000). New York: Springer.

Prochaska, J. O., & DiClemente, C. C. (1983). *The transtheoretical approach: Crossing traditional boundaries of change.* Homewood, IL: Dow Jones Irving.

Prochaska, J. O., Velicer, W. F., DiClemente, C. C., & Fava, J. L. (1988). Measuring the processes of change: Applications to the cessation of smoking. *Journal of Consulting and Clinical Psychology, 56,* 520–528.

Storr, C. L., Pacek, L. R., & Martins, S. S. (2012). Substance use disorders and adolescent psychopathology. *Public Health Reviews, 34*(2). Retrieved from *www.publichealthreviews.eu/upload/pdf_files/12/00_Storr.pdf.*

Substance Abuse and Mental Health Services Administration. (2014). Screening, brief intervention, and referral to treatment (SBIRT). Retrieved from *http://beta.samhsa.gov/sbirt.*

Tanner-Smith, E. E., & Lipsey, M. W. (2015). Brief alcohol interventions for adolescents and young adults: A systematic review and meta-analysis. *Journal of Substance Abuse Treatment, 51,* 1–18.

Toumbourou, J. W., Stockwell, T., Neighbors, C., Marlatt, G. A., Sturge, J., & Rehm, J. (2007). Interventions to reduce harm associated with adolescent substance use. *Lancet, 369,* 1391–1401.

Volkow, N. D., Compton, W. M., & Weiss, S. R. (2014). Adverse health effects of marijuana use. *New England Journal of Medicine, 371,* 879.

Wendel, M. (2016). Drinking over the lifespan: Focus on early adolescents and youth. *Alcohol Research: Current Reviews, 38*(1), 95–101.

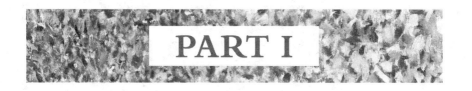

PART I

ETIOLOGY AND DEVELOPMENTAL CONTEXT

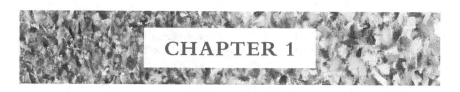

CHAPTER 1

Development Matters

Taking the Long View on Substance Use during Adolescence and the Transition to Adulthood

John Schulenberg, Julie Maslowsky,
Jennifer L. Maggs, and Robert A. Zucker

*I*t would be difficult to argue against taking a developmental perspective on adolescent substance use. To do so would be to attempt to assert, for example, that age and other markers of developmental status (e.g., pubertal development, adult role acquisition) do not contribute importantly to our understanding of the onset and course of substance use, either directly or as moderators of risk factors. But what does it mean to take a developmental perspective on the etiology and prevention of substance use during adolescence? And what are some advantages of doing so for research and intervention? We address these and related questions in this chapter.

To set the stage, consider Figure 1.1, a lithograph from 1895 entitled *The Smokers*, by K. Wilkowski. On the surface, this is simply a nostalgic illustration of two boys who are about to light up, one a cigarette and the other a little corncob pipe, both presumably containing tobacco. At another level, this shared experience can be seen as advancing the friendship between these two boys. Indeed, it appears that this is a first-time experience for the younger one on the right with the tentative look and short pants. Perhaps the older one, who is lighting the match, is initiating his younger friend. According to Sullivan (1947), forming a "chumship" or special intimate friendship during early adolescence is critical for continued social and identity development—young adolescents clearly understand the social purposes of substance use (Jackson et al., 2014). More generally, substance use during adolescence may be associated with some positive developmentally advantageous purposes, like social integration, in addition to many serious negative consequences (Chassin, Presson, & Sherman, 1989; Crosnoe, 2011; Maggs & Hurrelmann, 1998). Thus, in this illustration, a consequential "bonding experience" is occurring for which substance use may be a catalyst, despite the likely sequelae of negative health outcomes.

This example illustrates one of the key features of a developmental perspective—that is, to understand substance use in relation to adolescents' various developmental tasks and transitions (Brown et al., 2008; Masten, Faden, Zucker, & Spear, 2008; Newcomb, 1997; Schulenberg & Maggs, 2002; Schulenberg, Maggs, & Hurrelmann, 1997; Schulenberg, Patrick, Maslowsky, & Maggs, 2014). The second key feature is to examine individual courses of change over time in substance use and abuse and related risk factors. The single snapshot of *The Smokers* leaves us wondering what led up to this moment and what happened next. What individual and contextual characteristics set the stage for these two young people to use tobacco? How did this shared moment fit into the underlying course of their friendship and substance use? How did this and subsequent substance use influence their future health and well-being?

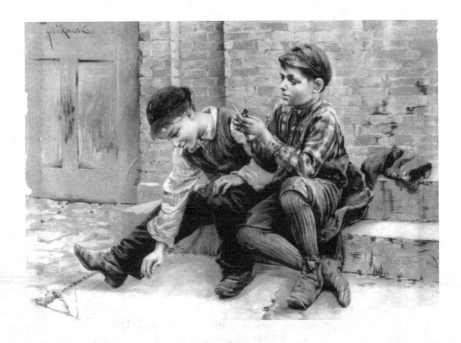

FIGURE 1.1. *The Smokers.*

In this chapter, we expand on these two key and interrelated features of a developmental perspective on substance use during adolescence and discuss the implications of this developmental perspective for understanding risk and protective factors and for conceptualizing prevention and intervention efforts.

SUBSTANCE USE IN RELATION TO ADOLESCENTS' CHANGING LIVES

In this section we offer a brief overview of adolescent development and consider the ways in which substance use can be viewed in relation to the numerous changes that typically occur during adolescence. We begin with a selective overview of advances in the study of adolescence, followed by a discussion of the potentially pivotal importance of adolescence in the life course. We then consider the fundamental changes and major domains of transitions during adolescence and conclude this section with a consideration of conceptual models for linking substance use (and risks to health and well-being more generally) to the various normative and non-normative developmental transitions during adolescence.

Advances in the Study of Adolescence

G. Stanley Hall, the founder of the scientific study of adolescence (Muuss, 1996), gave us the enduring image of adolescence as a time of unavoidable "storm and stress." According to Hall's (1916) biologically based theory, individual development (ontogeny) recapitulates species development (phylogeny), with adolescence reflecting the turbulent transition in human history from savagery to civilization. Nothing can be done to ease adolescents' turmoil because developmental maturation is fully controlled by biology and thus unaffected by culture or context. A century later, Hall's mythical image of the adolescent is still reflected in popular culture, if not in the scientific literature (Hollenstein & Lougheed, 2013).

Hall was not alone in his beliefs on this subject. Sigmund Freud's psychoanalytic theory viewed turmoil as an unavoidable and even essential component of adolescence. According to Freud, puberty brings on the genital stage of psychosexual development, during which the strengthening of sexual desire and the necessity of severing emotional dependence on parents leads to inner and interpersonal turmoil (Freud, 1958). Anna Freud, Sigmund's daughter and a prominent child psychoanalyst, called adolescence a "developmental disturbance," meaning it was a necessary and time-limited perturbation of upheaval that does not represent true psychopathology (Freud, 1969). Other neopsychoanalytic theorists also highlighted the inevitability of adolescent turmoil, although they were sensitive to the social and cultural factors that contributed to this (Erikson, 1968; Sullivan, 1947).

In addition to these organismic and psychoanalytic roots of current images of adolescence, there are mechanistic and contextual roots as well (cf. Pepper, 1942). Margaret Mead (1950) and Ruth Benedict (1950) argued that "storm and stress" is primarily a cultural phenomenon caused by the discontinuity in roles and responsibilities between childhood and adulthood in modern societies. Kurt Lewin (1939) attributed adolescent difficulties to adolescents' ambiguous life space rather than to their individual characteristics. Robert Havighurst (1952) identified culturally defined developmental tasks that individuals needed to accomplish during certain age ranges. He viewed difficulties that arose during adolescence in terms of inability or unwillingness to accomplish the necessary tasks.

Although some diversity in present-day scientific images of adolescence remains, reflecting strong roots in both biology and culture, broad-based empirical studies of adolescents have given no support for the notion that adolescence is *necessarily* a time of storm and stress (Lerner, 2008). Notions of biologically based stages and developmental determinism have given way to probabilistic conceptualizations of person–context interactions and multilevel mechanisms (Jessor, 1993; Lerner, 2006; Sameroff, 2010; Steinberg, 2015). Consistent with lifespan, life course, and ecological perspectives (Baltes, 1987; Bronfenbrenner, 1979; Elder & Shanahan, 2006), the typical answer from those who study adolescence to any question about the impact of some characteristic or event on adolescent development has become "It depends." A common view now is "Adolescence is characterized by change, and is challenging, but it need not be tumultuous and problematic unless societal conditions prompt it" (Petersen & Leffert, 1995, p. 3).

There is not one unified, agreed-upon developmental theory or conceptual framework. Indeed, developmental scientists often disagree about the very meaning of development, and this disagreement stems from differences in philosophical assumptions about humans and their nature and nurture. The developmental perspective we offer in this chapter is consistent with a developmental–contextual framework that emphasizes multilevel, multidimensional, and multidirectional development across the lifespan, with stability and change occurring as a function of the ongoing interaction between individuals and their contexts (Baltes, 1987; Lerner, 2006; Sameroff, 2010; Zucker, Hicks, & Heitzeg, 2016). This perspective has much in common with approaches in adjacent fields including life course or developmental epidemiology (Kellam & Van Horn, 1997; Kuh, Ben-Shlomo, Lynch, Hallqvist, & Power, 2003), developmental evolutionary psychology (Ellis et al., 2012), and life course theory in sociology (Elder, Kirkpatrick Johnson, & Crosnoe, 2003). Although genetic and other biological factors play a primary role in development, they do so in conjunction with contextual forces. Even physical maturation, which is heavily driven by biological factors, is partially regulated by the context structure that enhances and dampens the organism's basic genetic template, as well as assigns developmental and social meaning to the physical changes (Lynne-Landsman,

Graber, & Andrews, 2010; Schriber & Guyer, 2015). In relation to the etiology of substance use, developmental stability and change are viewed as ongoing interactions between individual and context. Not only does the etiology depend on individual characteristics that are given to developmental change but it also depends on features of the context (e.g., availability of a given drug, regulatory and expectancy structures that govern its use, friends' use), as well as on the strong and ongoing interactions between individuals and contexts.

Why Focus on Adolescence?

When asked why he robbed banks, Willie Sutton allegedly answered, "because that's where the money is." Likewise, when considering substance use etiology and interventions, one obvious reason to focus on adolescence is "because that's where the drugs are." Rarely is substance use initiated prior to or after the second decade of life (Johnston, O'Malley, Bachman, Schulenberg, & Miech, 2015). For some young people, the various psychosocial changes of adolescence set the stage for the manifestation of risky trajectories rooted in childhood (or earlier)—for others, the many transitions of adolescence contribute to some (statistically) normative venturing into problem behaviors in general and into experimentation with substance use in particular (Jessor, 1993; Schulenberg et al., 2014).

There is no other time in the lifespan at which both individual and contextual changes are as rapid and pervasive as they are during adolescence. Although the rates of physical and cognitive growth are more rapid during infancy than during adolescence, unlike infants, adolescents are keenly aware of their physical and cognitive changes (Silbereisen & Kracke, 1997). For some young people, the immediacy and simultaneity of these changes may contribute to decreased health and well-being. Likewise, the varying tempo and timing of these changes can also threaten the health and well-being of adolescents (Graber, 2013). For instance, once they are physically able, many young people engage in sexual intercourse before they acquire the motivations and skills to protect themselves and their partners (Dir, Coskunpinar, & Cyders, 2014; Donohew et al., 2000). Similarly, they may gain access to automobiles or firearms without appreciating their own limited experience or the dangers involved. Such discrepancies between adolescents' repertoire of behaviors and their cognitive, emotional, and social development result in some disturbing outcomes (Moffitt, 1993; Steinberg, 2008). Indeed, the top causes of adolescent mortality—accidental injury, homicide, and suicide—are often direct sequelae of risk behavior (Heron, 2016). Alcohol and other drug use begins amid the biological, cognitive, emotional, and social changes of adolescence. The onset and escalation of substance use likely amplify other concurrent threats to health and well-being.

One of the most compelling reasons to focus on adolescents is that successful interventions are likely to have long-term benefits across the lifespan

(Catalano et al., 2012; Gonzales et al., 2014; Hale, Fitzgerald-Yau, & Viner, 2014; Koning et al., 2013; Spoth et al., 2013). The primary causes of mortality and morbidity during adolescence are related to preventable social, environmental, and behavioral factors (Global Burden of Disease Pediatrics Collaboration, 2016; Heron, 2016). Many physical and mental health problems of adulthood (and the chronic diseases that mark their endpoint status) have their origin in habits that are formed during adolescence (e.g., smoking, exercise, eating habits; Kann et al., 2014), as well as in maladaptive coping styles (e.g., emotion-focused, rather than problem-focused coping) that are consolidated during this time (Eitle & Eitle, 2014; Hampel & Peterman, 2006; Thorsteinsson, Ryan, & Sveinbjornsdottir, 2013). In addition, during adolescence and young adulthood, many consequential life decisions are made concerning educational attainment, occupational choices, relationship and family formation, and lifestyle options, making this a formative period in regard to health and well-being across the lifespan (Institute of Medicine, 2014). Thus, adolescence can be viewed as a potential sensitive period for interventions that can have lifelong impact (Catalano et al., 2012; Fink et al., 2016; Maggs, Schulenberg, & Hurrelmann, 1997; Schulenberg & Maslowsky, 2015).

Developmental Transitions during Adolescence

Many obvious developmental transitions occur during adolescence, such as puberty and moving from primary to secondary (middle to high) school. Many more developmental transitions are less obvious but still central in defining the transformation from child to adult: cognitive shifts that set the stage for more abstract identities and future orientations, changes in parent–child relationships such that the adolescent gains more privacy and freedom, and heightened peer-group involvement followed by individualized friendships and dating relationships. These developmental transitions are "the paths that connect us to transformed physical, mental, and social selves" (Schulenberg et al., 1997, p. 1). They offer young people opportunities to compound or disrupt the strengths and difficulties acquired earlier in life and thus represent both continuity and discontinuity in functioning and adjustment (Beauchaine & McNulty, 2013; Dodge et al., 2009; Rutter, 1996; Schulenberg, Maslowsky, Patrick, & Martz, 2016). The challenge is how to influence young people's negotiations of developmental transitions such that health-enhancing characteristics of the individual and surrounding context are maintained and strengthened across adolescence, and health-compromising characteristics are diminished.

The meaning of developmental transitions originates in the interaction of physical maturational processes, cultural influences and expectations, and personal values and goals. Individuals shape their own developmental transitions as they act on and are acted on by the social and physical environment (Lerner, 1982; Sameroff, 2010). As with other developmental processes, these transitions are embedded in a sociocultural context, and therefore may vary by gender, class, culture, and historical period (Settersten, Furstenberg, & Rumbaut, 2005). Culturally based age-related expectations shape developmental transitions in that they provide a normative social timetable for role transitions (e.g., employment, parenthood). There are also significant interindividual variations in the order and importance of the various transitions, depending on personal goals and life situations (Nurmi, 1997).

Developmental transitions can be grouped into the following categories: (1) fundamental changes of pubertal, neural, and cognitive development; (2) affiliative transitions (e.g., changes in relationships with parents, peers, romantic partners); (3) achievement transitions (e.g., school and work transitions); and (4) identity transitions (e.g., changes in self-definition, increased self-regulation; Schulenberg et al., 1997).

Models Relating Developmental Transitions to Substance Use

Health risks tend to increase during adolescence. These risks do not accrue automatically with age but rather as direct and indirect functions of the numerous developmental transitions. There are several ways in which various developmental transitions during adolescence relate to risks to health and well-being and specifically to substance use (Cicchetti & Rogosch, 2002; Schulenberg & Maggs, 2002). We summarize five relevant conceptual models based on some of our work (Schulenberg et al., 1997, 2014, 2016). Note that these models are not mutually exclusive—given the multiplicity of developmental transitions, as well as of health risks and opportunities, all five models are likely to operate across individuals in a given population and within individuals over time. As we briefly discuss, each of these models has implications regarding substance abuse interventions (Maggs et al., 1997).

The Overload Model

In the overload model, health risks are viewed as a potential result of experiencing developmental transitions. When developmental transitions overwhelm current coping capabilities, health and well-being are likely to suffer, and health-risk behaviors (such as substance use) may become an alternative strategy for coping, which in turn may undermine more effective coping strategies (Brown et al., 2008; Wingo, Baldessarini, & Windle, 2015). Given the major and multiple transitions that occur during adolescence, existing coping strategies may be challenged (Sontag, Graber, Brooks-Gunn, & Warren, 2008). This view is consistent with Coleman's (1978) focal theory, in which he argues that decrements in well-being during adolescence result not from hormone-induced "storm and stress" but instead from the multiple and simultaneous transitions that occur in a relatively short period of time. Potential interventions based on this model include attempting to increase adolescents' coping capacities (Hoyt,

Chase-Lansdale, McDade, & Adam, 2012; Sibinga, Webb, Ghazarian, & Ellen, 2016), as well as attempting to stagger the timing of various transitions (Eccles, Lord, Roeser, Barber, & Jozefowicz, 1997; Seidman & French, 2004), avoiding, for instance, having young people change schools just as puberty manifests.

The Developmental Match/Mismatch Model

In the developmental match/mismatch model, health risks and opportunities are viewed as a result of the impact of developmental transitions on the developmental match (Eccles et al., 1993, 1997) or goodness of fit (Lerner, 1982, 2006) between individuals and their contexts. Developing individuals are embedded within changing ecological niches. For example, consider a young adolescent who is in the midst of pubertal and cognitive changes who moves to middle school and gains a new sibling all at the same time. The match between this adolescent's developmental needs and what the context provides is itself dynamic. When developmental transitions can lead to an improved match between adolescents' needs and what the context provides, healthy development is likely to be enhanced. For example, becoming a middle school student and an older sibling could provide developmentally appropriate challenges and experiences, feelings of competence, and increased well-being (Schulenberg & Maggs, 2002). On the other hand, when developmental transitions reduce the match between adolescents' needs and contextual supports and demands, health may be adversely affected. For example, if parental monitoring became inadequate during this combined school and family transition, a young adolescent might not cope well if newly exposed to deviant peer influences. To the extent that we can increase the synchrony between developmental needs and contextual affordances, we may be able to diminish health risks associated with developmental transitions (Gutman & Eccles, 2007; Maggs et al., 1997).

The Increased Heterogeneity Model

In the increased heterogeneity model, developmental transitions are viewed as moderators of ongoing health risk status. Developmental transitions can serve to increase interindividual variability in functioning and adjustment and in this way can be viewed as important junctures along one's health status trajectory. Evidence from a variety of studies indicates that divergence increases throughout adolescence between those who cope effectively with various stressors and those who do not (McLaughlin & King, 2015; Reinke, Eddy, Dishion, & Reid, 2012). For example, the transition to junior high/middle school is worse for young people who are already experiencing difficulties with behavior problems and adjustment to school, and likewise, adolescents who have difficulties with the transition are likely to have increasingly severe difficulties in high school (Booth & Gerard, 2014; Eccles et al., 1997).

This "pathways" perspective (Cairns & Cairns, 1994; Crockett & Crouter,

1995) is consistent with Erikson's (1968) psychosocial theory of life course development, in which the individual's resolution of one developmental crisis (e.g., adolescent identity vs. identity confusion) is dependent on how he or she resolved previous crises (e.g., preadolescent industry vs. inferiority) and has implications for the resolution of subsequent crises (e.g., young adulthood intimacy vs. isolation; see also Havighurst, 1952; Sullivan, 1947). There are likely to be several mechanisms that serve to exacerbate a trajectory of ongoing health risks, including ineffective coping strategies and unhealthy lifestyles (Nurmi, 1997). Contexts (e.g., low social supports, contact with a deviant peer group) can also facilitate such a trajectory of risk development. Living in a context that lacks social support to alter, and an abundance of support to maintain, a trajectory of ongoing risky behaviors will sustain and may even exacerbate such an unhealthy risk trajectory (Draper, Grobler, Micklesfield, & Norris, 2015). The prevention implications of this model include, for example, altering self-defeating coping strategies and enhancing social network contacts that discourage risky behavior for youth who are following worrisome trajectories (Maslowsky et al., 2016; Pinkerton & Dolan, 2007; Valente et al., 2007). Furthermore, as with the mismatch model, interventions aimed at providing adolescents with alternative positive experiences and opportunities for success are likely to have long-term beneficial health effects.

The Transition Catalyst Model

According to the transition catalyst model, substance use and risk taking in general can be viewed as important components of negotiating certain developmental transitions. The idea that a certain amount of adolescent risk taking is normative is supported by high prevalence rates across species, animal and human studies of adolescent brain development, and by evidence that it often accompanies healthy personality development in humans (Baumrind, 1987; Bukobza, 2009; Casey, Jones, & Hare, 2008). According to Chassin et al. (1989), risk taking and deviance can serve constructive, as well as destructive, functions in adolescents' health and development—a point echoed by many others in the literature (e.g., Crosnoe, 2011; Maggs, Almeida, & Galambos, 1995; Maslowsky, Buvinger, Keating, Steinberg, & Cauffman, 2011; Rawn & Vohs, 2011; Spear, 2000; Willoughby, Good, Adachi, Hamza, & Tavernier, 2013). For example, risk taking appears to be an important aspect of negotiating greater autonomy from parents (Irwin & Millstein, 1992) and may serve the evolutionary function of helping adolescents to move beyond the family home and establish stronger links with the outside world (Casey et al., 2008; Spear, 2000). Likewise, alcohol use and sexual behaviors during the transition to college may help adolescents achieve valued social goals, such as making friends in a new environment, although these behaviors may also pose important risks for health (Maggs, 1997; Patrick, Maggs, & Abar, 2007). Undergirding these potential developmental benefits of substance use is the evolutionary pressure to leave the protective influence of the family of origin to seek out mates and establish a territory of one's own. From this perspective also, risk taking and opposition to one's parents can be seen as the extreme end of a dimension involving the drive toward adult capability and its concomitant rewards.

According to the identity literature, experimentation with alternative identities may involve some increased risk taking. Given that failing to explore options may lead to premature identity foreclosure (Erikson, 1968; Marcia, 1994), some risk taking can be viewed as an important component of developmental transitions associated with identity formation. This highlights an important dilemma with this model when considering intervention implications. To the extent that risk taking plays an essential role in identity formation, as well as in negotiating peer-related and other developmental transitions (Patrick & Lee, 2010; Patrick et al., 2007), attempts to eliminate risk taking may in turn have adverse consequences for identity development in particular and optimal development in general (Baumrind, 1987; Dumas, Ellis, & Wolfe, 2012; Wilkerson, Brooks, & Ross, 2010). Of course, health-enhancing behaviors may also be components of negotiating developmental transitions. For example, reduced substance use often corresponds with the transition to marriage (Martin, Blozis, Boeninger, Masarik, & Conger, 2014; Staff et al., 2010).

The Heightened Vulnerability to Chance Events Model

The heightened vulnerability to chance events model is based on the role of chance in altering the courses of individuals' lives. Random, unpredicted events can include unexpected encounters with individuals, contexts, or situations. Bandura (1982) suggests that such chance events are ubiquitous: people meet in an elevator and end up marrying, others die from freak accidents, and so on. Yet chance events, large and small, are often less random than they may first appear (Bandura, 1998). The couple that met in an elevator likely shared lifestyles, interests, or professions that led them both to be on that particular elevator at that time, and both were likely to be receptive to this chance meeting.

Just as there are individual differences in receptivity to chance events, there are also intraindividual (or within-person) changes in this receptivity, with certain periods during the lifespan being more conducive to chance effects. As we have argued, major developmental transitions that involve new contexts, such as the transition to college, may be particularly conducive periods because they engender heightened sensitivity to and exploratory behavior of the new context and the self in relation to the new context (Maggs, 1997; Schulenberg & Maggs, 2002; Schulenberg et al., 2016). Young people undergoing such transitions may seek out and be open to the effects of novel experiences. As they explore their niche in the context, chance events may take on special significance. Thus, developmental transitions can increase one's contact with novel experiences and heighten one's vulnerability to the positive and negative effects of chance events. Just as there are likely to be unexpected salutary effects that result from these significant chance events and encounters, there are likely to be some health-compromising effects, including increased substance use and increased negative consequences of such use.

Intervening in such chance events and encounters typically is viewed as being beyond the reach of prevention efforts. Nevertheless, resilience to some of the negative effects of chance events and encounters is possible. There is some evidence to indicate that early exposure to moderate stress can have a "steeling" or buffering effect against later difficulties (Rutter, 2012; Shapero et al., 2015). Similarly, programs that aim to build basic social skills may also enable young people to take advantage of promising opportunities that arise by chance.

EXAMINING THE COURSE
OF SUBSTANCE USE AND RELATED FACTORS

As we illustrated in the previous section, a key feature of a developmental perspective on alcohol and other drug use is the consideration of substance use in relation to the numerous developmental transitions of adolescence. Examining change and stability in substance use and related factors within individuals over time is the second key feature of a developmental perspective. We start this section with a brief discussion of the necessity for and advantages of longitudinal research. We then consider strategies for examining change over time and include illustrations from some of our etiological and intervention research.

Why Conduct Multiwave Longitudinal Studies?

Longitudinal studies follow individuals across years of the life course to track individual change. Such multiwave prospective panel studies are expensive in terms of funding, effort, and respondent burden; are complicated in terms of measurement and analysis; and tend to be compromised by differential attrition. So why do we need them?

At a general level, longitudinal designs are necessary for addressing the primary goals of developmental research: the description and explanation of intraindividual (or within-person) developmental change and of interindividual (or between-person) differences and similarities in patterns of intraindividual developmental change (Baltes, Reese, & Nesselroade, 1977; Menard, 2007). Developmental change may occur in smooth or abrupt quantitative increments; or it may involve discontinuous, qualitative transformations in which one behavior is superseded by another; or it may involve changes in patterns of relationships among variables. Although cross-sectional data can be used to estimate age changes at the group level, they are inadequate to determine the nature, magnitude, and structure of such changes. Furthermore, longitudinal data provide information about the determinants and consequences of intraindividual change and about individual differences in these processes. Hypotheses about time-ordered antecedents and consequences require the relevant variables to be measured in the sequence in which they occur. Within-time correlations among relevant variables may in fact reflect spurious associations that are due to a third, shared, determining variable. With longitudinal data, it becomes possible to ask whether hypothesized causes precede their effects, as well as to examine long-term treatment outcomes, discontinuous phenomena (e.g., sleeper effects), and multidirectional processes (Rutter, 1994).

To help developmental scientists address the most important questions we face about substance use etiology and intervention, following the same individuals over several points in time represents the best, and arguably only, strategy. Particularly during adolescence, when pervasive multidimensional change is the backdrop, knowing a young person's substance use at only one point in time tells us little if anything about its likely course, causes, and consequences.

Furthermore, although it is far better to have two waves of data than just a single wave, longitudinal data that span three or more waves are especially informative. Multiple waves of data permit the consideration of more complex mediational and reciprocal models aimed at understanding how relationships between risk factors and substance use unfold (Sher & Wood, 1997). In addition, multiple waves of longitudinal data make it possible to identify different trajectories of substance use in terms of the timing of onset and pattern of change over time—information that is essential for determining the type and severity of substance use problems (Dodge et al., 2009; Jester, Wong, Cranford, Fitzgerald, & Zucker, 2015; Terry-McElrath et al., 2017).

Short-term multiwave longitudinal data are useful for examining processes among temporally proximal risk factors and substance use, especially during major developmental transitions such as the transition to middle school (e.g., Eccles et al., 1997) or college (e.g., Rhoades & Maggs, 2006). Intensive measurement using frequent (e.g., weekly, daily, momentary, or even continuous) assessment has dramatically increased our knowledge of the processes underlying the pairing of situational and proximal risk factors with substance use in real-world settings (e.g., Del Boca, Darkes, Greenbaum, & Goldman, 2004; Howard, Patrick, & Maggs, 2015; Jackson, Colby, & Sher, 2010; Quinn & Fromme, 2012). This is also being applied in event-specific prevention targeting specific developmental and other peak periods of risk such as high school graduation, spring break, and 21st birthdays (Neighbors et al., 2007).

Longer intervals between waves make it difficult to capture the sometimes rapid changes and influences that occur during these transitions, such as making new friends and escalating binge drinking. However, long-term multiwave panel data are essential for understanding how distal influences relate to proximal ones (e.g., Maslowsky, Schulenberg, & Zucker, 2014; McCabe, Veliz, & Schulenberg, 2016; Schulenberg et al., 2015). In particular, early delinquent activity during adolescence is one of the strongest predictors of both the early onset of substance use and later problem substance use (Dishion, Capaldi, & Yoerger, 1999; Donovan, 2004; Maslowsky & Schulenberg, 2013; Maslowsky, Schulenberg, O'Malley, & Kloska, 2014; Zucker, Donovan, Masten, Mattson, & Moss, 2008), and long-term longitudinal studies suggest even earlier distal influences. For example, in a longitudinal study of children of alcoholics, Mayzer, Fitzgerald, and Zucker (2009) traced the source of the effect found between adolescent delinquency and substance use back to differences in behavioral undercontrol observed at age 3. This long-term follow-up of preschool-age children suggests that adolescent delinquent activity serves less as a stand-alone causative agent and more as a mediator (or ongoing extension) of earlier behavior difficulties. Without long-term panel data, this distal causal connection would be overlooked, a meaningful oversight given the alternative intervention implications.

Perhaps one of the most compelling reasons for longitudinal studies on substance use is to identify why great numbers of individuals do not develop serious substance abuse problems despite exposure to significant risk factors and, likewise, why many individuals do develop problems despite little exposure to risk factors (Rutter, 1990). The concepts of equifinality and multifinality are relevant to this point (Cicchetti & Rogosch, 1996). As discussed in the next section, equifinality refers to the multiple pathways that can lead to a similar outcome. For example, Jester, Buu, and Zucker (2016) reported that among adults with symptoms of alcohol abuse, some had a lengthy history of persistent and severe difficulties, whereas others had only recent difficulties. In this example, the trajectories of problem use and the ramifications of being on a particular trajectory pathway vary substantially (Zucker et al., 2016). Multifinality pertains to multiple alternative outcomes that stem from a given initial level of adaptation. Whereas some adolescents who misuse substances are likely to experience difficulty during the transition to early adulthood, many others exhibit patterns of misuse that will subside with the onset of early adulthood (Schulenberg & Maggs, 2002). Clearly, as these examples show, relying only on a "snapshot" at one point in time to capture the multiplicity of antecedent and consequent pathways of substance use during adolescence would be inadequate at best and very likely misleading.

Strategies for Studying Individual–Level Change and Stability

There has been a perennial tension in psychology between the nomothetic goals of science (i.e., to find general laws of behavior that apply to all) and the idiographic goals (i.e., to describe and explain a given individual's behavior; Allport, 1937; Molenaar, 2004; Nesselroade, 1992). Almost a half-century ago, Jack Block (1971) argued for an intermediate position: "A greater lawfulness may be discerned (when) what is general and undifferentiated is partitioned into smaller but more homogeneous classes for study. . . . This conceptual recognition demands a respect for the possibility of different courses of character evolution without a denial of what indeed may be universal for all persons" (p. 11). Finding and maintaining an appropriate balance between nomothetic and idiographic perspectives should be an important goal for developmental science. Recent methodological and statistical advances have made it possible to better embrace this goal.

Figure 1.2 is an adaptation of Raymond Cattell's (1988) classic three-dimensional data box. This cube includes three key dimensions of developmentally based research: persons, variables, and occasions. Although this data box originated decades ago, it still provides a highly useful way to categorize current data collection and analysis strategies (Beltz, Wright, Sprague, & Molenaar, 2016; Ram & Gerstorf, 2009). The interrelatedness of the three dimensions has general implications for how we collect and analyze data, including how we define and sample from "the population"—that is, populations should be thought of not only in terms of persons but also in terms of variables and occasions. This model also has specific implications for how we conceptualize and analyze individual-level change over time (Molenaar & Campbell, 2009). These implications are considered below as we examine the three two-dimensional "slices" in Figure 1.2.

R/Q Techniques

The R/Q slice represents a sample of variables collected from a sample of individuals at one occasion. The R technique refers to aggregating variables across persons in order to examine interindividual differences and variability in the variables at one point in time (e.g., to examine the correlation between risk taking and substance use). Cross-sectional studies that include different ages/grade levels can provide age/grade-level differences in the levels and relationships of the variables (e.g., how the risk taking–substance use correlation is different across age), but with the one-measurement occasion, there is no consideration of intraindividual change and stability prospectively over time, nor is there any consideration of the fact that environments simultaneously are changing prospectively as well.

The Q technique refers to aggregating persons across variables in order to identify types of people according to their common constellations of scores on variables at one point in time (e.g., to distinguish a subgroup of adolescents with high scores on both risk taking and substance use from a subgroup with high scores on risk taking and low scores on substance use). This strategy began to gain greater popularity in the developmental literature in the 1980s and 1990s, represented by what was often called "person-centered" or "pattern-centered" (typically cluster analytic) approaches championed by, for example, David Magnusson (e.g., Magnusson, 1997; Magnusson & Bergman, 1988) and Robert Cairns (Cairns & Cairns, 1994). Now, latent class analysis is a commonly used strategy for identifying types of people at one measurement occasion.

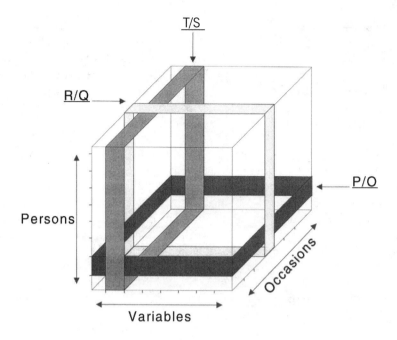

FIGURE 1.2. Adaptation of Cattell's original data box. From Cattell (1988). Copyright © 1998 Plenum Press. Adapted with permission of Springer.

Multiple R/Q slices can be taken to examine change over time. In the case of multiwave R technique, the typical focus is interindividual differences in terms of rank-order stability over time and static predictors of such change (e.g., in a cross-lag panel analysis). For example, in a structural equation model, one could examine how risk taking at Time 1 predicts change in drug use between Time 1 and Time 2. In the case of multiwave Q technique, such as repeated-measures cluster analysis (Bergman, 2000) or latent transition analysis (Collins, Graham, Rousculp, & Hansen, 1997; Collins & Lanza, 2013), change and stability in types or subgroups of individuals (based on constellations of scores) can be examined to consider, for example, whether the classes were the same across time or whether one class at Time 1 broke into two classes at Time 2. Despite a lack of emphasis on intraindividual change trajectories (discussed below regarding T/S techniques), such strategies are useful for examining types of individuals and tracking their change from one point in time to another.

P/O Techniques

The P/O slice represents a sample of variables collected across a sample of multiple occasions from a single person. The P technique refers to aggregating variables across occasions in order to examine how variables vary and covary over time within an individual (e.g., to examine the extent to which risk taking and substance use co-occur within a given individual)—a strategy ideal for identifying moods, states, and other day-to-day changes within individuals (Molenaar & Campbell, 2009; Nesselroade, 1992). The O technique refers to aggregating occasions across variables in order to examine how occasions group together on variables within an individual (e.g., to examine what sorts of occasions elicit risk taking and substance use within a given individual). P/O-technique research is relatively rare in the literature. Birkett and Cattell (1978) conducted a P-technique study to examine the day-to-day variability in symptoms in an alcohol-dependent patient. Clearly, P-technique strategies are idiographic, but they can also be made more nomothetic by conducting multiple P-technique studies and determining the extent of interindividual differences and similarities in the state dimensions (analogous steps could be taken with the O technique). Extensions of more nomothetic P-technique strategies include dynamic factor analysis (Molenaar, 1985) and pooled time-series analyses (Velicer & Colby, 1997), allowing for specific consideration of interindividual differences in intraindividual change (Beltz et al., 2016; Nesselroade & Ghisletta, 2000; Ram & Gerstorf, 2009).

T/S Techniques

The T/S slice represents a single variable (or set of variables) collected from a sample of individuals across several occasions. T and S techniques permit some blending of nomothetic and idiographic perspectives, providing a balance between the two for many purposes.

The T technique refers to aggregating occasions across persons in order to determine, for example, the average rate of change in one variable (or set of variables) over time, as well as interindividual differences in the average rate of change (e.g., to examine the average trajectory of increased alcohol use during adolescence, as well as interindividual variations from the average trajectory). T technique, as represented by growth curve modeling (Bryk & Raudenbush, 1987; Muthén & Curran, 1997; Raudenbush, 2001), allows researchers to focus on group-level and individual trajectories of change over time and to examine static and time-varying predictors of interindividual variations in the average trajectory of change (e.g., to determine whether initially high or increasing levels of risk taking contribute to a faster than average increase in substance use during adolescence). As powerful as these T-technique strategies are for understanding group and individual trajectories of substance use and more generally the etiology and prevention of substance use (see also Jester et al., 2008; Maggs & Schulenberg, 1998; Patton et al., 2007), one important limitation from a developmental perspective is that such techniques tend to assume a single developmental "ideal" trajectory, with individual variations being viewed in terms of departures from the single developmental ideal trajectory.

In contrast, the S technique assumes multiple developmental ideal trajectories. The S technique refers to aggregating persons across occasions in order to examine what we call developmental typologies—that is, grouping individuals according to how they change over time on a developmentally important variable or set of variables. By forming relatively few homogeneous categories of individuals according to how they change over time, it is possible to obtain important information about distinctive patterns of change over time without becoming overwhelmed with the nearly infinite variations of individual-level change. S-technique research can be useful when distinctly different developmental trajectories are expected, for example, in regard to theoretical groups that are hypothesized to differ in their course of substance use (Cloninger, 1987; Zucker, 1987) or when diversity in paths is expected across developmental transitions (Schulenberg et al., 2014, 2016). Such differentiations are not only useful as descriptors of developmental variation in substance use but they also have the potential to show different precursive behavioral patterns that may themselves be harbingers of the later developmental pathway (see, e.g., Jester, 2016).

Over the past decade, there have been important advances in strategies for forming trajectory groups, including growth mixture modeling (Muthén & Asparouhov, 2008) and repeated measures latent class analysis (Collins & Lanza, 2013), highlighting the utility of the S technique in the literature. To illustrate how it can be useful, we draw what is now a classic example from previous work with Monitoring the Future. Schulenberg and colleagues (Schulenberg, O'Malley, Bachman, Wadsworth, & Johnston, 1996; Schulenberg, Wadsworth, O'Malley, Bachman, & Johnston, 1996) identified six distinct trajectories of binge drinking during the transition from adolescence to young adulthood (guided by theory, initially using cluster analysis, confirmed more recently with growth mixture modeling; Schulenberg & Patrick, 2011). Five of these trajectories (chronic, decrease, increase, fling, and rare) are illustrated in Figure 1.3 (the "never" group [36%] is excluded from the figure, as well as the 10% of the sample that did not fit any trajectory group). Perhaps what is most striking in this figure is how much information is lost when considering only the normative trends of binge drinking. There are examples of equifinality (i.e., several pathways to a given outcome), including the three different pathways into low levels of binge drinking at age 24 (decrease, fling, and rare; see Figure 1.3). Examples of multifinality (i.e., several alternative pathways originating from a given initial status) are also represented in many diverging trajectories (e.g., increase, fling, and rare; see Figure 1.3).

Once trajectories or developmental typologies are identified, it is then possible to predict membership as a function of initial risk factors (especially among initially similar but subsequently diverging trajectories), as well as to predict from the different trajectories to various outcomes. For example, Schulenberg, Wadsworth, and colleagues (1996) found that general self-efficacy at Wave 1 (age 18) predicted subsequent divergence between the chronic (lower

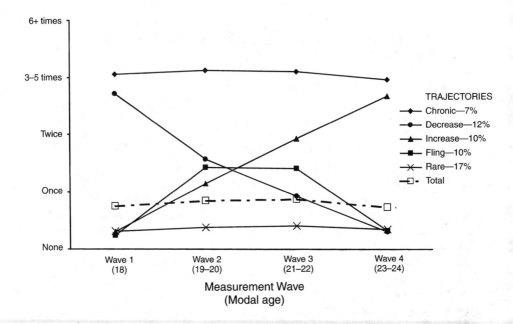

FIGURE 1.3. Mean score for five or more drinks in a row in past 2 weeks by binge-drinking trajectory. Data from Schulenberg, O'Malley, Bachman, Wadsworth, and Johnston (1996).

efficacy) and decrease (higher efficacy) trajectories. In addition, despite the general lack of Wave 1 predictors of the subsequent divergences among the increase, fling, and rare trajectories, the increase trajectory group was found to have more psychosocial difficulties at age 30 than the other two trajectories (Schulenberg & Patrick, 2011). By using S-technique analyses, these findings offer insights into types of change patterns in alcohol use during adolescence (in contrast to a single normative change trajectory), as well as into the timing and robustness of various risk and protective mechanisms that are not available via other analytic strategies.

As this illustrative discussion of the various techniques (along with a far-from-comprehensive list of available representative analytic strategies) shows, the data box can be a useful heuristic tool for developmentally minded researchers. Some of the distinctions drawn among the techniques may not always hold up, and, indeed, one would not want to restrict one's focus to a single slice in the data box (but rather to gather data along all three dimensions). Nevertheless, the key to advancing our understanding of the etiology of and effective interventions for substance use during adolescence is a primary focus on individual trajectories of substance use, a focus that requires the inclusion of multiple occasions of data on individuals and effective analytic strategies that consider multiwave data for samples of individuals.

IMPLICATIONS FOR UNDERSTANDING RISK AND PROTECTIVE FACTORS

A more developmentally sensitive understanding of risk and protective factors provides a stronger foundation for addressing fundamental questions about substance use etiology and intervention. Much effort over the past half-century has identified and catalogued risk and protective factors, and these successful efforts have yielded a useful, albeit overwhelming, array of relevant individual and contextual factors (e.g., Chassin, Colder, Hussong, & Sher, 2016; Donovan, 2004; Hawkins, Catalano, & Miller, 1992; Petraitis, Flay, & Miller, 1995; Zucker et al., 2016). This large and growing list of potential multilevel risk and protective factors sets the stage for specifying the processes that link risk and protective factors with substance use within individuals over time and across contexts (e.g., Chassin et al., 2016; Dodge et al., 2009; Zucker et al., 2016). In this section, in an effort to assist the relevant literature in continuing to move toward a more developmental understanding of linkages among risk and protective factors with substance use over time, we offer a series of conceptual guideposts.

Normative and More Nuanced Conceptualizations of Causality

The first guidepost pertains to conceptualizations about causality in studies examining risk and protective factors. Despite major advances in statistical modeling, establishing causality remains primarily an issue of research design, not statistical analysis, with randomized experiments remaining the gold standard for ruling out important alternative hypotheses, such as selection effects or reverse causality. Of course, practical and ethical considerations often make randomized experiments (and even randomized controlled trials) impossible for understanding the vast array of multidimensional influences underlying substance use and its effects across the lifespan. Much current research on risk and protective factors involves correlational and quasi-experimental studies that implicitly or explicitly views causality in terms of relatively simplistic and normative temporally ordered antecedent–consequent relations (A causes B causes C). Often, the purpose of such analyses is to draw conclusions about the normative sequencing of risk factors and mediational relationships. Yet it is important to recognize that this sequential view of causality refers only to the normative sequence. Although it might describe what happens among adolescents at the population level (e.g., that those who do poorly in school are more likely to initiate substance use), the opposite sequence can occur for some individuals (e.g., substance use may precede and contribute to drops in school performance). Understanding the normative temporal order in reference to potential causality is an important goal of our research. But alternative conceptualizations that focus on the diversity of causal connections deserve consideration as well (Laird, Pettit, Bates, & Dodge, 2003; Malmberg et al., 2013; Roebroek & Koning, 2016; Schulenberg, 2006), particularly ones that attend to reciprocal and co-occurring relations. Indeed, determining that two variables "move together" within individuals over time may be as important as determining that one variable tends to trigger the other in general, especially when we are focusing on risk and protective factors that are proximal to substance use.

As we summarize above, the concepts of equifinality and multifinality are of particular importance for examining more distal risk and protective factors (Cicchetti & Rogosch, 1996). When considering how risk and protective factors might contribute to later substance use, several different types of risk factors can lead to the same outcome (i.e., equifinality). For example, as discussed previously, among adults with symptoms of alcohol use disorders, two likely pathways are represented by those with an early and enduring history of substance abuse and those who began drinking heavily in adulthood (Jester et al., 2016). Each of these histories reflects different developmental trajectories that involve two distinct constellations of risk and protective factors (Moffitt, 1993). With regard to multifinality, certain risk factors can also serve as protective factors for some individuals in some circumstances. For example, children whose parents have alcohol use disorders are at heightened risk for alcohol use disorders themselves (Sher, 1991); nevertheless, they also have a higher than average chance of abstaining from alcohol. As these examples suggest, because of variation across individuals in temporal ordering of risk factors as well as equifinality and multifinality, modeling nomothetic antecedent–consequent relationships between risk factors and outcomes may yield findings that prove inconsistent across different samples.

Relationship between Risk and Protective Factors

A second guidepost involves the relationship between risk and protective factors. One common approach is to view risk and protective factors as opposite ends of the same continuum. Thus, a variable such as behavioral undercontrol in childhood can heighten one's risk for drinking if it is high, or reduce one's risk if it is low. Using this approach, labeling something as either a risk factor or a protective factor merely depends on which end of the scale is emphasized. The benefit of this conceptualization is in its straightforwardness and interpretability. It precludes the need to consider risk and protective factors separately and fits nicely into statistical models that assume linear relationships among continuous/ordinal variables. At the same time, the low level of a risk factor is not automatically the obverse of it—it just is an indicator that this particular

risk factor is not present. For example, a low level of parent–adolescent relationship conflict does not necessarily indicate the presence of positive relationship dynamics, but simply a lack of negative dynamics.

One alternative conceptualization is that protective factors serve to moderate or buffer the effects of risk factors (e.g., Brook et al., 1997; Garmezy,
Masten, & Tellegen, 1984; Hawkins et al., 1992; Jolliffe, Farrington, Loeber,
& Pardini, 2016; Luthar, Cicchetti, & Becker, 2000; Rutter, 1990; Sameroff,
2010), such that protective factors operate only in the presence of risk factors
whose effects they moderate. A supportive family environment, for example,
might be especially protective for young people prone to risk taking or deviant
peer susceptibility (Dever et al., 2012; Maslowsky et al., 2016). Although this
interactive model affords a more sophisticated theoretical description of risk,
it is more difficult to test empirically. Rutter (1990) also warns that statistical
interaction effects may not always capture the protective processes they are
intended to represent. Protective factors, for instance, may not only moderate
the effect of risk factors but may actually reduce the presence of risk factors to
begin with. In other words, protective factors can be mediated by moderate risk
factors. For instance, a supportive family environment may reduce the likelihood of exposure to negative peer influences (mediation)—in addition, once
the young person is exposed to negative peer influences, a supportive family
environment can reduce the effects of negative peer influences (moderation).

Recent work using more sophisticated statistical analyses involving multiple levels of analysis points to an even greater complexity in the operation of
these effects. This work has shown that for some individuals, protective factors
are not protective (i.e., they have no effect), and for others, there is particular
sensitivity to the protective factor's presence or absence (e.g., Brody, Chen, &
Beach, 2013; Latendresse et al., 2011). Studies of Gene × Environment interaction effects have observed these outcomes for a number of different risk factors
and protective environments. For individuals with one genotype, environmental effects have essentially no impact in reducing vulnerability, while for others
with a different allelic combination of the same gene, presence of the protective
environment leads to a lower level of the risky behavior, but absence of the
environmental protection leads to greater than average risky behavior (i.e., the
vulnerability is enhanced). This has been termed a *susceptibility effect* (Belsky
& Pluess, 2009). To provide but one example, Trucco, Villafuerte, Heitzeg,
Burmeister, and Zucker (2016) observed that for youth who shared the minor
allelic variant (GG) of the GABA receptor subunit alpha-2 (GABRA2), living
in families with high levels of parental monitoring was associated with lower
externalizing behavior among the children, whereas low levels of parental
monitoring were associated with higher externalizing behavior. In contrast,
children who were carriers of the major allele (AA and AG genotypes) did not
differ in level of externalizing behavior, irrespective of whether they were living
in high or low parental monitoring families.

Robustness and Continuity of Risk and Protective Factors

Ideally, risk and protective factors predict a likely outcome in advance, providing us with essential information about who is likely to encounter difficulties and who is not. Longitudinal panel studies from early childhood through adulthood suggest that some risk and protective factors first appear during childhood or earlier, well before the onset of any substance use (e.g., Dubow, Boxer, & Huesmann, 2008; Maggs, Patrick, & Feinstein, 2008; Maggs, Staff, Patrick, Wray-Lake, & Schulenberg, 2015; Pitkänen, Kokko, Lyyra, & Pulkkinen, 2008; Staff, Whichard, Sienneck, & Maggs, 2015; Zucker et al., 2016) and related difficulties (e.g., Caspi, Moffitt, Newman, & Silva, 1996; Fergusson, Boden, & Horwood, 2015; Moffitt et al., 2011). Although such factors as genetic susceptibility to substance use, inept parenting, or early behavioral undercontrol do not necessarily doom a child to a life of substance use and failure, they do offer researchers and clinicians early indicators of a child's heightened vulnerability. Either directly or indirectly, these factors continue to contribute to a young person's vulnerability despite the many transitions he or she will experience during adolescence and young adulthood (Moffitt, 1993).

Risk and protective factors can be grouped according to whether they are robust (i.e., predict both current levels of and future changes in substance use), emergent (i.e., predict future changes in, but not current levels of, substance use), or concurrent (i.e., predict current levels of, but not changes in, substance use). For example, in Schulenberg, Wadsworth, and colleagues (1996) we found that male gender and the motivation of drinking "to get drunk" at age 18 were robust risk factors because both predicted current binge drinking, as well as increased binge drinking during the transition to young adulthood. In addition, general self-efficacy at age 18 was an emergent protective factor because, although it did not predict current binge drinking, it did predict less drinking during the transition to young adulthood.

In longitudinal studies of substance use that span the transition from adolescence to adulthood, many risk and protective factors have been found to be only concurrent (Bates & Labouvie, 1997; Schulenberg, Wadsworth, et al., 1996), which is not surprising given the difficulties of predicting change over time and the fact that risk and protective factors also change over time. It is important to distinguish between two types of concurrent risk and protective factors. *Time-varying* risk and protective factors change in unison with changes in substance use and reflect the continuous association of these variables (Kandel & Raveis, 1989). For example, Schulenberg, Wadsworth, and colleagues (1996) found that risk taking is a moving concurrent risk factor for binge drinking during the transition to young adulthood—that is, risk taking is related to binge drinking throughout adolescence and young adulthood. *Developmentally limited* risk and protective factors cease to change or change independently from substance use—in other words, they are of importance for only a limited time period. In Schulenberg, Wadsworth, and colleagues' (1996) study, for example, overt hostility was associated with binge drinking in high school but not during young adulthood, suggesting some discontinuity in the web of influences related to this behavior.

The constellation of risk and protective factors that move together over time with substance use also may reflect the reciprocal nature of their relationship. Just as high self-efficacy in refusal skills can protect against substance use, abstaining from substances may increase self-efficacy in refusal skills. The same phenomenon exists for more distal influences as well. For example, personality traits such as sensation seeking and impulsivity that contribute to the initiation and development of a pattern of hazardous substance use can be exacerbated once an individual begins using drugs (Malmberg et al., 2013). So long as these relationships remain intact, individuals likely will maintain a developmental trajectory that continues to elicit hazardous substance use.

INTERVENTION IMPLICATIONS OF DEVELOPMENTAL PERSPECTIVE

From a developmental perspective, two primary goals of intervention are to (1) redirect potentially risky trajectories, such that unhealthy behavioral patterns are replaced by more positive ones; and (2) alter the web of influence, such that initial risk factors lose their impact and do not inevitably lead to undesirable outcomes (Maggs et al., 1997).

To achieve these two goals, universal, selected, and indicated preventive interventions may be employed. At the population level, it is essential to reduce risky behaviors that become widely prevalent during the adolescent years, such as binge drinking, unprotected sex, and unsafe driving. However, in addition to, or as part of universal interventions that aim to promote healthy behaviors among all adolescents, attention should be given to those individuals who are already manifesting signs of problematic behavioral trajectories (Conduct Disorders Prevention Research Group, 2010; Gonzales et al., 2012). Selected and indicated preventive interventions may be necessary to assist adolescents to quit smoking, to successfully parent an unplanned child, or to finish high school after dropping out.

Strategically, common developmental transitions, such as puberty, identity quests, moving into middle or high school, and starting a part-time job, may provide opportune windows for successful intervention. As noted earlier in this chapter, developmental transitions can be stressful due to powerful needs to adapt to changes in the environment, in the individual, and in their interaction. Thus, these periods in the life course represent potential times of vulnerability. At the same time, change and discontinuity represent opportunities for individuals to develop new healthy habits, skills, and relationships. For example, the move from high school to college may allow an adolescent who was a frequent binge drinker to make new friends who have more healthful and balanced social interactions. In this way, developmental transitions may be sensitive periods for intervention; intervention programmers can take advantage of these naturally occurring windows of disequilibrium.

A developmental perspective also reminds us of the importance of taking the long view on intervention and health promotion. Positive short-term effects of preventive or clinical efforts are certainly of consequence, particularly as they relate to avoiding immediate health risks—nonetheless, long-term impact is often of greater interest. It is sometimes the case that no measurable changes in behavior are visible immediately after the conclusion of a preventive intervention—for example, a middle school program to prevent later onset and escalation of substance use (Dielman, 1994). However, minor alterations in the slope of a developmental trajectory can result in consequential changes as they accumulate over a period of years (Kellam et al., 2008; Poduska et al., 2008). This important long-term impact would be missed if data were collected only at the time of, and shortly after, the program's operation.

Finally, intervention research has much to offer developmental theory and research by providing opportunities to address fundamental questions about causal relationships in adolescent development in general and substance use in particular. Etiological theories can be put to rigorous test by attempts to alter the constellation of risk factors and observing whether hypothesized changes in targeted behaviors occur (Bronfenbrenner, 1979; Catalano et al., 2012; Coie et al., 1993; Dishion, McCord, & Poulin, 1999; Dodge, 2007; Gonzales et al., 2012).

SUMMARY AND CONCLUSIONS

As we have discussed in this chapter, alcohol and other drug use among young people is embedded within the many developmental transitions that take place during adolescence and the transition to young adulthood. This makes it essential to examine substance use in relation to adolescents' changing lives and changing contexts, as well as to follow individuals over time. Developmental transitions during adolescence and young adulthood include the fundamental changes of pubertal and cognitive development, affiliative transitions, achievement transitions, and identity transitions. As we have argued, increased health risks, including substance use, are best understood in relation to these developmental transitions. The understanding of how substance use relates to developmental transitions, including how individual characteristics and contextual features serve to moderate these relationships, offers an important foundation for attempts to contribute to lasting change in young people. The many transitions that occur during adolescence represent windows of opportunity to intervene to change courses of behavior that are already changing. By redirecting potentially risky trajectories, successful developmental interventions may not only assist in the resolution of immediate difficulties but also set the stage for continued enhanced health and well-being across the lifespan. Finally, as is becoming clearer with more long-term follow-ups of intervention studies, intervention research can assist in the understanding of basic developmental processes, letting us see what in the naturally occurring environment can contribute to long-term optimal development.

ACKNOWLEDGMENTS

Effort on this chapter for John Schulenberg and Jennifer L. Maggs was funded in part by grants from the National Institute on Drug Abuse (Nos. R01 DA001411 to Richard Miech, and R01 DA016575 to John Schulenberg). Julie Maslowsky is a Faculty Research Associate of the Population Research Center at the University of Texas at Austin, which is supported by the Eunice Kennedy Shriver National Institute of Child Health and Human Development Grant No. 5 R24 HD042849. Jennifer L. Maggs's effort was also supported by a grant from the National Institute on Alcohol Abuse and Alcoholism (No. R01 AA019606). Robert A. Zucker's effort was supported in part by grants from the National Institute on Alcohol Abuse and Alcoholism (Nos. R01 AA07065 and R01 AA12217) to Robert A. Zucker and Mary M. Heitzeg. The content here is solely the responsibility of the authors and does not necessarily represent the official views of the sponsors. We wish to thank Deborah Kloska and Virginia Laetz for their assistance with the manuscript and the editors and reviewers for their helpful comments.

REFERENCES

Allport, G. W. (1937). *Pattern and growth in personality*. New York: Holt, Rinehart & Winston.

Baltes, P. B. (1987). Theoretical propositions of life-span developmental psychology: On the dynamics between growth and decline. *Developmental Psychology, 23,* 611–626.

Baltes, P. B., Reese, H. W., & Nesselroade, J. R. (1977). *Life-span developmental psychology: Introduction to research methods*. Hillsdale, NJ: Erlbaum.

Bandura, A. (1982). The psychology of chance encounters and life paths. *American Psychologist, 37,* 747–755.

Bandura, A. (1998). Exploration of fortuitous determinants of life paths. *Psychological Inquiry, 9,* 95–98.

Bates, M. E., & Labouvie, E. W. (1997). Adolescent risk factors and the prediction of persistent alcohol and drug use into adulthood. *Alcoholism: Clinical and Experimental Research, 21,* 944–950.

Baumrind, D. (1987). A developmental perspective on adolescent risk taking in contemporary America. In C. E. Irwin, Jr. (Ed.), *Adolescent social behavior and health* (pp. 93–125). San Francisco: Jossey-Bass.

Beauchaine, T. P., & McNulty, T. (2013). Comorbidities and continuities as ontogenic processes: Toward a developmental spectrum model of externalizing psychopathology. *Development and Psychopathology, 25*(4, Pt. 2), 1505–1528.

Belsky, J., & Pluess, M. (2009). Beyond diathesis stress: Differential susceptibility to environmental influences. *Psychological Bulletin, 135,* 885–908.

Beltz, A. M., Wright, A. C., Sprague, B. N., & Molenaar, P. M. (2016). Bridging the nomothetic and idiographic approaches to the analysis of clinical data. *Assessment, 23*(4), 447–458.

Benedict, R. (1950). *Patterns of culture.* New York: New American Library.

Bergman, L. R. (2000). The application of a person-oriented approach: Types and clusters. In L. R. Bergman & R. B. Cairns (Eds.), *Developmental science and the holistic approach* (pp. 137–154). Mahwah, NJ: Erlbaum.

Birkett, H., & Cattell, R. B. (1978). Diagnosis of the dynamic roots of a clinical symptom by P-technique: A case of episodic alcoholism. *Multivariate Experimental Clinical Research, 3,* 173–194.

Block, J. (1971). *Lives through time.* Berkeley, CA: Bancroft Books.

Booth, M. Z., & Gerard, J. M. (2014). Adolescents' stage–environment fit in middle and high school: The relationship between students' perceptions of their schools and themselves. *Youth and Society, 46*(6), 735–755.

Brody, G. H., Chen, Y., & Beach, S. R. (2013). Differential susceptibility to prevention: GABAergic, dopaminergic, and multilocus effects. *Journal of Child Psychology and Psychiatry, 54,* 863–871.

Bronfenbrenner, U. (1979). *The ecology of human development: Experiments by nature and design.* Cambridge, MA: Harvard University Press.

Brook, J. S., Balka, E. B., Gursen, M. D., Brook, D. W., Shapiro, J., & Cohen, P. (1997). Young adults' drug use: A 17-year longitudinal inquiry of antecedents. *Psychological Reports, 80,* 1235–1251.

Brown, S. A., McGue, M., Maggs, J. L., Schulenberg, J. E., Hingson, R., Swartzwelder, S., et al. (2008). A developmental perspective on alcohol and youths 16 to 20 years of age. *Pediatrics, 121,* S290–S310.

Bryk, A. S., & Raudenbush, S. W. (1987). Application of hierarchical linear models to assessing change. *Psychological Bulletin, 101,* 147–158.

Bukobza, G. (2009). Relations between rebelliousness, risk-taking behavior, and identity status during emerging adulthood. *Identity, 9*(2), 159–177.

Cairns, R. B., & Cairns, B. D. (1994). *Lifelines and risks: Pathways of youth in our time.* New York: Cambridge University Press.

Casey, B. J., Jones, R. M., & Hare, T. A. (2008). The adolescent brain. *Annals of the New York Academy of Sciences, 1124,* 111–126.

Caspi, A., Moffitt, T. E., Newman, D. L., & Silva, E. A. (1996). Behavioral observations at age 3 years predict adult psychiatric disorders: Longitudinal evidence from a birth cohort. *Archives of General Psychiatry, 53,* 1033–1039.

Catalano, R. F., Fagan, A. A., Gavin, L. E., Greenberg, M. T., Irwin, C. E., Jr., Ross, D. A., et al. (2012). Worldwide application of prevention science in adolescent health. *The Lancet, 379*(9826), 1653–1664.

Cattell, R. B. (1988). The data box: Its ordering of total resources in terms of possible relational systems. In J. R. Nesselroade & R. B. Cattell (Eds.), *Handbook of multivariate experimental psychology* (2nd ed., pp. 69–130). New York: Plenum Press.

Chassin, L., Colder, C. R., Hussong, A., & Sher, K. J. (2016). Substance use and substance use disorders. In D. Cicchetti (Ed.), *Developmental psychopathology: Vol. 3. Maladaptation and psychopathology* (3rd ed., pp. 833–897). Hoboken, NJ: Wiley.

Chassin, L., Presson, C. C., & Sherman, S. J. (1989). "Constructive" vs. "destructive" deviance in adolescent heath-related behaviors. *Journal of Youth and Adolescence, 18,* 245–262.

Cicchetti, D., & Rogosch, F. A. (1996). Equifinality and multifinality in developmental psychopathology. *Development and Psychopathology, 8,* 597–600.

Cicchetti, D., & Rogosch, F. A. (2002). A developmental psychopathology perspective on adolescence. *Journal of Consulting and Clinical Psychology, 70*(1), 6–20.

Cloninger, C. R. (1987). Neurogenetic adaptive mechanisms and alcoholism. *Science, 236,* 410–416.

Coie, J. D., Watt, N. F., West, S. G., Hawkins, J. D., Asarnow, J. R., Markman, H. J., et al. (1993). The science of prevention: A conceptual framework and some directions for a national research program. *American Psychologist, 48,* 1013–1022.

Coleman, J. (1978). Current contradictions in adolescent theory. *Journal of Youth and Adolescence, 7,* 1–11.

Collins, L. M., Graham, J. W., Rousculp, S. S., & Hansen, W. B. (1997). Heavy caffeine use and the beginning of the substance use onset process: An illustration of latent transition analysis. In K. J. Bryant, M. Windle, & S. G. West (Eds.), *The science of prevention: Methodological advances from alcohol and substance abuse research* (pp. 79–99). Washington, DC: American Psychological Association.

Collins, L. M., & Lanza, S. T. (2013). *Latent class and latent transition analysis: With applications in the social, behavioral, and health sciences.* Hoboken, NJ: Wiley.

Conduct Disorders Prevention Research Group. (2010). Fast Track intervention effects on youth arrests and delinquency. *Journal of Experimental Criminology, 6,* 131–157.

Crockett, L. J., & Crouter, A. C. (Eds.). (1995). *Pathways through adolescence: Individual development in relation to social contexts.* Mahwah, NJ: Erlbaum.

Crosnoe, R. (2011). *Fitting in, standing out: Navigating the social challenges of high school to get an education.* New York: Cambridge University Press.

Del Boca, F. K., Darkes, J., Greenbaum, P. E., & Goldman, M. S. (2004). Up close and personal: Temporal variability in the drinking of individual college students during their first year. *Journal of Consulting and Clinical Psychology, 72,* 155–164.

Dever, B. V., Schulenberg, J. E., Dworkin, J. B., O'Malley, P. M., Kloska, D. D., & Bachman, J. G. (2012). Predicting risk-taking with and without substance use: The effects of parental monitoring, school bonding, and sports participation. *Prevention Science, 13*(6), 605–615.

Dielman, T. E. (1994). School-based research on the prevention of adolescent alcohol use and misuse: Methodological issues and advances. *Journal of Research on Adolescence, 4,* 271–293.

Dir, A. L., Coskunpinar, A., & Cyders, M. A. (2014). A meta-analytic review of the relationship between adolescent risky sexual behavior and impulsivity across gender, age, and race. *Clinical Psychology Review, 34*(7), 551–562.

Dishion, T. J., Capaldi, D. M., & Yoerger, K. (1999). Middle childhood antecedents to progressions in male adolescent substance use: An ecological analysis of risk and protection. *Journal of Adolescent Research, 14,* 175–205.

Dishion, T. J., McCord, J., & Poulin, F. (1999). When interventions harm: Peer groups and problem behavior. *American Psychologist, 54,* 755–764.

Dodge, K. A. (2007). Fast Track randomized controlled trial to prevent externalizing psychiatric disorders: Findings from grades 3 to 9. *Journal of the Academy of Child and Adolescent Psychiatry, 46,* 1250–1262.

Dodge, K. A., Malone, P. S., Lansford, J. E., Miller, S., Pettit, G. S., & Bates, J. E.

(2009). A dynamic cascade model of the development of substance use onset. *Monographs of the Society for Research in Child Development, 74*(3), 1–120.

Donohew, L., Zimmerman, R., Cupp, P. S., Novak, S., Colon, S., & Abell, R. (2000). Sensation seeking, impulsive decision-making, and risky sex: Implications for risk-taking and design of interventions. *Personality and Individual Differences, 28*(6), 1079–1091.

Donovan, J. E. (2004). Adolescent alcohol initiation: A review of psychosocial risk factors. *Journal of Adolescent Health, 35*, 7–18.

Draper, C. E., Grobler, L., Micklesfield, L. K., & Norris, S. A. (2015). Impact of social norms and social support on diet, physical activity and sedentary behaviour of adolescents: A scoping review. *Child: Care, Health and Development, 41*(5), 654–667.

Dubow, E. F., Boxer, P., & Huesmann, L. R. (2008). Childhood and adolescent predictors of early and middle adulthood alcohol use and problem drinking: The Columbia County Longitudinal Study. *Addiction, 103*(Suppl. 1), 36–47.

Dumas, T. M., Ellis, W. E., & Wolfe, D. A. (2012). Identity development as a buffer of adolescent risk behaviors in the context of peer group pressure and control. *Journal of Adolescence, 35*(4), 917–927.

Eccles, J. S., Lord, S. E., Roeser, R. W., Barber, B. L., & Jozefowicz, D. M. H. (1997). The association of school transitions in early adolescence with developmental trajectories through high school. In J. Schulenberg, J. L. Maggs, & K. Hurrelmann (Eds.), *Health risks and developmental transitions during adolescence* (pp. 283–320). New York: Cambridge University Press.

Eccles, J. S., Midgley, C., Wigfield, A., Buchanan, C. M., Reuman, D., Flanagan, C., et al. (1993). Development during adolescence: The impact of stage–environment fit on young adolescents' experiences in schools and in families. *The American Psychologist, 48*, 90–101.

Eitle, T. M., & Eitle, D. (2014). Race, coping strategies, and substance use behaviors: A preliminary analysis examining white and American Indian adolescents. *Substance Use and Misuse, 49*(3), 315–325.

Elder, G. H., Jr., Kirkpatrick Johnson, M., & Crosnoe, R. (2003). The emergence and development of life course theory. In J. T. Mortimer & M. J. Shanahan (Eds.), *Handbook of the life course* (pp. 3–19). New York: Kluwer Academic/Plenum.

Elder, G. H., Jr., & Shanahan, M. J. (2006). The life course and human development. In W. Damon & R. M. Lerner (Series Eds.) & R. M. Lerner (Vol. Ed.), *Handbook of child psychology: Vol. 1. Theoretical models of human development* (6th ed., pp. 665–715). Hoboken, NJ: Wiley.

Ellis, B. J., Del Giudice, M., Dishion, T. J., Figueredo, A. J., Gray, P., Griskevicius, V., et al. (2012). The evolutionary basis of risky adolescent behavior: Implications for science, policy, and practice. *Developmental Psychology, 48*, 598–623.

Erikson, E. H. (1968). *Identity, youth and crisis.* New York: Norton.

Fergusson, D. M., Boden, J. M., & Horwood, L. J. (2015). Psychosocial sequelae of cannabis use and implications for policy: Findings from the Christchurch Health and Development Study. *Social Psychiatry and Psychiatric Epidemiology, 50*(9), 1317–1326.

Fink, D. S., Gallaway, M. S., Tamburrino, M. B., Liberzon, I., Chan, P., Cohen, G. H., et al. (2016). Onset of alcohol use disorders and comorbid psychiatric disorders in a military cohort: Are there critical periods for prevention of alcohol use disorders? *Prevention Science, 17*, 347–356.

Freud, A. (1958). Adolescence. *Psychoanalytic Study of the Child, 13,* 255–278.

Freud, A. (1969). Adolescence as a developmental disturbance. In G. Caplan & S. Lebovici (Eds.), *Adolescence: Psychosocial perspectives* (pp. 5–10). New York: Basic Books.

Garmezy, N., Masten, A. S., & Tellegen, A. (1984). The study of stress and competence in children: A building block for developmental psychopathology. *Child Development, 55,* 97–111.

Global Burden of Disease Pediatrics Collaboration. (2016). Global and national burden of diseases and injuries among children and adolescents between 1990 and 2013: Findings from the Global Burden of Disease 2013 study. *JAMA Pediatrics, 170*(3), 267–287.

Gonzales, N. A., Dumka, L. E., Millsap, R. E., Gottschall, A., McClain, D. B., Wong, J. J., et al. (2012). Randomized trial of a broad preventive intervention for Mexican American adolescents. *Journal of Consulting and Clinical Psychology, 80*(1), 1–16.

Gonzales, N. A., Wong, J. J., Toomey, R. B., Millsap, R., Dumka, L. E., & Mauricio, A. M. (2014). School engagement mediates long term prevention effects for Mexican American adolescents. *Prevention Science, 15,* 929–939.

Graber, J. A. (2013). Pubertal timing and the development of psychopathology in adolescence and beyond. *Hormones and Behavior, 64*(2), 262–269.

Gutman, L. M., & Eccles, J. S. (2007). Stage–environment fit during adolescence: Trajectories of family relations and adolescent outcomes. *Developmental Psychology, 43*(2), 522–537.

Hale, D. R., Fitzgerald-Yau, N., & Viner, R. M. (2014). A systematic review of effective interventions for reducing multiple health risk behaviors in adolescence. *American Journal of Public Health, 104*(5), e19–e41.

Hall, G. S. (1916). *Adolescence* (Vols. 1–2). New York: Appleton.

Hampel, P., & Petermann, F. (2006). Perceived stress, coping, and adjustment in adolescents. *Journal of Adolescent Health, 38*(4), 409–415.

Havighurst, R. (1952). *Developmental tasks and education.* New York: McKay.

Hawkins, J. D., Catalano, R. F., & Miller, J. Y. (1992). Risk and protective factors for alcohol and other drug problems in adolescence and early adulthood: Implications for substance abuse prevention. *Psychological Bulletin, 112,* 64–105.

Heron, M. (2016). Deaths: Leading causes for 2013. *National Vital Statistics System, 65*(2), 1–95.

Hollenstein, T., & Lougheed, J. P. (2013). Beyond storm and stress: Typicality, transactions, timing, and temperament to account for adolescent change. *The American Psychologist, 68*(6), 444–454.

Howard, A. L., Patrick, M. E., & Maggs, J. L. (2015). College student affect and heavy drinking: Variable associations across days, semesters, and people. *Psychology of Addictive Behaviors, 29,* 430–443.

Hoyt, L. T., Chase-Lansdale, P. L., McDade, T. W., & Adam, E. K. (2012). Positive youth, healthy adults: Does positive well-being in adolescence predict better perceived health and fewer risky health behaviors in young adulthood? *Journal of Adolescent Health, 50*(1), 66–73.

Institute of Medicine. (2014). *Investing in the health and well-being of young adults.* Washington, DC: National Academies Press. Retrieved from *http://iom.edu/Reports/2014/Investing-in-the-Health-and-Well-Being-of-Young-Adults.aspx.*

Irwin, C. E., Jr., & Millstein, S. G. (1992). Risk-taking behaviors and biopsychosocial development during adolescence. In E. J. Susman, L. V. Feagans, & W. J. Ray (Eds.), *Emotion, cognition, health, and development in children and adolescents* (pp. 75–102). Hillsdale, NJ: Erlbaum.

Jackson, K. M., Colby, S. M., & Sher, K. J. (2010). Daily patterns of conjoint smoking and drinking in college student smokers. *Psychology of Addictive Behaviors, 24,* 424–435.

Jackson, K. M., Roberts, M. E., Colby, S. M., Barnett, N. P., Abar, C. C., & Merrill, J. E. (2014). Willingness to drink as a function of peer offers and peer norms in early adolescence. *Journal of Studies on Alcohol and Drugs, 75,* 404–414.

Jessor, R. (1993). Successful adolescent development among youth in high-risk settings. *The American Psychologist, 48,* 117–126.

Jester, J. M., Buu, A., & Zucker, R. A. (2016). Longitudinal phenotypes for alcoholism: Heterogeneity of course, early identifiers, and life course correlates. *Development and Psychopathology, 28*(4, Pt. 2), 1531–1546.

Jester, J. M., Nigg, J. T., Buu, A., Puttler, L. I., Glass, J. M., Heitzig, M. M., et al. (2008). Trajectories of childhood aggression and inattention/hyperactivity: Differential effects on substance abuse in adolescence. *Journal of the American Academy of Child and Adolescent Psychiatry, 47*(10), 1158–1165.

Jester, J. M., Wong, M. M., Cranford, J. A., Fitzgerald, H. E., & Zucker, R. A. (2015). Alcohol expectancies in childhood: Changes with the onset of drinking and ability to predict adolescent drunkenness and binge drinking. *Addiction, 110,* 71–79.

Johnston, L. D., O'Malley, P. M., Bachman, J. G., Schulenberg, J. E., & Miech, R. A. (2015). *Monitoring the Future national survey results on drug use, 1975–2014: Vol. II. College students and adults age 19–55.* Ann Arbor: Institute for Social Research, University of Michigan.

Jolliffe, D., Farrington, D. P., Loeber, R., & Pardini, D. (2016). Protective factors for violence: Results from the Pittsburgh Youth Study. *Journal of Criminal Justice, 45*(C), 32–40.

Kandel, D. B., & Raveis, V. H. (1989). Cessation of illicit drug use in young adulthood. *Archives of General Psychiatry, 46,* 109–116.

Kann, L., Kinchen, S., Shanklin, S. L., Flint, K. H., Kawkins, J., Harris, W. A., et al. (2014). Youth risk behavior surveillance—United States, 2013. *MMWR Surveillance Summary, 63*(Suppl. 4), 1–168.

Kellam, S. G., Brown, C. H., Poduska, J. M., Ialongo, N. S., Wang, W., Toyinbo, P., et al. (2008). Effects of a universal classroom behavior management program in first and second grades on young adult behavioral, psychiatric, and social outcomes. *Drug and Alcohol Dependence, 95*(Suppl. 1), S5–S28.

Kellam, S. G., & Van Horn, Y. V. (1997). Life course development, community epidemiology, and preventive trials: A scientific structure for prevention research. *American Journal of Community Psychology, 25,* 177–188.

Koning, I. M., van den Eijnden, R. J., Verdurmen, J. E., Engels, R. C., & Vollebergh, W. A. (2013). A cluster randomized trial on the effects of a parent and student intervention on alcohol use in adolescents four years after baseline: No evidence of catching-up behavior. *Addictive Behaviors, 38*(4), 2032–2039.

Kuh, D., Ben-Schlomo, Y., Lynch, J., Hallqvist, J., & Power, C. (2003). Life course epidemiology. *Journal of Epidemiology and Community Health, 57,* 778–783.

Laird, R. D., Pettit, G. S., Bates, J. E., & Dodge, K. A. (2003). Parents' monitoring-relevant knowledge and adolescents' delinquent behavior: Evidence of correlated developmental changes and reciprocal influences. *Child Development, 74*(3), 752–768.

Latendresse, S. J., Bates, J. E., Goodnight, J. A., Lansford, J. E., Budde, J. P., Goate, A., et al. (2011). Differential susceptibility to adolescent externalizing trajectories: Examining the interplay between CHRM2 and peer group antisocial behavior. *Child Development, 82,* 1797–1814.

Lerner, R. M. (1982). Children and adolescents as producers of their own development. *Developmental Review, 2,* 342–370.

Lerner, R. M. (2006). Developmental science, developmental systems, and contemporary theories of human development. In W. Damon & R. M. Lerner (Series Eds.) & R. M. Lerner (Vol. Ed.), *Handbook of child psychology: Vol. 1. Theoretical models of human development* (6th ed., pp. 1–17). Hoboken, NJ: Wiley.

Lerner, R. M. (2008). *The good teen: Rescuing adolescence from the myths of the storm and stress years.* New York: Harmony.

Lewin, K. (1939). The field theory approach to adolescence. *American Journal of Sociology, 44,* 868–897.

Luthar, S. S., Cicchetti, D., & Becker, B. (2000). The construct of resilience: A critical evaluation and guidelines for future work. *Child Development, 71*(3), 543–562.

Lynne-Landsman, S. D., Graber, J. A., & Andrews, J. A. (2010). Do trajectories of household risk in childhood moderate pubertal timing effects on substance initiation in middle school? *Developmental Psychology, 46*(4), 853–868.

Maggs, J. L. (1997). Alcohol use and binge drinking as goal-directed action during the transition to postsecondary education. In J. Schulenberg, J. L. Maggs, & K. Hurrelmann (Eds.), *Health risks and developmental transitions during adolescence* (pp. 345–371). New York: Cambridge University Press.

Maggs, J. L., Almeida, D. M., & Galambos, N. L. (1995). Risky business: The paradoxical meaning of problem behavior for young adolescents. *Journal of Early Adolescence, 15,* 339–357.

Maggs, J. L., & Hurrelmann, K. (1998). Do substance use and delinquency have differential associations with adolescents' peer relations? *International Journal of Behavioral Development, 22,* 367–388.

Maggs, J. L., Patrick, M. E., & Feinstein, L. (2008). Childhood and adulthood predictors of alcohol use and problems in adolescence and adulthood in the National Child Development Study. *Addiction, 103*(Suppl. 1), 7–22.

Maggs, J. L., & Schulenberg, J. (1998). Reasons to drink and not to drink: Altering trajectories of drinking through an alcohol misuse prevention program. *Applied Developmental Science, 2,* 48–60.

Maggs, J. L., Schulenberg, J., & Hurrelmann, K. (1997). Developmental transitions during adolescence: Health promotion implications. In J. Schulenberg, J. L. Maggs, & K. Hurrelmann (Eds.), *Health risks and developmental transitions during adolescence* (pp. 522–546). New York: Cambridge University Press.

Maggs, J. L., Staff, J., Patrick, M. E., Wray-Lake, L., & Schulenberg, J. (2015). Alcohol use at the cusp of adolescence: A prospective, national birth cohort study of prevalence and risk factors. *Journal of Adolescent Health, 56,* 639–645.

Magnusson, D. (Ed.). (1997). *The lifespan development of individuals: Behavioral, neurobiological, and psychosocial perspectives: A synthesis.* New York: Cambridge University Press.

Magnusson, D., & Bergman, L. R. (1988). Individual and variable-based approaches to longitudinal research on early risk factors. In M. Rutter (Ed.), *Studies of psychosocial risk* (pp. 45–61). Cambridge, UK: Cambridge University Press.

Malmberg, M., Kleinjan, M., Overbeek, G., Vermulst, A. A., Lammers, J., & Engels, R. C. (2013). Are there reciprocal relationships between substance use risk personality profiles and alcohol or tobacco use in early adolescence? *Addictive Behaviors, 38*(12), 2851–2859.

Marcia, J. (1994). Identity and psychotherapy. In S. L. Archer (Ed.), *Interventions for adolescent identity development* (pp. 29–46). Thousand Oaks, CA: SAGE.

Martin, M. J., Blozis, S. A., Boeninger, D. K., Masarik, A. S., & Conger, R. D. (2014). The timing of entry into adult roles and changes in trajectories of problem behaviors during the transition to adulthood. *Developmental Psychology, 50*(11), 2473–2484.

Maslowsky, J., Buvinger, E., Keating, D. P., Steinberg, L., & Cauffman, E. (2011). Cost–benefit analysis mediation of the relationship between sensation seeking and risk behavior among adolescents. *Personality and Individual Differences, 51*(7), 802–806.

Maslowsky, J., & Schulenberg, J. E. (2013). Interaction matters: Quantifying conduct problem × depressive symptoms interaction and its association with adolescent alcohol, cigarette, and marijuana use in a national sample. *Development and Psychopathology, 25*(4, Pt. 1), 1029–1043.

Maslowsky, J., Schulenberg, J., Chiodo, L. M., Hannigan, J. H., Greenwald, M. K., Janisse, J., et al. (2016). Parental support, mental health, and alcohol and marijuana use in national and high-risk African-American adolescent samples. *Substance Abuse: Research and Treatment, 9*(Suppl. 1), 11–20.

Maslowsky, J., Schulenberg, J. E., O'Malley, P. M., & Kloska, D. D. (2014). Depressive symptoms, conduct problems, and risk for polysubstance use among adolescents: Results from U.S. national surveys. *Mental Health and Substance Use, 7*(2), 157–169.

Maslowsky, J., Schulenberg, J. E., & Zucker, R. A. (2014). Influence of conduct problems and depressive symptomatology on adolescent substance use: Developmentally proximal versus distal effects. *Developmental Psychology, 50*(4), 1179–1189.

Masten, A. S., Faden, V. B., Zucker, R. A., & Spear, L. P. (2008). Underage drinking: A developmental framework. *Pediatrics, 121*(Suppl. 4), S235–S251.

Mayzer, R., Fitzgerald, H. E., & Zucker, R. A. (2009). Anticipating problem drinking risk from preschoolers' antisocial behavior: Evidence for a common delinquency-related diathesis model. *Journal of the American Academy of Child and Adolescent Psychiatry, 48*(8), 820–827.

McCabe, S. E., Veliz P., & Schulenberg J. E. (2016). Adolescent context of exposure to prescription opioids and substance use disorder symptoms at age 35: A national longitudinal study. *Pain, 157*(10), 2173–2178.

McLaughlin, K. A., & King, K. (2015). Developmental trajectories of anxiety and depression in early adolescence. *Journal of Abnormal Child Psychology, 43*, 311–323.

Mead, M. (1950). *Coming of age in Samoa.* New York: New American Library.

Menard, S. (Ed.). (2007). *Handbook of longitudinal research: Design, measurement, and analysis.* Burlington, MA: Academic Press.

Moffitt, T. E. (1993). Adolescence-limited and life-course-persistent antisocial behavior: A developmental taxonomy. *Psychological Review, 100*, 674–701.

Moffitt, T. E., Arseneault, L., Belsky, D., Dickson, N., Hancox, R. J., Harrington, H. L., et al. (2011). A gradient of childhood self control predicts health, wealth, and public safety. *Proceedings of the National Academy of Sciences of the USA, 108*(7), 2693–2698.

Molenaar, P. C. M. (1985). A dynamic factor model for the analysis of multivariate time series. *Psychometrika, 50,* 181–202.

Molenaar, P. C. M. (2004). A manifesto on psychology as idiographic science: Bringing the person back into scientific psychology, this time forever. *Measurement, 2,* 201–218.

Molenaar, P. C. M., & Campbell, C. G. (2009). The new person-specific paradigm in psychology. *Current Directions in Psychological Science, 18*(20), 112–128.

Muthén, B., & Asparouhov, T. (2008). Growth mixture modeling: Analysis with non-Gaussian random effects. *Longitudinal Data Analysis,* 143–165.

Muthén, B. O., & Curran, P. J. (1997). General longitudinal modeling of individual differences in experimental designs: A latent variable framework for analysis and power estimation. *Psychological Methods, 2,* 371–402.

Muuss, R. E. (1996). *Theories of adolescence* (6th ed.). New York: Random House.

Neighbors, C., Walters, S. T., Lee, C. M., Vader, A. M., Vehige, T., Szigethy, T., et al. (2007). Event-specific prevention: Addressing college student drinking during known windows of risk. *Addictive Behaviors, 32,* 2667–2680.

Nesselroade, J. R. (1992). Adult personality development: Issues in assessing constancy and change. In R. A. Zucker, A. I. Rabin, J. Aronoff, & S. Frank (Eds.), *Personality structure in the life course* (pp. 221–275). New York: Springer.

Nesselroade, J. R., & Ghisletta, P. (2000). Beyond static concepts in modeling behavior. In L. R. Bergman & R. B. Cairns (Eds.), *Developmental science and the holistic approach* (pp. 121–135). Mahwah, NJ: Erlbaum.

Newcomb, M. D. (1997). Psychosocial predictors and consequences of drug use: A developmental perspective within a prospective study. *Journal of Addictive Diseases, 16,* 51–89.

Nurmi, J. E. (1997). Self-definition and mental health during adolescence and young adulthood. In J. Schulenberg, J. L. Maggs, & K. Hurrelmann (Eds.), *Health risks and developmental transitions during adolescence* (pp. 395–419). New York: Cambridge University Press.

Patrick, M. E., & Lee, C. M. (2010). Sexual motivations and engagement in sexual behavior during the transition to college. *Archives of Sexual Behavior, 39*(3), 674–681.

Patrick, M. E., Maggs, J. L., & Abar, C. C. (2007). Reasons to have sex, personal goals, and sexual behavior during the transition to college. *Journal of Sex Research, 44*(3), 240–249.

Patton, G. C., Coffey, C., Lynskey, M. T., Reid, S., Hemphill, S., Carlin, J. B., et al. (2007). Trajectories of adolescent alcohol and cannabis use into young adulthood. *Addiction, 102,* 607–615.

Pepper, S. C. (1942). *World hypotheses: A study of evidence.* Berkeley: University of California Press.

Petersen, A. C., & Leffert, N. (1995). What is special about adolescence? In M. Rutter (Ed.), *Psychosocial disturbances in young people: Challenges for prevention* (pp. 3–36). New York: Cambridge University Press.

Petraitis, J., Flay, B. R., & Miller, T. Q. (1995). Reviewing theories of adolescent substance use: Organizing pieces of the puzzle. *Psychological Bulletin, 117,* 67–86.

Pinkerton, J., & Dolan, P. (2007). Family support, social capital, resilience and adolescent coping. *Child and Family Social Work, 12*(3), 219–228.

Pitkänen, T., Kokko, K., Lyyra, A.-L., & Pulkkinen, L. (2008). A developmental approach to alcohol drinking behavior in adulthood: A follow-up study from age 8 to age 42. *Addiction, 103*(Suppl. 1), 48–68.

Poduska, J. M., Kellam, S. G., Wang, W., Brown, C. H., Ialongo, N. S., & Toyinbo, P. (2008). Impact of the Good Behavior Game, a universal classroom-based behavior intervention, on young adult service use for problems with emotions, behavior, or drugs or alcohol. *Drug and Alcohol Dependence, 95*(Suppl. 1), S29–S44.

Quinn, P. D., & Fromme, K. (2012). Event-level associations between objective and subjective alcohol intoxication and driving after drinking across the college years. *Psychology of Addictive Behaviors, 26*(3), 384–392.

Ram, N., & Gerstorf, D. (2009). Methods for the study of development: Developing methods. *Research in Human Development, 6*(2–3), 61–73.

Raudenbush, S. W. (2001). Toward a coherent framework for comparing trajectories of individual change. In L. M. Collins & A. G. Sayer (Eds.), *New methods for the analysis of change*. Washington, DC: American Psychological Association.

Rawn, C. D., & Vohs, K. D. (2011). When people strive for self-harming goals: Sacrificing personal health for interpersonal success. In K. D. Vohs & R. F. Baumeister (Eds.), *Handbook of self-regulation: Research, theory, and applications* (2nd ed., pp. 374–389). New York: Guilford Press.

Reinke, W. M., Eddy, J. M., Dishion, T. J., & Reid, J. B. (2012). Joint trajectories of symptoms of disruptive behavior problems and depressive symptoms during early adolescence and adjustment problems during emerging adulthood. *Journal of Abnormal Child Psychology, 40*(7), 1123–1136.

Rhoades, B. L., & Maggs, J. L. (2006). Do academic and social goals predict planned alcohol use among college-bound high school graduates? *Journal of Youth and Adolescence, 35*, 913–923.

Roebroek, L., & Koning, I. M. (2015). The reciprocal relation between adolescents' school engagement and alcohol consumption, and the role of parental support. *Prevention Science, 17*(2), 218–226.

Rutter, M. (1990). Psychosocial resilience and protective mechanisms. In J. Rolf, A. Mastern, D. Cicchetti, K. H. Nuechterlein, & S. Weintraub (Eds.), *Risk and protective factors in the development of psychopathology* (pp. 181–214). Cambridge, UK: Cambridge University Press.

Rutter, M. (1994). Beyond longitudinal data: Causes, consequences, changes, and continuity. *Journal of Consulting and Clinical Psychology, 62*, 928–940.

Rutter, M. (1996). Transitions and turning points in developmental psychopathology: As applied to the age span between childhood and mid-adulthood. *International Journal of Behavioral Development, 19*, 603–626.

Rutter, M. (2012). Resilience as a dynamic concept. *Development and Psychopathology, 24*(2), 335–344.

Sameroff, A. (2010). A unified theory of development: A dialectic integration of nature and nurture. *Child Development, 81*, 6–22.

Schriber, R. A., & Guyer, A. E. (2015). Adolescent neurobiological susceptibility to social context. *Developmental Cognitive Neuroscience, 19*, 1–18.

Schulenberg, J. E. (2006). Understanding the multiple contexts of adolescent risky behavior and positive development: Advances and future directions. *Applied Developmental Science, 10,* 107–113.

Schulenberg, J. E., & Maggs, J. L. (2002). A developmental perspective on alcohol use and heavy drinking during adolescence and the transition to young adulthood. *Journal of Studies on Alcohol Supplement, 14,* 54–70.

Schulenberg, J., Maggs, J. L., & Hurrelmann, K. (1997). Negotiating developmental transitions during adolescence and young adulthood: Health risks and opportunities. In J. Schulenberg, J. L. Maggs, & K. Hurrelmann (Eds.), *Health risks and developmental transitions during adolescence* (pp. 1–19). New York: Cambridge University Press.

Schulenberg, J. E., & Maslowsky, J. (2015). Contribution of adolescence to the life course: What matters most in the long run? [Special issue: R. A. Settersten, Jr., & M. McClelland (Eds.), *Just one wish for the study of human development*]. *Research in Human Development 12*(3–4), 319–326.

Schulenberg, J. E., Maslowsky, J., Patrick, M. E., & Martz, M. (2016). Substance use in the context of adolescent development. In R. Zucker and S. Brown (Eds.), *The Oxford handbook of adolescent substance abuse.* New York: Oxford University Press.

Schulenberg, J., O'Malley, P. M., Bachman, J. G., Wadsworth, K. N., & Johnston, L. D. (1996). Getting drunk and growing up: Trajectories of frequent binge drinking during the transition to young adulthood. *Journal of Studies on Alcohol, 57*(3), 289–304.

Schulenberg, J. E., Patrick, M. E., Kloska, D. D., Maslowsky, J., Maggs, J. L., & O'Malley, P. M. (2015). Substance use disorder in early midlife: A national prospective study on health and well-being correlates and long-term predictors. *Substance Abuse: Research and Treatment, 9*(Suppl. 1), 41–57.

Schulenberg, J. E., & Patrick, M. E. (2011). Historical and developmental patterns of alcohol and drug use among college students: Framing the problem. In H. R. White & D. L. Rabiner (Eds.), *College drinking and drug use* (pp. 13–35). New York: Guilford Press.

Schulenberg, J. E., Patrick, M. E., Maslowsky, J., & Maggs, J. L. (2014). The epidemiology and etiology of adolescent substance use in developmental perspective. In M. Lewis & K. Rudolph (Eds.), *Handbook of developmental psychopathology* (3rd ed., pp. 601–620). New York: Springer.

Seidman, E., & French, S. E. (2004). Developmental trajectories and ecological transitions: A two-step procedure to aid in the choice of prevention and promotion interventions. *Development and Psychopathology, 16*(4), 1141–1159.

Schulenberg, J., Wadsworth, K. N., O'Malley, P. M., Bachman, J. G., & Johnston, L. D. (1996). Adolescent risk factors for binge drinking during the transition to young adulthood: Variable and pattern-centered approaches to change. *Developmental Psychology, 32,* 659–674.

Settersten, R. A., Furstenberg, F. F., Jr., & Rumbaut, R. G. (2005). *On the frontier of adulthood: Theory, research, and public policy.* Chicago: University of Chicago Press.

Shapero, B. G., Hamilton, J. L., Stange, J. P., Liu, R. T., Abramson, L. Y., & Alloy, L. B. (2015). Moderate childhood stress buffers against depressive response to proximal stressors: A multi-wave prospective study of early adolescents. *Journal of Abnormal Child Psychology, 43*(8), 1403–1413.

Sher, K. J. (1991). *Children of alcoholics: A critical appraisal of theory and research.* Chicago: University of Chicago Press.

Sher, K. J., & Wood, P. K. (1997). Methodological issues in conducting prospective research on alcohol-related behavior: A report from the field. In K. J. Bryant, M. Windle, & S. G. West (Eds.), *The science of prevention: Methodological advances from alcohol and substance abuse research* (pp. 3–41). Washington, DC: American Psychological Association.

Sibinga, E. M. S., Webb, L., Ghazarian, S. R., & Ellen, J. M. (2016). School-based mindfulness instruction: An RCT. *Pediatrics, 137*(1), 1–8.

Silbereisen, R. K., & Kracke, B. (1997). Self-reported maturational timing and adaptation in adolescence. In J. Schulenberg, J. L. Maggs, & K. Hurrelmann (Eds.), *Health risks and developmental transitions during adolescence* (pp. 85–109). New York: Cambridge University Press.

Sontag, L. M., Graber, J. A., Brooks-Gunn, J., & Warren, M. P. (2008). Coping with social stress: Implications for psychopathology in young adolescent girls. *Journal of Abnormal Child Psychology, 36*(8), 1159–1174.

Spear, L. P. (2000). The adolescent brain and age-related behavioral manifestations. *Neuroscience and Behavioral Reviews, 24,* 417–463.

Spoth, R., Trudeau, L., Shin, C., Ralston, E., Redmond, C., Greenberg, M., et al. (2013). Longitudinal effects of universal preventive intervention on prescription drug misuse: Three randomized controlled trials with late adolescents and young adults. *American Journal of Public Health, 103*(4), 665–672.

Staff, J., Schulenberg, J. E., Maslowsky, J., Bachman, J. G., O'Malley, P. M., Maggs, J. L., et al. (2010). Substance use changes and social role transitions: Proximal developmental effects on ongoing trajectories from late adolescence through early adulthood. *Development and Psychopathology, 22*(4), 917–932.

Staff, J., Whichard, C., Siennick, S. E., & Maggs, J. (2015). Early life risks, antisocial tendencies, and preteen delinquency. *Criminology, 53,* 677–701.

Steinberg, L. (2008). A social neuroscience perspective on adolescent risk-taking. *Developmental Review, 28,* 78–106.

Steinberg, L. (2015). *Age of opportunity: Lessons from the new science of adolescence.* Boston: Eamon Dolan/Mariner Books.

Sullivan, H. S. (1947). *Conceptions of modern psychiatry.* Washington, DC: William Alanson White Psychiatric Foundation.

Terry-McElrath, Y. M., O'Malley, P. M., Johnston, L. D., Bray, B. C., Patrick, M. E., & Schulenberg, J. E. (2017). Longitudinal patterns of marijuana use across ages 18–50 in a U.S. national sample: A descriptive examination of predictors and health correlates of repeated measures latent class membership. *Drug and Alcohol Dependence, 171,* 70–83.

Thorsteinsson, E. B., Ryan, S. M., & Sveinbjornsdottir, S. (2013). The mediating effects of social support and coping on the stress–depression relationship in rural and urban adolescents. *Open Journal of Depression, 2*(1), 1–6.

Trucco, E. M., Villafuerte, S., Heitzeg, M. M., Burmeister, M., & Zucker, R. A. (2016). Susceptibility effects of GABR receptor subunit alpha-2 (GABRA2) variants and parental monitoring on externalizing behavior trajectories: Risk and protection conveyed by the minor allele. *Development and Psychopathology, 28,* 15–26.

Valente, T. W., Ritt-Olson, A., Stacy, A., Unger, J. B., Okamoto, J., & Sussman, S. (2007). Peer acceleration: Effects of a social network tailored substance abuse prevention program among high-risk adolescents. *Addiction, 102*(11)*,* 1804–1815.

Velicer, W. F., & Colby, S. M. (1997). Time series analysis for prevention and treatment research. In K. J. Bryant, M. Windle, & S. G. West (Eds.), *The science of prevention: Methodological advances from alcohol and substance abuse research* (pp. 211–249). Washington, DC: American Psychological Association.

Wilkerson, J. M., Brooks, A. K., & Ross, M. W. (2010). Sociosexual identity development and sexual risk taking of acculturating collegiate gay and bisexual men. *Journal of College Student Development, 51*(3), 279–296.

Willoughby, T., Good, M., Adachi, P. J. C., Hamza, C., & Tavernier, R. (2013). Examining the link between adolescent brain development and risk taking from a social–developmental perspective. *Brain and Cognition, 83*(3), 315–323.

Wingo, A. P., Baldessarini, R. J., & Windle, M. (2015). Coping styles: Longitudinal development from ages 17 to 33 and associations with psychiatric disorders. *Psychiatry Research, 225*(3), 299–304.

Zucker, R. A. (1987). The four alcoholisms: A developmental account of the etiologic process. In P. C. Rivers (Ed.), *Nebraska Symposium on Motivation, 1987: Alcohol and addictive behavior* (pp. 27–83). Lincoln: University of Nebraska Press.

Zucker, R. A., Donovan, J. E., Masten, A. S., Mattson, M. E., & Moss, H. B. (2008). Early developmental processes and the continuity of risk for underage drinking and problem drinking. *Pediatrics, 121*(Suppl. 4), S252–S272.

Zucker, R. A., Hicks, B. M., & Heitzeg, M. H. (2016). Alcohol use and the alcohol use disorders over the life course: A cross-level developmental review. In D. Cicchetti (Ed.), *Developmental psychopathology: Vol. 3. Maladaptation and psychopathology* (3rd ed., pp. 793–833). Hoboken, NJ: Wiley.

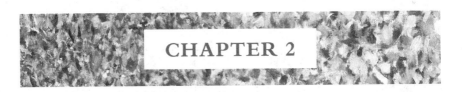

CHAPTER 2

The Neurocognitive Impact of Alcohol and Marijuana Use on the Developing Adolescent and Young Adult Brain

Krista M. Lisdahl, Skyler Shollenbarger,
Kelly A. Sagar, and Staci A. Gruber

*W*orldwide, most people start experimenting with drugs during the teenage years (Degenhardt et al., 2008). Alcohol is the most popular drug among youth, with 21% of 12th graders and 40% of young adults reporting recent binge drinking (Johnston, O'Malley, et al., 2017), which is defined as five standard drinks for males and four standard drinks for females per occasion. Although alcohol is typically initiated in adolescence, peak binge use occurs in the young adult years (Schulenberg & Maggs, 2002). The majority of adolescent drinkers (58%) also use marijuana (Martin, Kaczynski, Maisto, & Tarter, 1996), resulting in significant comorbidity between alcohol use disorder (AUD) and cannabis use disorder (CUD; Agosti, Nunes, & Levin, 2002). Of concern, during the past decade marijuana use is on the rise in youth in the United States, with 23% of high school seniors and approximately 20% of college students reporting past-year use (Johnston et al., 2017).

Adolescence is a period with an increase in risk-taking behaviors, such as experimentation with substances, which coincide with significant neurodevelopmental changes (Casey, Getz, & Galvan, 2008; Casey, Giedd, & Thomas, 2000; Eaton et al., 2006; Gardner & Steinberg, 2005). Gray matter continues to mature, with areas associated with executive functioning, including the prefrontal cortex (PFC), maturing into the mid-20s (Giedd et al., 1996; Gogtay et al., 2004; Houston, Herting, & Sowell, 2014; Lenroot & Giedd, 2006; Mills, Goddings, Clasen, Giedd, & Blakemore, 2014; Schmitt et al., 2014; Sowell, Thompson, Holmes, Jernigan, & Toga, 1999; Sowell et al., 2004; Sowell, Trauner, Gamst, & Jernigan, 2002). Preclinical animal studies have suggested that compared with adults, adolescent animals show increased neurotoxic effects following alcohol exposure (see Barron et al., 2005; Monti et al., 2005). Taken together, findings from preclinical studies (Rubino et al., 2009; see Rubino, Zamberletti, & Parolaro, 2012, for a review) have demonstrated greater microcellular changes associated with delta-9-tetrahydrocannabinol (THC) exposure, the primary psychoactive constituent in marijuana, during adolescence compared with adulthood. Therefore, the neurocognitive effects of chronic alcohol or marijuana exposure in youth are of great interest. In this chapter, we provide an overview of studies that examined the impact of adolescent and young adult binge drinking, AUD, and regular marijuana exposure. We also examine potential clinical and public health implications of these findings.

ADOLESCENT SUBSTANCE USE EXPOSURE AND RISKS FOR SUBSTANCE USE DISORDERS

Converging lines of evidence suggest that adolescence may represent a sensitive period during which exposure to substances increases the risk of substance use disorders (SUDs) and neurocognitive impairments compared with adult exposure (Brown & Tapert, 2004; Spear, 2015; Spear & Swartzwelder, 2014). Several studies have reported that adolescent alcohol exposure is associated with increased risk for developing an AUD (Dawson, Goldstein, Chou, Ruan, & Grant, 2008; DeWit, Adlaf, Offord, & Ogborne, 2000; Hingson, Heeren, & Winter, 2006; McGue, Iacono, Legrand, Malone, & Elkins, 2001; Robins & Przybeck, 1985; Winters & Lee, 2008). For example, one study reported that the odds of developing an AUD are decreased by 14% with each increasing year of age of alcohol use onset (Grant & Dawson, 1997). Earlier age of marijuana use has also been associated with increased risk for developing a CUD. In one study, Anthony (2006) reported that 17% of those who tried marijuana prior to age 17 became dependent, and a later survey study indicated that 11.5% of adults who reported having tried marijuana prior to age 14 met DSM-5 criteria for CUD as compared with only 2.6% of those who tried marijuana after age 18 (Substance Abuse and Mental Health Services Administration, 2013). Further, earlier onset of marijuana use has also been associated with higher rates of alcohol dependence as well as other SUDs (Brook, Brook, Zhang, Cohen, & Whiteman, 2002; Lynskey, Heath, Bucholz, & Slutske, 2003). Together, these findings support the hypothesis that adolescence is a vulnerable developmental period in which individuals have a higher risk of developing an SUD following exposure to alcohol and marijuana.

NEUROCOGNITIVE CONSEQUENCES OF ADOLESCENT BINGE DRINKING

Binge drinking is typically defined as four or more standard alcohol drinks on an occasion for females and five or more drinks for males. In humans, converging evidence has also suggested that adolescent onset of regular alcohol exposure is associated with increased risk for neurocognitive deficits (see Jacobus & Tapert, 2013; Lisdahl, Gilbart, Wright, & Shollenbarger, 2013; Squeglia, Jacobus, & Tapert, 2009; Squeglia et al., 2015, for reviews). Below we provide an overview of the cognitive and brain structural and functional findings associated with human adolescent and young adult binge drinking.

Cognition

As previously reported in our work (Lisdahl, Gilbart, et al., 2013) and in several additional studies, adolescent and young adult binge drinking is associated with cognitive deficits across numerous domains. Youth who engage in binge drinking have been found to exhibit poorer verbal working memory (Parada et al., 2012), spatial working memory (Scaife & Duka, 2009; Townshend & Duka, 2005), sustained attention (Hartley, Elsabagh, & File, 2004), memory (Hartley et al., 2004; Parada et al., 2011; Scaife & Duka, 2009), perseverative responding (Parada et al., 2012), and decision making (Malone et al., 2014). In addition, poorer response inhibition and rule acquisition has been noted in adolescent female binge drinkers (Scaife & Duka, 2009; Townshend & Duka, 2005). Although slower psychomotor speed was also observed in one study (Hartley et al., 2004), two later studies reported faster motor speed (Scaife & Duka, 2009; Townshend & Duka, 2005; see Table 2.1).

For example, in a monozygotic co-twin controlled investigation, Malone and colleagues (2014) reported that among twin pairs who were discordant for alcohol use, adolescent binge drinkers demonstrated significantly poorer decision making on the Iowa Gambling Task; these differences were directly related to alcohol use status among twins, suggesting a causal effect of alcohol (Malone et al., 2014). In contrast, a longitudinal investigation (TRAILS) following 11- to 19-year-olds did not find executive functioning deficits (inhibition, working memory, sustained attention) associated with drinking status (nondrinkers compared with chronic heavy drinkers; Boelema et al., 2015). The authors suggested previous findings may be due to premorbid differences (i.e., differences that existed prior to drinking onset) that placed adolescents at risk for binge drinking. However, a 3-year longitudinal study (Jacobus et al., 2015) found that adolescents with concomitant alcohol and marijuana use

TABLE 2.1. Human Studies Reporting Neuropsychological Effects of Regular Alcohol and Marijuana Exposure in Adolescents and Emerging Adults

Authors	Teen onset worse?[a]	Cognitive findings (bingers vs. controls)
Binge-drinking studies		
Boelema et al. (2015)		No differences in executive functioning
Hartley, Elsabagh, & File (2004)		↓ sustained attention, memory, and psychomotor speed
Malone et al. (2014)		↓ executive functioning
Parada et al. (2011)		↓ verbal memory, working memory, and executive functioning
Scaife & Duka (2009)		↓ verbal memory, spatial working memory, and executive functioning
Townshend & Duka (2009)		↓ spatial working memory and executive functioning; ↑ motor speed
AUD studies		
Hicks, Durbin, Blonigen, Iacono, & McGue (2012)	Yes	↑ behavioral disinhibition
Lyvers, Czerczyk, Follent, & Lodge (2009)	Yes	↑ reward sensitivity and disinhibition
Lyvers, Duff, & Hasking (2011)	Yes	↑ reward sensitivity and disinhibition
White et al. (2011)		↓ executive functioning; ↑ disinhibition
Brown, Tapert, Granholm, & Delis (2000)		↓ verbal memory
Hanson, Medina, Padula, Tapert, & Brown (2011)		↓ verbal memory, visuospatial ability, and executive functioning
Thoma et al. (2011)		↓ processing speed
Koskinen et al. (2011)		↓ attention
Tapert & Brown (1999)		↓ attention
Giancola, Mezzich, & Tarter (1998)		↓ visuospatial ability
Sher, Martin, Wood, & Rutledge (1997)		↓ visuospatial ability
Tapert, Granholm, Leedy, & Brown (2002)		↓ visuospatial ability
Moss, Kirisci, Gordon, & Tarter (1994)		↓ language

(continued)

TABLE 2.1. (*continued*)

Authors	Teen onset worse?[a]	Cognitive findings (bingers vs. controls)
	Marijuana studies	
Meier et al. (2012)	Yes	↓ IQ, complex attention, verbal learning, psychomotor speed, and executive functioning
Pope et al. (2003)	Yes	↓ IQ
Ehrenreich et al. (1999)	Yes	↓ working memory
Dougherty et al. (2013)	Yes	↑ impulsivity; ↓ short-term memory
Dahlgren, Sagar, Racine, Dreman, & Gruber (2016)		↓ executive functioning
Fontes et al. (2011)	Yes	↓ executive functioning
Gonzalez et al. (2012)		↓ executive functioning
Grant, Chamberlain, Schreiber, & Odlaug (2012)		↓ executive functioning
Gruber & Yurgelun-Todd (2005)		↓ executive functioning
Gruber, Sagar, Dahlgren, Racine, & Lukas (2012)	Yes	↓ executive functioning and processing speed
Hanson, Thayer, & Tapert (2014)	Yes	↑ risk taking; ↓ executive functioning
Jacobus et al. (2015)	Yes	↓ executive functioning and processing speed
Sagar et al. (2015)	Yes	↓ executive functioning
Schuster, Crane, Mermelstein, & Gonzalez (2012)		↓ executive functioning; ↑ risky sexual behavior
Solowij et al. (2012)	Yes	↓ executive functioning
Tamm et al. (2013)	Yes	↓ executive functioning
Hanson, Winward, et al. (2010)		↓ complex attention, verbal memory, and executive functioning
Harvey, Sellman, Porter, & Frampton (2007)		↓ complex attention, verbal memory, and executive functioning
Lisdahl & Price (2012)		↓ complex attention, processing speed, sequencing ability, and cognitive inhibition
Medina, Hanson, et al. (2007)		↓ complex attention, processing speed, verbal memory, and executive functioning

TABLE 2.1. (*continued*)

Authors	Teen onset worse?[a]	Cognitive findings (bingers vs. controls)
Mathias et al. (2011)		↓ complex attention and executive functioning
Tapert, Baratta, Abrantes, & Brown (2002)		↓ complex attention
Becker, Collins, & Luciana (2014)	Yes	↓ verbal memory, spatial working memory, spatial planning, and executive functioning
Crane, Schuster, & Gonzalez (2013)		↓ episodic memory (females) and executive functioning (males)
Crane, Schuster, Mermelstein, & Gonzalez (2015)	Yes	↓ episodic memory and IQ
Fried, Watkinson, & Gray (2005)		↓ verbal memory and processing speed
McHale & Hunt (2008)		↓ verbal memory and executive functioning
Schwartz, Gruenwald, Klitzner, & Fedio (1989)		↓ verbal memory
Solowij et al. (2011)		↓verbal memory and executive functioning
Tait, Mackinnon, & Christensen (2011)		↓ verbal memory
Thoma et al. (2011)		↓ verbal memory
Winward, Hanson, Tapert, & Brown (2014)	Yes	↓ verbal memory, psychomotor speed, and inhibition
Cousijn, Watson, et al. (2013)		↑ attentional bias to marijuana-related words
Takagi et al. (2011)		No differences reported
Comorbid marijuana + alcohol		
Jacobus et al. (2015)	Yes	↓ complex attention, memory, processing speeding, and visuospatial functioning
Winward et al. (2014)	Yes	↓ executive functioning, verbal memory, and working memory

[a] If "yes," analysis revealed that teenage age of onset (<16, 17, or 18 years of age) was associated with significantly poorer neurocognitive outcome; if "no," onset was not associated with outcome; if left blank, age-of-onset analysis was not conducted in this study.

performed significantly more poorly than controls in the neuropsychological domains of complex attention, memory, processing speed, and visuospatial functioning across three time points.

Brain Structure

Studies examining the impact of binge or heavy drinking on brain morphometry have generally found reduced gray matter volume, abnormal cortical thickness, and reduced white matter integrity in multiple brain regions (Lisdahl, Gilbart, et al., 2013). Specifically, increased alcohol use in adolescents has been linked with reduced cerebellar (Medina, Nagel, & Tapert, 2010; Lisdahl, Thayer, Squeglia, McQueeny, & Tapert, 2013); orbitofrontal cortex (Malone et al., 2014); ventromedial PFC and inferior frontal gyrus (Whelan et al., 2014); PFC, lateral frontal, and temporal cortex (Squeglia et al., 2015); total, PFC, and temporal gray matter volumes (Pfefferbaum et al., 2016); and larger middorsolateral PFC volume (Doallo et al., 2014). Other studies have reported abnormal cortical thickness, including increased cortical thickness in prefrontal, parietal, and temporal regions (Jacobus, Squeglia, Sorg, Nguyen-Louie, & Tapert, 2014) and thinner right-middle frontal gyrus (Luciana, Collins, Muetzel, & Lim, 2013); total, frontal, and temporal cortices (Pfefferbaum et al., 2016); and cingulate cortex (Mashhoon et al., 2014) in young binge drinkers. One longitudinal investigation (Squeglia et al., 2015) compared brain structure in 75 adolescents who transitioned into heavy drinking and 50 who remained light to nondrinkers over approximately 3.5 years—they found that the heavy-drinking adolescents demonstrated accelerated gray matter reductions in PFC and temporal volumes. Several studies to date have also demonstrated reduced white matter volume and integrity in young binge drinkers (Bava, Jacobus, Thayer, & Tapert, 2013; Jacobus et al., 2009; Jacobus, Squeglia, Infante, Bava, & Tapert, 2013; Luciana et al., 2013; McQueeny et al., 2009; Pfefferbaum et al., 2016; Squeglia et al., 2015). Notably, McQueeny et al. (2009) found that increased hangover symptoms and greater estimated peak blood alcohol concentration estimates were significantly correlated with poorer white matter quality in frontocerebellar tracts.

Brain Function

Studies have reported abnormal functional magnetic resonance imaging (fMRI) response in adolescent binge drinkers to spatial working memory (Squeglia et al., 2012; Squeglia, Schweinsburg, Pulido, & Tapert, 2011), decision-making (Gilman, Ramchandani, Crouss, & Hommer, 2012; Xiao et al., 2013), inhibitory control (Ahmadi et al., 2013, 2014; Wetherill, Squeglia, Yang, & Tapert, 2013), verbal memory (Schweinsburg, McQueeny, Nagel, Eyler, & Tapert, 2010), and figural memory (Dager et al., 2014) tasks. For example, Schweinsburg and colleagues (2010) reported that adolescent binge drinkers, when compared with nondrinkers, failed to engage the hippocampus during a novel verbal encoding fMRI task. Two longitudinal investigations revealed that baseline differences in fMRI response to an inhibitory control and visual working memory task predicted initiation of heavy alcohol drinking in that adolescents who transitioned to heavy alcohol use showed blunted fMRI response at baseline in frontal and parietal regions (Squeglia et al., 2012; Wetherill, Squeglia, et al., 2013).

Taken together, these findings suggest that large doses of alcohol (binges) during the adolescent years are associated with cognitive, structural, and functional abnormalities. However, additional large-scale longitudinal studies are needed to confirm causation. These neurocognitive consequences, combined with other alcohol-related consequences (e.g., legal issues, poor sleep, hangover, emotional stress, interpersonal conflict), may significantly impact performance in the classroom, as previous research has reported that binge drinking is predictive of poorer end-of-semester grade-point averages (Read, Merrill, Kahler, & Strong, 2007).

NEUROCOGNITIVE CONSEQUENCES OF AUDS IN ADOLESCENTS

An estimated 2.7% of adolescents (ages 12–17) and 12.3% of young adults (ages 18–25) met past-year criteria for an AUD in 2014 (Center for Behavioral Health Statistics and Quality, 2015). Several studies have now shown that despite fewer years of drinking and less overall alcohol exposure than adults, adolescents and young adults with AUD demonstrate significant neurocognitive deficits.

Cognition

Studies examining the neuropsychological functioning in adolescents and young adults with AUD have demonstrated several cognitive deficits, including poorer verbal memory (Brown, Tapert, Granholm, & Delis, 2000; Hanson, Medina, Padula, Tapert, & Brown, 2011), attention (Koskinen et al., 2011; Tapert & Brown, 1999; Thoma et al., 2011), psychomotor speed (Thoma et al., 2011), language function (Moss, Kirisci, Gordon, & Tarter, 1994), visuospatial ability (Giancola, Mezzich, & Tarter, 1998; Hanson et al., 2011; Sher, Martin, Wood, & Rutledge, 1997; Tapert, Granholm, Leedy, & Brown, 2002), and executive functioning (Hanson et al., 2011; White et al., 2011). Further, three studies have reported that adolescent onset of binge drinking was associated with worsened executive functioning (disinhibition) and increased reward sensitivity (Hicks, Durbin, Blonigen, Iacono, & McGue, 2012; Lyvers, Czerczyk, Follent, & Lodge, 2009; Lyvers, Duff, & Hasking, 2011; see Table 2.1.) Consistent with McQueeny et al. (2009), withdrawal symptoms have predicted poorer memory retrieval and visuospatial performance (Brown et al., 2000; Hanson et al., 2011; Tapert & Brown, 1999; Tapert, Granholm, et al., 2002), suggesting that drinking to the point of experiencing withdrawal may be related to an increased likelihood of neurocognitive deficits.

Brain Structure

Converging lines of evidence have shown structural abnormalities in adolescents with AUD, including smaller PFC (De Bellis et al., 2005; Medina et al., 2008), hippocampal (De Bellis et al., 2000; Medina, Schweinsburg, Cohen-Zion, Nagel, & Tapert, 2007; Nagel, Schweinsburg, Phan, & Tapert, 2005), and temporal and parietal (Fein et al., 2013) volumes. A recent study by Brooks and colleagues (2014) found that teens with AUD demonstrated reduced superior temporal gyrus brain volume, although AUD did not predict reductions in other areas, such as the hippocampus, after controlling for childhood trauma (Brooks et al., 2014), suggesting that reduced hippocampal volumes reported in other studies may partially be due to childhood trauma. Additional studies are therefore needed to examine the impact of childhood trauma and other related variables on structural brain findings.

Brain Function

FMRI studies in adolescents and young adults with AUD have revealed abnormal cortical activation during spatial working memory in girls (Tapert et al., 2001) (Caldwell et al., 2005) and verbal working memory tasks in males (Park et al., 2011). In summary, adolescents and young adults with AUD demonstrate mild to moderate neurocognitive impairments, especially in the executive function, memory, and visuospatial domains. They also have reduced cortical and subcortical volumes and abnormal brain activation to working memory tasks. These findings parallel what is seen in adults with AUD, despite youth having fewer drinking years and less overall exposure.

IMPACT OF ADOLESCENT
MARIJUANA USE ON NEUROCOGNITION

The endogenous endocannabinoid (eCB) system has been shown to have an integral role in developmental brain processes, most importantly neuroplasticity, including neurogenesis and activity-dependent distinction and specificity of neuronal connections (Díaz-Alonso, Guzmán, & Galve-Roperh, 2012; Lee & Gorzalka, 2012; Nyilas et al., 2008). Several recent studies have reported a relationship between the eCB system and cognition and behavior, noting that increased eCB signaling is associated with improved executive functioning, reduced stress response, increased endogenous reward signaling, and improved emotional regulation (Befort, 2015; Egerton, Allison, Brett, & Pratt, 2006; Filbey & DeWitt, 2012; Hill & McEwen, 2010; Hill & Tasker, 2012; Hillard, Weinlander, & Stuhr, 2012; Hurd, Michaelides, Miller, & Jutras-Aswad, 2014; Lee & Gorzalka, 2012; Pazos et al., 2013). However, exposure to *exogenous* cannabinoids, including delta-9-THC (or THC), a CB_1 agonist with strong binding affinity, has been shown to have deleterious effects on the brain. In particular, changes following THC exposure may alter the function and structure of brain regions rich in CB_1 cannabinoid receptors, especially during adolescence.

Cognition

As reported in recent reviews (Jacobus & Tapert, 2014; Lisdahl, Gilbart, et al., 2013; Lisdahl, Wright, Kirchner-Medina, Maple, & Shollenbarger, 2014), teen-age onset of marijuana use is associated with greater neurocognitive deficits relative to those who begin marijuana use in adulthood. Increased frequency of marijuana use (weekly or more often) prior to age 18 has been associated with reduced performance on measures of IQ (Crane, Schuster, Mermelstein, & Gonzalez, 2015; Meier et al., 2012; Pope et al., 2003), spatial working memory (Becker, Collins, & Luciana, 2014; Cousijn, Watson, et al., 2013), visual scanning (Ehrenreich et al., 1999), memory (Becker et al., 2014; Crane, Schuster, & Gonzalez, 2013; Crane et al., 2015; Dougherty et al., 2013; Winward, Hanson, Tapert, & Brown, 2014), psychomotor speed (Jacobus et al., 2015; Winward et al., 2014), and executive functioning (Becker et al., 2014; Crane et al., 2013; Dahlgren, Sagar, Racine, Dreman, & Gruber, 2016; Dougherty et al., 2013; Fontes et al., 2011; Gruber, Dahlgren, Sagar, Gönenç, & Killgore, 2012; Hanson, Thayer, & Tapert, 2014; Jacobus et al., 2015; Sagar et al., 2015; Solowij et al., 2012; Tamm et al., 2013; Winward et al., 2014).

Longitudinal studies have also assessed the association between marijuana use and cognitive performance in order to clarify the potential impact of adolescent marijuana use. While one study demonstrated that poorer inhibitory functioning at ages 12–14 was predictive of more frequent marijuana use at ages 17 and 18 (Squeglia, Jacobus, Nguyen-Louie, & Tapert, 2014), other longitudinal investigations have linked adolescent marijuana use to deficits in attention (Jacobus et al., 2015; Tapert, Granholm, et al., 2002), memory (Jacobus et al., 2015; Tait, Mackinnon, & Christensen, 2011), processing speed, and visuospatial functioning (Jacobus et al., 2015). Further, Jacobus and colleagues (2015) reported that *earlier onset* of marijuana use was associated with poorer processing speed and executive functioning at follow-up 3 years later. In a large prospective study (Meier et al., 2012), individuals assessed from childhood into adulthood diagnosed with marijuana dependence at three or more study visits exhibited an average loss of 5.8 IQ points; individuals with more persistent and early marijuana use demonstrated the greatest reduction in IQ. Although the final sample size for persistent marijuana dependence was small ($n = 23$), after controlling for potential confounding variables the authors also found that deficits in executive functioning, sustained attention, verbal list learning, and psychomotor speed were associated with persistent marijuana dependence. Two more recent longitudinal studies have recently challenged the reported association between marijuana use and reduced IQ, however, suggesting that observed differences in IQ between marijuana users and nonusers may in fact be due to familial (Jackson et al., 2016) or other confounding factors (e.g., cigarette use; Mokrysz et al., 2016). Cross-sectional studies focused on examining marijuana-using youth and emerging adults have reported marijuana-related cognitive deficits with only one exception (Takagi et al., 2011). Overall, studies have reported an association between marijuana use and reduced processing speed (Fried, Watkinson, & Gray, 2005; Gruber, Dahlgren, Sagar, Gönenç, & Killgore, 2012; Jacobus et al., 2015; Lisdahl & Price, 2012; Medina, Hanson, et al., 2007), complex attention (Hanson, Winward, et al., 2010; Harvey et al., 2007; Lisdahl & Price, 2012; Mathias et al., 2011; Medina, Hanson, et al., 2007; Tapert, Baratta, et al., 2002), verbal memory (Becker et al., 2014; Dougherty et al., 2013; Fried et al., 2005; Hanson, Winward, et al., 2010; Harvey et al., 2007; McHale & Hunt, 2008; Medina, Hanson, et al., 2007; Schwartz, Gruenewald, Klitzner, & Fedio, 1989; Solowij et al., 2011; Tait, Mackinnon, & Christensen, 2011; Thoma et al., 2011; Winward et al., 2014), executive functioning (Becker et al., 2014; Crane et al., 2013; Dahlgren et al., 2016; Dougherty et al., 2013; Gonzalez et al., 2012; Grant, Chamberlain, Schreiber, & Odlaug, 2012; Gruber, Dahlgren, et al., 2012; Gruber & Yurgelun-Todd, 2005; Hanson et al., 2014; Hanson, Winward, et al., 2010; Harvey et al., 2007; Jacobus et al., 2015; Lisdahl & Price, 2012; Mathias et al., 2011; McHale & Hunt, 2008; Medina, Hanson, et al., 2007; Sagar et al., 2015; Schuster, Crane, Mermelstein, & Gonzalez, 2012; Solowij et al., 2012; Winward et al., 2014), attentional bias to marijuana cues (Cousijn, Watson, et al., 2013), and risky sexual behavior (Schuster et al., 2012; see Table 2.1.).

Brain Structure

Consistent with research documenting the association between cognitive deficits and adolescent onset of marijuana use, numerous cross-sectional studies have also observed structural alterations in those with adolescent marijuana onset, with few exceptions (Block et al., 2000; Weiland et al., 2015). Across studies, results are bidirectional in terms of increased or decreased gray matter, and findings are often dependent on the brain region under examination (see Batalla et al., 2013, for a review). Nonetheless, numerous studies document alterations among adolescent and early-onset users (Ashtari et al., 2011; Battistella et al., 2014; Gilman et al., 2012; Lisdahl et al., 2016; Mashhoon, Sava, Sneider, Nickerson, & Silveri, 2015; McQueeny et al., 2011; Schacht, Hutchison, & Filbey, 2012), which persist after 1 month of closely monitored abstinence (Medina et al., 2010). Moreover, several studies have linked gray matter alterations to increased executive dysfunction (Churchwell, Lopez-Larson, &

Yurgelun-Todd, 2010; Medina et al., 2009, 2010; Price et al., 2015), mood symptoms (McQueeny et al., 2011), poor verbal memory (Ashtari et al., 2011), and novelty seeking (Churchwell, Carey, Ferrett, Stein, & Yurgelun-Todd, 2012).

Studies assessing cortical thickness in adolescent and young adult marijuana users have also reported bidirectional findings (Jacobus et al., 2014, 2015; Lisdahl et al., 2016; Mashhoon et al., 2015) that appear to be dependent on the brain region under study (Lopez-Larson et al., 2011) and age of onset of use. For example, an examination of cortical architecture in early- and late-onset marijuana users revealed that among early-onset users, continued years of marijuana use (i.e., longer duration of use) and increased current levels of marijuana use (in grams) were associated with thicker cortex measurements, while late-onset users who initiated use after age 16 exhibited thinner cortex measurements within the anterior dorsolateral prefrontal cortex (Filbey, McQueeny, DeWitt, & Mishra, 2015). Additional research is needed to clarify the impact of cortical thickness on cognitive functioning or other related variables.

Finally, recent studies have also investigated the extent of gyrification, folds in the cerebral cortex, or cortical curvature as a measure of gray matter architecture. Studies have reported reduced cortical curvature (Mata et al., 2010), decreased local gyrification in early- relative to late-onset users (Filbey et al., 2015), and reduced PFC gyrification (Shollenbarger, Price, Wieser, & Lisdahl, 2015a). Further, Shollenbarger and colleagues (2015a) found that this reduced cortical folding complexity was linked with poorer working memory in the cannabis users.

Although CB_1 cannabinoid receptors are primarily found on neurons, they also exist on myelinating glial cells and are thought to play a significant role in structural connectivity (Moldrich & Wenger, 2000). Perhaps not surprisingly, marijuana use during adolescence appears to affect the trajectory of white matter development. Structural (Medina, Nagel, Park, McQueeny, & Tapert, 2007) and microstructural (Arnone et al., 2008; Ashtari et al., 2009; Bava et al., 2009, 2013; Gruber, Dahlgren, Sagar, Gönenç, & Lukas, 2014; Gruber, Silveri, Dahlgren, & Yurgelun-Todd, 2011; Shollenbarger, Price, Wieser, & Lisdahl, 2015b) reductions in white matter have been observed both in adolescent marijuana users, as well as in adults who initiated marijuana use during adolescence. With only one exception (Delisi et al., 2006), several studies have reported reduced white matter quality in several PFC, limbic, parietal, and cerebellar tracts in adolescent and emerging adult marijuana users (Arnone et al., 2008; Ashtari et al., 2009; Bava et al., 2009; Clark, Chung, Thatcher, Pajtek, & Long, 2012; Epstein & Kumra, 2015; Gruber et al., 2011). Alterations in white matter have been identified as a potential risk factor for psychological dysregulation and CUD-related symptoms (Clark et al., 2012). In one of our own studies (Gruber et al., 2014), analyses revealed that lower white matter integrity was inversely correlated with higher impulsivity scores, specifically within early-onset marijuana smokers (marijuana use prior to age 16); this relationship was *not* detected within the late-onset marijuana group (marijuana use after age 16), underscoring the importance of early intervention and education to help prevent adverse consequences associated with early-onset marijuana use.

Brain Function

With one exception (Cousijn et al., 2014), several studies have also reported altered brain activation patterns in young marijuana users (see Batalla et al., 2013; Jacobus & Tapert, 2014; Lisdahl, Gilbart, et al., 2013, for reviews). FMRI studies designed to examine brain activation patterns in adolescent marijuana users have reported abnormal PFC, orbitofrontal, cingulate, parietal, insular, subcortical/limbic, and cerebellar activation during attentional control (Abdullaev, Posner, Nunnally, & Dishion, 2010), implicit memory (Ames et al., 2013), spatial working memory (Schweinsburg et al., 2005), verbal working memory (Jacobsen, Mencl, Westerveld, & Pugh, 2004; Jacobsen, Pugh, Constable, Westerveld, & Mencl, 2007), verbal learning (Becker, Wagner, Gouzoulis-Mayfrank, Spuentrup, & Daumann, 2010), affective processing (Gruber, Rogowska, & Yurgelun-Todd, 2009), and reward processing tasks (Chung, Paulsen, Geier, Luna, & Clark, 2015; De Bellis et al., 2013; Jager, Block, Luijten, & Ramsey, 2013). Further, several recent papers specifically highlight altered activation patterns during the performance of executive functioning tasks in early-onset marijuana users relative to healthy controls, including decision making (Behan et al., 2014; Cousijn, Wiers, et al., 2013; De Bellis et al., 2013; Vaidya et al., 2012) and inhibitory control (Gruber, Sagar, Dahlgren, Racine, & Lukas, 2012; Sagar et al., 2015; Tapert et al., 2007) tasks. The majority of studies suggest that early marijuana exposure may result in the brain attempting to compensate via recruitment of additional neuronal regions, resulting in altered functional connectivity relative to healthy controls. However, this compensatory function may fail when challenged with increasing task complexity, as marijuana users often demonstrate reduced performance on more difficult tasks designed to assess processing speed, verbal memory, inhibitory control, working memory, and attention (Lisdahl, Gilbart, et al., 2013; Sagar et al., 2015).

Taken together, studies conducted to date suggest that regular exposure to eCBs may disrupt healthy neurodevelopment, especially in the PFC and parietal cortices, areas underlying higher-order cognitive functioning. These changes have been associated with poor neuronal efficiency and cognitive impairment across multiple domains. In particular, psychomotor speed, executive functioning, emotional control, learning, and memory appear to be most affected, even after a month of monitored abstinence from marijuana use. This is consistent with the finding that increased school difficulty, reduced grades, higher absenteeism, lower SAT scores, and reduced college degree attainment have been observed in marijuana-using teens and young adults (Maggs et al., 2015; Medina, Hanson, et al., 2007; Meier, Hill, Small, & Luthar, 2015). Early initiation of marijuana use may therefore impact the typical neurodevelopmental trajectory, resulting in millions of youth who may not reach their full intellectual potential.

DOES CONTENT OF MARIJUANA (ESPECIALLY CANNABIDIOL VS. THC) MATTER?

Marijuana comprises hundreds of chemicals, including numerous distinct phytocannabinoids that modulate the endocannabinoid system. Different cannabinoids have unique effects on both physiological and psychological functioning, and the relative amount and ratio of each cannabinoid is especially important. THC is the major psychoactive constituent of marijuana and is mainly responsible for the subjective "high" felt by recreational marijuana users. Over the past two decades, while THC levels have steadily increased, levels of the major nonpsychoactive constituent of marijuana, cannabidiol (CBD), shown to have a variety of potential therapeutic and medicinal properties, have decreased (Burgdorf, Kilmer, & Pacula, 2011; ElSohly et al., 2016). Literature focused on *acute* exposure suggests that higher levels of CBD, as opposed to THC, may mitigate some of the negative effects of use (Niesink & van Laar, 2013), such as anxiety (Fusar-Poli et al., 2009; Winton-Brown et al., 2011), psychotic-like symptoms (Bhattacharyya et al., 2010; Englund et al., 2013; Winton-Brown et al., 2011), and memory impairment (Englund et al., 2013; Morgan, Schafer, Freeman, & Curran, 2010). Further, some suggest that CBD may moderate the effects of THC on affective processing (Bhattacharyya et al., 2010; Fusar-Poli et al., 2009), verbal memory and response inhibition (Bhattacharyya et al., 2010), and visual and auditory processing (Bhattacharyya et al., 2010; Winton-Brown et al., 2011). In addition, CBD may serve to mitigate some of the structural and neurochemical alterations related to THC (Lorenzetti, Solowij, & Yücel,, 2016; Yücel et al., 2016).

These findings are particularly salient given reports of sharply rising potency of recreational marijuana in the United States. The potency of recreational marijuana, expressed as the percentage of THC present, is estimated to have increased from 4% in 1995 to 12% in 2014 (ElSohly et al., 2016), raising concern about whether marijuana users may experience more pronounced cognitive deficits and alterations in brain structure and function. Further, data suggests that CBD content in recreational marijuana products has dropped precipitously; it is now estimated that the average ratio of THC to CBD in recreational marijuana strains has gone from 14:1 to 80:1 (ElSohly et al., 2016). National trends have also revealed an increase in the use of concentrates, including butane hash oil (BHO), as well as shatter, budder, and wax, particularly among younger populations, which can contain up to 90% THC (Bell et al., 2015). Further studies are needed to investigate the specific impact of high THC-containing compounds as they may confer additional risk, particularly among young recreational marijuana consumers. Similarly, studies should assess the impact of CBD, both alone and in conjunction with THC, to determine whether it exerts protective properties and/or potentially mitigates the adverse effects associated with THC exposure.

"NORMALIZATION" WITH EXTENDED ABSTINENCE?

While some investigations of cognitive function in adolescents who drink alcohol or use marijuana report improvement in function following relatively brief abstinence periods (Fried et al., 2005; Pope, Gruber, & Yurgelun-Todd, 2001), little research is available to determine whether *extended* abstinence from alcohol and marijuana results in recovery of cognitive function and/or normalization of structural brain changes. However, findings to date appear promising. In binge drinkers, increased duration of abstinence has been associated with larger bilateral cerebellar volumes (Lisdahl, Thayer, et al., 2013). Hanson and colleagues (2011) also reported that increased days of abstinence from alcohol and drugs at a 10-year follow-up was associated with improved executive functioning, even after controlling for baseline executive functioning and education. Within adolescent marijuana users, short-term memory improved following 3–6 weeks of marijuana abstinence (Hanson, Winward, et al., 2010; Schwartz et al., 1989), while another study found that adolescent marijuana users who abstained for a minimum of 3 months demonstrated similar cognitive performance as healthy controls (Fried et al., 2005). Taken together, these data suggest that altered neurocognition observed in young marijuana users may begin to normalize after several weeks of abstinence. It is possible that extended periods of abstinence may allow for further reversal of the adverse consequences associated with early onset of alcohol and marijuana use. However, additional prospective research using longer periods of abstinence is necessary to more thoroughly examine the extent of recovery of neurocognitive function and reversal of structure abnormalities in adolescents. Nonetheless, these findings can be utilized to help increase motivation for abstinence in alcohol- and marijuana-using youth, as it is likely that continued abstinence will result in at least minimal improvements in attention, verbal memory, and neuronal processing speed.

POTENTIAL LIMITATIONS OF THE EXISTING LITERATURE

Although converging lines of evidence are increasingly convincing that adolescent and young adult alcohol and marijuana use are associated with neurocognitive deficits, limitations of the research to date must be considered. Several of the aforementioned studies did balance or statistically control for potential confounding factors, such as family history of SUD or subclinical symptoms of depression or other mood problems, and most excluded participants with comorbid psychiatric disorders. However, it is still difficult to disentangle the impact of premorbid factors (differences prior to onset of use) from causal drug exposure influence. Indeed, risk factors associated with substance use initiation (e.g., inhibitory control, conduct disorder, attention problems, and family history of SUD) are also related to neurocognitive abnormalities (Aronowitz et al., 1994; Kelly et al., 2016; Hanson, Medina, et al., 2010; Hill, Kostelnik, et al., 2007; Hill, Muddasani, et al., 2007; Nigg et al., 2004; Ridenour et al., 2009; Schweinsburg et al., 2004, 2008; Spadoni, Norman, Schweinsburg, & Tapert, 2008; Tapert, Baratta, et al., 2002; Tapert & Brown, 2000), and some evidence exists that preexisting brain structural and functional abnormalities predate and predict the onset of regular drug exposure (e.g., Cheetham et al., 2012; Squeglia et al., 2014; Wetherill, Castro, Squeglia, & Tapert, 2013). It is notable, however, that prospective longitudinal studies have provided evidence for additional cognitive and brain abnormalities following the onset of regular alcohol or marijuana use that extend beyond premorbid differences in personality, cognition, and brain structure (Hicks et al., 2012; Maurage, Pesenti, Philippot, Joassin, & Campanella, 2009; Meier et al., 2012; Squeglia et al., 2012; Wetherill, Squeglia, et al., 2013; White et al., 2011). Reversal effects also support causal relations, as do marijuana constituent (THC vs. CBD) studies. Still, additional prospective, longitudinal, twin-informed studies are needed to truly determine whether exposure to alcohol and marijuana causes these neurocognitive abnormalities.

CONCLUSIONS AND RECOMMENDATIONS

Summary: It's Worth the Wait

Adolescence is considered the "gateway to adult health outcomes" (Raphael, 2013). From a public health perspective, this is worrisome, as alarming numbers of youth regularly binge drink and use marijuana (Johnston et al., 2017) despite evidence that alcohol and marijuana use during this critical period of neurodevelopment negatively impacts cognition, brain structure, and function in otherwise healthy teens and emerging adults. In fact, the research presented in this chapter suggests that binge drinking, AUD, and chronic marijuana use during the teenage and emerging adult years results in gray and white matter micro- and macrostructural abnormalities that have often correlated with cognitive deficits. The current body of research should also be utilized to inform public health policy. The issue of adolescent alcohol and marijuana use is not solely confined to cognition and brain health, but is likely to have overarching affects on adolescents' lives. The combined negative impact of both drug- and alcohol-related consequences—which include sleep deprivation/disruption (Cohen-Zion et al., 2009), hangovers, emotional stress, and intoxication while at school—may result in problems related to school functioning and emotional well-being. Information presented in class or "on the job" may be missed or misinterpreted as a result of reduced learning or processing speed, as well as difficulties with attention and working memory. Research study findings are consistent with this theory, as youth who use substances have lower than expected academic performance, increased school problems, risky decision making, and poorer emotional regulation (Kloos, Weller, Chan, & Weller, 2009; Lynskey & Hall, 2000; Medina, Hanson, et al., 2007).

In moving forward with prevention strategies, we know that the "just say no" policy was unsuccessful. It is imperative to shift the outdated message of pure refusal or abstinence to a more realistic stance, especially in light of shifting attitudes regarding marijuana. Instead, the focus should be on *delaying* the onset of use, in order to allow the most vulnerable period of neurodevelopment to pass. Although "just say no" was not well received by our nation's youth, "just not yet" is likely a more easily adopted and embraced message, especially if paired with meaningful data that resonate personally with adolescents.

Increase Screening and Personalized Feedback

In order to reduce the likelihood of regular alcohol or marijuana use, it is critical to disseminate research findings to high school and college students, young military enlistees, therapists, teachers, child psychiatrists, pediatricians, parents, and consumers across the nation. Materials focused on the effects of alcohol and drugs on the brain, including pamphlets specifically designed for teens and young adults, are readily available at no cost through government institutes (National Institute on Drug Abuse, National Institute on Alcohol Abuse and Alcoholism) as well as teen-centered (*www.thecoolspot.gov*, *www. drugfreeamerica.org*) and university websites such as Teen Safe (*www.Teen-Safe. org*), which also includes an excellent parent resource center. In addition to providing general information and related statistics, personalized feedback regarding the effects of alcohol and marijuana that is tailored to individuals is likely to improve outcomes among youth (see Larimer & Cronce, 2007). Further, screening for youth utilizing measures such as the CRAFFT screening tool (Knight, Sherritt, Shrier, Harris, & Chang, 2002), which asks subjects six questions and reveals a teen's risk for problematic, abusive, or dependent use patterns (*www.ceasar.org/teens/test.php*), should be widely implemented. After utilizing the screening tool, physicians and therapists could then employ brief motivational interviewing (described in Part II of this volume) to help educate youth further about the potential negative effects of alcohol and marijuana use. Additionally, therapists or other practitioners could employ neuropsychological testing, tailored specifically to the cognitive domains known to be most affected by alcohol and/or marijuana use, which would provide personalized feedback regarding the youth's cognitive status. Current prevention, screening, and treatment programs should leverage the invaluable data acquired from cognitive neuroscience and general psychoeducation, coupled with personalized feedback regarding the potential effects of chronic drug use on cognition and brain health. Most importantly, empirically validated interventions aimed at delaying, decreasing, and ultimately preventing alcohol and marijuana use in youth must be consistently implemented to optimize neurodevelopmental trajectories and minimize the impact of alcohol and marijuana use on the developing brain.

ACKNOWLEDGMENTS

During manuscript preparation, Krista M. Lisdahl was supported by grant No. R01DA030354 and Staci A. Gruber by Grant No. R01DA032646 from the National Institute of Drug Abuse.

REFERENCES

Abdullaev, Y., Posner, M. I., Nunnally, R., & Dishion, T. J. (2010). Functional MRI evidence for inefficient attentional control in adolescent chronic cannabis abuse. *Behavioural Brain Research, 215*(1), 45–57.

Agosti, V., Nunes, E., & Levin, F. (2002). Rates of psychiatric comorbidity among U.S. residents with lifetime cannabis dependence. *American Journal of Drug and Alcohol Abuse, 28*(4), 643–652.

Ahmadi, A., Pearlson, G. D., Meda, S. A., Dager, A., Potenza, M. N., Rosen, R., et al. (2013). Influence of alcohol use on neural response to go/no-go task in college drinkers. *Neuropsychopharmacology, 38*(11), 2197–2208.

Ames, S. L., Grenard, J. L., Stacy, A. W., Xiao, L., He, Q., Wong, S. W., et al. (2013). Functional imaging of implicit marijuana associations during performance on an Implicit Association Test (IAT). *Behavioural Brain Research, 256*, 494–502.

Ames, S. L., Wong, S. W., Bechara, A., Cappelli, C., Dust, M., Grenard, J. L., et al. (2014). Neural correlates of a go/no-go task with alcohol stimuli in light and heavy young drinkers. *Behavioural Brain Research, 274*, 382–389.

Anthony, J. C. (2006). The epidemiology of cannabis dependence. In R. A. Roffman & R. S. Stephens (Eds.), *Cannabis dependence: Its nature, consequences and treatment* (pp. 58–105). Cambridge, UK: Cambridge University Press.

Arnone, D., Barrick, T. R., Chengappa, S., Mackay, C. E., Clark, C. A., & Abou-Saleh, M. T. (2008). Corpus callosum damage in heavy marijuana use: Preliminary evidence from diffusion tensor tractography and tract-based spatial statistics. *NeuroImage, 41*(3), 1067–1074.

Aronowitz, B., Liebowitz, M., Hollander, E., Fazzini, E., Durlach-Misteli, C., Frenkel, M., et al. (1994). Neuropsychiatric and neuropsychological findings in conduct disorder and attention-deficit hyperactivity disorder. *Journal of Neuropsychiatry and Clinical Neurosciences, 6*(3), 245–249.

Ashtari, M., Avants, B., Cyckowski, L., Cervellione, K. L., Roofeh, D., Cook, P., et al. (2011). Medial temporal structures and memory functions in adolescents with heavy cannabis use. *Journal of Psychiatric Research, 45*(8), 1055–1066.

Ashtari, M., Cervellione, K., Cottone, J., Ardekani, B. A., Sevy, S., & Kumra, S. (2009). Diffusion abnormalities in adolescents and young adults with a history of heavy cannabis use. *Journal of Psychiatric Research, 43*(3), 189–204.

Barron, S., White, A., Swartzwelder, H. S., Bell, R. L., Rodd, Z. A., Slawecki, C. J., et al. (2005). Adolescent vulnerabilities to chronic alcohol or nicotine exposure: Findings from rodent models. *Alcoholism-Clinical and Experimental Research, 29*(9), 1720–1725.

Batalla, A., Bhattacharyya, S., Yücel, M., Fusar-Poli, P., Crippa, J. A., Nogué, S., et al. (2013). Structural and functional imaging studies in chronic cannabis users: A systematic review of adolescent and adult findings. *PLOS ONE, 8*(2), e55821.

Battistella, G., Fornari, E., Annoni, J. M., Chtioui, H., Dao, K., Fabritius, M., et al. (2014). Long-term effects of cannabis on brain structure. *Neuropsychopharmacology, 39*(9), 2041–2048.

Bava, S., Frank, L. R., McQueeny, T., Schweinsburg, B. C., Schweinsburg, A. D., & Tapert, S. F. (2009). Altered white matter microstructure in adolescent substance users. *Psychiatry Research, 173*(3), 228–237.

Bava, S., Jacobus, J., Thayer, R. E., & Tapert, S. F. (2013). Longitudinal changes in white matter integrity among adolescent substance users. *Alcoholism: Clinical and Experimental Research, 37*(Suppl. 1), E181–E189.

Becker, B., Wagner, D., Gouzoulis-Mayfrank, E., Spuentrup, E., & Daumann, J. (2010). The impact of early-onset cannabis use on functional brain correlates of working memory. *Progress in Neuro-Psychopharmacology and Biological Psychiatry , 34*(6), 837–845.

Becker, M. P., Collins, P. F., & Luciana, M. (2014). Neurocognition in college-aged daily marijuana users. *Journal of Clinical and Experimental Neuropsychology, 36*(4), 379–398.

Befort, K. (2015). Interactions of the opioid and cannabinoid systems in reward: Insights from knockout studies. *Frontiers in Pharmacology, 6*, 6.

Behan, B., Connolly, C. G., Datwani, S., Doucet, M., Ivanovic, J., Morioka, R., et al. (2014). Response inhibition and elevated parietal-cerebellar correlations in chronic adolescent cannabis users. *Neuropharmacology, 84*, 131–137.

Bell, C., Slim, J., Flaten, H. K., Lindberg, G., Arek, W., & Monte, A. A. (2015). Butane hash oil burns associated with marijuana liberalization in Colorado. *Journal of Medical Toxicology, 11*(4), 422–425.

Bhattacharyya, S., Morrison, P. D., Fusar-Poli, P., Martin-Santos, R., Borgwardt, S., Winton-Brown, T., et al. (2010). Opposite effects of delta-9-tetrahydrocannabinol and cannabidiol on human brain function and psychopathology. *Neuropsychopharmacology, 35*(3), 764–774.

Block, R. I., O'Leary, D. S., Ehrhardt, J. C., Augustinack. J. C., Ghoneim, M. M., Arndt, S., et al. (2000). Effects of frequent marijuana use on brain tissue volume and composition. *NeuroReport, 28*(3), 491–496.

Boelema, S. R., Harakeh, Z., van Zandvoort, M. J., Reijneveld, S. A., Verhulst, F. C., Ormel, J., et al. (2015). Adolescent heavy drinking does not affect maturation of basic executive functioning: Longitudinal findings from the TRAILS study. *PLOS ONE, 10*(10), e0139186.

Brook, D. W., Brook, J. S., Zhang, C., Cohen, P., & Whiteman, M. (2002). Drug use and the risk of major depressive disorder, alcohol dependence, and substance use disorders. *Archives of General Psychiatry, 59*(11), 1039–1044.

Brooks, S. J., Dalvie, S., Cuzen, N. L., Cardenas, V., Fein, G., & Stein, D. J. (2014). Childhood adversity is linked to differential brain volumes in adolescents with alcohol use disorder: A voxel-based morphometry study. *Metabolic Brain Disease, 29*(2), 311–321.

Brown, S. A., & Tapert, S. F. (2004). Adolescence and the trajectory of alcohol use: Basic to clinical studies. *Annals of the New York Academy of Sciences, 1021*, 234–244.

Brown, S. A., Tapert, S. F., Granholm, E., & Delis, D. C. (2000). Neurocognitive functioning of adolescents: Effects of protracted alcohol use. *Alcoholism: Clinical and Experimental Research, 24*(2), 164–171.

Burgdorf, J. R., Kilmer, B., & Pacula, R. L. (2011). Heterogeneity in the composition of marijuana seized in California. *Drug and Alcohol Dependence, 117*(1), 59–61.

Caldwell, L. C., Schweinsburg, A. D., Nagel, B. J., Barlett, V. C., Brown, S. A., & Tapert, S. F. (2005). Gender and adolescent alcohol use disorders on BOLD (blood oxygen level dependent) response to spatial working memory. *Alcohol and Alcoholism, 40*(3), 194–200.

Casey, B. J., Getz, S., & Galvan, A. (2008). The adolescent brain. *Developmental Review, 28*(1), 62–77.

Casey, B. J., Giedd, J. N., & Thomas, K. M. (2000). Structural and functional brain development and its relation to cognitive development. *Biological Psychology, 54*(1–3), 241–257.

Center for Behavioral Health Statistics and Quality. (2015). Behavioral health trends in the United States: Results from the 2014 National Survey on Drug Use and Health (HHS Publication No. SMA 15-4927, NSDUH Series H-50). Retrieved from *www.samhsa.gov/data*.

Cheetham, A., Allen, N. B., Whittle, S., Simmons, J. G., Yücel, M., & Lubman, D. I. (2012). Orbitofrontal volumes in early adolescence predict initiation of cannabis use: A 4-year longitudinal and prospective study. *Biological Psychiatry, 71*(8), 684–692.

Chung, T., Paulsen, D. J., Geier, C. F., Luna, B., & Clark, D. B. (2015). Regional brain activation supporting cognitive control in the context of reward is associated with treated adolescents' marijuana problem severity at follow-up: A preliminary study. *Developmental Cognitive Neuroscience, 16*, 93–100.

Churchwell, J. C., Carey, P. D., Ferrett, H. L., Stein, D. J., & Yurgelun-Todd, D. A. (2012). Abnormal striatal circuitry and intensified novelty seeking among adolescents who abuse methamphetamine and cannabis. *Developmental Neuroscience, 34*(4), 310–317.

Churchwell, J. C., Lopez-Larson, M., & Yurgelun-Todd, D. A. (2010). Altered frontal cortical volume and decision making in adolescent cannabis users. *Frontiers in Psychology, 1*, 225.

Clark, D. B., Chung, T., Thatcher, D. L., Pajtek, S., & Long, E. C. (2012). Psychological dysregulation, white matter disorganization and substance use disorders in adolescence. *Addiction, 107*(1), 206–214.

Cohen-Zion, M., Drummond, S. P., Padula, C. B., Winward, J., Kanady, J., Medina, K. L., et al. (2009). Sleep architecture in adolescent marijuana and alcohol users during acute and extended abstinence. *Addictive Behaviors, 34*(11), 976–979.

Cousijn, J., Watson, P., Koenders, L., Vingerhoets, W. A., Goudriaan, A. E., & Wiers, R. W. (2013). Cannabis dependence, cognitive control and attentional bias for cannabis words. *Addictive Behaviors, 38*(12), 2825–2832.

Cousijn, J., Wiers, R. W., Ridderinkhof, K. R., van den Brink, W., Veltman, D. J., & Goudriaan, A. E. (2014). Effect of baseline cannabis use and working-memory network function on changes in cannabis use in heavy cannabis users: A prospective fMRI study. *Human Brain Mapping, 35*(5), 2470–2482.

Cousijn, J., Wiers, R. W., Ridderinkhof, K. R., van den Brink, W., Veltman, D. J., Porrino, L. J., et al. (2013). Individual differences in decision making and reward processing predict changes in cannabis use: A prospective functional magnetic resonance imaging study. *Addiction Biology, 18*(6), 1013–1023.

Crane, N. A., Schuster, R. M., & Gonzalez, R. (2013). Preliminary evidence for a sex-specific relationship between amount of cannabis use and neurocognitive performance in young adult cannabis users. *Journal of the International Neuropsychological Society, 19*(9), 1009–1015.

Crane, N. A., Schuster, R. M., Mermelstein, R. J., & Gonzalez, R. (2015). Neuropsychological sex differences associated with age of initiated use among young adult cannabis users. *Journal of Clinical and Experimental Neuropsychology, 37*(4), 389–401.

Dager, A. D., Jamadar, S., Stevens, M. C., Rosen, R., Jiantonio-Kelly, R. E., Sisante, J. F., et al. (2014). fMRI response during figural memory task performance in college drinkers. *Psychopharmacology (Berlin), 231*(1), 167–179.

Dahlgren, M. K., Sagar, K. A., Racine, M. T., Dreman, M. W., & Gruber, S. A. (2016). Marijuana use predicts cognitive performance on tasks of executive function. *Journal of Studies on Alcohol and Drugs, 77*, 298–308.

Dawson, D. A., Goldstein, R. B., Chou, S. P., Ruan, W. J., & Grant, B. F. (2008). Age at first drink and the first incidence of adult-onset DSM-IV alcohol use disorders. *Alcoholism: Clinical and Experimental Research, 32*(12), 2149–2160.

De Bellis, M. D., Clark, D. B., Beers, S. R., Soloff, P. H., Boring, A. M., Hall, J., et al. (2000). Hippocampal volume in adolescent-onset alcohol use disorders. *American Journal of Psychiatry, 157*(5), 737–744.

De Bellis, M. D., Narasimhan, A., Thatcher, D. L., Keshavan, M. S., Soloff, P., & Clark, D. B. (2005). Prefrontal cortex, thalamus, and cerebellar volumes in adolescents and young adults with adolescent-onset alcohol use disorders and comorbid mental disorders. *Alcoholism: Clinical and Experimental Research, 29*(9), 1590–1600.

De Bellis, M. D., Wang, L., Bergman, S. R., Yaxley, R. H., Hooper, S. R., & Huettel, S. A. (2013). Neural mechanisms of risky decision-making and reward response in adolescent onset cannabis use disorder. *Drug and Alcohol Dependence, 133*(1), 134–145.

Degenhardt, L., Chiu, W. T., Sampson, N., Kessler, R. C., Anthony, J. C., Angermeyer, M., et al. (2008). Toward a global view of alcohol, tobacco, cannabis, and cocaine use: Findings from the WHO World Mental Health Surveys. *PLOS Medicine, 5*(7), e141.

Delisi, L. E., Bertisch, H. C., Szulc, K. U., Majcher, M., Brown, K., Bappal, A., et al. (2006). A preliminary DTI study showing no brain structural change associated with adolescent cannabis use. *Harm Reduction Journal, 3*, 17.

DeWit, D. J., Adlaf, E. M., Offord, D. R., & Ogborne, A. C. (2000). Age at first alcohol use: A risk factor for the development of alcohol disorders. *American Journal of Psychiatry, 157*(5), 745–750.

Díaz-Alonso, J., Guzmán, M., & Galve-Roperh, I. (2012). Endocannabinoids via CB_1 receptors act as neurogenic niche cues during cortical development. *Philosophical*

Transactions of the Royal Society of London, Series B: Biological Sciences, 367(1607), 3229–3241.

Doallo, S., Cadaveira, F., Corral, M., Mota, N., López-Caneda, E., & Holguín, S. R. (2014). Larger mid-dorsolateral prefrontal gray matter volume in young binge drinkers revealed by voxel-based morphometry. *PLOS ONE, 9*(5), e96380.

Dougherty, D. M., Mathias, C. W., Dawes, M. A., Furr, R. M., Charles, N. E., Liguori, A., et al. (2013). Impulsivity, attention, memory, and decision-making among adolescent marijuana users. *Psychopharmacology (Berlin), 226*(2), 307–319.

Eaton, D. K., Kann, L., Kinchen, S., Ross, J., Hawkins, J., Harris, W. A., et al. (2006). Youth risk behavior surveillance: United States, 2005. *Morbidity and Mortality Weekly Report Surveillance Summaries, 55*(5), 1–108.

Egerton, A., Allison, C., Brett, R. R., & Pratt, J. A. (2006). Cannabinoids and prefrontal cortical function: Insights from preclinical studies. *Neuroscience and Biobehavioral Reviews, 30*(5), 680–695.

Ehrenreich, H., Rinn, T., Kunert, H. J., Moeller, M. R., Poser, W., Schilling, L., et al. (1999). Specific attentional dysfunction in adults following early start of cannabis use. *Psychopharmacology, 142*(3), 295–301.

ElSohly, M. A., Mehmedic, Z., Foster, S., Gon, C., Chandra, S., & Church, J. C. (2016). Changes in cannabis potency over the last 2 decades (1995–2014): Analysis of current data in the United States. *Biological Psychiatry, 79*(7), 613–619.

Englund, A., Morrison, P. D., Nottage, J., Hague, D., Kane, F., Bonaccorso, S., et al. (2013). Cannabidiol inhibits THC-elicited paranoid symptoms and hippocampal-dependent memory impairment. *Journal of Psychopharmacology, 27*(1), 19–27.

Epstein, K. A., & Kumra, S. (2015). Altered cortical maturation in adolescent cannabis users with and without schizophrenia. *Schizophrenia Research, 162*(1–3), 143–152.

Fein, G., Greenstein, D., Cardenas, V. A., Cuzen, N. L., Fouche, J. P., Ferrett, H., et al. (2013). Cortical and subcortical volumes in adolescents with alcohol dependence but without substance or psychiatric comorbidities. *Psychiatry Research, 214*(1), 1–8.

Filbey, F. M., & DeWitt, S. J. (2012). Cannabis cue-elicited craving and the reward neurocircuitry. *Progress in Neuro-Psychopharmacology and Biological Psychiatry, 38*(1), 30–35.

Filbey, F. M., McQueeny, T., DeWitt, S. J., & Mishra, V. (2015). Preliminary findings demonstrating latent effects of early adolescent marijuana use onset on cortical architecture. *Developmental Cognitive Neuroscience, 16,* 16–22.

Fontes, M. A., Bolla, K. I., Cunha, P. J., Almeida, P. P., Jungerman, F., Laranjeira, R. R., et al. (2011). Cannabis use before age 15 and subsequent executive functioning. *British Journal of Psychiatry, 198*(6), 442–447.

Fried, P. A., Watkinson, B., & Gray, R. (2005). Neurocognitive consequences of marihuana: A comparison with pre-drug performance. *Neurotoxicology Teratology, 27*(2), 231–239.

Fusar-Poli, P., Crippa, J. A., Bhattacharyya, S., Borgwardt, S. J., Allen, P., Martin-Santos, R., et al. (2009). Distinct effects of {delta}9-tetrahydrocannabinol and cannabidiol on neural activation during emotional processing. *Archives of General Psychiatry, 66*(1), 95–105.

Gardner, M., & Steinberg, L. (2005). Peer influence on risk taking, risk preference, and risky decision making in adolescence and adulthood: An experimental study. *Developmental Psychology, 41*(4), 625–635.

Giancola, P. R., Mezzich, A. C., & Tarter, R. E. (1998). Disruptive, delinquent and aggressive behavior in female adolescents with a psychoactive substance use disorder: Relation to executive cognitive functioning. *Journal of Studies on Alcohol, 59*, 560–567.

Giedd, J. N., Snell, J. W., Lange, N., Rajapakse, J. C., Casey, B. J., Kozuch, P. L., et al. (1996). Quantitative magnetic resonance imaging of human brain development: Ages 4–18. *Cerebral Cortex, 6*(4), 551–560.

Gilman, J. M., Ramchandani, V. A., Crouss, T., & Hommer, D. W. (2012). Subjective and neural responses to intravenous alcohol in young adults with light and heavy drinking patterns. *Neuropsychopharmacology, 37*(2), 467–477.

Gogtay, N., Giedd, J. N., Lusk, L., Hayashi, K. M., Greenstein, D., Vaituzis, A. C., et al. (2004). Dynamic mapping of human cortical development during childhood through early adulthood. *Proceedings of the National Academy of Sciences of the USA, 101*(21), 8174–8179.

Gonzalez, R., Schuster, R. M., Mermelstein, R. J., Vassileva, J., Martin, E. M., & Diviak, K. R. (2012). Performance of young adult cannabis users on neurocognitive measures of impulsive behavior and their relationship to symptoms of cannabis use disorders. *Journal of Clinical and Experimental Neuropsychology, 34*(9), 962–976.

Grant, B. F., & Dawson, D. A. (1997). Age at onset of alcohol use and its association with DSM-IV alcohol abuse and dependence: Results from the National Longitudinal Alcohol Epidemiologic Survey. *Journal of Substance Abuse, 9*, 103–110.

Grant, J. E., Chamberlain, S. R., Schreiber, L., & Odlaug, B. L. (2012). Neuropsychological deficits associated with cannabis use in young adults. *Drug and Alcohol Dependence, 121*(1–2), 159–162.

Gruber, S. A., Dahlgren, M. K., Sagar, K. A., Gönenç, A., & Killgore, W. D. (2012). Age of onset of marijuana use impacts inhibitory processing. *Neuroscience Letters, 511*(2), 89–94.

Gruber, S. A., Dahlgren, M. K., Sagar, K. A., Gönenç, A., & Lukas, S. E. (2014). Worth the wait: Effects of age of onset of marijuana use on white matter and impulsivity. *Psychopharmacology (Berlin), 231*(8), 1455–1465.

Gruber, S. A., Rogowska, J., & Yurgelun-Todd, D. A. (2009). Altered affective response in marijuana smokers: An FMRI study. *Drug and Alcohol Dependence, 105*(1–2), 139–153.

Gruber, S. A., Sagar, K. A., Dahlgren, M. K., Racine, M., & Lukas, S. E. (2012). Age of onset of marijuana use and executive function. *Psychology of Addictive Behaviors, 26*(3), 496–506.

Gruber, S. A., Silveri, M. M., Dahlgren, M. K., & Yurgelun-Todd, D. (2011). Why so impulsive?: White matter alterations are associated with impulsivity in chronic marijuana smokers. *Experimental and Clinical Psychopharmacology, 19*(3), 231–242.

Gruber, S. A., & Yurgelun-Todd, D. A. (2005). Neuroimaging of marijuana smokers during inhibitory processing: A pilot investigation. *Brain Research: Cognitive Brain Research, 23*(1), 107–118.

Hanson, K. L., Medina, K. L., Nagel, B. J., Spadoni, A. D., Gorlick, A., & Tapert, S. F. (2010). Hippocampal volumes in adolescents with and without a family history of alcoholism. *American Journal of Drug and Alcohol Abuse, 36*(3), 161–167.

Hanson, K. L., Medina, K. L., Padula, C. B., Tapert, S. F., & Brown, S. A. (2011). Impact of adolescent alcohol and drug use on neuropsychological functioning in young adulthood: 10-year outcomes. *Journal of Child and Adolescent Substance Abuse, 20*(2), 135–154.

Hanson, K. L., Thayer, R. E., & Tapert, S. F. (2014). Adolescent marijuana users have elevated risk-taking on the balloon analog risk task. *Journal of Psychopharmacology, 28*(11), 1080–1087.

Hanson, K. L., Winward, J. L., Schweinsburg, A. D., Medina, K. L., Brown, S. A., & Tapert, S. F. (2010). Longitudinal study of cognition among adolescent marijuana users over three weeks of abstinence. *Addictive Behaviors, 35*(11), 970–976.

Hartley, D. E., Elsabagh, S., & File, S. E. (2004). Binge drinking and sex: Effects on mood and cognitive function in healthy young volunteers. *Pharmacology Biochemistry and Behavior, 78*(3), 611–619.

Harvey, M. A., Sellman, J. D., Porter, R. J., & Frampton, C. M. (2007). The relationship between non-acute adolescent cannabis use and cognition. *Drug and Alcohol Review, 26*(3), 309–319.

Hicks, B. M., Durbin, C. E., Blonigen, D. M., Iacono, W. G., & McGue, M. (2012). Relationship between personality change and the onset and course of alcohol dependence in young adulthood. *Addiction, 107*(3), 540–548.

Hill, M. N., & McEwen, B. S. (2010). Involvement of the endocannabinoid system in the neurobehavioural effects of stress and glucocorticoids. *Progress in Neuro-Psychopharmacology and Biological Psychiatry, 34*(5), 791–797.

Hill, M. N., & Tasker, J. G. (2012). Endocannabinoid signaling, glucocorticoid-mediated negative feedback, and regulation of the hypothalamic–pituitary–adrenal axis. *Neuroscience, 204*, 5–16.

Hill, S. Y., Kostelnik, B., Holmes, B., Goradia, D., McDermott, M., Diwadkar, V., et al. (2007). fMRI BOLD response to the eyes task in offspring from multiplex alcohol dependence families. *Alcoholism: Clinical and Experimental Research, 31*(12), 2028–2035.

Hill, S. Y., Muddasani, S., Prasad, K., Nutche, J., Steinhauer, S. R., Scanlon, J., et al. (2007). Cerebellar volume in offspring from multiplex alcohol dependence families. *Biological Psychiatry, 61*(1), 41–47.

Hillard, C. J., Weinlander, K. M., & Stuhr, K. L. (2012). Contributions of endocannabinoid signaling to psychiatric disorders in humans: Genetic and biochemical evidence. *Neuroscience, 204*, 207–229.

Hingson, R. W., Heeren, T., & Winter, M. R. (2006). Age at drinking onset and alcohol dependence: Age at onset, duration, and severity. *Archives of Pediatrics and Adolescent Medicine, 160*(7), 739–746.

Houston, S. M., Herting, M. M., & Sowell, E. R. (2014). The neurobiology of childhood structural brain development: Conception through adulthood. *Current Topics in Behavioral Neuroscience, 16*, 3–17.

Hurd, Y. L., Michaelides, M., Miller, M. L., & Jutras-Aswad, D. (2014). Trajectory of adolescent cannabis use on addiction vulnerability. *Neuropharmacology, 76*(Pt. B), 416–424.

Jackson, N. J., Isen, J. D., Khoddamn, R., Irons, D., Tuvblad, C., Iacono, W. G., et al. (2016). Impact of adolescent marijuana use on intelligence: Results from two longitudinal twin studies. *Proceedings of the National Academy of Sciences of the USA, 113*(5), E500–E508.

Jacobsen, L. K., Mencl, W. E., Westerveld, M., & Pugh, K. R. (2004). Impact of cannabis use on brain function in adolescents. *Annals of New York Academy of Sciences, 1021,* 384–390.

Jacobsen, L. K., Pugh, K. R., Constable, R. T., Westerveld, M., & Mencl, W. E. (2007). Functional correlates of verbal memory deficits emerging during nicotine withdrawal in abstinent adolescent cannabis users. *Biological Psychiatry, 61*(1), 31–40.

Jacobus, J., McQueeny, T., Bava, S., Schweinsburg, B. C., Frank, L. R., Yang, T. T., et al. (2009). White matter integrity in adolescents with histories of marijuana use and binge drinking. *Neurotoxicology Teratology, 31*(6), 349–355.

Jacobus, J., Squeglia, L. M., Bava, S., & Tapert, S. F. (2013). White matter characterization of adolescent binge drinking with and without co-occurring marijuana use: A 3-year investigation. *Psychiatry Research, 214*(3), 374–381.

Jacobus, J., Squeglia, L. M., Infante, M. A., Bava, S., & Tapert, S. F. (2013). White matter integrity pre- and post marijuana and alcohol initiation in adolescence. *Brain Sciences, 3*(1), 396–414.

Jacobus, J., Squeglia, L. M., Infante, M. A., Castro, N., Brumback, T., Meruelo, A. D., et al. (2015). Neuropsychological performance in adolescent marijuana users with co-occurring alcohol use: A three-year longitudinal study. *Neuropsychology, 29*(6), 829–843.

Jacobus, J., Squeglia, L. M., Sorg, S. F., Nguyen-Louie, T. T., & Tapert, S. F. (2014). Cortical thickness and neurocognition in adolescent marijuana and alcohol users following 28 days of monitored abstinence. *Journal of Studies on Alcohol and Drugs, 75*(5), 729–743.

Jacobus, J., & Tapert, S. F. (2013). Neurotoxic effects of alcohol in adolescence. *Annual Review of Clinical Psychology, 9,* 703–721.

Jacobus, J., & Tapert, S. F. (2014). Effects of cannabis on the adolescent brain. *Current Pharmaceutical Design, 20*(13), 2186–2193.

Jager, G., Block, R. I., Luijten, M., & Ramsey, N. F. (2013). Tentative evidence for striatal hyperactivity in adolescent cannabis-using boys: A cross-sectional multicenter fMRI study. *Journal of Psychoactive Drugs, 45*(2), 156–167.

Johnston, L. D., O'Malley, P. M., Miech, R. A., Bachman, J. G., & Schulenberg, J. E. (2017). *Monitoring the future national survey results on drug use, 1975–2016: Overview of key findings on adolescent drug use.* Ann Arbor: Institute for Social Research, University of Michigan.

Kelly, C., Castellanos, F. X., Tomaselli, O., Lisdahl, K., Tamm, L., Jernigan, T., et al. (2016). Distinct effects of childhood ADHD and cannabis use on brain functional architecture in young adults. *Neuroimage: Clinical, 13,* 188–200.

Kloos, A., Weller, R. A., Chan, R., & Weller, E. B. (2009). Gender differences in adolescent substance abuse. *Current Psychiatry Reports, 11*(2), 120–126.

Knight, J. R., Sherritt, L., Shrier, L. A., Harris, S. K., & Chang, G. (2002). Validity of the CRAFFT substance abuse screening test among adolescent clinic patients. *Archives of Pediatrics and Adolescent Medicine, 156*(6), 607–614.

Koskinen, S. M., Ahveninen, J., Kujala, T., Kaprio, J., O'Donnell, B. F., Osipova, D., et al. (2011). A longitudinal twin study of effects of adolescent alcohol abuse on the neurophysiology of attention and orienting. *Alcoholism: Clinical and Experimental Research, 35*(7), 1339–1350.

Larimer, M. E., & Cronce, J. M. (2007). Identification, prevention, and treatment revisited: Individual-focused college drinking prevention strategies 1999–2006. *Addictive Behaviors, 32*(11), 2439–2468.

Lee, T. T., & Gorzalka, B. B. (2012). Timing is everything: Evidence for a role of corti-colimbic endocannabinoids in modulating hypothalamic–pituitary–adrenal axis activity across developmental periods. *Neuroscience, 204*, 17–30.

Lenroot, R. K., & Giedd, J. N. (2006). Brain development in children and adolescents: Insights from anatomical magnetic resonance imaging. *Neuroscience and Biobehavioral Reviews, 30*(6), 718–729.

Lisdahl, K. M., Gilbart, E. R., Wright, N. E., & Shollenbarger, S. (2013). Dare to delay?: The impacts of adolescent alcohol and marijuana use onset on cognition, brain structure, and function. *Frontiers in Psychiatry, 4*, 53.

Lisdahl, K. M., & Price, J. S. (2012). Increased marijuana use and gender predict poorer cognitive functioning in adolescents and emerging adults. *Journal of the International Neuropsychological Society, 18*(4), 678–688.

Lisdahl, K. M., Tamm, L., Epstein, J. N., Jernigan, T., Molina, B. S., Hinshaw, S. P., et al. (2016). The impact of ADHD persistence, recent cannabis use, and age of regular cannabis use onset on subcortical volume and cortical thickness in young adults. *Drug and Alcohol Dependence, 161*, 135–146.

Lisdahl, K. M., Thayer, R., Squeglia, L. M., McQueeny, T. M., & Tapert, S. F. (2013). Recent binge drinking predicts smaller cerebellar volumes in adolescents. *Psychiatry Research, 211*(1), 17–23.

Lisdahl, K. M., Wright, N. E., Kirchner-Medina, C., Maple, K. E., & Shollenbarger, S. (2014). Considering cannabis: The effects of regular cannabis use on neurocognition in adolescents and young adults. *Current Addiction Reports, 1*(2), 144–156.

Lopez-Larson, M. P., Bogorodzki, P., Rogowska, J., McGlade, E., King, J. B., Terry, J., et al. (2011). Altered prefrontal and insular cortical thickness in adolescent marijuana users. *Behavioural Brain Reseearch, 220*(1), 164–172.

Lorenzetti, V., Solowij, N., & Yücel, M. (2016). The role of cannabinoids in neuroanatomic alterations in cannabis users. *Biological Psychiatry, 79*(7), e17–e31.

Luciana, M., Collins, P. F., Muetzel, R. L., & Lim, K. O. (2013). Effects of alcohol use initiation on brain structure in typically developing adolescents. *American Journal of Drug and Alcohol Abuse, 39*(6), 345–355.

Lynskey, M., & Hall, W. (2000). The effects of adolescent cannabis use on educational attainment: A review. *Addiction, 95*(11), 1621–1630.

Lynskey, M. T., Heath, A. C., Bucholz, K. K., Slutske, W. S., Madden, P. A. F., Nelson, E. C., et al. (2003). Escalation of drug use in early-onset cannabis users vs co-twin controls. *Journal of the American Medical Association, 289*(4), 427–433.

Lyvers, M., Czerczyk, C., Follent, A., & Lodge, P. (2009). Disinhibition and reward sensitivity in relation to alcohol consumption by university undergraduates. *Addiction Research and Theory, 17*(6), 668–677.

Lyvers, M., Duff, H., & Hasking, P. (2011). Risky alcohol use and age at onset of regular alcohol consumption in relation to frontal lobe indices, reward sensitivity and rash impulsiveness. *Addiction Research and Theory, 19*(3), 251–259.

Maggs, J. L., Staff, J., Kloska, D. D., Patrick, M. E., O'Malley, P. M., & Schulenberg, J. (2015). Predicting young adult degree attainment by late adolescent marijuana use. *Journal of Adolescent Health, 57*(2), 205–211.

Malone, S. M., Luciana, M., Wilson, S., Sparks, J. C., Hunt, R. H., Thomas, K. M., et al. (2014). Adolescent drinking and motivated decision-making: A cotwin-control investigation with monozygotic twins. *Behavior Genetics, 44*(4), 407–418.

Martin, C. S., Kaczynski, N. A., Maisto, S. A., & Tarter, R. E. (1996). Polydrug use in adolescent drinkers with and without DSM-IV alcohol abuse and dependence. *Alcoholism: Clinical and Experimental Research, 20*(6), 1099–1108.

Mashhoon, Y., Czerkawski, C., Crowley, D. J., Cohen-Gilbert, J. E., Sneider, J. T., & Silveri, M. M. (2014). Binge alcohol consumption in emerging adults: Anterior cingulate cortical "thinness" is associated with alcohol use patterns. *Alcoholism: Clinical and Experimental Research, 38*(7), 1955–1964.

Mashhoon, Y., Sava, S., Sneider, J. T., Nickerson, L. D., & Silveri, M. M. (2015). Cortical thinness and volume differences associated with marijuana abuse in emerging adults. *Drug and Alcohol Dependence, 155,* 275–283.

Mata, I., Perez-Iglesias, R., Roiz-Santiañez, R., Tordesillas-Gutierrez, D., Pazos, A., Gutierrez, A., et al. (2010). Gyrification brain abnormalities associated with adolescence and early-adulthood cannabis use. *Brain Research, 1317,* 297–304.

Mathias, C. W., Blumenthal, T. D., Dawes, M. A., Liguori, A., Richard, D. M., Bray, B., et al. (2011). Failure to sustain prepulse inhibition in adolescent marijuana users. *Drug and Alcohol Dependence, 116*(1–3), 110–116.

Maurage, P., Pesenti, M., Philippot, P., Joassin, F., & Campanella, S. (2009). Latent deleterious effects of binge drinking over a short period of time revealed only by electrophysiological measures. *Journal of Psychiatry and Neuroscience, 34*(2), 111–118.

McGue, M., Iacono, W. G., Legrand, L. N., Malone, S., & Elkins, I. (2001). Origins and consequences of age at first drink: I. Associations with substance-use disorders, disinhibitory behavior and psychopathology, and P3 amplitude. *Alcoholism: Clinical and Experimental Research, 25*(8), 1156–1165.

McHale, S., & Hunt, N. (2008). Executive function deficits in short-term abstinent cannabis users. *Human Psycholpharmacology, 23*(5), 409–415.

McQueeny, T., Padula, C. B., Price, J., Medina, K. L., Logan, P., & Tapert, S. F. (2011). Gender effects on amygdala morphometry in adolescent marijuana users. *Behavioural Brain Research, 224*(1), 128–134.

McQueeny, T., Schweinsburg, B. C., Schweinsburg, A. D., Jacobus, J., Bava, S., Frank, L. R., & Tapert, S. F. (2009). Altered white matter integrity in adolescent binge drinkers. *Alcoholis: Clinical and Experimental Research, 33*(7), 1278–1285.

Medina, K. L., Hanson, K. L., Schweinsburg, A. D., Cohen-Zion, M., Nagel, B. J., & Tapert, S. F. (2007). Neuropsychological functioning in adolescent marijuana users: Subtle deficits detectable after a month of abstinence. *Journal of the International Neuropsychological Society, 13*(5), 807–820.

Medina, K. L., McQueeny, T., Nagel, B. J., Hanson, K. L., Schweinsburg, A. D., & Tapert, S. F. (2008). Prefrontal cortex volumes in adolescents with alcohol use disorders: Unique gender effects. *Alcoholism: Clinical and Experimental Research, 32*(3), 386–394.

Medina, K. L., McQueeny, T., Nagel, B. J., Hanson, K. L., Yang, T. T., & Tapert, S. F. (2009). Prefrontal cortex morphometry in abstinent adolescent marijuana users: Subtle gender effects. *Addiction Biology, 14*(4), 457–468.

Medina, K. L., Nagel, B. J., Park, A., McQueeny, T., & Tapert, S. F. (2007). Depressive symptoms in adolescents: Associations with white matter volume and marijuana use. *Journal of Child Psychology and Psychiatry, 48*(6), 592–600.

Medina, K. L., Nagel, B. J., & Tapert, S. F. (2010). Abnormal cerebellar morphometry in abstinent adolescent marijuana users. *Psychiatry Research, 182*(2), 152–159.

Medina, K. L., Schweinsburg, A. D., Cohen-Zion, M., Nagel, B. J., & Tapert, S. F. (2007). Effects of alcohol and combined marijuana and alcohol use during adolescence on hippocampal volume and asymmetry. *Neurotoxicology Teratology, 29*(1), 141–152.

Mehmedic, Z., Chandra, S., Slade, D., Denham, H., Foster, S., Patel, A. S., et al. (2010). Potency trends of D 9-THC and other cannabinoids in confiscated cannabis preparations from 1993 to 2008. *Journal of Forensic Sciences, 55*(5), 1209–1217.

Meier, M. H., Caspi, A., Ambler, A., Harrington, H., Houts, R., Keefe, R. S., et al. (2012). Persistent cannabis users show neuropsychological decline from childhood to midlife. *Proceedings of the National Academy of Sciences of the USA, 109*(40), E2657–E2664.

Meier, M. H., Hill, M. L., Small, P. J., & Luthar, S. S. (2015). Associations of adolescent cannabis use with academic performance and mental health: A longitudinal study of upper middle class youth. *Drug and Alcohol Dependence, 156*, 207–212.

Mills, K. L., Goddings, A. L., Clasen, L. S., Giedd, J. N., & Blakemore, S. J. (2014). The developmental mismatch in structural brain maturation during adolescence. *Developmental Neuroscience, 36*(3–4), 147–160.

Mokrysz, C., Landy, R., Gage, S. H., Munafo, M. R., Roiser, J. P., & Curran, H. V. (2016). Are IQ and educational outcomes in teenagers related to their cannabis use?: A prospective cohort study. *Journal of Psychopharmacology, 30*(2), 159–168.

Moldrich, G., & Wenger, T. (2000). Localization of the CB_1 cannabinoid receptor in the rat brain: An immunohistochemical study. *Peptides, 21*(11), 1735–1742.

Monti, P. M., Miranda, R., Nixon, K., Sher, K. J., Swartzwelder, H. S., Tapert, S. F., et al. (2005). Adolescence: Booze, brains, and behavior. *Alcoholism: Clinical and Experimental Research, 29*(2), 207–220.

Morgan, C. J., Schafer, G., Freeman, T. P., & Curran, H. V. (2010). Impact of cannabidiol on the acute memory and psychotomimetic effects of smoked cannabis: Naturalistic study [corrected]. *British Journal of Psychiatry, 197*(4), 285–290.

Moss, H. B., Kirisci, L., Gordon, H. W., & Tarter, R. E. (1994). A neuropsychologic profile of adolescent alcoholics. *Alcoholism: Clinical and Experimental Research, 18*(1), 159–163.

Nagel, B. J., Schweinsburg, A. D., Phan, V., & Tapert, S. F. (2005). Reduced hippocampal volume among adolescents with alcohol use disorders without psychiatric comorbidity. *Psychiatry Research, 139*(3), 181–190.

Niesink, R. J., & van Laar, M. W. (2013). Does cannabidiol protect against adverse psychological effects of THC? *Frontiers in Psychiatry, 4*, 130.

Nigg, J. T., Glass, J. M., Wong, M. M., Poon, E., Jester, J. M., Fitzgerald, H. E., et al. (2004). Neuropsychological executive functioning in children at elevated risk for alcoholism: Findings in early adolescence. *Journal of Abnormal Psychology, 113*(2), 302–314.

Nyilas, R., Dudok, B., Urbán, G. M., Mackie, K., Watanabe, M., Cravatt, B. F., et al. (2008). Enzymatic machinery for endocannabinoid biosynthesis associated with calcium stores in glutamatergic axon terminals. *Journal of Neuroscience, 28*(5), 1058–1063.

Parada, M., Corral, M., Caamaño-Isorna, F., Mota, N., Crego, A., Holguín, S. R., et al. (2011). Binge drinking and declarative memory in university students. *Alcoholism: Clinical and Experimental Research, 35*(8), 1475–1484.

Parada, M., Corral, M., Mota, N., Crego, A., Rodríguez Holguín, S., & Cadaveira, F.

(2012). Executive functioning and alcohol binge drinking in university students. *Addictive Behaviors, 37*(2), 167–172.

Park, M. S., Sohn, S., Park, J. E., Kim, S. H., Yu, I. K., & Sohn, J. H. (2011). Brain functions associated with verbal working memory tasks among young males with alcohol use disorders. *Scandinavian Journal of Psychology, 52*(1), 1–7.

Pazos, M. R., Mohammed, N., Lafuente, H., Santos, M., Martínez-Pinilla, E., Moreno, E., et al. (2013). Mechanisms of cannabidiol neuroprotection in hypoxic–ischemic newborn pigs: Role of 5HT(1A) and CB_2 receptors. *Neuropharmacology, 71*, 282–291.

Pfefferbaum, A., Rohlfing, T., Pohl, K. M., Lane, B., Chu, W., Kwon, D., et al. (2016). Adolescent development of cortical and white matter structure in the NCANDA sample: Role of sex, ethnicity, puberty, and alcohol drinking. *Cerebral Cortex, 26*(10), 4101–4121.

Pope, H. G., Gruber, A. J., Hudson, J. I., Cohane, G., Huestis, M. A., & Yurgelun-Todd, D. (2003). Early-onset cannabis use and cognitive deficits: What is the nature of the association? *Drug and Alcohol Dependence, 69*(3), 303–310.

Pope, H. G., Gruber, A. J., & Yurgelun-Todd, D. (2001). Residual neuropsychologic effects of cannabis. *Current Psychiatry Reports, 3*(6), 507–512. Retrieved from *www.ncbi.nlm.nih.gov/pubmed/11707165*.

Price, J. S., McQueeny, T., Shollenbarger, S., Browning, E. L., Wieser, J., & Lisdahl, K. M. (2015). Effects of marijuana use on prefrontal and parietal volumes and cognition in emerging adults. *Psychopharmacology (Berlin), 232*(16), 2939–2950.

Raphael, D. (2013). Adolescence as a gateway to adult health outcomes. *Maturitas, 75*(2), 137–141.

Read, J. P., Merrill, J. E., Kahler, C. W., & Strong, D. R. (2007). Predicting functional outcomes among college drinkers: Reliability and predictive validity of the Young Adult Alcohol Consequences Questionnaire. *Addictive Behaviors, 32*(11), 2597–2610.

Ridenour, T. A., Tarter, R. E., Reynolds, M., Mezzich, A., Kirisci, L., & Vanyukov, M. (2009). Neurobehavior disinhibition, parental substance use disorder, neighborhood quality and development of cannabis use disorder in boys. *Drug and Alcohol Dependence, 102*(1–3), 71–77.

Robins, L. N., & Przybeck, T. R. (1985). Age of onset of drug use as a factor in drug and other disorders. *NIDA Research Monograph, 56*, 178–192.

Rubino, T., Realini, N., Braida, D., Guidi, S., Capurro, V., Viganò, D., et al. (2009). Changes in hippocampal morphology and neuroplasticity induced by adolescent THC treatment are associated with cognitive impairment in adulthood. *Hippocampus, 19*(8), 763–772.

Rubino, T., Zamberletti, E., & Parolaro, D. (2012). Adolescent exposure to cannabis as a risk factor for psychiatric disorders. *Journal of Psychopharmacology, 26*(1), 177–188.

Sagar, K. A., Dahlgren, M. K., Gönenç, A., Racine, M. T., Dreman, M. W., & Gruber, S. A. (2015). The impact of initiation: Early onset marijuana smokers demonstrate altered Stroop performance and brain activation. *Developmental Cognitive Neuroscience, 16*, 84–92.

Scaife, J. C., & Duka, T. (2009). Behavioural measures of frontal lobe function in a population of young social drinkers with binge drinking pattern. *Pharmacology Biochemistry and Behavior, 93*(3), 354–362.

Schacht, J. P., Hutchison, K. E., & Filbey, F. M. (2012). Associations between canna-binoid receptor-1 (CNR1) variation and hippocampus and amygdala volumes in heavy cannabis users. *Neuropsychopharmacology, 37*(11), 2368–2376.

Schmitt, J. E., Neale, M. C., Fassassi, B., Perez, J., Lenroot, R. K., Wells, E. M., et al. (2014). The dynamic role of genetics on cortical patterning during childhood and adolescence. *Proceedings of the National Academy of Sciences of the USA, 111*(18), 6774–6779.

Schulenberg, J. E., & Maggs, J. L. (2002). A developmental perspective on alcohol use and heavy drinking during adolescence and the transition to young adulthood. *Journal of Studies on Alcohol Supplement, 14*, 54–70.

Schuster, R. M., Crane, N. A., Mermelstein, R., & Gonzalez, R. (2012). The influence of inhibitory control and episodic memory on the risky sexual behavior of young adult cannabis users. *Journal of the International Neuropsychological Society, 18*(5), 827–833.

Schwartz, R. H., Gruenewald, P. J., Klitzner, M., & Fedio, P. (1989). Short-term mem-ory impairment in cannabis-dependent adolescents. *American Journal of Diseases of Children, 143*(10), 1214–1219.

Schweinsburg, A. D., McQueeny, T., Nagel, B. J., Eyler, L. T., & Tapert, S. F. (2010). A preliminary study of functional magnetic resonance imaging response during verbal encoding among adolescent binge drinkers. *Alcohol, 44*(1), 111–117.

Schweinsburg, A. D., Nagel, B. J., Schweinsburg, B. C., Park, A., Theilmann, R. J., & Tapert, S. F. (2008). Abstinent adolescent marijuana users show altered fMRI response during spatial working memory. *Psychiatry Research, 163*(1), 40–51.

Schweinsburg, A. D., Paulus, M. P., Barlett, V. C., Killeen, L. A., Caldwell, L. C., Pulido, C., et al. (2004). An FMRI study of response inhibition in youths with a family history of alcoholism. *Annals of the New York Academy of Sciences of the USA, 1021*, 391–394.

Schweinsburg, A. D., Schweinsburg, B. C., Cheung, E. H., Brown, G. G., Brown, S. A., & Tapert, S. F. (2005). fMRI response to spatial working memory in adolescents with comorbid marijuana and alcohol use disorders. *Drug and Alcohol Depen-dence, 79*(2), 201–210.

Sher, K. J., Martin, E. D., Wood, P. K., & Rutledge, P. C. (1997). Alcohol use disorders and neuropsychological functioning in first-year undergraduates. *Experimental and Clinical Psychopharmacology, 5*(3), 304–315.

Shollenbarger, S. G., Price, J., Wieser, J., & Lisdahl, K. (2015a). Impact of cannabis use on prefrontal and parietal cortex gyrification and surface area in adolescents and emerging adults. *Developmental Cognitive Neuroscience, 16*, 46–53.

Shollenbarger, S. G., Price, J., Wieser, J., & Lisdahl, K. (2015b). Poorer frontolimbic white matter integrity is associated with chronic cannabis use, FAAH genotype, and increased depressive and apathy symptoms in adolescents and young adults. *Neuroimage: Clinical, 8*, 117–125.

Solowij, N., Jones, K. A., Rozman, M. E., Davis, S. M., Ciarrochi, J., Heaven, P. C., et al. (2011). Verbal learning and memory in adolescent cannabis users, alcohol users and non-users. *Psychopharmacology (Berlin), 216*(1), 131–144.

Solowij, N., Jones, K. A., Rozman, M. E., Davis, S. M., Ciarrochi, J., Heaven, P. C., et al. (2012). Reflection impulsivity in adolescent cannabis users: A comparison with alcohol-using and non-substance-using adolescents. *Psychopharmacology (Berlin), 219*(2), 575–586.

Sowell, E. R., Thompson, P. M., Holmes, C. J., Jernigan, T. L., & Toga, A. W.(1999). In vivo evidence for post-adolescent brain maturation in frontal and striatal regions. *Nature Neuroscience, 2*(10), 859–861.

Sowell, E. R., Thompson, P. M., Leonard, C. M., Welcome, S. E., Kan, E., & Toga, A. W. (2004). Longitudinal mapping of cortical thickness and brain growth in normal children. *Journal of Neuroscience, 24*(38), 8223–8231.

Sowell, E. R., Trauner, D. A., Gamst, A., & Jernigan, T. L. (2002). Development of cortical and subcortical brain structures in childhood and adolescence: A structural MRI study. *Developmental Medicine and Child Neurology, 44*(1), 4–16.

Spadoni, A. D., Norman, A. L., Schweinsburg, A. D., & Tapert, S. F. (2008). Effects of family history of alcohol use disorders on spatial working memory BOLD response in adolescents. *Alcoholism: Clinical and Experimental Research, 32*(7), 1135–1145.

Spear, L. P. (2015). Adolescent alcohol exposure: Are there separable vulnerable periods within adolescence? *Physiology and Behavior, 148,* 122–130.

Spear, L. P., & Swartzwelder, H. S. (2014). Adolescent alcohol exposure and persistence of adolescent-typical phenotypes into adulthood: A mini-review. *Neuroscience and Biobehavioral Reviews, 45,* 1–8.

Squeglia, L. M., Jacobus, J., Nguyen-Louie, T. T., & Tapert, S. F. (2014). Inhibition during early adolescence predicts alcohol and marijuana use by late adolescence. *Neuropsychology, 28*(5), 782–790.

Squeglia, L. M., Jacobus, J., & Tapert, S. F. (2009). The influence of substance use on adolescent brain development. *Clinical EEG Neuroscience, 40*(1), 31–38.

Squeglia, L. M., Pulido, C., Wetherill, R. R., Jacobus, J., Brown, G. G., & Tapert, S. F. (2012). Brain response to working memory over three years of adolescence: Influence of initiating heavy drinking. *Journal of Studies on Alcohol and Drugs, 73*(5), 749–760.

Squeglia, L. M., Schweinsburg, A. D., Pulido, C., & Tapert, S. F. (2011). Adolescent binge drinking linked to abnormal spatial working memory brain activation: Differential gender effects. *Alcoholism: Clinical and Experimental Research, 35*(10), 1831–1841.

Squeglia, L. M., Tapert, S. F., Sullivan, E. V., Jacobus, J., Meloy, M. J., Rohlfing, T., et al. (2015). Brain development in heavy-drinking adolescents. *American Journal of Psychiatry, 172*(6), 531–542.

Substance Abuse and Mental Health Services Administration. (2014). *Results from the 2013 National Survey on Drug Use and Health: Summary of national findings* (NSDUH Series H-48, HHS Publication No. [SMA] 14-4863). Rockville, MD: Author.

Tait, R. J., Mackinnon, A., & Christensen, H. (2011). Cannabis use and cognitive function: 8-year trajectory in a young adult cohort. *Addiction, 106*(12), 2195–2203.

Takagi, M., Lubman, D. I., Cotton, S., Fornito, A., Baliz, Y., Tucker, A., et al. (2011). Executive control among adolescent inhalant and cannabis users. *Drug and Alcohol Review, 30*(6), 629–637.

Tamm, L., Epstein, J. N., Lisdahl, K. M., Molina, B., Tapert, S., Hinshaw, S. P., et al. (2013). Impact of ADHD and cannabis use on executive functioning in young adults. *Drug and Alcohol Dependence, 133,* 607–614.

Tapert, S. F., Baratta, M. V., Abrantes, A. M., & Brown, S. A. (2002). Attention dysfunction predicts substance involvement in community youths. *Journal of the American Academy of Child and Adolescent Psychiatry, 41*(6), 680–686.

Tapert, S. F., Brown, G. G., Kindermann, S. S., Cheung, E. H., Frank, L. R., Brown, S. A. (2001). fMRI measurement of brain dysfunction in alcohol-dependent young women. *Alcoholism, Clinical and Experimental Research, 25*(2), 236–245.

Tapert, S. F., & Brown, S. A. (1999). Neuropsychological correlates of adolescent substance abuse: Four year outcomes. *Journal of the International Neuropsychological Society, 5*(6), 481–493.

Tapert, S. F., & Brown, S. A. (2000). Substance dependence, family history of alcohol dependence and neuropsychological functioning in adolescence. *Addiction, 95*(7), 1043–1053.

Tapert, S. F., Granholm, E., Leedy, N. G., & Brown, S. A. (2002). Substance use and withdrawal: Neuropsychological functioning over 8 years in youth. *Journal of the International Neuropsychological Society, 8*(7), 873–883.

Tapert, S. F., Schweinsburg, A. D., Drummond, S. P., Paulus, M. P., Brown, S. A., Yang, T. T., et al. (2007). Functional MRI of inhibitory processing in abstinent adolescent marijuana users. *Psychopharmacology (Berlin), 194*(2), 173–183.

Thoma, R. J., Monnig, M. A., Lysne, P. A., Ruhl, D. A., Pommy, J. A., Bogenschutz, M., et al. (2011). Adolescent substance abuse: The effects of alcohol and marijuana on neuropsychological performance. *Alcoholism: Clinical and Experimental Research, 35*(1), 39–46.

Townshend, J. M., & Duka, T. (2005). Binge drinking, cognitive performance and mood in a population of young social drinkers. *Alcoholism: Clinical and Experimental Research, 29*(3), 317–325.

Vaidya, J. G., Block, R. I., O'Leary, D. S., Ponto, L. B., Ghoneim, M. M., & Bechara, A. (2012). Effects of chronic marijuana use on brain activity during monetary decision-making. *Neuropsychopharmacology, 37*(3), 618–629.

Weiland, B. J., Thayer, R. E., Depue, B. E., Sabbineni, A., Bryan, A. D., & Hutchison, K. E. (2015). Daily marijuana use is not associated with brain morphometric measures in adolescents or adults. *Journal of Neuroscience, 35*(4), 1505–1512.

Wetherill, R. R., Castro, N., Squeglia, L. M., & Tapert, S. F. (2013). Atypical neural activity during inhibitory processing in substance-naïve youth who later experience alcohol-induced blackouts. *Drug and Alcohol Dependence, 128*(3), 243–249.

Wetherill, R. R., Squeglia, L. M., Yang, T. T., & Tapert, S. F. (2013). A longitudinal examination of adolescent response inhibition: Neural differences before and after the initiation of heavy drinking. *Psychopharmacology (Berlin), 230*(4), 663–671.

Whelan, R., Watts, R., Orr, C. A., Althoff, R. R., Artiges, E., Banaschewski, T., et al. (2014). Neuropsychosocial profiles of current and future adolescent alcohol misusers. *Nature, 512*(7513), 185–189.

White, H. R., Marmorstein, N. R., Crews, F. T., Bates, M. E., Mun, E. Y., & Loeber, R. (2011). Associations between heavy drinking and changes in impulsive behavior among adolescent boys. *Alcoholism: Clinical and Experimental Research, 35*(2), 295–303.

Winters, K. C., & Lee, C. Y. (2008). Likelihood of developing an alcohol and cannabis use disorder during youth: Association with recent use and age. *Drug and Alcohol Dependence, 92*(1–3), 239–247.

Winton-Brown, T. T., Allen, P., Bhattacharyya, S., Borgwardt, S. J., Fusar-Poli, P., Crippa, J. A., et al. (2011). Modulation of auditory and visual processing by delta-9-tetrahydrocannabinol and cannabidiol: An FMRI study. *Neuropsychopharmacology, 36*(7), 1340–1348.

Winward, J. L., Hanson, K. L., Tapert, S. F., & Brown, S. A. (2014). Heavy alcohol use, marijuana use, and concomitant use by adolescents are associated with unique and shared cognitive decrements. *Journal of the International Neuropsychological Society, 20*(8), 784–795.

Xiao, L., Bechara, A., Gong, Q., Huang, X., Li, X., Xue, G., et al. (2013). Abnormal affective decision making revealed in adolescent binge drinkers using a functional magnetic resonance imaging study. *Psychology of Addictive Behaviors, 27*(2), 443–454.

Yücel, M., Lorenzetti, V., Suo, C., Zalesky, A., Fornito, A., Takagi, M. J., et al. (2016). Hippocampal harms, protection and recovery following regular cannabis use. *Translational Psychiatry, 6,* e710.

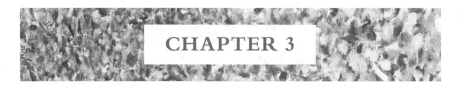

CHAPTER 3

Assessing Adolescent Substance Use Problems and Other Areas of Functioning

State of the Art

Ken C. Winters, Andria M. Botzet, and Susanne Lee

The use of alcohol and other drugs (hereafter referred to simply as "drugs") by adolescents continues to be a public health problem in the United States. Such use often occurs in conjunction with other types of problems, including school difficulties, family disruption, risky sexual behavior, and delinquency (Khan, Berger, Wells, & Cleland, 2012). Based on the 2014 nationwide survey conducted by the University of Michigan (Monitoring the Future; Miech, Johnston, O'Malley, Bachman, & Schulenberg, 2015; Schulenberg, Maslowsky, Maggs, & Zucker, Chapter 1, this volume), alcohol has been tried by 27% of 8th graders, 49% of 10th graders, and 66% of 12th graders. The annual prevalence of any illicit drug (including marijuana) was 15% (8th graders), 30% (10th graders), and 39% (12th graders; Miech et al., 2015). Adolescence is also a developmental period characterized by relatively high rates of substance use disorders (SUDs), as defined by official diagnostic criteria. Based on the 2008 National Survey on Drug Use and Health (NSDUH) dataset, 7.6% of 12- to 17-year–olds met criteria for at least one DSM-IV (American Psychiatric Association, 1994) SUD in the past year, and an additional 17% of teenagers, while not meeting an abuse diagnosis, still reported one or two substance-dependence criteria (Martin, Chung, & Langenbucher, 2008). Moreover, the onset of drug use during adolescence greatly increases the likelihood of developing an SUD into adulthood (Brown et al., 2008), and emerging studies point to the potential risk that teenage drug use may alter brain maturation and contribute to cognitive deficits, school failure, trouble with the law, and mental illness in a vulnerable person (Lisdahl, Shollenbarger, Sagar, & Gruber, Chapter 2, this volume; Volkow, Baler, Compton, & Weiss, 2014).

On the positive side, many youth make it through high school drug-free. A recent analysis of Monitoring the Future survey data indicates that among 12th graders, the percentage of students who never used alcohol, tobacco, marijuana, or other drugs in their lifetimes rose from 2.9% in 1983 to 25% in 2013 (Institute for Behavioral Health, 2016). Also, the majority of adolescents who use drugs do not develop an SUD—that is, they do not meet official DSM-5 criteria for this disorder (American Psychiatric Association, 2013). It is more common that youth who use drugs do so at a level of chronicity and intensity that falls short of meeting criteria for an SUD (Chung & Martin, 2011), and if problems occur, they would be of a subclinical nature (e.g., a one-time argument with a parent after discovering the teenager's drinking, feeling uneasy the day after a night of drinking). To put the range of drug use and possible resulting problems in perspective, we later discuss stages of drug involvement representing the continuum of adolescent use.

An accurate understanding of a teenager's drug involvement benefits from a valid and timely screening and assessment process. This chapter describes principles of adolescent assessment, including the assessment process and brief interventions, clinical content, distinguishing normative from hazardous or harmful use, and an overview of measurement tools.

PRINCIPLES OF ADOLESCENT ASSESSMENT

There are two main types of assessment: screening and comprehensive assessment (Allen, 1991). Numerous examples of psychometrically sound instruments, including interviews and computer-administered and paper-and-pencil questionnaires, are available (some of which are in the public domain). It behooves a drug treatment program to use at least one standardized, adolescent-specific and psychometrically sound screening instrument and assessment instrument as part of its intake. Later, we provide summaries of both types of instruments.

A screening process is often the first step when the task is to determine whether a teenager may be using drugs and is experiencing drug-related problems. A good screening tool is brief, easy to use, and accurate. It is common for screening tools in this field to consist of questions pertaining to recent drug use quantity and frequency, adverse consequences of use (e.g., school and social problems), and the context of the teenager's use (e.g., Use alone? Use in social situations?).

Yet even the most accurate screening tool should not be the basis for a definitive diagnosis nor as the only basis to determine whether treatment is needed. The results from a screening should be used to inform the need for a comprehensive assessment. Such an in-depth assessment would involve a detailed review of the extent and nature of the drug involvement, diagnostic-related symptoms, psychosocial functioning (e.g., home and school), other mental or behavioral disorders, the motivation to change, treatment needs, and personal strengths (e.g., hobbies, how one spends free time, what he or she is proud of). Multiple sources (client report, parent report, archival records) and methods (e.g., self-administered and interview formats) should be included. Thus, this assessment procedure requires a multidimensional framework. An important task of comprehensive assessment is establishing clarity as to whether the signs of drug use are bona fide symptoms of drug use or are actually symptoms of a behavioral problem or disorder that occurs during adolescence, such as conduct disorder (CD), attention-deficit/hyperactivity disorder (ADHD), or trauma. Toward this end, the assessor should thoroughly review the past and present history of psychiatric symptoms, and if present, whether onset was prior or subsequent to the possible use of drugs (Riggs & Davies, 2002).

ASSESSMENT PROCESS AND BRIEF INTERVENTIONS

It is typical that eligibility for a brief intervention is determined by a screening. Several screening protocols and psychometrically sound tools exist. We favor an adaptation of the model described by Levy and Shrier (2014). This approach involves leading off with a small number of drug use frequency questions, and if recent use of any kind is reported, then the adolescent is directed to answer a handful of questions that are indicative of a drug problem. In our example, we recommend the six-item CRAFFT (Knight, Sherritt, Shrier, Harris, & Chang, 2002). It is advisable for the counselor to implement a brief intervention if the adolescent endorses two or more problems on the CRAFFT. An exception is if the teenager endorsed all items (score of 6)—this may reflect a severe-end drug problem and it may be advisable to refer him or her for a comprehensive assessment and consideration of a more intensive treatment. An example of this screening model follows:

> We ask all our adolescents to complete this form, because alcohol and other drug use can affect physical and mental health. Please answer all the questions. Your answers will be confidential.

> *During the past 12 months, have you . . .*

> Q1. Drank any alcohol (more than a few sips)?
> _____ No   _____ Yes
> Q2. Smoked marijuana or hashish?
> _____ No   _____ Yes

Q3.   Use anything else to get high?

_____ No   _____ Yes

("Anything else" includes illegal drugs, over-the-counter and prescription drugs, and things that you sniff or huff.)

If you answered yes to any of the above (Q1–Q3), answer Q4–Q9.

Q4.   Have you ever ridden in a **CAR** driven by someone (including yourself) who was "high" or had been using alcohol or drugs?

_____ No   _____ Yes

Q5.   Do you ever use alcohol or drugs to **RELAX**, feel better about yourself, or fit in?

_____ No   _____ Yes

Q6.   Do you ever use alcohol or drugs while you are by yourself, **ALONE**?

_____ No   _____ Yes

Q7.   Do your **FAMILY** or **FRIENDS** ever tell you that you should cut down on your drinking or drug use?

_____ No   _____ Yes

Q8.   Do you ever **FORGET** things you did while using alcohol or drugs?

_____ No   _____ Yes

Q9.   Have you gotten into **TROUBLE** while you were using alcohol or drugs?

_____ No   _____ Yes

CLINICAL CONTENT

Understanding the emotional and behavioral problems associated with adolescents' drug use requires a comprehensive assessment of a wide range of variables. The variables can be organized into two main domains. The first area pertains to the details of a person's use problem severity and resulting symptoms. This domain is the primary focus when a screening process is used to help determine whether a brief intervention is warranted. The second domain is the biopsychosocial factors that are presumed to have contributed to the onset, maintenance, and progression of the drug involvement, and may have implications in the planning of treatment services.

Drug Use Problem Severity

Several factors related to drug use problem severity have been identified as important to assess comprehensively: age of first drug use and age of transition to regular drug use; lifetime and more recent (e.g., prior 6 months) pattern of use, including frequency, quantity, and duration for individual drugs; which drug or drugs are preferred; the functional value of the drug use for the adolescent (e.g., social benefits, psychological benefits); and the presence of DSM-based symptoms of a drug use disorder. The latter component merits further discussion.

Drug use that goes beyond experimentation and progresses into problematic involvement is formally delineated by various classification systems, with the primary system being the fifth edition of the *Diagnostic and Statistical Manual of Mental Disorders* (DSM-5; American Psychiatric Association, 2013). The diagnosis of an SUD is based on significant behavioral and physiological impairment associated with drug use. SUDs are diagnosed when a person displays two or more symptoms out of a set of 11 symptoms pertaining to inability to control one's use, health problems, social impairment, and failure to fulfill major responsibilities at home, school, or work. Individuals would be assigned a diagnosis based on how many symptom criteria the individual met: no disorder (zero to one), mild (two to three), moderate (four to five), or severe (six or more).

DSM-5 criteria include some positive changes for defining SUDs among adolescents. One set of criteria to diagnose a single SUD makes sense for youth. The prior distinction of abuse and dependence in DSM-IV (American Psychiatric Association, 1994) was not a valid differentiation for adolescents (Martin, Chung, Kirisci, & Langenbucher, 2006), and factor and latent class analyses revealed a single dimension of problems linked to drug involvement (Chung & Martin, 2001, 2005; Martin et al., 2006). Also, the elimination of the "legal problems" symptom from DSM-5 is also a developmentally appropriate decision given that for adolescents this symptom was highly related to coexisting CD (Martin et al., 2006).

Given the frequent comorbidity of SUDs and other psychiatric disorders (Grella, Hser, Joshi, & Rounds-Bryant, 2001), it is important that the assessor comprehensively review via a timeline the past and present history of possible psychiatric symptoms. This type of detailed interview can help sort out the course of the onset of SUD symptoms and symptoms related to a mental or behavioral disorder (Riggs & Davies, 2002). Table 3.1 provides a list of several comprehensive diagnostic interviews that provide the structure for this type of assessment.

Biopsychosocial Risk and Protective Factors

Biopsychosocial factors refer to the range of personal, environmental, and biological factors that influence the onset, development, and maintenance of drug use behaviors. Examples of biopsychosocial factors include family functioning, family history of drug use, peer drug use, school functioning, and coexisting psychological disorders. These factors work together to either increase (via the presence of factors that pose a risk for drug use, such as presence of peer drug use) or decrease (via the presence of factors that protect against drug use, such as effective parental monitoring) an individual's propensity to use drugs (Clark

TABLE 3.1. Select Comprehensive Assessment Tools for Adolescent Drug Use

Instrument name	Authors	Type	Length	Content	Source for psychometrics
Adolescent Diagnostic Interview (ADI)	Winters & Henly (1993)	Interview	—	Drug involvement, psychosocial functioning, screen for psychiatric disorders	Winters & Henly (1993); Winters, Stinchfield, Fulkerson, & Henly (1993)
Adolescent Problem Severity Index (APSI)	Metzger, Kushner, & McLellan (1991)	Interview	—	Drug involvement, psychosocial functioning	Metzger et al. (1991)
Adolescent Self-Assessment Profile—II (ASAP-II)	Wanberg (2006)	Questionnaire	225 items	Drug involvement, psychosocial functioning	Wanberg (2006)
Comprehensive Addiction Severity Index for Adolescents (CASI-A)	Meyers (1991)	Interview	—	Drug involvement, psychosocial functioning	Meyers (1991)
Diagnostic Interview Schedule for Children—Version 2.3 (DISC-2.3)	Shaffer et al. (1996)	Interview	—	Drug involvement, psychiatric disorders, psychosocial functioning	Shaffer et al. (1996); Fisher et al. (1993); Roberts, Solovitz, Chen, & Casat (1996)
Global Appraisal of Individual Needs (GAIN)	Dennis, Titus, White, Unsicker, & Hodgkins (2002)	Interview	—	Drug involvement, psychiatric disorders, psychosocial functioning	Dennis et al. (2002)
Personal Experience Inventory (PEI)	Winters & Henly (1989)	Questionnaire	276 items	Drug involvement, psychosocial factors, response distortion	Winters & Henly (1989); Botzet, Winters, & Stinchfield (2006)

(continued)

TABLE 3.1. *(continued)*

Instrument name	Authors	Type	Length	Content	Source for psychometrics
Substance Use Disorders Diagnostic Schedule (SUDDS)	Hoffmann & Harrison (1989)	Interview	—	Drug involvement, psychosocial factors	Hoffmann & Harrison (1989); Davis, Hoffmann, Morse, & Luehr (1992)
Teen Addiction Severity Index (T-ASI)	Kaminer, Bukstein, & Tarter (1991)	Interview	—	Drug involvement, psychiatric disorders, psychosocial factors	Kaminer et al. (1991)

& Winters, 2002; Petraitis, Flay, & Miller, 1995). For youth already using drugs, identifying and addressing these factors can help to personalize interventions and treatments and, thus, optimize effectiveness of behavior change efforts (Shoham & Insel, 2011). Here we provide a brief overview of four biopsychosocial factors that are strongly related to adolescent drug use problems: family history of an SUD, parenting practices, peer influences, and coexisting mental/behavioral disorders.

Family History of a Drug Problem and Family Functioning

Children of parents with a positive history of an SUD have increased liability for an SUD (McGue, 1999; Zucker, Donovan, Masten, Mattson, & Moss, 2008), and this liability represents both a heritable as well as an environmental risk, both directly and through effects on family functioning. Many phenotypic characteristics relevant to developing an SUD likely have a significant heritable component, such as disinhibitory traits (Elkins, McGue, & Iacono, 2007; Nestler & Landsman, 2001). Family discord, as evidenced by poor parenting or by parental mental illness, particularly parental antisocial behavior history (e.g., Cadoret, Yates, Troughton, Woodworth, & Stewart, 1995), contribute to environmental risk. Poor global family functioning and poor quality of parent–child relationships are associated with more alcohol and drug involvement (Bahr & Hoffmann, 2010).

Parenting Practices

Positive parenting can have a profound impact on the development of healthy adolescents, such as by providing security and emotional support for the child and by supporting the teenager's psychosocial development and competency to cope with everyday life stressors. Parents continue to exert considerable influence on their child's drug use during adolescence and young adulthood (Abar & Turrisi, 2008). Among parenting-related variables, parental support and monitoring have the most important influences on development. Parental support and connectedness to the child, and monitoring of his or her whereabouts, are associated with reduced use, whereas lack of nurturance and poor monitoring are linked to increased drug involvement (Clark, Thatcher, & Maisto, 2005; LaBrie & Cail, 2011). A plausible explanation for these findings is that adolescents from nonsupportive homes characterized by hostility and lack of affection may have problems with self-regulation and engage with deviant peers to gain social support, which are linked to increased risk of drug use (Brody & Ge, 2001; Simons & Robertson, 1989). High levels of monitoring can insulate children and adolescents from misbehaviors and drug use. Closely monitored adolescents may be protected against starting to use drugs, even when they have been exposed to friends who use (Chilcoat & Anthony, 1996; Steinberg, Fletcher, & Darling, 1994).

Peer Effects

Extensive literature demonstrates that peers influence adolescent substance use (Donovan, 2004; Ramirez, Hinman, Sterling, Weisner, & Campbell, 2012; Simons-Morton & Farhat, 2010). Adolescents who associate with drug-using peers are more likely to initiate use and report higher levels of use than those who do not report peer use (D'Amico & McCarthy, 2006; Farrell & Danish, 1993). Peer relationships are complex given that peer influences can be reciprocal and membership of peer networks can change frequently. The nature of the association between drug use and peers could be due to the increased likelihood that drug-using individuals seek out other drug-using peers for socializing and for access to drugs. Other factors that have been linked to adolescent drug involvement are prodrug attitudes among peers and the extent of the youth's peer attachment to peer groups with prodrug attitudes (Dishion, Capaldi, Spracklen, & Fuzhong, 1995; Patterson, Forgatch, Yoerger, & Stoolmiller, 1998).

Coexisting Behavioral/Mental Disorders

Clinical and epidemiological studies demonstrate that drug-involved adolescents are likely to have one or more coexisting disorders (Deas, 2006). The behavioral and mental disorders that commonly coexist with an SUD represent complex constructs that are relevant to understanding the etiology of drug involvement and also provide insights into the prevention and treatment of an SUD (Clark & Winters, 2002). One major category of coexisting disorders is conceptualized as externalizing disorders. These are characterized by behavioral dysregulation (impulsive decision making) and include CD, oppositional defiant disorder (ODD), and ADHD. Another prominent category is internalizing disorders, which includes anxiety disorders (e.g.., social phobia), mood disorders (e.g., major depression) and posttraumatic stress disorder (PTSD). A common feature among this group of disorders is that the person's emotional states compromise his or her level of functioning. Other disorders such as eating disorders and bipolar disorder have been shown from cross-sectional research to be highly prevalent among youth with an SUD (Pisetsky, Chao, Dierker, May, & Striegel-Moore, 2008; Wilens, Biederman, Abrantes, & Spencer, 1997).

Prospective studies on externalizing disorders (CD, ODD, and ADHD) and SUDs show that externalizing behaviors, particularly antisocial behaviors in late childhood (ages 8–11), are highly linked to the initiation of drug use in early adolescence and to the development of a later SUD (August et al., 2006; Lee, Humphreys, Flory, Liu, & Glass, 2011; Mirza & Bukstein, 2011). Complicating our understanding of the causal relation between externalizing disorders and an SUD are studies indicating that an SUD increases the presence of externalizing behaviors (Clark & Bukstein, 1998; Lynskey & Fergusson, 1995). Thus, a youth with minimal conduct problems who then gets involved with drugs may eventually develop a CD.

Internalizing disorders (depression and anxiety disorders) are the second most commonly diagnosed comorbid condition in youth with an SUD following externalizing disorders (see Esposito-Smythers, Rallis, Machell, Williams, & Fisher, Chapter 7, this volume; O'Neil, Conner, & Kendall, 2011, for reviews). Numerous studies report elevated rates of internalizing disorders and related symptoms among adolescents with an SUD, especially among females compared with male adolescents with an SUD (Martin, Lynch, Pollock, & Clark, 2000). The association does not, however, *establish* that the childhood internalizing disorder causes the later involvement with drugs. Similarly with externalizing disorders and SUDs, there is mixed evidence about the temporal order of onset of internalizing disorders and SUDs in youth. Some studies show that internalizing disorders temporally precede SUDs (Costello, Erkanli, Federman, & Angold, 1999), whereas other studies suggest the opposite pattern in adolescent samples (Rohde, Lewinsohn, & Seeley, 1991).

Cognitive Variables

Research on the cognitive precursors of drug use behaviors has been largely directed at demonstrating that cognitions have an impact either on drug use patterns (Aarons, Goldman, Greenbaum, & Coovert, 2003) or on the likelihood of future use (Smith, Goldman, Greenbaum, & Christiansen, 1995). Naturally, developmental considerations are important with respect to assessing cognitive factors. Cognitive capacities for abstract thinking begin to take a more prominent role during early adolescence, yet older adolescents are better equipped to consider the future consequences of their actions (Dahl, 2004).

Also, cognitions may be significantly influenced during adolescence by contextual factors, such as peers (Gardner & Steinberg, 2005).

We discuss below four cognitive variables that have been prominent in the literature with respect to the onset or maintenance of adolescent drug use: reasons for drug use, expectancies about behavioral outcomes (and the related construct of risk perception), readiness to change, and confidence in personal ability (or self-efficacy).

REASONS FOR DRUG USE

Research suggests that use by adolescents may be associated with several reasons, including recreational benefits (e.g., use to have fun), social conformity, mood enhancement, and coping with stress (Clark & Winters, 2002; Lopez et al., 2001; Petraitis et al., 1995). There is some evidence that youth with an SUD ascribe greater benefits associated with the social conformity and mood enhancement effects of drug involvement compared with nondependent adolescents (Henly & Winters, 1988).

EXPECTANCIES ABOUT BEHAVIORAL OUTCOMES

Drug use-related expectancies in adolescents have been shown to be associated with negative physical effects, negative psychosocial effects, future health concerns, positive social effects, and reduction of negative affect (e.g., Brown, Christiansen, & Goldman, 1987; Smith et al., 1995). Another expectancy variable discussed in the literature pertains to perception of risk cost of drug use versus perceived psychological or social benefit of drug use (Miller & Rollnick, 2004). Many individuals who have knowledge about hazard and its risk nonetheless deny that they personally are at risk. This denial can lead to two cognitive processes: (1) belief perseverance in which individuals selectively attend to messages that support their belief (Festinger, 1957) and exhibit counterarguments when faced with disconfirming evidence (Nisbett & Ross, 1980), and (2) optimistic bias or erroneous beliefs that personal risk is less than the risk faced by others (Janis & Mann, 1977; Prochaska et al., 1994). Some variables relevant for measurement of expectancies and risk perception include perceived vulnerability to, and knowledge about, the health risk of drug use, perceived personal vulnerability to drug-related consequences, the person's belief that quitting drug use will reduce his or her personal risk for such consequences, and the way the individual communicates susceptibility to risk (Leigh, 1989). Also, there may be merit in measuring what has been referred to as "optimistic bias" for personal risk. Subjects can be asked to rate their chances of developing certain consequences of drug use behaviors (e.g., much lower than average, lower than average, above average) and their responses can be compared with estimates of actual consequences obtained from national data (Weinstein & Klein, 1995).

READINESS TO CHANGE

This motivation-based construct involves a range of concepts: problem rec-ognition, readiness for change, treatment suitability, and external influences on treatment seeking (Prochaska, DiClemente, & Norcross, 1992). The deter-minants of and interplay between these motivational variables with respect to behavior change in adolescents is not well understood (Clark & Winters, 2002). Adolescents may be subject to many of the same underlying motiva-tional forces that influence behavior change in adults, such as the phenomenon when an individual recognizes that the negative personal effects of drug use may outweigh perceived personal benefits (Shaffer & Simoneau, 2001). How-ever, adolescents may be less inclined than adults to project the consequences of their drug use into the future (Winters & Arria, 2011). To further aggra-vate the change process, adolescents may have experienced coercive pressure to seek and continue treatment. There are no empirical studies that provide reliable estimates of the extent and type of coercion that occurs in the pro-cess of youth seeking and receiving drug treatment, but conventional wisdom suggests that many adolescents have explicitly or implicitly been coerced into treatment. Coercive influences can take several forms, such as exclusion from the decision-making process about seeking treatment, use of force and deceit to impose treatment, and use of restraint to retain the person in treatment (Monahan et al., 1995). Consequently, at the outset of treatment, counselors must be sensitive to motivational barriers that may be linked to such circum-stances.

CONFIDENCE IN PERSONAL ABILITY (SELF-EFFICACY)

Self-efficacy, or confidence in personal ability, has a central role in many con-ceptualizations about behavioral control and change (e.g., Bandura, 1977). Self-efficacy not only affects one's choice of activities, such as behavior change goals, but also how much effort is expended in such activities and how long one will persist despite adversity. This construct has been shown to predict a variety of health behavior outcomes, including alcohol treatment outcome (Miller & Rollnick, 2012). Self-efficacy measures should be accompanied by measures of goal setting and achievement, as well as other constructs believed to underlie self-efficacy, such as the adolescent's perceptions of his or her ability to overcome barriers to change (Miller & Rollnick, 2012).

DISTINGUISHING NORMATIVE USE
FROM HARMFUL USE

As suggested by research (Lisdahl et al., Chapter 2, this volume), risk-taking and impulsive or peer-driven behaviors, including alcohol and other drug use, are common during adolescence (Collado, Felton, MacPherson, & Lejuez, 2014; Steinberg, 2007). Respectful to the developmental normalcy, many experts have categorized adolescent drug use according to its severity or intensity. We propose the following levels of severity, with recognition of the new language in DSM-5 for levels of an SUD (American Psychiatric Association, 2013):

1. Abstinence: never uses any illicit drug or alcohol (more than a few sips).
2. Experimentation: represents the first few times that a drug is used, when the adolescent is learning the experience of intoxication.
3. Limited use: signifies social use in relatively low-risk situations.
4. Mild: use occurs in high-risk situations, and/or results in minor or infrequent school, family, or legal consequences.
5. Moderate: use results in recurrent problems or interferes with functioning.
6. Severe: use results in loss of control and compulsive drug use (Levy & Kokotailo, 2011).

Though this spectrum is based on DSM-IV criteria for an SUD (American Psychiatric Association, 1994), these general stages are congruent with the current DSM-5 criteria (American Psychiatric Association, 2013). Whereas minimal research has been published on the validity of DSM-5 criteria for an SUD as applied to adolescents (Winters, 2013), we noted earlier that several changes in DSM-5 are developmentally appropriate (e.g., eliminating the legal criteria; Winters, Martin, & Chung, 2011).

Because some drug use is statistically normative during adolescence (Schulenberg et al., Chapter 1, this volume), it may be difficult for parents and clinicians to discern the line from which "normative use" becomes harmful or problematic use. Often, parents and other caregivers are unaware whether their adolescent has initiated alcohol or drug use (experimental stage) or falls in the limited use category, as symptoms of use during these stages are short-lived and commonly concealed for fear of punishment. Behavioral symptoms are the first signs that the drug use may be a problem. Common behavioral symptoms include withdrawal from previously enjoyed activities (e.g., quitting a sports team), an increase in academic problems (e.g., skipping school, lower achievement/grades), increased mental health problems (e.g., depression, anxiety), increased social concerns (e.g., isolating oneself, poor social skills, changing peer group), and increased legal involvement (e.g., possession, minor consumption; Bukstein et al., 2005).

Brief Interventions

As severity of the problem increases, the quantity, frequency, and/or intensity of the aforementioned behavioral symptoms also tend to increase, and are more likely to raise awareness in parents, teachers, and other concerned persons. There is considerable debate as to what level of adolescent drug problem severity is a good clinical fit for a brief intervention (Hingson & Compton, 2014). Based on the research, there appears to be an overwhelming tendency for adolescent brief interventions to be applied most commonly to youth who are at the early stages of their drug use and are experiencing a mild-to-moderate drug problem severity picture (Winters, Tanner-Smith, Bresani, & Meyers; 2014). Based on our earlier discussions on measuring and conceptualizing drug use severity, a brief intervention for adolescents would be appropriate for youth who score a 2 or more on the CRAFFT, or those who fit a DSM-5 SUD diagnosis at either a mild or moderate level.

MEASURING ADOLESCENT DRUG INVOLVEMENT

Because use occurs on such a broad spectrum, effective measurement is necessary to gain insight regarding where the adolescent falls on that spectrum. Knowledge can better equip the provider to make recommendations for additional services, as appropriate. As with other health concerns, risky use can be more effectively managed and addressed when identified early.

Screening Tools

Because the early stages of drug use are not typically observed by parents and other concerned adults, a routine screening of all youth seen at school health and other clinics is advisable, in an attempt to address all stages of drug involvement. Screening tools are designed to be short (ideally 10 minutes or less) self-reported snapshots of current (or recent) drug use. A recent screener consists of just two age-specific core questions: one question focuses on the teenager's drinking frequency and the other question on peer drinking frequency (Chung et al., 2012). Screens are designed to identify *potential* problems and areas to address. Providers and other professionals working with adolescents must be sensitive to the fact that a screener is *not* an assessment. Definitive judgments about diagnoses should not be made based solely on results from a screening measure.

Formats vary for screening tools; they commonly include the interview format, self-administered questionnaire, or computer-assisted format (including mobile devices). Research on the psychometrics of these techniques suggests that, in most cases, the validity of disclosure is similar across formats (e.g., Dillon, Turner, Robbins, & Szapocznik, 2005; Newman et al., 2002). More recent research suggests that adolescents may prefer electronic or computer-assisted screenings due to the cultural and generational comfort with this format (Harris & Knight, 2014). Table 3.2 provides a summary of common screening tools that address drug use. The tools listed in this table were developed and normed for adolescents, and they inquire about both alcohol and other drugs. Other screening tools exist, but many are developed for adults or for a specific drug.

As mentioned above, universal screening is ideal, when possible and appropriate, for a variety of reasons, including early detection and as an aid to help destigmatize the topic of drug use among adolescents. If a screening tool is routinely administered "to all teens who walk through the door," teens may be less likely to feel singled out and limit their response bias due to social desirability. In addition, screening often, rather than sporadically, can help to address the fluctuating behaviors of adolescents and may become more reliable as their trust in the provider and the system or routine increases. Multiple variables can influence the reliability of a screening tool, including cognitive process (e.g., comprehension, recall), social desirability, attention seeking, perceived lack of confidentiality, and situational factors (e.g., trust in the provider, fear of reprisal; Brener, Billy, & Grady, 2003). Thus, confidential universal screening and frequent screening likely optimize early detection of problems related to drug use.

In administering a screening tool to adolescents, and entrusting them to respond honestly, the provider should convey a message of concern and appreciation—not acknowledging the results may negatively affect the provider–client relationship and reduce trust in the provider, or in the field, in general. Negative screens can be addressed with positive reinforcement, such as using statements like "Keep up the good work!" or "I'm pleased to see that alcohol use hasn't been an issue for you." Screening results that indicate some level of alcohol or other drug use should be followed by a more comprehensive assessment, such as the ones mentioned in the following section.

COMPREHENSIVE ASSESSMENT TOOLS

This type of assessment tool is intended to address use more comprehensively, take more time to administer, and is generally rooted in DSM-based criteria. These tools are designed to measure the *nature* and *extent* of the specific drug(s) being used. Administration time is longer than for screening tools, though it varies across tools. Typically, these tools are administered using an interviewer format, taking approximately 45–60 minutes, though some assessments are conducted using self-administered and computer-assisted formats.

Most comprehensive assessments are structured, meaning items are to be read verbatim, follow a decision-tree format, and responses consist of a few pre-defined options. Diagnostic assessments are conducted by well-trained professionals experienced with adolescent use issues, such as a psychologist, mental health professional, school counselor, social worker, or an addiction counselor (Winters, Fahnhorst, Botzet, Stinchfield, & Nicholson, 2017).

Diagnostic assessments include more detailed investigation of each drug used, including the age of onset; progression of use; context of use (e.g., the

TABLE 3.2. Select Screening Instruments for Adolescent Drug Use

Instrument name	Authors	Type	Length	Content	Source for psychometrics
Brief Screener for Tobacco, Alcohol, and Other Drugs (BSTAD)	Kelly et al. (2014)	3-item questionnaire	1 minute	Drug involvement	Kelly et al. (2014)
CAGE-AID	Brown & Rounds (1994)	5-item questionnaire	3 minutes	Drug involvement	Brown & Rounds (1994)
Client Substance Index—Short (CSI-S)	Thomas (1990)	15-item questionnaire	10 minutes	Drug involvement	Thomas (1990)
CRAFFT	Knight, Sherritt, Shrier, Harris, & Chang (2002)	6-item questionnaire	3 minutes	Drug involvement	Knight et al. (2002)
Global Appraisal of Individual Needs—Short Screener (GAIN-SS)	Dennis, Chan, & Funk (2006)	20-item questionnaire	10 minutes	Drug involvement, co-occurring problems	Dennis et al. (2006)
Personal Experience Screening Questionnaire (PESQ)	Winters (1992)	40-item questionnaire	10 minutes	Drug involvement, co-occurring problems, response distortion	Winters (1992)

usual times and places of drug use); consequences of the use; and personal, social, and cultural antecedents that are associated with the adolescent's drug use (e.g., peer involvement, risky sexual behavior, mental health, physical health; Winters et al., 2014). This in-depth information assists the provider in determining courses of action and/or treatment approaches that might best suit the adolescent. See Table 3.1 for a summary of select comprehensive and diagnostic assessment instruments that were developed for adolescents and are associated with favorable psychometric properties. Also, Table 3.3 lists other instruments that may be suitable for a comprehensive assessment—these instruments address cognition- and motivation-related variables (e.g., problem recognition, self-efficacy).

SUMMARY AND FUTURE DIRECTIONS

Drug use is still prevalent among American teenagers—of particular concern is that for some grade levels there is a recent increase in marijuana. Whereas adolescent drug use has routinely been linked to health concerns, emerging evidence now sharpens the view that drug involvement while the adolescent brain is still developing may have lasting negative impacts (Volkow et al., 2014).

Accurately identifying those adolescents has been aided by over two decades of assessment research. Service providers and researchers have a range of adolescent screening and comprehensive assessment tools from which to choose. A recent online catalogue, the PhenX Toolkit (*www.phenxtoolkit.org*), provides a compendium of rigorously vetted measures for a broad range of research domains, including drug use, underlying factors that trigger and maintain drug use, diagnostic symptoms, and co-occurring problems. We conclude that a range of self-administered and interview-based, developmentally appropriate, and psychometrically sound screening and comprehensive assessment tools exist, and that brief intervention programs will benefit from this relatively strong and diverse assessment field. The development of very brief and accurate screening tools is particularly helpful in the use of brief interventions in health settings where there may be only 5–10 minutes of time to screen for drug use (e.g., pediatric clinic).

Where should future research focus its efforts? More work is needed to develop accurate biological assays—one challenge in this area is the need for an accurate roadside assessment of one's possible impairment resulting from smoking or ingesting marijuana. Also, the use of mobile technology to support behavior change will benefit from the use of these technologies for assessing the change process. For example, handheld personal digital assistants are a promising strategy to more precisely assess how specific situations, stressors, and cognitions may impact drug use (Shrier, Rhoads, Burke, Walls, & Blood, 2014). A welcomed development is research on assessment tools and measures of theory-driven treatment processes and outcomes. One salient example is the measurement of "change talk" and interviewing styles that maximize change talk (D'Amico & Ewing, Chapter 14, this volume). The extent that an adolescent talks about change is a significant predictor of treatment outcome (Baer et al., 2008) and there are motivational interviewing techniques that promote goal-directed change talk (Barnett et al., 2014). Other research needs include evaluating assessment tools in subpopulations of young people defined by age, race, and type of setting; evaluating tools as a measure of change; and how or

TABLE 3.3. Select Other Measures

Instrument name	Authors	Type	Length	Content	Source for psychometrics
Alcohol Expectancy Questionnaire— Adolescent (AEQ-A)	Brown, Christiansen, & Goldman (1987)	Questionnaire	90 items	Alcohol expectancies	Brown et al. (1987); Christiansen, Smith, Roehling, & Goldman (1989)
Circumstances, Motivation, Readiness and Suitability (CMRS)	Jainchill, Bhattacharya, & Yagelka (1995)	Questionnaire	25 items	Readiness for change and suitability for treatment	Jainchill et al. (1995)
Decisional Balance Scale	Migneault, Pallonen, & Velicer (1997)	Questionnaire	16 items	Pros and cons of drinking	Migneault et al. (1997)
Drinking Motives Questionnaire— Revised (DMQ-R)	Cooper (1994)	Questionnaire or interview	20 items	Reasons for drinking alcohol	Cooper (1994)
Drug Avoidance Self-Efficacy Scale (DASES)	Martin, Wilkinson, & Poulos (1995)	Questionnaire	16 items	Self-efficacy in multiple-drug users	Martin et al. (1995)
Marijuana Effect Expectancy Questionnaire (MEEQ)	Aarons, Brown, Stice, & Coe (2001)	Questionnaire	78 items	Marijuana expectancies	Aarons et al. (2001)
Marijuana Motives Measure (MMM)	Simons, Correia, Carey, & Borsari (1998)	Questionnaire or interview	25 items	Reasons for using marijuana	Simons et al. (1998); Lee, Neighbors, Hendershot, & Grossband (2009)
Problem Recognition Questionnaire (PRQ)	Cady, Winters, Jordan, & Solheim (1996)	Questionnaire	24 items	Readiness for change	Cady et al. (1996)
Self-Efficacy Questionnaire for Children (SEQ-C)	Muris (2001)	Questionnaire	24 items	Self-efficacy (academics, social, and coping)	Muris (2001)

to what extent environmental, personal, and contextual risk and protective factors are linked to drug use onset, escalation, and maintenance.

There is great potential for brief interventions to address adolescent drug involvement. With some exceptions, research in the past decade suggests that brief interventions are effective with youth. The vast assessment literature provides clinicians and researchers with numerous psychometrically sound options when determining the suitability for a brief intervention. Several research challenges still remain, but if progress is made with them, an already mature field will be further strengthened.

ACKNOWLEDGMENT

Preparation of this chapter was supported by Grant No. DA029785 from the National Institutes of Health.

REFERENCES

Aarons, G. A., Brown, S. A., Stice, E., & Coe, M. T. (2001). Psychometric evaluation of the marijuana and stimulant effect expectancy questionnaires for adolescents. *Addictive Behaviors, 26,* 219–236.

Aarons, G. A., Goldman, M. S., Greenbaum, P. E., & Coovert, M. D. (2003). Alcohol expectancies: Integrating cognitive science and psychometric approaches. *Addictive Behaviors, 28,* 947–961.

Abar, C., & Turrisi, R. (2008). How important are parents during the college years?: A longitudinal perspective of indirect influences their parents yield on their college teens' alcohol use. *Addictive Behaviors, 33,* 1360–1368.

Allen, J. P. (1991). The interrelationship of alcoholism assessment and treatment. *Alcohol Health Research World, 15,* 178–185.

American Psychiatric Association. (1994). *Diagnostic and statistical manual of mental disorders* (4th ed). Washington, DC: Author.

American Psychiatric Association. (2013). *Diagnostic and statistical manual of mental disorders* (5th ed). Arlington, VA: Author.

August, G. J., Winters, K. C., Realmuto, G. M., Fahnhorst, T., Botzet, A., & Lee, S. (2006). Prospective study of adolescent drug use among community samples of ADHD and non-ADHD participants. *Journal of the American Academy of Child and Adolescent Psychiatry, 45,* 824–832.

Baer, J. S., Beadnell, B., Garrett, S. B., Hartzler, B., Wells, E. A., & Peterson, P. L. (2008). Adolescent change language within a brief motivational intervention and substance use outcomes. *Psychology of Addictive Behaviors, 22,* 570–575.

Bahr, S. J., & Hoffmann, J. P. (2010). Parenting style, religiosity, peers, and adolescent heavy drinking. *Journal of Studies on Alcohol and Drugs, 71,* 539–543.

Bandura, A. (1977). Self-efficacy: Toward a unifying theory of behavioral change. *Psychological Review, 84,* 191–215.

Barnett, E., Spruijt-Metz, D., Moyers, T. B., Smith, C., Rohrbach, L. A., Sun, P., et al. (2014). Bidirectional relationships between client and counselor speech: The importance of reframing. *Psychology of Addictive Behaviors, 28,* 1212–1219.

Botzet, A. M., Winters, K. C., & Stinchfield, R. D. (2006). Gender differences in measuring adolescent drug abuse and related psychosocial problems. *Journal of Child and Adolescent Substance Abuse, 16,* 91–108.

Brener, N. D., Billy, J. O., & Grady, W. R. (2003). Assessment of factors affecting the validity of self-reported health-risk behavior among adolescents: Evidence from the scientific literature. *Journal of Adolescent Health, 33,* 436–457.

Brody, G. H., & Ge, X. (2001). Linking parenting processes and self-regulation to psychological functioning and alcohol use during early adolescence. *Journal of Family Psychology, 15,* 82–94.

Brown, R. L., & Rounds, L. A. (1994). Conjoint screening questionnaires for alcohol and other drug abuse: Criterion validity in a primary care practice. *Wisconsin Medical Journal, 94,* 135–140.

Brown, S. A., Christiansen, B. A., & Goldman, M. S. (1987). The Alcohol Expectancies Questionnaire: An instrument for the assessment of adolescent and adult alcohol expectancies. *Journal of the Studies on Alcohol, 48,* 483–491.

Brown, S. A., McGue, M., Maggs, J., Schulenberg, J., Hingson, R., Swartzwelder, S., et al. (2008). A developmental perspective on alcohol and youth ages 16–20. *Pediatrics, 121,* S290–S310.

Bukstein, O. G., Bernet, W., Arnold, V., Beitchman, J., Shaw, J., Benson, R. S., et al. (2005). Practice parameter for the assessment and treatment of children and adolescents with substance use disorders. *Journal of the American Academy of Child and Adolescent Psychiatry, 44,* 609–621.

Cadoret, R. J., Yates, W. R., Troughton, E., Woodworth, G., & Stewart, M. A. (1995). Adoption study demonstrating two genetic pathways to drug abuse. *Archives of General Psychiatry, 52,* 42–52.

Cady, M., Winters, K. C., Jordan, D., & Solheim, K. (1996). Motivation to change as a predictor of treatment outcome for adolescent substance abusers. *Journal of Child and Adolescent Substance Abuse, 5,* 73–91.

Chilcoat, H. D., & Anthony, J. C. (1996). Impact of parent monitoring on initiation of drug use through late childhood. *Journal of the American Academy of Child and Adolescent Psychiatry, 35,* 91–100.

Christiansen, B. A., Smith, G. T., Roehling, P. V., & Goldman, M. S. (1989). Using alcohol expectancies to predict adolescent drinking behavior after one year. *Journal of Consulting and Clinical Psychology, 57*(1), 93–99.

Chung, T., & Martin, C. S. (2001). Classification and course of alcohol problems among adolescents in addictions treatment programs. *Alcoholism: Clinical and Experimental Research, 25,* 1734–1742.

Chung, T., & Martin, C. S. (2005). What were they thinking?: Adolescents' interpretations of DSM-IV alcohol dependence symptom queries and implications for diagnostic validity. *Drug and Alcohol Dependence, 80,* 191–200.

Chung, T., & Martin, C. S. (2011). Adolescent substance use and substance use disorders: Prevalence and clinical course. In Y. Kaminer & K. C. Winters (Eds.), *Clinical manual of adolescent substance abuse treatment* (pp. 1–23). Washington, DC: American Psychiatric Association.

Chung, T., Smith, G. T., Donovan, J. E., Windle, M., Faden, V. B., Chen, C. M., et al. (2012). Drinking frequency as a brief screen for adolescent alcohol problems. *Pediatrics, 129,* 1–8.

Clark, D. B., & Bukstein, O. G. (1998). Psychopathology in adolescent alcohol abuse and dependence. *Alcohol Health and Research World, 22,* 117–121.

Clark, D. B., Thatcher, D. L., & Maisto, S. A. (2005). Supervisory neglect and adolescent alcohol use disorders: Effects on AUD onset and treatment outcome. *Addictive Behaviors, 30,* 1737–1750.

Clark, D. B., & Winters, K. C. (2002). Measuring risks and outcomes in substance use disorders prevention research. *Journal of Consulting and Clinical Psychology, 70,* 1207–1223.

Collado, A., Felton, J. W., MacPherson, L., & Lejuez, C. W. (2014). Longitudinal trajectories of sensation seeking, risk taking propensity, and impulsivity across early to middle adolescence. *Addictive Behaviors, 39,* 1580–1588.

Cooper, M. L. (1994). Motivations for alcohol use among adolescents: Development and validation of a four-factor model. *Psychological Assessment, 6,* 117–128.

Costello, E. J., Erkanli, A., Federman, E., & Angold, A. (1999). Development of psychiatric comorbidity with substance abuse in adolescents: Effects of timing and sex. *Journal of Clinical Child Psychology, 28,* 298–311.

Dahl, R. E. (2004). Adolescent brain development: A period of vulnerabilities and opportunities. Keynote address. *Annals of the New York Academy of Sciences, 1021,* 1–22.

D'Amico, E. J., & McCarthy, D. M. (2006). Escalation and initiation of younger adolescents' substance use: The impact of perceived peer use. *Journal of Adolescent Health, 39,* 481–487.

Davis, L. J., Hoffmann, N. G., Morse, R. M., & Luehr, J. G. (1992). Substance Use Disorder Diagnostic Schedule (SUDDS): The equivalence and validity of a computer-administered and interviewer-administered format. *Alcoholism: Clinical and Experimental Research, 16,* 250–254.

Deas, D. (2006). Adolescent substance abuse and psychiatric comorbidities. *Journal of Clinical Psychiatry, 67*(Suppl. 7), 18–23.

Dennis, M. L., Chan, Y.-F., & Funk, R. R. (2006). Development and validation of the GAIN Short Screener (GAIN-SS) for psychopathology and crime/violence among adolescents and adults. *American Journal on Addictions, 15,* S80–S91.

Dennis, M. L., Titus, J. C., White, M. K., Unsicker, J. I., & Hodgkins, D. (2002). *Global Appraisal of Individual Needs (GAIN): Administration guide for the GAIN and related measures.* Bloomington, IL: Chestnut Health Systems.

Dillon, F., Turner, C., Robbins, M., & Szapocznik, J. (2005). Concordance among biological interview and self-report measures of drug use among African American and Hispanic adolescents referred for drug abuse treatment. *Psychology of Addictive Medicine, 19,* 404–413.

Dishion, T. J., Capaldi, D., Spracklen, K. M., & Fuzhong, L. (1995). Peer ecology and male adolescent drug use. *Development and Psychopathology, 7,* 803–824.

Donovan, J. E. (2004). Adolescent alcohol initiation: A review of psychosocial risk factors. *Journal of Adolescent Health, 35,* 529.e7–529.e18.

Elkins, I. J., McGue, M., & Iacono, W. G. (2007). Prospective effects of ADHD, conduct disorder, and sex on adolescent substance use and abuse. *Archives of General Psychiatry, 64,* 1145–1152.

Farrell, A. D., & Danish, S. J. (1993). Peer drug associations and emotional restraint: Causes or consequences of adolescents' drug use? *Journal of Consulting and Clinical Psychology, 61,* 327–334.

Festinger, L. (1957). *A theory of cognitive dissonance.* Stanford, CA: Stanford University Press.

Fisher, P., Shaffer, D., Piacentini, J. C., Lapkin, J., Kafantaris, V., Leonard, H., et al. (1993). Sensitivity of the Diagnostic Interview Schedule for Children, 2nd edition (DISC-2.1) for specific diagnoses of children and adolescents. *Journal of the American Academy of Child and Adolescent Psychiatry, 32,* 666–673.

Gardner, M., & Steinberg, L. (2005). Peer influence on risk taking, risk preference, and risky decision making in adolescence and adulthood: An experimental study. *Developmental Psychology, 41,* 625–635.

Grella, C. E., Hser, Y. I., Joshi, V., & Rounds-Bryant, J. (2001). Drug treatment outcomes for adolescents with comorbid mental and substance use disorders. *Journal of Nervous and Mental Disease, 189,* 384–392.

Harris, S. K., & Knight, J. R. (2014). Putting the screen in screening: Technology-based alcohol screening and brief interventions in medical settings. *Alcohol Research: Current Reviews, 36,* 63–79.

Henly, G. A., & Winters, K. C. (1988). Development of problem severity scales for the assessment of adolescent alcohol and drug abuse. *International Journal of the Addictions, 23,* 65–85.

Hingson, R., & Compton, W. M. (2014). Screening and brief intervention and referral to treatment for drug use in primary care: Back to the drawing board. *JAMA, 312,* 488–489.

Hoffmann, N. G., & Harrison, P. A. (1989). *Substance Use Disorders Diagnostic Schedule* (SUDDS). St. Paul, MN: New Standards.

Institute for Behavioral Health. (2016). *Internet parenting advice for preventing adolescent substance use.* Rockville, MD: Author.

Jainchill, N., Bhattacharya, G., & Yagelka, J. (1995). Therapeutic communities for adolescents. In E. Rahdert & D. Czechowicz (Eds.), *Adolescent drug abuse: Clinical assessment and therapeutic interventions* (Research monograph series No. 156; pp. 190–217). Rockville, MD: National Institute on Drug Abuse.

Janis, I. L., & Mann, L. (1977). *Decision making: A psychological analysis of conflict, choice and committment.* New York: Free Press.

Kaminer, Y., Bukstein, O., & Tarter, R. E. (1991). The Teen-Addiction Severity Index: Rationale and reliability. *International Journal of Addictions, 26,* 219–226.

Kelly, S. M., Gryczynski, J., Mitchell, S. G., Kirk, A., O'Grady, K. E., & Schwartz, R. P. (2014). Validity of brief screening instrument for adolescent tobacco, alcohol, and drug use. *Pediatrics, 133,* 819–826.

Khan, M. R., Berger, A. T., Wells, B. E., & Cleland, C. M. (2012). Longitudinal associations between adolescent alcohol use and adulthood sexual risk behavior and sexually transmitted infection in the United States: Assessment of differences by race. *American Journal of Public Health, 102,* 867–876.

Knight, J. R., Sherritt, L., Shrier, L. A., Harris, S. K., & Chang, G. (2002). Validity of the CRAFFT substance abuse screening test among adolescent clinic patients. *Archives of Pediatrics and Adolescent Medicine, 156,* 607–614.

LaBrie, J. W., & Cail, J. (2011). The moderating effect of parental contact on the influence of perceived peer norms on drinking during the transition to college. *Journal of College Student Development, 52,* 610–621.

Lee, C. M., Neighbors, C., Hendershot, C. S., & Grossband, J. R. (2009). Development and preliminary validation of a comprehensive marijuana motives questionnaire. *Journal of Studies on Alcohol and Drugs, 70,* 279–287.

Lee, S. S., Humphreys, K. L., Flory, K., Liu, R., & Glass, K. (2011). Prospective association of childhood attention-deficit/hyperactivity disorder (ADHD) and substance use and abuse/dependence: A meta-analytic review. *Clinical Psychology Review 31*, 328–341.

Leigh, B. C. (1989). In search of the Seven Dwarves: Issues of measurement and meaning in alcohol expectancy research. *Psychological Bulletin, 105*, 361–373.

Levy, S. J., & Kokotailo, P. K. (2011). Substance use screening, brief intervention, and referral to treatment for pediatricians. *Pediatrics, 128*, e1330–e1340.

Levy, S., & Shrier, L. (2014). *Adolescent SBIRT toolkit for providers*. Boston: Boston Children's Hospital.

Lopez, J. S., Martínez, J. M., Martín, A., Martín, J. M., Martín, M. J., & Scandroglio, B. (2001). An exploratory multivariate approach to drug consumption patterns in young people based on primary socialization theory. *Substance Use and Misuse, 36*, 1611–1649.

Lynskey, M. T., & Fergusson, D. M. (1995). Childhood conduct problems and attention deficit behaviors and adolescent alcohol, tobacco and illicit drug use. *Journal of Abnormal Child Psychology, 23*, 281–302.

Martin, C. S., Chung, T., Kirisci, L., & Langenbucher, J. W. (2006). Item response theory analysis of diagnostic criteria for alcohol and cannabis use disorders in adolescents: Implications for DSM-V. *Journal of Abnormal Psychology, 115*, 807–814.

Martin, C. S., Chung, T., & Langenbucher, J. W. (2008). How should we revise diagnostic criteria for substance use disorders in the DSM-V? *Journal of Abnormal Psychology, 117*, 561–575.

Martin, C. S., Lynch, K. G., Pollock, N. K., & Clark, D. B. (2000). Gender differences and similarities in the personality correlates of adolescent alcohol problems. *Psychology of Addictive Behaviors, 14*, 121–133.

Martin, G. W., Wilkinson, D. A., & Poulos, C. X. (1995). The Drug Avoidance Self-Efficacy Scale. *Journal of Substance Abuse, 7*, 151–163.

McGue, M. (1999). Behavioral genetic models of alcoholism and drinking. In K. E. Leonard & H. T. Blane (Eds.), *Psychological theories of drinking and alcoholism* (2nd ed., pp. 372–421). New York: Guilford Press.

Metzger, D. S., Kushner, H., & McLellan, A. T. (1991). *Adolescent Problem Severity Index: Administration manual*. Philadelphia: Biomedical Computer Research Institute.

Meyers, K. (1991). *Comprehensive Addiction Severity Index for Adolescents*. Philadelphia: University of Pennsylvania.

Miech, R. A., Johnston, L. D., O'Malley, P. M., Bachman, J. G., & Schulenberg, J. E. (2015). *Monitoring the Future national survey results on drug use, 1975–2014: Vol. I. Secondary school students*. Ann Arbor: Institute for Social Research, University of Michigan.

Migneault, J. P., Pallonen, U. E., & Velicer, W. F. (1997). Decisional balance and stage of change for adolescent drinking. *Addictive Behaviors, 22*(3), 339–351.

Miller, W. R., & Rollnick, S. (2004). Talking oneself into change: Motivational interviewing, stages of change, and therapeutic process. *Journal of Cognitive Psychotherapy, 18*, 299–308.

Miller, W. R., & Rollnick, S. (2012). *Motivational interviewing: Helping people change* (3rd ed.). New York: Guilford Press.

Mirza, K. A. H., & Bukstein, O. (2011). Attention deficit-disruptive behavior disorders and substance use disorders in adolescents. In Y. Kaminer and K. C. Winters

(Eds.), *Clinical manual of adolescent substance abuse treatment* (pp. 283–305). Washington, DC: American Psychiatric Publishing.

Monahan, J., Hoge, S. K., Lidz, C., Roth, L. H., Bennett, N., Gardner, W., et al. (1995). Coercion and commitment: Understanding involuntary mental hospital admission. *International Journal of Law and Psychiatry, 18*, 249–263.

Muris, P. (2001). A brief questionnaire for measuring self-efficacy in youths. *Journal of Psychopathology and Behavioral Assessment, 23*, 145–149.

Nestler, E. J., & Landsman, D. (2001). Learning about addiction from the genome. *Nature, 409*, 834–835.

Newman, J. C., Des Jarlais, D. C., Turner, C. F., Gribble, J., Cooley, P., & Paone, D. (2002). The differential effects of face-to-face and computer interview modes. *American Journal of Public Health, 92*, 294–297.

Nisbett, R. E., & Ross, L. (1980). *Human inference: Strategies and shortcomings of social judgment.* Englewood Cliffs, NJ: Prentice Hall.

O'Neil, K. A., Conner, B. T., & Kendall, P. C. (2011). Internalizing disorders and substance use disorders in youth: Comorbidity, risk, temporal order, and implications for intervention. *Clinical Psychology Review, 31*, 104–112.

Patterson, G. R., Forgatch, M. S., Yoerger, K. L., & Stoolmiller, M. (1998). Variables that initiate and maintain an early-onset trajectory for juvenile offending. *Development and Psychopathology, 10*, 531–548.

Petraitis, J., Flay, B. R., & Miller, T. Q. (1995). Reviewing theories of adolescent substance abuse: Organizing pieces in the puzzle. *Psychological Bulletin, 117*, 67–86.

Pisetsky, E. M., Chao, Y., Dierker, L. C., May, A. M., & Striegel-Moore, R. H. (2008). Disordered eating and substance use in high school students: Results from the youth risk behavior surveillance system. *International Journal of Eating Disorders, 41*, 464–470.

Prochaska, J. O., DiClemente, C. C., & Norcross, J. C. (1992). In search of how people change: Applications to addictive behaviors. *American Psychologist, 47*, 1102–1114.

Prochaska, J. O., Velicer, W. F., Rossi, J. S., Goldstein, M. G., Marcus, B. H., Rakowski, W., et al. (1994). Stages of change and decisional balance for 12 problem behaviors. *Health Psychology, 13*, 39–46.

Ramirez, R., Hinman, A., Sterling, S., Weisner, C., & Campbell, C. (2012). Peer influences on adolescent alcohol and other drug use outcomes. *Journal of Nursing Scholarship, 44*, 36–44.

Riggs, P. D., & Davies, R. (2002). A clinical approach to treatment of depression in adolescents with substance use disorders and conduct disorder. *Journal of the American Academy of Child and Adolescent Psychiatry, 41*, 1253–1255.

Roberts, R. E., Solovitz, B. L., Chen, Y. W., & Casat, C. (1996). Retest stability of DSM-III-R diagnoses among adolescents using the Diagnostic Interview Schedule for Children (DISC-2.1C). *Journal of Abnormal Child Psychology, 24*, 349–362.

Rohde, P., Lewinsohn, P. M., & Seeley, J. R. (1991). Comorbidity of unipolar depression: II. Comorbidity with other mental disorders in adolescents and adults. *Journal of Abnormal Psychology, 100*, 214–222.

Shaffer, D., Fisher, P., Dulcan, M. K., Davies, M., Piacentini, J., Schwab-Stone, M. E., et al. (1996). The NIMH Diagnostic Interview Schedule for Children Version 2.3 (DISC-2.3): Description, acceptability, prevalence rates, and performance in the MECA study. *Journal of the American Academy of Child and Adolescent Psychiatry, 35*, 865–877.

Shaffer, H. J., & Simoneau, G. (2001). Reducing resistance and denial by exercising ambivalence during the treatment of addiction. *Journal of Substance Abuse Treatment, 20,* 99–105.

Shoham, V., & Insel, T. R. (2011). Rebooting for whom?: Portfolios, technology, and personalized intervention. *Perspectives on Psychological Science, 6,* 478–482.

Shrier, L. A., Rhoads, A., Burke, P., Walls, C., & Blood, E. A. (2014). Real-time, contextual intervention using mobile technology to reduce marijuana use among youth: A pilot study. *Addictive Behaviors, 39,* 173–180.

Simons, J., Correia, C. J., Carey, K. B., & Borsari, B. E. (1998). Validating a five-factor Marijuana Motives Measure: Relations with use, problems, and alcohol motives. *Journal of Counseling Psychology, 45,* 265–273.

Simons, R. L., & Robertson, J. F. (1989). The impact of parenting factors, deviant peers, and coping style upon adolescent drug use. *Family Relations, 38,* 273–281.

Simons-Morton, B., & Farhat, T. (2010). Recent findings on peer group influences on adolescent substance use. *Journal of Primary Prevention, 31,* 191–208.

Smith, G. T., Goldman, M. S., Greenbaum, P. E., & Christiansen, B. A. (1995). Expectancy for social facilitation from drinking: The divergent paths of high-expectancy and low-expectancy adolescents. *Journal of Abnormal Psychology, 104,* 32.

Steinberg, L. (2007). Risk taking in adolescence: New perspectives from brain and behavioral science. *Current Directions in Psychological Science, 16,* 55–59.

Steinberg, L., Fletcher, A., & Darling, N. (1994). Parental monitoring and peer influences on adolescent substance use. *Pediatrics, 93*(6), 1060–1064.

Thomas, D. W. (1990). *Substance abuse screening protocol for the juvenile courts.* Pittsburgh: National Center for Juvenile Justice.

Volkow, N. D., Baler, R. D., Compton, W. M., & Weiss, S. R. (2014). Adverse health effects of marijuana use. *New England Journal of Medicine, 370,* 2219–2227.

Wanberg, K. W. (2006). *Adolescent Self Assessment Profile–II.* Arvada, CO: Center for Alcohol/Drug Abuse Research and Evaluation.

Weinstein, N. D., & Klein, W. M. (1995). Resistance of personal risk perceptions to debiasing interventions. *Health Psychology, 14,* 132–140.

Wilens, T. E., Biederman, J., Abrantes, A. M., & Spencer, T. J. (1997). Clinical characteristics of psychiatrically referred adolescent outpatients with substance use disorder. *Journal of the American Academy of Child and Adolescent Psychiatry, 36,* 941–947.

Winters, K. C. (1992). Development of an adolescent alcohol and other drug abuse screening scale: Personal Experience Screening Questionnaire. *Addictive Behaviors, 17,* 479–490.

Winters, K. C. (2013). Advances in the science of adolescent drug involvement: Implications for assessment and diagnosis. *Current Opinion in Psychiatry, 26,* 318–324.

Winters, K. C., & Arria, A. M. (2011). Adolescent brain development and drugs. *The Prevention Researcher, 18,* 21–24.

Winters, K. C., Fahnhorst, T., Botzet, A., Stinchfield, R., & Nicholson, A. (2017). Assessing adolescent alcohol and other drug abuse. In R. Zucker & S. Brown (Eds.), *The Oxford handbook of adolescent substance abuse.* New York: Oxford University Press.

Winters, K. C., & Henly, G. A. (1989). *Personal Experience Inventory (PEI) Test and manual.* Los Angeles: Western Psychological Services.

Winters, K. C., & Henly, G. A. (1993). *Adolescent Diagnostic Interview Schedule and manual.* Los Angeles: Western Psychological Services.

Winters, K. C., Martin, C. S., & Chung, T. (2011). Commentary on O'Brien: Substance use disorders in DSM-5 when applied to adolescents. *Addiction, 106,* 882–884.

Winters, K. C., Stinchfield, R. D., Fulkerson, J., & Henly, G. A. (1993). Measuring alcohol and cannabis use disorders in an adolescent clinical sample. *Psychology of Addictive Disorders, 7,* 185–196.

Winters, K. C., Tanner-Smith, E., Bresani, E., & Meyers, K. (2014). Current advances in the treatment of adolescent substance use. *Adolescent Health, Medicine and Therapeutics, 5,* 199–210.

Zucker, R. A., Donovan, J. E., Masten, A. S., Mattson, M. M., & Moss, H. B. (2008). Early developmental processes and the continuity of risks for underage drinking and problem drinking. *Pediatrics, 121,* S252–S272.

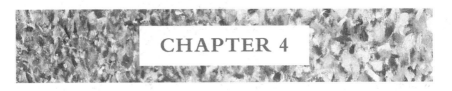

CHAPTER 4

Transactions among Personality and Psychosocial Learning Risk Factors for Adolescent Addictive Behavior

The Acquired Preparedness Model of Risk

Heather A. Davis, Elizabeth N. Riley,
and Gregory T. Smith

*A*dolescent addictive behavior represents, in part, the results of a complex interplay among genetic factors, personality traits, and psychosocial learning processes. In this chapter, we present our model describing one set of transactions among genetic-based personality traits and psychosocial learning that increase risk for adolescent engagement in addictive behaviors. Our model integrates dispositional and learning-based risk factors to allow for a more comprehensive account of the unfolding of the risk process for addictive behaviors in adolescents.

In the 15 years since our model, known as the acquired preparedness (AP) model, was presented in Smith and Anderson (2001), it has undergone a great deal of empirical scrutiny, first with cross-sectional studies and more recently using longitudinal designs. As we describe below, the core structure of the model relating personality to psychosocial learning has received consistent support. It is also true that advances in the basic science of personality research have led to substantive changes in the personality traits thought to be most central to the AP process. A visual depiction of the model as it relates to drinking risk is provided in Figure 4.1.

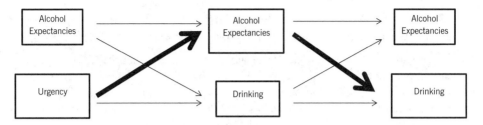

FIGURE 4.1. The AP model of risk for drinking. This model, applied to drinking behavior, holds that the personality trait urgency shapes high-risk psychosocial learning, which in turn leads to increased drinking. The implication of this model is that the influence of personality traits on subsequent drinking behavior should be mediated by learning. Thus, a significant portion of the influence of traits on drinking behavior should be through learning, as represented by the sequence of paths from urgency to expectancies and from expectancies to drinking. Controlling for prior levels of learned alcohol expectancies and drinking is a key component of modeling this effect. Therefore, this depiction of the model includes prior alcohol expectancies and prior drinking, which both lead to increased drinking and increased alcohol expectancies.

To introduce the model, we begin by providing an overview of the validity of both the personality and learning-based risk factors that are integrated into the AP model of risk. First, we briefly review advances in personality research and how they have informed our understanding of personality-based risk. Second, we describe the learning component of our theory. Third, we present the AP model by describing how high-risk personality traits and psychosocial learning combine to increase risk. In this section, we review the current version of the AP model and the empirical evidence supporting it. Fourth, we discuss treatment considerations from this proposed theoretical framework. Finally, we discuss the model in terms of sociocultural context.

INDIVIDUAL DIFFERENCES IN PERSONALITY AND ADDICTIVE BEHAVIOR RISK: PERSONALITY UNDERPINNINGS TO IMPULSIVE BEHAVIOR

Over time, it has become increasingly clear to personality researchers that numerous different personality processes have been included under the broad "impulsivity" umbrella. Indeed, Depue and Collins (1999) noted that "impulsivity comprises a heterogeneous cluster of lower-order traits that includes terms such as impulsivity, sensation seeking, risk-taking, novelty seeking, boldness, adventuresomeness, boredom susceptibility, unreliability, and unorderliness" (p. 495). This recognition led to efforts to develop measures of the multiple different traits that can contribute to impulsive behavior.

Substantive Advances in Identifying the Personality Dimensions That Contribute to Impulsive Behavior

Several authors have investigated the wide variety of personality traits that predict impulsive behavior (Evenden, 1999; Eysenck & Eysenck, 1977; Whiteside & Lynam, 2001). The approach taken by Whiteside and Lynam (2001) may be particularly useful, because it has provided theoretically clear results and is easily integrated with comprehensive models of personality. They gathered 10 commonly used personality measures involving impulsivity and conducted a factor analysis of the items of those measures, which led to the identification of four dimensions underlying the set of measures: sensation seeking (the tendency to seek out novel and thrilling experiences), lack of planning (the tendency to act without thinking), lack of perseverance (the inability to remain focused on a task), and urgency (the tendency to act rashly in response to distress, which is now referred to as negative urgency).

These four traits map onto different factors of the five-factor model (FFM) of personality, which is thought to be a comprehensive account of the major domains of personality functioning (Costa & McCrae, 1992). The FFM is comprised of five higher-order factors or domains (i.e., neuroticism, extraversion, openness to experience, agreeableness, and conscientiousness), each containing six subfactors, or facets (e.g., warmth, gregariousness, assertiveness, activity, excitement seeking, and positive emotion on the extraversion domain). Each of the four impulsigenic traits load onto the FFM (measured using the NEO Personality Inventory—Revised [NEO PI-R]; Costa & McCrae, 1992), with lack of planning reflecting low scores on the deliberation facet of conscientiousness, lack of perseverance reflecting low scores on the self-discipline facet of conscientiousness, sensation seeking reflecting high scores on the excitement-seeking facet of extraversion, and negative urgency reflecting high scores on the impulsiveness facet of neuroticism, as well as low conscientiousness and low agreeableness (Cyders & Smith, 2008; Seibert, Miller, Pryor, Reidy, & Zeichner, 2010; Whiteside & Lynam, 2001).

Whiteside and Lynam (2001) found intercorrelations among the four scales ranging from –.14 (between sensation seeking and lack of perseverance) through .00 (between sensation seeking and lack of planning) to a high of .45 (between lack of perseverance and lack of planning). Thus, the four scales appear to reflect different personality dimensions related to impulsive behavior. The primary advantage of this work is that it identified a core set of separate dimensions underlying the body of existing impulsivity measures, and showed how those dimensions fit into a more comprehensive model of personality.

Although these four dimensions summarized the content of existing impulsivity measures, they did not include impulsive behavior when experiencing intensely positive emotional states. Although positive affect is of course valuable in many ways (Isen, Niedenthal, & Cantor, 1992; Phillips, MacLean,

& Allen, 2002), strong positive affect can also (1) interfere with orientation toward the pursuit of one's long-term goals, (2) increase distractibility, (3) increase optimism about the positive outcomes of a situation (Dreisbach & Goschke, 2004), (4) lead to less discriminative use of information (Forgas, 1992), and (5) lead to poorer decision making (Slovic, Finucane, Peters, & MacGregor, 2004). For example, a group of adolescents who attend a high school football game in which their team wins in overtime may experience intense positive affect in response to this event and celebrate by binge drinking after the game. This may lead to poor decisions such as unprotected sex, driving under the influence, or using other substances. In short, intense positive affect can lead to behavior that is often described as impulsive.

The omission of positive emotion-based impulsivity was addressed by Cyders et al. (2007), who provided evidence for a fifth impulsivity-related personality trait. They called it positive urgency, or the tendency to act rashly when experiencing extremely positive emotion, and found that their measure of positive urgency was unidimensional, distinct from other impulsigenic personality constructs, and explained variance in risky behavior not explained by those other constructs.

Cyders and Smith (2007) provided evidence for the validity of the resulting five factors by conducting a multitrait–multimethod (MTMM) study, using interview and questionnaire measures of the five impulsigenic traits defined by Whiteside and Lynam (2001) and Cyders et al. (2007). They found good evidence for convergent validity for each of the five traits across assessment method, with correlations of the same trait measured with different methods ranging from .56 for lack of perseverance to .74 for sensation seeking. There was also good evidence for discriminant validity between traits within assessment method: Correlations among the five traits using questionnaire assessment ranged from –.06 to .49, with a median correlation of .21. For the interview method, correlations ranged from .01 to .46, with a median correlation of .20. Positive and negative urgency were the most highly correlated traits (.49 and .46, respectively, for the two methods). Lack of planning and lack of perseverance also correlated significantly (.34 by questionnaire and .31 by interview).

Cyders and Smith (2007) also examined the hierarchal structure of the five traits. The best-fitting model identified positive and negative urgency as facets of an overall urgency dimension, lack of planning and lack of perseverance as facets of an overall low conscientiousness dimension, and sensation seeking as a third dimension (see Figure 4.2).

The Importance of the Urgency Traits for Adolescent Addictive Behavior Involvement

An important distinction among the five traits is that positive and negative urgency are affect-based traits, in that they describe a disposition to behave rashly when highly emotional. Neither sensation seeking nor the two low-conscientiousness traits (lack of planning and lack of perseverance) are based on affective arousal. Cyders and Smith (2008) presented a theory of positive and negative urgency and proposed that, because of the affective basis of the traits, they would be particularly important in the risk process for adolescent addictive behavior. Adolescents in particular tend to experience heightened emotionality and are thus predisposed to rash action such as substance use—that is, impulsive actions for adolescents often occur when they are highly emotional. Consistent with this hypothesis, the urgency traits relate cross-sectionally and longitudinally to multiple forms of addictive behavior in children, adolescents, and adults.

Children and Adolescents

Zapolski, Stairs, Settles, Combs, and Smith (2010) and Zapolski and Smith (2013) developed preadolescent measures of the positive and negative urgency traits, demonstrated good convergent and discriminant validity for them when measured by different methods, and showed that they predicted behavior in ways consistent with urgency theory (more urgency, more drinking). An example item for positive urgency is "When I am very happy, I tend to do things that may cause problems in my life." For negative urgency, a sample item is "When I am upset I often act without thinking."

Settles, Zapolski, and Smith (2014) showed that positive urgency (but not negative urgency) measured in fifth grade predicted the onset of, and increases in, drinking behavior over the following 12 months. Pearson, Combs, Zapolski, and Smith (2012) showed that negative urgency (but not positive urgency), also measured in fifth grade, predicted the onset of and increases in the bulimic behaviors of binge eating and purging. Guller, Zapolski, and Smith (2015b) showed that the two urgency traits, again measured in children, predicted future smoking behavior as well.

Late Adolescence and Early Adulthood

In college students, the urgency traits also predict future alcohol use and problems. Problems with alcohol are assessed by asking participants if and how often they have experienced negative outcomes when drinking, such as having blackouts, having trouble with the law because of their drinking, getting into fights with loved ones while drinking, or experiencing hangovers after drinking. Positive urgency prospectively predicted increases in the quantity of alcohol consumed and the resulting negative outcomes experienced by college students (Cyders, Flory, Rainer, & Smith, 2009). Settles, Cyders, and Smith (2010) found that both positive and negative urgency predicted drinking quantity prospectively in first-year college students. In an experimental study, Cyders and colleagues (2010) found that positive urgency significantly

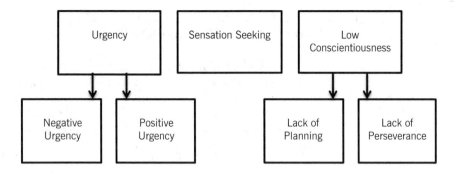

FIGURE 4.2. Relations among the five impulsigenic traits.

predicted negative outcomes on a risk-taking task and increases in beer consumption following a positive mood manipulation. Importantly, in multiple meta-analytic reviews of impulsivity-related traits, negative urgency showed the greatest association with addictive behavior involvement (Berg, Latzman, Bliwise, & Lilienfeld, 2015; Coskunpinar, Dir, & Cyders, 2013; Fischer, Smith, & Cyders, 2008; Stautz & Cooper, 2013).

One important question concerns whether positive and negative urgency play distinct roles. There are reasons to believe they do. Settles et al. (2010) mapped different predictive pathways to problem drinking for the two traits, such that positive urgency predicted increased drinking mediated by expectancies that alcohol provides positive arousing effects, and negative urgency predicted drinking quantity mediated by the motive to drink alcohol to cope with subjective distress. Cyders and Smith (2010) showed that positive urgency prospectively predicts rash acts, such as risky sex, when in a positive mood, while negative urgency prospectively predicts rash acts, such as binge eating, when in a negative mood. Additionally, Cyders et al. (2010) showed that positive urgency, but not negative urgency, predicted increases in beer consumption following a positive mood induction. With respect to disordered eating, negative urgency is predictive and positive urgency is not (Cyders et al., 2007). On the other hand, among young children the two traits correlate more highly than they do in adults (in one case the correlation was as high as .70: Combs, Spillane, Caudill, Stark, & Smith, 2012).

In sum, when considering the role of personality in the impulsive behavior of adolescent addictive behavior involvement, the urgency traits appear to be of particular importance. As we describe below, they play a central role in the AP model of risk. Of course, disposition alone cannot explain risk for substance use behavior. In the following section, we introduce the second significant component of our theory of risk: psychosocial learning as measured by expectancies.

PSYCHOSOCIAL LEARNING AND ADDICTIVE
BEHAVIOR RISK: EXPECTANCIES

One way to measure learning regarding addictive behaviors is to assess expectancies for reinforcement from engaging in such behaviors. Expectancies are thought to represent summaries of one's learning history about the outcomes of one's behavioral choices (Bolles, 1972; Tolman, 1932). There are different expectancy models. In the one we employ, reports of explicit expectancies are understood to provide markers of memory-based associative learning (Goldman, Darkes, & Del Boca, 1999; Goldman, Reich, & Darkes, 2006). For example, high scores on a scale reflecting the expectancy that alcohol facilitates positive social interactions are thought to reflect a strong learned association between drinking and positive social experiences. In an alternative model, explicit expectancies are understood to refer to planned or deliberative behavior (Ajzen & Fishbein, 1980)—part of what contributes to a drinking decision is the thought that drinking allows for a better social experience. Our model assigns less weight to deliberative action and more to learned associations of a behavior (such as drinking) and a reward (such as positive social experience). The association influences the behavior (Bolles, 1972; Tolman, 1932), and one may or may not experience oneself as choosing the behavior explicitly to obtain the expected outcome. Considerable support for this model, and for the explicit measurement of expectancies as markers of learned associations, has accrued over several decades (Bolles, 1972; Goldman, Brown, Christiansen, & Smith, 1991; Goldman et al., 1999; Hohlstein, Smith, & Atlas, 1998; Tolman, 1932).

Expectancies are thus understood to reflect summaries of an individual's psychosocial learning history concerning anticipated reinforcement from behaviors. Expectancy formation appears to occur not just through direct experience with a behavior, but also through observation of, or modeling by, parents, older siblings, teenagers, and the media; this occurs even in children with no prior involvement in the behavior, such as no drinking experience (Dunn & Goldman, 1996; Miller, Smith, & Goldman, 1990). Expectancies formed prior to experience predict the subsequent onset of, and increases in, addictive behaviors (e.g., Guller, Zapolski, & Smith, 2015a; Pearson et al., 2012; Smith, Goldman, Greenbaum, & Christiansen, 1995).

We emphasize five predictions from expectancy theory:

1. Researchers should be able to measure an individual's expectancies reliably and validly.
2. Expectancies for reinforcement from a behavior should predict the onset of the behavior.
3. Expectancies should mediate the influence of early engagement in the behavior on later increases in the behavior.
4. Manipulation of expectancies should shape future behavior.
5. There should be a reciprocal relationship between behavior and

expectancy endorsement—that is, expectancies developed through modeling behaviors should predict subsequent behavior, and the behavior should, in turn, modify a person's expectancies.

We briefly review empirical evidence for these six predictions before considering its relation to the AP model.

Measurement of Expectancies

Numerous measures of alcohol expectancies have been developed, and the content domains covered by them are broadly consistent. We will not review specifics of the different scales, but a consistent finding is that specific expected consequences of drinking can be measured reliably and with stable factor structures (see Brown, Goldman, Inn, & Anderson, 1980; Christiansen, Goldman, & Inn, 1982; Fromme, Stroot, & Kaplan, 1993; Leigh, 1987, for examples). Reviews of the alcohol expectancy concept and its measurement are available (Carter & Goldman, 2008; Goldman & Darkes, 2004; Goldman et al., 2006). We discuss specific alcohol expectancies below.

A measure of expectancies for reinforcement from eating and from dieting/thinness has been developed (Hohlstein et al., 1998) and has proven stable over time and internally consistent. The same is true for measures of expectancies for reinforcement from smoking (e.g., Lewis-Esquerre, Rodrigue, & Kahler, 2005).

Expectancies Predict Onset of Addictive Behavior

Longitudinal studies have consistently documented that alcohol expectancies held by nondrinking youth predict the subsequent onset of drinking. This finding has been observed among adolescents (Christiansen, Smith, Roeling, & Goldman, 1989; Smith et al., 1995) as well as in children as young as fifth and sixth grade (Goldberg, Halpern-Felsher, & Millstein, 2002; Settles et al., 2014).

Researchers have also examined the influence of alcohol expectancies on future levels of drinking behavior, controlling statistically for early levels of use. Many authors have found support for the hypothesis that, when controlling for prior levels of use, alcohol expectancies predict increases in drinking behavior (Christiansen et al., 1989; Goldberg et al., 2002; Ouellette, Gerrard, Gibbons, & Reis-Bergan, 1999; Settles et al., 2010, 2014; Smith et al., 1995). Each of these studies concerned preadolescents or adolescents. For the prediction of drinking onset, the expectancy that appears to be most predictive is the expectancy that drinking enhances social experience.

With respect to disordered eating, youth expectancies regarding eating and dieting/thinness predict the subsequent onset of binge eating and purging (Pearson et al., 2012), as well as trajectories of eating disorder symptom change across adolescence (Pearson & Smith, 2015). With respect to smoking, youth expectancies for reinforcement from smoking predict subsequent smoking onset (Guller et al., 2015a).

Expectancies Mediate Learning Influences on Adolescent Addictive Behavior

The concept of mediation refers to a causal sequence of events. Using drinking as an example, the claim that expectancies for reinforcement from drinking mediate the influence of family drinking on adolescent drinking involves the claims that (1) family drinking predicts and influences adolescent alcohol expectancies, (2) adolescent alcohol expectancies predict and influence adolescent drinking, and (3) family drinking predicts and influences adolescent drinking at least in part through its influence on adolescent alcohol expectancies. It is of course the case that correlational data, even using longitudinal designs, do not provide definitive tests of causal hypotheses. Instead, researchers can test whether the pattern of predictive influences is consistent with a causal model. To evaluate how compelling a correlational test is of a mediation hypothesis, one considers whether the design allows for prospective prediction over time or, alternatively, whether there are other good reasons to trust the temporal sequencing of the variables in the model.

To assess whether alcohol expectancies mediate the influence of early learning on adolescent drinking, researchers often assess variables that seem to indicate positive learning about the effects of alcohol. Variables that are thought to represent the probability of positive learning about alcohol include those that reflect familial attitudes and behaviors regarding alcohol use, such as frequency of parental alcohol consumption and parents' attitudes toward adult drinking. Other variables that may reflect modeling alcohol consumption in the pursuit of reinforcement include history of alcoholism in the family and even parents' experience of life problems associated with drinking (Smith, 1994). One can then test whether the predictive influence of such variables on adolescent drinking appears to be mediated by expectancies for reinforcement from drinking.

A few studies have provided evidence consistent with the hypothesis that alcohol expectancies mediate environmental/learning influences on adolescent drinking behavior. Smith (1994) provided a partially longitudinal test, by measuring family drinking (positive parental attitudes, parental drinking, positive family history of alcoholism) and adolescent alcohol expectancies at one wave of a longitudinal study and predicting drinking behavior 1 year later. Family drinking did predict adolescent drinking and its predictive influence was partially explained by adolescent alcohol expectancies as a putative mediator. Data from three cross-sectional designs are consistent with this conclusion: adolescent alcohol expectancies appear to mediate (1) the predictive influence of intrinsic religiosity on alcohol consumption (Galen & Rogers, 2004), (2) the predictive influence of a positive family history of alcoholism and behavioral undercontrol on late adolescent alcohol involvement (Sher, Walitzer, Wood, &

Brent, 1991), and (3) the predictive influence of masculine norms on drinking behavior (Iwamoto, Corbin, Lejuez, & MacPherson, 2014).

Similar findings have accrued with respect to disordered eating. Mac-Brayer, Smith, McCarthy, Demos, and Simmons (2001) found that the predictive influence of family of origin food-related experiences on bulimic symptomatology was mediated by expectancies for reinforcement from eating and from dieting/thinness.

Experimental Manipulation of Expectancies Reduces Addictive Behavior

The bulk of the experimental work has been done with alcohol consumption. Although longitudinal studies documenting alcohol expectancies' prediction of subsequent adolescent drinking are quite important, to provide stronger evidence that expectancies cause drinking behavior it is valuable to conduct controlled experiments. Darkes and Goldman (1993) studied a sample of heavy-drinking college students to test whether a manipulation of an individual's alcohol expectancies would promote actual change in drinking behavior. They found that (1) alcohol expectancies could indeed be manipulated, (2) decreases in the measured expectancies due to the manipulation paralleled decreases in drinking behavior over a 2-week time frame, and (3) these decreases in expectancies had the most profound impact on reducing drinking behavior in the heaviest (problem) drinkers (Darkes & Goldman, 1993).

The finding that experimental manipulation of alcohol expectancies was associated with reductions in drinking behavior provides strong evidence in support of alcohol expectancy theory. Together with basic science findings demonstrating expectancy effects on behavior dating back to Tolman (1932) and the existing, large body of longitudinal evidence that alcohol expectancies predict subsequent drinking (Christiansen et al., 1989; Goldberg et al., 2002; Ouellette et al., 1999; Settles et al., 2010, 2014; Smith et al., 1995), there is good reason to believe that expectancies are a critical mechanism that affects drinking behavior. Expected positive consequences from alcohol appear to be a central component of the alcohol use risk process in adolescents such that manipulations of the expectancies (reducing the positive perceived consequences of drinking) lead to reduced levels of alcohol consumption.

One similar study has been done with respect to eating disorders. Annus, Smith, and Masters (2008) experimentally reduced thinness and dieting expectancies, and found reductions in the cognitive symptoms of disordered eating. Further work in this area is necessary.

The Positive Feedback Loop of Reciprocal Influence between Expectancies and Behavior

Because expectancies are understood to represent summaries of learning histories, ongoing experience should be expected to influence subsequent expectancies. Because of the frequently replicated finding that adolescent alcohol expectancies predict subsequent drinking onset and drinking behavior, the possibility that drinking behavior itself shapes subsequent expectancies raises the possibility of a reciprocal relationship between alcohol expectancies and drinking behavior. If this is true, an important question is whether drinking experience serves a corrective function, reducing expectations for reinforcement from drinking, or instead further enhances such expectations.

Research on two longitudinal samples of adolescents has shown that (1) drinking behavior does predict subsequent expectancies, controlling for prior expectancies; and (2) that prediction is positive, such that drinking experience leads to further increases in expectancies for reinforcement from drinking (Settles et al., 2014; Smith et al., 1995). Thus, there is replicated evidence for a reciprocal relationship, in the form of a positive feedback loop, between alcohol expectancies and adolescent drinking behavior. Expected reinforcement from drinking predicts both the onset of and increases in drinking behavior, which predicts subsequent increases in positive expectancies of drinking, which in turn predict further increases in drinking. In both studies, the key expectancy predicted by prior drinking and predictive of future drinking was again the expectancy that drinking enhances social experience. Importantly, there was no evidence of a "corrective" feedback process in which drinking experiences served to reduce alcohol expectancies. This set of findings further highlights the risk associated with high levels of positive alcohol expectancies in youth.

Recently, researchers have found a similar process with respect to early adolescent smoking. Guller et al. (2015a) found reciprocal prediction between smoking expectancies and smoking behavior among early adolescents. Importantly, they also found a positive feedback loop and no evidence of a corrective process.

INTEGRATING PERSONALITY AND PSYCHOSOCIAL LEARNING: THE AP MODEL

The AP model is an extension of person–environment transaction theory (Caspi & Moffitt, 1993; Caspi & Roberts, 2001), which is an attempt to characterize the process by which personality traits combine with life events to influence behavior. One form of person–environment transaction is referred to as a reactive person–environment transaction. Two individuals exposed to the same environmental event will have different reactions to the event, due to differences in their personalities. For example, an event such as turbulence on an airplane may be perceived as highly stressful for a person high in neuroticism but as inconsequential to a person who is not.

To the degree that humans engage in reactive transactions, an objectively common learning event may not be experienced in the same way by different people (Hartup & Van Lieshout, 1995). It follows that two individuals may learn different things from the same event. In this way, their different personalities may lead them toward different behavioral choices, despite their common experience. The concept that personality differences can lead to differences in psychosocial learning experience is the AP extension of person–environment transaction theory.

The term *acquired preparedness* reflects the concept that different individuals are differentially prepared to acquire certain learning experiences as a function of their personalities. An analogue longitudinal laboratory study demonstrated that this process could occur (Smith, Williams, Cyders, & Kelley, 2006). College business students learned about stock market investing and engaged in mock investments each week for several weeks. The study was done online and, unbeknownst to the participants, each person experienced the same outcomes from his or her investments. Despite having the same outcomes, participants formed different expectancies for future anticipated outcomes from stock investing. The different expectancies they formed could be predicted by prior differences in their personalities.

In clinical field research, the AP model has been shown to be applicable to risk for multiple forms of addictive behavior. There have been a number of cross-sectional studies testing the AP model, but in this chapter we focus on longitudinal tests. Settles et al. (2010) reported on the first longitudinal test of the AP model applied to drinking behavior. They found two AP pathways in their three-wave study of first-year college students. The trait of positive urgency predicted increased expectancies for positive arousing effects of alcohol over time, and in turn this expectancy predicted subsequent increases in drinking quantity. The trait of negative urgency predicted increases in the motive to drink to cope with distress, which in part reflects the expectancy that drinking does help one manage distress, and the motive in turn predicted subsequent increases in drinking quantity. Also with college students, expectancies for reinforcement from drinking mediated the predictive influence of trait disinhibition (measured as sensation seeking, novelty seeking, and lack of planning) on drinking behavior over a 4-year period (Corbin, Iwamoto, & Fromme, 2011) and the predictive influence of a trait reflecting the inclination to act in pursuit of a reward (the behavioral activation system) on drinking over a 3-year period (Wardell, Read, Colder, & Merrill, 2012). These latter two findings suggest that the AP process is likely to operate for multiple impulsivity-related personality traits, not just for the urgency traits.

The AP model of drinking risk has also been supported in children making the transition from childhood to early adolescence: Settles et al. (2014) found that fifth-graders' positive urgency scores predicted increased drinking frequency at the end of sixth grade, and the prediction was mediated by increases in expectancies for positive social effects of drinking measured at the beginning of sixth grade. In addition, laboratory research has provided evidence that personality does appear to bias the learning process, as proposed by the AP model (Scott & Corbin, 2014). Scott and Corbin (2014) used a between-subjects design in which young adult drinkers received alcohol or a placebo and were asked about their experience. They found that regardless of whether they received alcohol or a placebo, participants high in the personality trait of sensation seeking reported a more positive experience.

With respect to disordered eating, Pearson et al. (2012) found that expectancies that eating helps one manage negative affect mediated the predictive influence of negative urgency on subsequent binge-eating behavior in youth making the transition to middle school. With respect to tobacco smoking, Doran and colleagues (2013) found that expectancies for negative reinforcement from smoking mediated the predictive influence of negative urgency on smoking initiation, and positive reinforcement expectancies mediated the predictive influence of sensation seeking on smoking initiation. Thus, the AP process appears to operate across behaviors; for each behavior studied to date, expectancies specific to that behavior mediate the influence of personality on engagement in the behavior.

One important benefit of the AP model is that, by clarifying the nature of the risk process, it can highlight targets for possible intervention. Both prevention and treatment models may benefit from addressing high-risk personality traits and learned expectancies.

TREATMENT IMPLICATIONS

In considering the implications of this theory for prevention and intervention methods, we first discuss the importance of identifying children with high-risk personality traits and high-risk expectancies. Following this, we consider treatments based on high-risk personality traits. We then review efforts regarding expectancy-based treatment.

Identifying High-Risk Youth

There are, of course, many dimensions to the risk process for early adolescent drinking. The AP model highlights two dimensions that may be useful for identifying youth at risk. The first is personality. In particular, elevations in positive and/or negative urgency are important for two reasons. The first is that the general disposition to act rashly when highly emotional heightens risk transdiagnostically—that is, for a number of negative outcomes. The second is that the traits predispose adolescents to be more susceptible to positive messages about the effects of a variety of addictive behaviors, including drinking, tobacco smoking, and binge eating, which in turn lead to increases in those behaviors.

At present, cutting scores (which are specific scores used to divide respondents on a questionnaire into groups) on personality scales that differentiate high-risk adolescents from low-risk adolescents have not yet been developed—the attempt to do so may represent an important avenue of research. There are both questionnaire and interview measures to assess the urgency traits, as well as to assess sensation seeking, lack of planning, and lack of perseverance (the measure is called the UPPS Impulsive Behavior Scale [UPPS-P] and is available from the authors Lynam, Smith, Cyders, Fischer, & Whiteside, 2007). In addition, a child version of the UPPS-P has been developed (Zapolski, Stairs, et al., 2010; Zapolski & Smith, 2013). The child version has been used with adolescents (Settles et al., 2014) and takes approximately 10 minutes to complete. Although the urgency traits appear to be most important to the risk process, each of the five traits correlate with addictive behaviors and we have reviewed evidence for the importance of sensation seeking and lack of planning to the AP risk process. Thus, use of the UPPS-P might help clarify the specific nature of a child's personality-based risk.

The second AP-based dimension useful for identifying high-risk adolescents is expectancies for reinforcement from engaging in a given addictive behavior. With respect to alcohol, Smith and Goldman (1994) provided cutting scores—that is, scores on the measure of the expectancy that alcohol can enhance or impede social behavior (from the Alcohol Expectancy Questionnaire—Adolescent Form [AEQ-A]; Christiansen et al., 1982), that identify youth at particular risk to begin drinking over the following 24 months. They found that use of the expectancy scale led to hit rates (which are the accurate identification of [1] the proportion of people who do begin to drink and [2] the proportion or people who do not) of 64% across the 2-year time lag, whereas prediction from family history of alcoholism predicted with a hit rate of 55%. This finding suggests that risk assessment based on learned expectancies for reinforcement from drinking may provide a useful addition to risk assessment protocols. To date, research on expectancies for other addictive behaviors, such as smoking and binge eating, has not investigated possible cutting scores on those measures.

Personality-Based Treatment

Because negative urgency, which involves the tendency to act rashly when distressed, overlaps heavily with behaviors associated with borderline personality disorder that are treated with dialectical behavior therapy (DBT; Linehan, 1993), Zapolski, Settles, Cyders, and Smith (2010) suggested employing DBT techniques for clients high in negative urgency. DBT emphasizes four categories of skills that are designed to manage distress and prevent rash action. These skills include distress tolerance, interpersonal effectiveness, emotion regulation, and mindfulness (Linehan, 1993). Inherent in this treatment is the goal of helping clients to tolerate their own distress and intense emotions without engaging in immediate action, communicate their emotions effectively to others, adjust their emotional reactions by considering the context, and learn to identify precipitating events or triggers to emotional reactivity and adjust their reactions accordingly. Efforts to adapt and apply DBT-based interventions to adolescent addictive behavior involvement are likely to be worthwhile. Because personality traits confer transdiagnostic risk, DBT-based interventions may have general value in relation to multiple addictive behaviors, including drinking, smoking, and binge eating.

It is less clear how one might intervene to reduce positive urgency-based risk. We believe excessive alcohol consumption due to positive urgency occurs as part of an extremely positive mood commonly experienced in celebratory contexts (such as gaining admission into college, sports wins, and parties with friends). Zapolski, Settles, and colleagues (2010) suggested the following possibilities for positive-urgency targeted treatment: (1) creative efforts to help individuals appreciate that maintenance of their positive mood might be helped by carefully considering the consequences of impulsive action; (2) teaching clients how to savor one's success in an integrative cognitive–affective way, by replaying or reviewing the success with family or friends; (3) working with clients to identify alternative, safer behaviors that can enhance one's existing positive mood; and (4) helping clients identify warning signs that they are at risk to behave impulsively, and develop reminder cues to help them remain cognizant of their long-term interests and goals. These possible interventions have not yet been tested empirically. Because positive urgency has been shown to predict subsequent increases in adolescent drinking and tobacco smoking, these interventions may be most useful for those behaviors.

Expectancy-Based Treatment

Because positive expectancies for engagement in a given addictive behavior predict earlier onset and more engagement in adolescents, a logical intervention goal is to reduce these positive expectancies. To date, the bulk of expectancy intervention work has been done with alcohol consumption, so we consider that research in some depth.

Darkes and Goldman (1993) challenged male college students' positive alcohol expectancies using two methods. First, heavy-drinking students were to participate in a drinking party and, upon finding out that some people had been given alcohol and others had been given a placebo, told to identify those who were drunk. Results revealed that students were unable to tell which of their peers were drunk and which were not drunk. The researchers then alerted them to this outcome and provided them with psychoeducation about expectancies and instructed them to record expectancy-relevant material they were exposed to from the media. This information communicated that many of the positive effects students thought were the results of alcohol were actually based on social expectations from drinking.

Outcome data revealed that students in the expectancy-treatment group showed (1) a significantly greater reduction in alcohol consumption than did students in either an alcohol reduction program or a no-treatment control group, and (2) reduced positive alcohol expectancies. This intervention also appeared to be the strongest for the heavier drinkers in the expectancy-treatment group. Multisession experiential expectancy challenges similar to this one have also been shown to be successful in reducing positive expectancies and alcohol consumption in young women when compared with a control group (Wiers & Kummeling, 2004).

Cruz and Dunn (2003) designed a study for fourth-grade children based on the methods used by Darkes and Goldman (1993, 1998). They examined two interventions: an expectancy modification intervention condition and a traditional alcohol information condition. The expectancy modification intervention involved showing the fourth graders clips from parties and informing them of the prevalence of positive messages about drinking that are not true. Interactive games and quizzes were used to ensure material comprehension. The traditional alcohol information condition emphasized the dangerous and negative effects of alcohol (the predominant message schools send to children in alcohol use-prevention programs). Results revealed that changes in expectancies were greater in the expectancy modification intervention condition than in the traditional alcohol education condition. These findings are suggestive of the potential for expectancy modification programs to decrease alcohol consumption in youth, as has been shown in adults (Darkes & Goldman, 1993, 1998).

A recent meta-analysis of alcohol expectancy challenge interventions with college students by Scott-Sheldon, Terry, Carey, Garey, and Carey (2012) identified 14 such studies. The studies differed in their intervention methods. Taken together, participants exposed to expectancy challenges reported lower positive alcohol expectancies, reduced alcohol use, and reduced frequency of heavy drinking. These effects operated within individuals exposed to expectancy challenges and they were not present in members of control groups. However, these effects were not maintained at follow-ups greater than 4 weeks. Among the possible conclusions from this review are (1) perhaps the specific nature of the expectancy challenge is important; (2) perhaps intervening earlier than the college years would be more effective; and (3) lasting interventions may well need to target multiple risk factors, not just expectancies.

Developing interventions that address both AP components of risk (disposition and psychosocial learning) may prove important. Interestingly, in the field of eating disorders, researchers have developed such a treatment. It is called integrative cognitive-affective therapy for bulimia nervosa (ICAT-BN: Wonderlich et al., 2014). ICAT-BN includes interventions that target negative urgency, emphasizing enhancing emotional awareness and emotion regulation through describing and labeling of emotions; identifying cues for emotional experiences; learning how to tolerate distress in the moment; increasing positive emotions; and learning alternative means of coping that do not harm oneself. This treatment also provides interventions to address cognitive risk factors, such as expectancies that eating helps alleviate distress and thinness brings overgeneralized life improvement. Early tests of the intervention are promising (Accurso et al., 2016; Wonderlich et al., 2014), and it may serve as a useful starting point for a similar alcohol-based intervention.

SOCIOCULTURAL CONSIDERATIONS

Sociocultural differences are an important consideration when studying the risk process for addictive behaviors in youth. Since our first publication of the AP model, several new studies have emerged using diverse samples. Notably, to date there is some evidence that the AP model applies to European Americans, African Americans, Hispanic Americans, and Asian Americans.

Among Chinese college students, the AP model of drinking risk was supported in a partially longitudinal design (Fu, Ko, Wu, Cherng, & Cheng, 2007). Using a cross-sectional design, McCarthy, Miller, Smith, and Smith (2001) found that, although African American college students scored lower than European American students on trait disinhibition, positive alcohol expectancies, and drinking behavior, the AP model applied in the same way for both groups. Meier, Slutske, Arndt, and Cadoret (2007) cross-sectionally examined the extent to which positive alcohol expectancies mediated the association between delinquency and alcohol use and whether that association was mediated by age, sex, or race in a sample of 85,301 schoolchildren from the sixth, eighth, and 11th grades. Delinquency predicted alcohol use, mediated by positive alcohol expectancies for each age, sex, and racial subgroup. Of course, delinquency is not a personality trait, so the Meier et al. (2007) findings, though consistent with the AP model, are not a direct test of it.

In terms of AP-based treatment for members of diverse groups, there is a great deal we do not yet know about what works best with different groups. It may be the case that expectancy challenge works well for men but less consistently with women (Scott-Sheldon et al., 2012), but this question requires further research. We know of no studies that have examined expectancy challenge with diverse ethnic groups. Though studies in the past 15 years have employed more diverse research samples, there is a need for more systematic empirical investigation of potential treatment and prevention methods for alcohol use in children of ethnic or racial status other than European American.

SUMMARY

We have described a model of adolescent risk for addictive behaviors that integrates personality disposition and psychosocial learning risk factors: the AP model. This model holds that adolescents with elevations in high-risk personality traits, particularly positive and negative urgency, are prepared to learn the reinforcing aspects of dangerous or deviant behaviors more strongly than others. When individuals high in this trait-based preparedness are exposed to extensive learning about a given addictive behavior, they are biased to form expectancies that the behavior provides reinforcement. Such expectancies predict adolescent addictive behavior onset, maintenance, and related problems. We believe that expectancies therefore mediate personality's influence on addictive behavior. We believe that research conducted over the past several decades represents compelling support for this assertion and provides a number of possible avenues for advancement in understanding of this model.

It may prove useful to develop interventions that target both facets of the AP model: high-risk personality traits and learned expectancies. Concerning personality trait-based intervention, early research taking such an approach for eating disorders has provided promising results. The apparent success of DBT is also encouraging. Concerning expectancy-based interventions, researchers have demonstrated some success with challenging positive alcohol expectancies in heavy-drinking college students. Expectancy challenge alone may not create lasting change in positive alcohol expectancies and drinking behavior in college student samples. Because AP-based risk processes are under way for a variety of addictive behaviors in children as young as fifth and sixth grade, interventions that address high-risk personality and learned expectancies targeted to preadolescent and early adolescent youth may be necessary.

REFERENCES

Accurso, E. C., Wonderlich, S. A., Crosby, R. D., Smith, T. L., Klein, M. H., Mitchell, J. E., et al. (2016). Predictors and moderators of treatment outcome in a randomized clinical trial for adults with symptoms of bulimia nervosa. *Journal of Consulting and Clinical Psychology, 84*(2), 178–184.

Ajzen, I., & Fishbein, M. (1980). *Understanding attitudes and predicting social behaviour.* London: Pearson.

Annus, A. M., Smith, G. T., & Masters, K. (2008). Manipulation of thinness and restricting expectancies: Further evidence for a causal role of thinness and restricting expectancies in the etiology of eating disorders. *Psychology of Addictive Behaviors, 22*(2), 278–287.

Berg, J. M., Latzman, R. D., Bliwise, N. G., & Lilienfeld, S. O. (2015). Parsing the heterogeneity of impulsivity: A meta-analytic review of the behavioral implications of the UPPS for psychopathology. *Psychological Assessment, 27*(4), 1129–1146.

Bolles, R. C. (1972). Reinforcement, expectancy, and learning. *Psychological Review, 79*(5), 394–409.

Brown, S. A., Goldman, M. S., Inn, A., & Anderson, L. R. (1980). Expectations of reinforcement from alcohol: Their domain and relation to drinking patterns. *Journal of Consulting and Clinical Psychology, 48*(4), 419–426.

Carter, A. C., & Goldman, M. S. (2008). Expectancies. In H. R. Kranzler & P. Korsmeyer (Eds.), *Encyclopedia of drugs, alcohol and addictive behavior* (3rd ed., Vol. 2 D–L, pp. 141–145). New York: Macmillan.

Caspi, A., & Moffitt, T. E. (1993). When do individual differences matter?: A paradoxical theory of personality coherence. *Psychological Inquiry, 4*(4), 247–271.

Caspi, A., & Roberts, B. W. (2001). Personality development across the life course: The argument for change and continuity. *Psychological Inquiry, 12*(2), 49–66.

Christiansen, B. A., Goldman, M. S., & Inn, A. (1982). Development of alcohol-related expectancies in adolescents: Separating pharmacological from social-learning influences. *Journal of Consulting and Clinical Psychology, 50*(3), 336–344.

Christiansen, B. A., Smith, G. T., Roehling, P. V., & Goldman, M. S. (1989). Using alcohol expectancies to predict adolescent drinking behavior after one year. *Journal of Consulting and Clinical Psychology, 57*(1), 93–99.

Combs, J. L., Spillane, N. S., Caudill, L., Stark, B., & Smith, G. T. (2012). The acquired preparedness risk model applied to smoking in 5th grade children. *Addictive Behaviors, 37*(3), 331–334.

Corbin, W. R., Iwamoto, D. K., & Fromme, K. (2011). A comprehensive longitudinal test of the acquired preparedness model for alcohol use and related problems. *Journal of Studies on Alcohol and Drugs, 72*(4), 602–610.

Coskunpinar, A., Dir, A. L., & Cyders, M. A. (2013). Multidimensionality in impulsivity and alcohol use: A meta-analysis using the UPPS model of impulsivity. *Alcoholism: Clinical and Experimental Research, 37*(9), 1441–1450.

Costa, P. T., & McCrae, R. R. (1992). Four ways five factors are basic. *Personality and Individual Differences, 13*(6), 653–665.

Cruz, I. Y., & Dunn, M. E. (2003). Lowering risk for early alcohol use by challenging alcohol expectancies in elementary school children. *Journal of Consulting and Clinical Psychology, 71*(3), 493–503.

Cyders, M. A., Flory, K., Rainer, S., & Smith, G. T. (2009). The role of personality dispositions to risky behavior in predicting first-year college drinking. *Addiction, 104*(2), 193–202.

Cyders, M. A., & Smith, G. T. (2007). Mood-based rash action and its components: Positive and negative urgency. *Personality and Individual Differences, 43*(4), 839–850.

Cyders, M. A., & Smith, G. T. (2008). Emotion-based dispositions to rash action: Positive and negative urgency. *Psychological Bulletin, 134*(6), 807–828.

Cyders, M. A., & Smith, G. T. (2010). Longitudinal validation of the urgency traits over the first year of college. *Journal of Personality Assessment, 92*(1), 63–69.

Cyders, M. A., Smith, G. T., Spillane, N. S., Fischer, S., Annus, A. M., & Peterson, C. (2007). Integration of impulsivity and positive mood to predict risky behavior: Development and validation of a measure of positive urgency. *Psychological Assessment, 19*(1), 107–118.

Cyders, M. A., Zapolski, T. C., Combs, J. L., Settles, R. F., Fillmore, M. T., & Smith, G. T. (2010). Experimental effect of positive urgency on negative outcomes from risk taking and on increased alcohol consumption. *Psychology of Addictive Behaviors, 24*(3), 367–375.

Darkes, J., & Goldman, M. S. (1993). Expectancy challenge and drinking reduction: Experimental evidence for a mediational process. *Journal of Consulting and Clinical Psychology, 61*(2), 344–353.

Darkes, J., & Goldman, M. S. (1998). Expectancy challenge and drinking reduction: Process and structure in the alcohol expectancy network. *Experimental and Clinical Psychopharmacology, 6*(1), 64–76.

Depue, R. A., & Collins, P. F. (1999). Neurobiology of the structure of personality: Dopamine, facilitation of incentive motivation, and extraversion. *Behavioral and Brain Sciences, 22*(3), 491–517.

Doran, N., Khoddam, R., Sanders, P. E., Schweizer, C. A., Trim, R. S., & Myers, M. G. (2013). A prospective study of the acquired preparedness model: The effects of impulsivity and expectancies on smoking initiation in college students. *Psychology of Addictive Behaviors, 27*(3), 714–722.

Dreisbach, G., & Goschke, T. (2004). How positive affect modulates cognitive control: Reduced perseveration at the cost of increased distractibility. *Journal of Experimental Psychology: Learning, Memory, and Cognition, 30*(2), 343–353.

Dunn, M. E., & Goldman, M. S. (1996). Empirical modeling of an alcohol expectancy memory network in elementary school children as a function of grade. *Experimental and Clinical Psychopharmacology, 4*(2), 209–217.

Evenden, J. L. (1999). Varieties of impulsivity. *Psychopharmacology, 146*(4), 348–361.

Eysenck, S. B., & Eysenck, H. J. (1977). The place of impulsiveness in a dimensional system of personality description. *British Journal of Social and Clinical Psychology, 16*(1), 57–68.

Fischer, S., Smith, G. T., & Cyders, M. A. (2008). Another look at impulsivity: A meta-analytic review comparing specific dispositions to rash action in their relationship to bulimic symptoms. *Clinical Psychology Review, 28*(8), 1413–1425.

Forgas, J. P. (1992). Mood and the perception of unusual people: Affective asymmetry in memory and social judgments. *European Journal of Social Psychology, 22*(6), 531–547.

Fromme, K., Stroot, E. A., & Kaplan, D. (1993). Comprehensive effects of alcohol: Development and psychometric assessment of a new expectancy questionnaire. *Psychological Assessment, 5*(1), 19–26.

Fu, A. T., Ko, H. C., Wu, J. Y. W., Cherng, B. L., & Cheng, C. P. (2007). Impulsivity and expectancy in risk for alcohol use: Comparing male and female college students in Taiwan. *Addictive Behaviors, 32*(9), 1887–1896.

Galen, L. W., & Rogers, W. M. (2004). Religiosity, alcohol expectancies, drinking motives and their interaction in the prediction of drinking among college students. *Journal of Studies on Alcohol and Drugs, 65*(4), 469–476.

Goldberg, J. H., Halpern-Felsher, B. L., & Millstein, S. G. (2002). Beyond invulnerability: The importance of benefits in adolescents' decision to drink alcohol. *Health Psychology, 21*(5), 477–484.

Goldman, M. S., Brown, S. A., Christiansen, B. A., & Smith, G. T. (1991). Alcoholism and memory: Broadening the scope of alcohol-expectancy research. *Psychological Bulletin, 110*(1), 137–146.

Goldman, M. S., & Darkes, J. (2004). Alcohol expectancy multiaxial assessment: A memory network-based approach. *Psychological Assessment, 16*(1), 4–15.

Goldman, M. S., Darkes, J., & Del Boca, F. K. (1999). Expectancy mediation of biopsychosocial risk for alcohol use and alcoholism. *Experimental and Clinical Psychopharmacology, 12*(1), 27–38.

Goldman, M. S., Reich, R. R., & Darkes, J. (2006). Expectancy as a unifying construct in alcohol-related cognition. In R. Weirs & A. W. Stacy (Eds.), *Handbook of implicit cognition in substance use* (pp. 105–120). Thousand Oaks, CA: SAGE.

Guller, L., Zapolski, T. C. B., & Smith, G. T. (2015a). Longitudinal test of a reciprocal model of smoking expectancies and smoking experience in youth. *Psychology of Addictive Behaviors, 29*(1), 201–210.

Guller, L., Zapolski, T. C. B., & Smith, G. T. (2015b). Personality measured in elementary school predicts middle school addictive behavior involvement. *Journal of Psychopathology and Behavioral Assessment, 37,* 523–532.

Hartup, W. W., & Van Lieshout, C. F. (1995). Personality development in social context. *Annual Review of Psychology, 46*(1), 655–687.

Hohlstein, L. A., Smith, G. T., & Atlas, J. G. (1998). An application of expectancy theory to eating disorders: Development and validation of measures of eating and dieting expectancies. *Psychological Assessment, 10*(1), 49–58.

Isen, A. M., Niedenthal, P. M., & Cantor, N. (1992). An influence of positive affect on social categorization. *Motivation and Emotion, 16*(1), 65–78.

Iwamoto, D. K., Corbin, W., Lejuez, C., & MacPherson, L. (2014). College men and alcohol use: Positive alcohol expectancies as a mediator between distinct masculine norms and alcohol use. *Psychology of Men and Masculinity, 15*(1), 29–39.

Leigh, B. C. (1987). Evaluations of alcohol expectancies: Do they add to prediction of drinking patterns? *Psychology of Addictive Behaviors, 1*(3), 135–139.

Lewis-Esquerre, J. M., Rodrigue, J. R., & Kahler, C. W. (2005). Development and validation of an adolescent smoking consequences questionnaire. *Nicotine and Tobacco Research, 7*(1), 81–90.

Linehan, M. M. (1993). *Cognitive-behavioral treatment of borderline personality disorder.* New York: Guilford Press.

Lynam, D., Smith, G. T., Cyders, M. A., Fischer, S., & Whiteside, S. A. (2007). *The UPPS-P: A multidimensional measure of risk for impulsive behavior.* Unpublished technical report.

MacBrayer, E. K., Smith, G. T., McCarthy, D. M., Demos, S., & Simmons, J. (2001). The role of family of origin food-related experiences in bulimic symptomatology. *International Journal of Eating Disorders, 30*(2), 149–160.

McCarthy, D. M., Miller, T. L., Smith, G. T., & Smith, J. A. (2001). Disinhibition and expectancy in risk for alcohol use: Comparing black and white college samples. *Journal of Studies on Alcohol and Drugs, 62*(3), 313–321.

Meier, M. H., Slutske, W. S., Arndt, S., & Cadoret, R. J. (2007). Positive alcohol expectancies partially mediate the relation between delinquent behavior and alcohol use: Generalizability across age, sex, and race in a cohort of 85,000 Iowa schoolchildren. *Psychology of Addictive Behaviors, 21*(1), 25–34.

Miller, P. M., Smith, G. T., & Goldman, M. S. (1990). Emergence of alcohol expectancies in childhood: A possible critical period. *Journal of Studies on Alcohol and Drugs, 51*(4), 343–349.

Ouellette, J. A., Gerrard, M., Gibbons, F. X., & Reis-Bergan, M. (1999). Parents, peers, and prototypes: Antecedents of adolescent alcohol expectancies, alcohol consumption, and alcohol-related life problems in rural youth. *Psychology of Addictive Behaviors, 13*(3), 183–197.

Pearson, C. M., Combs, J. L., Zapolski, T. C., & Smith, G. T. (2012). A longitudinal transactional risk model for early eating disorder onset. *Journal of Abnormal Psychology, 121*(3), 707–718.

Pearson, C. M., & Smith, G. T. (2015). Bulimic symptom onset in young girls: A longitudinal trajectory analysis. *Journal of Abnormal Psychology, 124*(4), 1003–1013.

Phillips, L. H., MacLean, R. D., & Allen, R. (2002). Age and the understanding of emotions: Neuropsychological and sociocognitive perspectives. *Journals of Gerontology Series B: Psychological Sciences and Social Sciences, 57*(6), P526–P530.

Scott, C., & Corbin, W. R. (2014). Influence of sensation seeking on response to alcohol versus placebo: Implications for the acquired preparedness model. *Journal of Studies on Alcohol and Drugs, 75*(1), 136–144.

Scott-Sheldon, L. A., Terry, D. L., Carey, K. B., Garey, L., & Carey, M. P. (2012). Efficacy of expectancy challenge interventions to reduce college student drinking: A meta-analytic review. *Psychology of Addictive Behaviors, 26*(3), 393–405.

Seibert, L. A., Miller, J. D., Pryor, L. R., Reidy, D. E., & Zeichner, A. (2010). Personality and laboratory-based aggression: Comparing the predictive power of the five-factor model, BIS/BAS, and impulsivity across context. *Journal of Research in Personality, 44*(1), 13–21.

Settles, R. F., Cyders, M., & Smith, G. T. (2010). Longitudinal validation of the acquired preparedness model of drinking risk. *Psychology of Addictive Behaviors, 24*(2), 198–208.

Settles, R. E., Zapolski, T. C., & Smith, G. T. (2014). Longitudinal test of a developmental model of the transition to early drinking. *Journal of Abnormal Psychology, 123*(1), 141–151.

Sher, K. J., Walitzer, K. S., Wood, P. K., & Brent, E. E. (1991). Characteristics of children of alcoholics: Putative risk factors, substance use and abuse, and psychopathology. *Journal of Abnormal Psychology, 100*(4), 427–448.

Slovic, P., Finucane, M. L., Peters, E., & MacGregor, D. G. (2004). Risk as analysis and risk as feelings: Some thoughts about affect, reason, risk, and rationality. *Risk Analysis, 24*(2), 311–322.

Smith, G. T. (1994). Psychological expectancy as mediator of vulnerability to alcoholism. *Annals of the New York Academy of Sciences, 708*(1), 165–171.

Smith, G. T., & Anderson, K. G. (2001). Personality and learning factors combine to create risk for adolescent problem drinking: A model and suggestions for intervention. In P. M. Monti, S. M. Colby, & T. A. O'Leary (Eds.), *Adolescents, alcohol, and substance abuse: Reaching teens through brief interventions* (pp. 109–141). New York: Guilford Press.

Smith, G. T., & Goldman, M. S. (1994). Alcohol expectancy theory and the identification of high-risk adolescents. *Journal of Research on Adolescence, 4*(2), 229–247.

Smith, G. T., Goldman, M. S., Greenbaum, P. E., & Christiansen, B. A. (1995). Expectancy for social facilitation from drinking: The divergent paths of high-expectancy and low-expectancy adolescents. *Journal of Abnormal Psychology, 104*(1), 32–40.

Smith, G. T., Williams, S. F., Cyders, M. A., & Kelley, S. (2006). Reactive personality-environment transactions and adult developmental trajectories. *Developmental Psychology, 42*(5), 877–887.

Stautz, K., & Cooper, A. (2013). Impulsivity-related personality traits and adolescent alcohol use: A meta-analytic review. *Clinical Psychology Review, 33*(4), 574–592.

Tolman, E. C. (1932). *Purposive behavior in animals and men.* Berkeley: University of California Press.

Wardell, J. D., Read, J. P., Colder, C. R., & Merrill, J. E. (2012). Positive alcohol expectancies mediate the influence of the behavioral activation system on alcohol use: A prospective path analysis. *Addictive Behaviors, 37*(4), 435–443.

Whiteside, S. P., & Lynam, D. R. (2001). The five factor model and impulsivity: Using a structural model of personality to understand impulsivity. *Personality and Individual Differences, 30*(4), 669–689.

Wiers, R. W., & Kummeling, R. H. (2004). An experimental test of an alcohol expectancy challenge in mixed gender groups of young heavy drinkers. *Addictive Behaviors, 29*(1), 215–220.

Wonderlich, S. A., Peterson, C. B., Crosby, R. D., Smith, T. L., Klein, M. H., Mitchell, J. E., et al. (2014). A randomized controlled comparison of integrative cognitive-affective therapy (ICAT) and enhanced cognitive-behavioral therapy (CBT-E) for bulimia nervosa. *Psychological Medicine, 44*(3), 543–553.

Zapolski, T. C., Settles, R. E., Cyders, M. A., & Smith, G. T. (2010a). Borderline personality disorder, bulimia nervosa, antisocial personality disorder, ADHD, substance use: Common threads, common treatment needs, and the nature of impulsivity. *Independent Practitioner, 30*(1), 20–23.

Zapolski, T. C., & Smith, G. T. (2013). Comparison of parent versus child-report of child impulsivity traits and prediction of outcome variables. *Journal of Psychopathology and Behavioral Assessment, 35*(3), 301–313.

Zapolski, T. C., Stairs, A. M., Settles, R. F., Combs, J. L., & Smith, G. T. (2010b). The measurement of dispositions to rash action in children. *Assessment, 17*(1), 116–125.

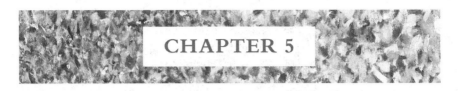

CHAPTER 5

Expanding the Reach of Brief Interventions to Address Unmet Treatment Needs

SBIRT-A (Screening, Brief Intervention, and Referral to Treatment for Adolescents)

Sara J. Becker, Timothy J. Ozechowski, and Aaron Hogue

One of the most pressing public health problems in the United States is the gap between those adolescents in need of treatment for a substance use disorder (SUD) and those who receive effective intervention. The National Survey on Drug Use and Health (NSDUH) annually assesses the prevalence, patterns, and consequences of alcohol and illicit drug use among adolescents in the United States. Data from the most recent NSDUH (Center for Behavioral Health Statistics and Quality, 2015) demonstrated that among adolescents ages 12–17, 11.5% reported current alcohol use, 9.4% reported current illicit drug use, and 5.0% met diagnostic criteria for an SUD during the past year. Among the 1.3 million adolescents who met diagnostic criteria for an SUD during the past year, only 122,000 (9.1% of those with a diagnosis) received specialty substance use treatment, leaving 1.2 million adolescents with an unmet need for treatment. Given the propensity for untreated SUD among adolescents to persist into adulthood, this pervasive level of unmet need is associated with a cascade of long-term health consequences and enormous economic costs to society (National Drug Intelligence Center, 2011).

Although the scope and severity of the adolescent SUD treatment gap has not appreciably diminished over the past decade, sensibilities about how to address the problem have evolved considerably. In particular, there has been increased recognition of the potential of brief intervention models, such as those described in Part II of this volume, to serve as an effective means of intervening with large numbers of adolescents at modest cost. This recognition was bolstered in the early 2000s by the publication of a set of landmark reports by the surgeon general (U.S. Department of Health and Human Services, 1999), the Institute of Medicine (2001), and the President's New Freedom Commission on Mental Health (2003). Collectively, these reports provided a stark assessment of prevailing levels of disorganization, fragmentation, and inefficiency characterizing the nation's behavioral health care system. Subsequent reports by McLellan and Myers (2004) and the Institute of Medicine (2006) levied similar critiques regarding SUD treatment for adults and adolescents in the United States. Priorities and recommendations for reform laid out across these reports emphasized the need for (1) proactive screening of individuals with behavioral health problems, (2) increased accessibility of brief evidence-based behavioral health interventions in community settings, (3) integrated systems linking screening and brief evidence-based interventions with referral activities, and (4) robust financing and other policy-level supports to expand capacity to meet population behavioral health care needs.

This impetus toward reform of mental and behavioral health care in the United States reverberated strongly within the child and adolescent service sectors (Green-Hennessy, 2010). Scholars in this area broadly endorsed emerging *systems of care* and *wraparound* models of service delivery as organizing frameworks for more coordinated, streamlined, patient- and family-centered services (Stroul & Blau, 2008). Around the same time, scholars articulated the need to better understand the common pathways by which youth access treatment. This led to emergence of the *gateway provider* model as a framework for clarifying the various factors that influence the likelihood that individuals coming into contact with youth—including both informal connections (i.e., family and friends) and formal providers (i.e., teachers, primary care practitioners, social workers, juvenile justice staff)—will identify youth at risk of behavioral health problems and channel such youth toward appropriate treatment (Stiffman, Pescosolido, & Cabassa, 2004). These and related innovations laid the foundation for new approaches to engineering youth services across all sectors of health care with the common themes of coordinated care, patient centeredness, and collaborative involvement among diverse stakeholders (see Green-Hennessy, 2010). Another key theme across these innovations was the need to address population health through brief evidence-based treatment models that could be widely implemented across settings and populations.

Evolving out of the systems-of-care, wraparound, and gateway provider frameworks came the most widely endorsed public health model for addressing the SUD treatment gap among both adolescents and adults (Substance Abuse and Mental Health Services Administration, 2013): Screening, Brief Intervention, and Referral to Treatment (SBIRT). SBIRT is a set of procedures for detecting individuals in the general population at risk of SUD and administering appropriate prevention, early intervention, and/or treatment referral. A primary reason that the SBIRT model gained traction so rapidly in the substance use field was the bold promise of the brief intervention component for promoting substantive changes in treatment motivation and substance use outcomes with modest resources.

Prior to the SBIRT model, brief interventions were predominantly evaluated among those who had presented to or were referred to treatment. The model represented a paradigm shift that dramatically extended the reach of brief interventions through the integration of two key components: universal screening and referral to treatment. Universal screening of individuals' level of risk of SUDs was incorporated as a means of proactively detecting those individuals in need of brief intervention. Formal decision rules were then introduced to differentiate between three groups of individuals: (1) those who did not require brief intervention, (2) those for whom brief intervention as a stand-alone intervention would be sufficient, and (3) those for whom brief intervention should be paired with referral to more intensive treatment. Under a conventional SBIRT model, all adolescents presenting to a service setting such as a primary care office, school, or juvenile justice facility are asked a series of questions to determine their level of health risk. Depending on their level of risk, adolescents are then provided with either positive reinforcement, a brief intervention, or a brief intervention paired with referral to treatment. From a public health perspective, the goal of combining these intervention components is to reduce the treatment gap by reaching a more substantial proportion of the population at risk of SUDs (see Substance Abuse and Mental Health Services Administration, 2013).

To date, SBIRT has been implemented predominantly with adults in primary care and emergency rooms, with data from several clinical trials supporting the model's effectiveness among adults with risky alcohol use (see Substance Abuse and Mental Health Services Administration, 2013). The U.S Preventive Services Task Force (USPSTF) has deemed the evidence base sufficient to recommend the routine use of SBIRT to identify risky alcohol consumption among adults in primary care (see Moyer, 2013). Data on SBIRT's effectiveness among adults with relatively severe alcohol use or illicit drug use are less compelling, however (Roy-Byrne et al., 2014; Saitz et al., 2014).

For adolescents, the evidence in support of the SBIRT model is more scant. A 2013 review of SBIRT trials with adolescents (Mitchell, Gryczynski, O'Grady, & Schwartz, 2013) identified a total of seven randomized clinical trials conducted in emergency departments and seven conducted in schools, with the majority of studies finding little or inconclusive evidence of the benefits of SBIRT over control or comparison conditions (e.g., assessment only, brief advice). In 2013, the USPSTF reviewed the evidence base in support of SBIRT and deemed it insufficient to recommend routine use of the model in pediatric primary care—according to the report, existing trials were too few in number and differences between SBIRT and usual care were too small to justify a formal recommendation. Nonetheless, reviews of SBIRT have acknowledged the model's potential benefits to increase the detection of substance use problems within this age group (see Mitchell et al., 2013), and scholars have argued that SBIRT is a pragmatic means of integrating basic substance use services into settings where teens spend a great deal of time. For these reasons, SBIRT has been uniformly championed for use with adolescents by virtually every major behavioral health organization, including the American Academy of Pediatrics, American Medical Association, National Institute on Alcohol Abuse and Alcoholism, National Institute on Drug Abuse, and Substance Abuse and Mental Health Services Administration.

ADAPTING SBIRT FOR ADOLESCENTS

Despite widespread enthusiasm for SBIRT across service settings, questions persist regarding the model's effectiveness, feasibility, and developmental appropriateness for adolescents under age 18 (see Mitchell et al., 2013). In light of such concerns, this chapter recommends a set of adaptations to the conventional SBIRT model for treatment providers seeking to serve adolescent populations more optimally. These recommendations are based on extant empirical studies of SBIRT and brief intervention, developmental theory, and documented barriers to implementing evidence-based practices. Collectively, we refer to the set of recommendations as SBIRT-A (see Ozechowski, Becker, & Hogue, 2016). Key themes across the recommended adaptations include reliance upon proactive methods to identify at-risk youth, innovation in service delivery aimed at improving the consistency and reach of brief interventions, and engagement of caregivers. For each component of the SBIRT model, we provide general suggestions that can be applied across a variety of gateway service settings in which adolescents and their caregivers are encountered (e.g., schools, child welfare, juvenile justice, primary care, and emergency departments). Table 5.1 presents an overview of the key areas of differentiation between the conventional SBIRT model and the SBIRT-A framework.

Screening (S)

Screening is the first component of the SBIRT-A model and provides the foundation for the other components. As noted by Winters, Botzet, and Lee (Chapter 3, this volume), state-of-the-art screening methods are essential to ensure accurate detection of adolescents at risk of SUDs, and a number of psychometrically sound screening measures exist. With universal substance use screening initiatives, briefer measures are generally preferred due to the time constraints faced by busy gateway service providers and the desire to reserve more lengthy assessments for adolescents at elevated levels of risk (see Levy &

TABLE 5.1. Comparison of Conventional SBIRT Model with SBIRT-A Framework

	Component	Conventional SBIRT	SBIRT-A
Screening	Delivery	Informal or pencil and paper	Technology delivered
	Focus	Teen self-report	Teen and caregiver report
	Timing	Varies, ad hoc	Predetermined
Brief Intervention	*Preventive stand-alone BI* Delivery	Face-to-face, manualized	Computerized, user responsive
	Content for teens	Education, normative feedback, decisional balance, change planning	Education, normative feedback, change planning
	Content for caregivers	Varies, ad hoc	Education
	Transitional BI Focus	Adolescent motivation building	Family-based treatment engagement
Referral to Treatment	Referral process	Provider gives referrals to adolescent	Provider facilitates warm hand-off, engages adolescent and caregiver
	Follow-up	Varies, ad hoc	Routinized

Kokotailo, 2011). Other prevailing recommendations for universal screening include the use of developmentally appropriate tools that can be administered with minimal staff burden to easily identify which adolescents are in need of further intervention (see Wissow et al., 2013). A recent study by Levy and colleagues (2014) found that a single screening question (i.e., "How often have you used [specific drug] over the past year . . . ?") was as effective as longer screening tools in triaging adolescents into different risk categories. Such a brief screening strategy is consistent with the single-item screening approach recommended among adults (see Saitz et al., 2014) and with the National Institute on Alcohol Abuse and Addiction's (2011) youth alcohol screening guide, which recommends using a single question about frequency of past-year alcohol use to determine adolescents' level of risk.

Current guidelines also emphasize the importance of embedding screening into routine practice. The American Academy of Pediatrics (Levy & Kokotailo, 2011) recommends that substance use screening be conducted during *every* primary care visit with the teen—whether for a wellness visit, an acute care appointment, or a sports physical. This approach is well suited for settings where adolescents receive services intermittently (e.g., medical and correctional settings), whereas settings where adolescents receive services more regularly (e.g., schools, therapy clinics) may prefer to administer screens at consistent, predetermined intervals.

While universal screening is becoming increasingly common in medical settings (see Wissow et al., 2013), it is far from the norm in school, child welfare, or juvenile justice settings. Even within pediatric primary care, where there are widely disseminated guidelines encouraging universal screening (Levy & Kokotailo, 2011), survey data suggest that less than half of physicians routinely screen adolescents for substance use using psychometrically valid tools (Harris, Herr-Zaya, et al., 2012). These low screening rates underscore a myriad of provider-level barriers to universal screening of both adolescents and adults, including time constraints, logistical hurdles, discomfort with the approach, low self-efficacy, and lack of motivation (see Sterling, Kline-Simon, Wibbelsman, Wong, & Weisner, 2012).

At least two adolescent-specific barriers further diminish the potential effectiveness of SUD risk screening. First, adolescents are likely to experience heightened concerns regarding the confidentiality of information revealed during SUD risk screening and therefore may be prone to underreport or deny substance use behavior and involvement (Delaney-Black et al., 2010). Second, predominant SBIRT approaches rely solely on adolescent report, despite evidence indicating that utilizing multiple sources of information to detect substance use among adolescents is more accurate than relying on any single source (see Brener, Bill, & Grady, 2003). These barriers suggest that even psychometrically sound screening tools, such as those described in Winters et al. (Chapter 3, this volume), may underestimate the proportion of adolescents at risk of SUDs. We therefore recommend the following two adolescent-specific adaptations to screening.

S Recommendation 1: Use Technology

To encourage accurate reporting, the SBIRT-A framework encourages the use of technology to administer screening tools via desktop or laptop computers, smart pads, or handheld devices. Evidence suggests that adolescents perceive computer-administered substance use screens to be more confidential than paper-and-pencil and/or interview screening formats (Pedersen, Grow, Duncan, Neighbors, & Larimer, 2012). Indeed, adolescents tend to report higher levels of substance use frequency using computer-administered assessment tools compared with more traditional screening methods and modalities, and this sensitivity to screening mode is more pronounced in adolescents than in adults (see Brener et al., 2003). Computer-administered screening is likely to be especially attractive to adolescents given the generally high levels of comfort and skill with technology in this age group (Lenhart, 2015). For gateway service providers, the use of electronically administered screening may reduce administrative burden, decrease the likelihood of missed or inaccurate screens, facilitate incorporation of screening results into existing records (including the electronic medical record if applicable), and enable instantaneous scoring that can inform the brief intervention and referral to treatment components of the framework (e.g., Buntin, Burke, Hoaglin, & Blumenthal, 2011).

S Recommendation 2: Involve Caregivers

Caregivers are vital sources of information about adolescent substance use risk. While the traditional SBIRT model recommends that only adolescents participate in screening, the SBIRT-A framework recommends that caregivers complete brief screening instruments to provide collateral reports of adolescent substance use. This conjoint approach to screening serves to increase the likelihood of case detection (see Delaney-Black et al., 2010) and to set the stage for caregiver involvement in subsequent components of the SBIRT-A framework.

There has been limited research on the accuracy of caregiver reports of adolescent substance use, although parental reports appear to be fair-to-good proxy measures of adolescent substance use behavior (McGillicuddy, Rychtarik, Morsheimer, & Burke-Storer, 2012). As such, administering empirically validated substance use screening tools to caregivers could help to assign adolescents more accurately to risk categories and increase early identification of adolescents at risk of SUDs. Few well-validated caregiver measures of adolescent substance use currently exist, rendering caregiver screening a priority for future research on the SBIRT-A framework.

Brief Intervention (BI)

The goal of the screening component of the model is to triage adolescents efficiently into specific risk categories in order to inform subsequent intervention. Consistent with the guidelines from the American Academy of Pediatrics (Levy & Kokotailo, 2011), the SBIRT-A framework recommends that adolescents reporting no history of substance use (corroborated by caregiver report) receive positive feedback to reinforce continued abstinence, whereas all other adolescents receive some type of brief intervention. Adolescents at mild-to-moderate SUD risk (defined as substance use less than once per month over the past year) should receive a preventive (stand-alone) brief intervention to increase motivation to reduce or abstain from substance use, whereas those at moderate-to-severe SUD risk (defined as substance use once or more per month over the past year) should receive a transitional brief intervention paired with linkage to more extensive services. Chapters in Part II of this volume discuss an array of considerations to improve the implementation of brief interventions with adolescents from varied populations across a range of diverse settings. The remainder of this section describes three broad recommendations to enhance the developmental fit of brief intervention procedures for adolescents when applied as part of a universal early intervention approach.

BI Recommendation 1: Use Technology-Assisted Intervention Platforms

To ensure that adolescents efficiently progress from screening to brief intervention and that the model is implemented with fidelity, administrators are advised to adopt technology-assisted intervention platforms. Face-to-face brief intervention sessions grounded in motivational interviewing techniques require about 30–45 minutes (Clark & Moss, 2010). Technology-assisted brief interventions are designed to reduce administration burden, minimize administrator differences in implementation fidelity, maximize information processing efficiency, and allow self-guided and response-sensitive intervention delivery (Carey, Scott-Sheldon, Elliot, Garey, & Carey, 2012). The initial wave of effectiveness studies on technology-assisted SBIRT for teens indicates that computerized brief interventions perform comparably to face-to-face versions, producing beneficial effects on substance use in some but not all studies (see Tanner-Smith & Lipsey, 2015).

In addition to reduced administration burden, the largest potential benefit of technology-assisted brief intervention is the capacity to tailor the selection and duration of brief intervention components based on real-time adolescent response to ongoing intervention. Although the added value of tailored versus nontailored brief intervention has not been rigorously tested in any age group, the possibilities are highly appealing. For example, animated substance use psychoeducation programs can selectively deliver variations in advice-giving options or role-play scenarios depending on successive respondent choices (e.g., Braciszewski & Havlicek, Chapter 9, this volume; Walton et al., 2013), so that each adolescent experiences a personalized and dynamic curriculum. Technology can also potentially be used to deliver personalized intervention content between visits to reinforce the effects of preventive brief interventions. Booster content can be delivered in a multitude of formats, ranging from brief text messages to interactive video messaging (Jones, 2014), and can even incorporate assessment functions to monitor changes in substance use disorder risk (Kumar et al., 2013). The use of technology to bolster and personalize brief intervention content is developmentally well suited for adolescents, but represents an emerging area in need of further research.

BI Recommendation 2: Emphasize Psychoeducation

Cumulative wisdom from brief intervention studies in adolescents, consistent with those targeting adults, recommends that certain brief intervention elements be emphasized in locations other than substance use specialty treatment. A mainstay, cost-effective feature of youth behavioral health interventions of all kinds is psychoeducation about the nature of the disorder, individual and family factors that impact the disorder, and clarification about service needs and options (Hoagwood, 2010). Psychoeducation for adolescents typically features normative feedback (comparing a given teen's consumption to meaningful norms in similar-age peers) and didactics on neurobiological effects and developmental risks (Turner, Spithoff, & Kahan, 2014). As demonstrated by many of the brief intervention models discussed in Part II, normative feedback can include national or state norms, or can be tailored to specific settings (e.g., school districts, medical practices), interest groups (e.g., sports players), or special populations (e.g., youth in foster care). Psychoeducation with personalized feedback is a pillar of one-session brief interventions that has shown effects for deterring substance use in multiple contexts, including schools (Carney, Myers, Louw, & Okwundu, 2014) and pediatric care (Harris, Csémy, et al., 2012). Another brief intervention staple, *decisional balance,* has mixed support. Decisional balance interventions prompt patients to carefully consider the positive and negative personal impacts of substance use and specify the cost/benefit ratio that leads to consumption (Mitchell et al., 2013). One recent meta-analysis of interventions for college drinking (Carey et al., 2012) found that decisional balance was one of few motivational interviewing components associated with poor outcomes, whereas a second focused on high school-age drinking (Tanner-Smith & Lipsey, 2015) determined that decisional balance and goal setting were as potent as personalized feedback and norm referencing. For these reasons, we recommend prioritizing psychoeducation with normative feedback and using decisional balance judiciously, especially in medical settings that may have fewer than 15 allotted minutes per session (Walton et al., 2013).

BI Recommendation 3: Involve Caregivers

Caregivers confer important risk and protective factors for adolescent substance use that are not addressed in prevailing SBIRT models. A handful of studies on family-focused brief interventions in high school settings (e.g., Winters, Fahnhorst, Botzet, Lee, & Lalone, 2012; Winters, Leitten, Wagner, & O'Leary Tevyaw, 2007) and pediatric settings (Gayes & Steele, 2014) demonstrate that brief interventions incorporating caregivers have added value over adolescent-only brief interventions. To balance the value of caregiver involvement with the need for adolescent confidentiality, we recommend expanding brief interventions to caregivers by providing them with basic psychoeducation on substance use (though not feedback about their adolescent's SUD risk). A computerized caregiver psychoeducation module would present minimal burden to administrators as well as set the stage for family involvement in transitional brief interventions for adolescents whose high-risk status warrants treatment referral (described in the next section). As with adolescents, the content could be made personal and dynamic based on caregiver data from the screening phase and their interaction with the psychoeducation module. To our knowledge, no computerized programs are currently available that cover all of the recommended screening and brief intervention content described here, suggesting that development of such a program is a priority for future tests of the SBIRT-A framework.

In summary, the brief intervention adaptations recommended above yield the following two intervention paths: (1) computer-based preventive, stand-alone brief intervention modules for low/moderate-risk adolescents, featuring user-responsive psychoeducation for adolescents and caregivers; or (2) transitional brief interventions folded into referral to treatment procedures for moderate/severe-risk adolescents.

Referral to Treatment (RT)

The referral to treatment component of SBIRT-A is implemented for those adolescents at moderate/severe SUD risk. The goal of this component is not simply to refer these high-risk adolescents to treatment, but also to ensure that they enroll in and actually receive treatment (Substance Abuse and Mental Health Services Administration, 2013). The screening and brief intervention components of SBIRT-A rely on electronic delivery with minimal provider involvement, whereas the referral to treatment component relies directly on provider participation. Yet relative to the screening and brief intervention components, protocols for executing referral to treatment with adolescents are considerably less well established (Mitchell et al., 2013). A general directive for implementing referral to treatment with high-risk populations is for gateway service providers to establish relationships and referral procedures with treatment programs in the local community (Substance Abuse and Mental Health Services Administration, 2013). Beyond such global prescriptions, however, few guidelines are in place to inform the typically complex process of channeling high-risk adolescents into treatment (see Mitchell et al., 2013). The absence of procedural guidelines by which frontline gateway service providers should put core components of empirically based interventions into practice, such as the referral to treatment component of SBIRT, hampers the implementation and sustainability of such interventions in community settings (see Wandersman, Chien, & Katz, 2012).

Delivery of referral to treatment in gateway service settings is also challenged by adolescent-specific considerations. It is well-known that adolescents are unlikely to receive treatment unless coerced by an external agency such as the school or juvenile justice system, especially in the absence of a comorbid disorder or precipitating crisis event that could signal the presence of a substance use problem (Ozechowski & Waldron, 2010). As such, we believe that effective referral to treatment procedures require engaging both the adolescent and caregiver in order to foster "buy in" in the treatment referral process (see Yatchmenoff, 2005). Although a fully detailed set of procedural guidelines is beyond the scope of this chapter, below we offer three overarching recommendations to help implement referral to treatment with adolescents in community-based gateway service settings.

RT Recommendation 1: Use a Strengths-Based Approach to Engage the Adolescent

Adolescents tracked into the referral to treatment phase should be engaged by frontline service providers in ways that lay essential groundwork for enrollment in substance use treatment. In particular, adolescents at moderate/severe SUD risk should be helped to recognize the health risks of substance use, the benefits of abstaining from (or at least substantially cutting down) substance use, and the potential value of seeking substance use treatment. In addition, adolescents should be supportively encouraged to talk directly with caregivers about their substance use involvement as a first step toward help seeking and behavior change (Ford, English, & Sigman, 2004).

Adolescents are most likely to disclose substance use behavior with gateway service providers when providers are perceived as credible sources of health information who are genuinely concerned for their personal well-being (Kadivar et al., 2014). Service providers are best positioned to convey these messages by interacting with adolescents in one-on-one sessions from a youth-centered, strength-based perspective during which they convey interest in adolescents' personal characteristics and potential for success (Sanders & Munford, 2014). A strengths-based approach would require providers to spend time learning about those personal attributes and accomplishments that adolescents most value about themselves. For example, a provider could begin an interview with questions such as "What achievements are you most proud of in your life? How did you make those achievements happen?" Providers could then use the answers to these questions to convey confidence in adolescents' capacity to manage their lives productively (e.g., "It sounds like when you put your mind to something, you are able to achieve it"), including making rational decisions regarding substance use involvement and treatment.

Adolescents are also more likely to engage with providers when confidentiality is ensured (Ford, Millstein, Halpern-Felsher, & Irwin, 1997). Providers in health care settings should remind adolescents of any state or federal regulations that protect their confidentiality (see Ford, et al., 2004), whereas providers in non-health care settings should specify the limits of confidentiality up-front. All providers should leverage strength-based alliances to encourage adolescent assent to disclose substance use problems to those caregivers who have the capacity to provide guidance and support with such issues.

RT Recommendation 2: Use a Strengths-Based Approach to Engage the Caregiver

It is widely recognized that persuading adolescents to enroll in treatment typically requires substantial family influence and involvement (Logan & King, 2001). Unfortunately, there is often a myriad of challenges to engaging family caregivers in this process (Ozechowski & Waldron, 2010). Such obstacles include caregiver unawareness or minimization of adolescent substance use severity, skepticism about the value of treatment, fear of being judged for adolescent substance use problems, discomfort about one's own substance use, and hopelessness about the possibility of change. The referral to treatment component of SBIRT-A calls for service providers to use a strengths-based approach to engage caregivers in order to address these challenges.

Service providers' interactions with caregivers should address three objectives. First, the provider should facilitate caregiver awareness and understanding of adolescent substance use problems by sharing the SUD risk data collected during the screening and brief intervention phases (only with adolescent assent, as described above) and explaining the corresponding risks. Second, providers should minimize the likelihood that caregivers will feel blamed for their adolescent's substance use involvement by adapting an empathetic and validating stance (see Kemp, Marcenko, Lyons, & Kruzich, 2014). Such a stance may entail acknowledging caregivers' past efforts to cope with the adolescent's substance use and associated behavior, reflecting caregivers' desire to safeguard their child from harm, reinforcing the vital importance of caregiver involvement on adolescent well-being, and reassuring that change is possible (though not guaranteed) with strong caregiver participation in efforts to deter and protect the adolescent from engaging in substance use. Finally, providers should attempt to join with caregivers in talking directly with adolescents about the risks of substance use involvement and the potential benefits of treatment, while being sensitive to caregivers who opt not to participate in such discussions or who wish not to have their concerns shared with their adolescent children. For instance, a provider might tell a caregiver:

> "It sounds like you really want the best for your son and you have been working hard to help him stay safe. I would like to have a conversation with your son about some options to help him make better choices about his use of alcohol and other drugs. It's clear to me that your son really values your opinion and in my experience, teenagers are more open to the idea of treatment if their parents are on board. Would you be willing to join me in talking with your son?"

Strength-based strategies such as these are consistent with established family-based treatment engagement procedures for adolescent substance use and associated problems (e.g., Alexander, Waldron, Robbins, & Neeb, 2013; Liddle, 2002; Szapocznik, Zarate, Duff, & Muir, 2013) as well as recommended procedures to mobilize caregiver support and encourage highly resistant adolescents to enroll in substance use treatment (see Ozechowski & Waldron, 2010).

RT Recommendation 3: Initiate the Referral in Person

Within the SBIRT-A framework, effective referral to treatment hinges on adolescent and caregiver engagement in the referral process. Ideally, frontline gateway service providers should initiate the process by contacting substance use treatment providers in the presence of adolescents and caregivers. This contact can serve to facilitate opportunities for personal introductions and to elicit adolescent and caregiver questions, concerns, and input regarding substance use treatment. If gateway and substance use treatment services are colocated (i.e., occurring in the same location) or integrated, these conversations can occur face-to-face. Otherwise, conference phone calls or videoconferences (e.g., Skype) can be used. The end goal of family involvement is to ensure successful handoff and procure treatment engagement. Enlisting service recipients as active partners in health care discussions is a hallmark of patient-centered approaches to health care delivery (Bechtel & Ness, 2010), which are themselves associated with better health outcomes, lower rates of subsequent and more intensive service utilization, and reduced costs (Hibbard, Greene, & Overton, 2013).

CONCLUSIONS

This chapter describes a set of developmentally informed adaptations to the SBIRT model, collectively called SBIRT-A, as a means of expanding the reach of brief interventions to adolescents across service settings and populations. Relative to the conventional SBIRT model, the SBIRT-A framework incorporates more proactive, assertive, and family-focused strategies for addressing the clinical needs of adolescents with substance use problems that are otherwise likely to go unnoticed in gateway service settings. Pairing brief interventions with comprehensive, developmentally informed identification and engagement strategies represents a timely and sorely needed strategy to meaningfully reduce the adolescent substance use treatment gap (see Ozechowski & Waldron, 2010).

The proposed developmental adaptations encompassed within SBIRT-A are aligned with broad-based shifts in health care policy and practice emphasizing collaboration among behavioral health, general medical, and other non-health care service providers (Institute of Medicine, 2006). Historically, those seeking to bridge disparate treatment systems have had to choose from a broad array of interventions under the rubric of collaborative care. Indeed, a report by the Canadian Collaborative Mental Health Initiative observed that "there are as many ways of 'doing' collaborative care as there are people writing about it" (Macfarlane, 2005, p. 11). Generally speaking, however, there are three basic distinctions among contemporary collaborative models: coordinated, colocated, and integrated (see Collins, Hewson, Munger, & Wade, 2010). Care by substance use and other providers can be *coordinated* across separate health care settings via formal linkages to facilitate patient referrals; exchange patient health information (e.g., through shared electronic medical records); schedule patient appointments; and track patient follow-through, treatment progress, and needs for additional services. Coordinated care delivery can also be *colocated* (occurring in the same location) or *integrated* (occurring under one unified and collaborative treatment plan). Colocated care models typically encompass all the elements of coordinated care, whereas integrated care models encompass all the elements of coordinated and colocated care. The SBIRT-A framework can be viewed as a component of a coordinated care model that promotes tighter and more routine linkages across systems. SBIRT-A is also compatible with colocated and integrated treatment models—in these cases, the referral to treatment component still places significant emphasis on family engagement, but the process of handing off the patient to a new provider is significantly streamlined.

The SBIRT-A framework was proposed to address adolescent-specific barriers to implementation of the conventional SBIRT model including inability to detect substance use accurately, burdensome training requirements, and lack of systematic guidelines to collaborate with other service providers (see Ozechowski et al., 2016). The recommendations contained within SBIRT-A may also serve to address universal barriers to implementation such as provider time constraints, self-efficacy, and motivation to learn new approaches (see Sterling et al., 2012). Due to the demanding realities of gateway service settings, many providers lack the time, confidence, and training needed to screen and intervene with adolescents at risk of SUDs. For this reason, the screening and brief intervention components of the adapted SBIRT-A framework rely heavily upon electronic delivery formats that require minimal provider expertise or time investment.

The only component of SBIRT-A that requires significant provider involvement is referral to treatment, which has been adapted to include *more* proactive and potentially time-intensive linkages to service providers than the conventional SBIRT model. However, as previously noted, contemporary innovations in substance use treatment delivery such as colocated and integrated care (see Collins et al., 2010) have the potential to expedite the referral process and decrease the time investment required to execute SBIRT-A. Furthermore, if gateway providers working directly with adolescents do not have time to execute the referral to treatment component of SBIRT-A, many of the components can potentially be shifted to ancillary staff members with proper training. For instance, Stoner, Mikko, and Carpenter (2014) showed that physicians, nurse practitioners, and physician assistants could all be trained to implement SBIRT with equivalent levels of proficiency using self-administered online tutorials and instructional materials. This approach is consistent with the emerging public health service policy and practice known as "task shifting" by which ancillary workers are trained to provide basic health care services in the face of provider shortages and other constraints on service providers' time (Kazdin & Rabbitt, 2013). Task shifting with regard to SBIRT-A is likely to be a viable and practical service delivery option that merits further investigation.

A key question to be addressed is how the recommended clinical components and procedures encompassed within SBIRT-A affect costs relative to the traditional SBIRT model. To date, the costs of implementing SBIRT with adolescents have not been quantified, though at least two investigations are currently in progress: Mitchell and colleagues (2016) are currently comparing the cost-effectiveness of two SBIRT approaches (generalist model delivered by physician vs. specialist model delivered by a behavioral health practitioner) for adolescents in federally qualified health centers (i.e., medical centers that receive federal funding for providing comprehensive services to underserved populations), while Gryczynski (2015) is currently comparing the cost effectiveness of two approaches (nurse-practitioner delivered vs. computer delivered) in schools. These investigations will help to inform the extent to which delivery method affects costs, and will provide a reasonable baseline estimate of the cost of traditional SBIRT in two critically important gateway service settings. In the meantime, there are some data on SBIRT costs among adults. Zarkin, Bray, Hinde, and Saitz (2015, p. 226) estimated the total cost of SBIRT per adult in outpatient medical settings—the cost of substance use screening was $15.61; a 15-minute preventive brief intervention was $38.94; and a complete transitional brief intervention session (perhaps followed by referral to treatment) was $252.26 (in 2001 dollars, with all components implemented by nonphysician behavioral health clinicians). The costs of the corresponding screening and brief intervention components of SBIRT-A are likely to be comparable to or lower than those for adults due to the emphasis on technology-assisted delivery, whereas referral to treatment is bound to be more costly given the level of time and effort entailed in orchestrating coordinated interactions among adolescents, caregivers, and substance use treatment providers. These implementation costs could be recovered numerous times over, however, if SBIRT-A were proven to prevent a substantial proportion of at-risk youth from progressing toward SUD in young adulthood and beyond (see National Drug Intelligence Center, 2011). Among adult SBIRT recipients in medical settings, cost benefits have been documented in the form of reduced health care service utilization and other costs to society (see Barbosa, Cowell, Bray, & Aldridge, 2015). In recognition of these types of public health benefits, financial coverage for SBIRT in medical settings is a priority under the Affordable Care Act (Ghitza & Tai, 2014). In like manner, reimbursement for SBIRT-A services in medical and nonmedical settings would likely be a prudent public health investment for policy makers as well as health insurance companies and managed care organizations.

This chapter provides a fairly broad overview of the SBIRT-A framework. Moving forward, the proposed SBIRT-A adaptations will require more detailed specification, manualization, and training materials to facilitate systematic application in specific settings. In particular, the validation of caregiver screening measures and the development of software programs for implementing the screening and stand-alone brief intervention components are critical next steps for the dissemination and implementation of SBIRT-A. In addition, experimental studies are needed to evaluate the effectiveness of SBIRT-A relative to conventional SBIRT in several areas: (1) improving the detection of adolescents at risk for SUD, (2) promoting intervention access and utilization, and (3) preventing the escalation of substance use-related problems among those adolescents who have initiated substance use. Empirical evaluations of SBIRT-A are also needed to determine which elements of the framework are essential, optimal strategies for implementation, and cost-effectiveness of the model. For the time being, we hope this chapter stimulates further thinking regarding novel and clinically resourceful ways to expand the reach of the brief intervention models described in Part II of this volume.

REFERENCES

Alexander, J. F., Waldron, H. B., Robbins, M. S., & Neeb, A. A. (2013). *Functional family therapy for adolescent behavior problems.* Washington, DC: American Psychological Association.

Barbosa, C., Cowell, A., Bray, J., & Aldridge, A. (2015). The cost-effectiveness of alcohol screening, brief intervention, and referral to treatment (SBIRT) in emergency and outpatient medical settings. *Journal of Substance Abuse Treatment, 53,* 1–8.

Bechtel, C., & Ness, D. L. (2010). If you build it, will they come?: Designing truly patient-centered health care. *Health Affairs, 29,* 914–920.

Brener, N. D., Billy, J. O., & Grady, W. R. (2003). Assessment of factors affecting the validity of self-reported health-risk behavior among adolescents: Evidence from the scientific literature. *Journal of Adolescent Health, 33*(6), 436–457.

Buntin, M. B., Burke, M. F., Hoaglin, M. C., & Blumenthal, D. (2011). The benefits of health information technology: A review of the recent literature shows predominantly positive results. *Health Affairs, 30*(3), 464–471.

Carey, K. B., Scott-Sheldon, L. A., Elliott, J. C., Garey, L., & Carey, M. P. (2012). Face-to-face versus computer-delivered alcohol interventions for college drinkers: A meta-analytic review, 1998 to 2010. *Clinical Psychology Review, 32,* 690–703.

Carney, T., Myers, B. J., Louw, J., & Okwundu, C. I. (2014). Brief school-based interventions and behavioural outcomes for substance-using adolescents. *Cochrane Database of Systematic Reviews, 2.*

Center for Behavioral Health Statistics and Quality. (2015). Behavioral health trends in the United States: Results from the 2014 National Survey on Drug Use and Health (HHS Publication No. SMA 15-4927, NSDUH Series H-50). Retrieved from *www.samhsa.gov/data.*

Clark, D. B., & Moss, H. B. (2010). Providing alcohol-related screening and brief interventions to adolescents through health care systems: Obstacles and solutions. *PLOS Medicine, 7*(3), e1000214.

Collins, C., Hewson, D. J., Munger, R., & Wade, T. (2010). Evolving models of behavioral health integration in primary care. Millibank Memorial Fund. Retrieved December 3, 2015, from *www.milbank.org/publications/milbank-reports/32-reports-evolving-models-of-behavioral-health-integration-in-primary-care.*

Delaney-Black, V., Chiodo, L. M., Hannigan, J. H., Greenwald, M. K., Janisse, J., Patterson, G., et al. (2010). Just say "I don't": Lack of concordance between teen report and biological measures of drug use. *Pediatrics, 126*(5), 887–893.

Ford, C., English, A., & Sigman, G. (2004). Confidential health care for adolescents:

A position paper of the Society for Adolescent Medicine. *Journal of Adolescent Health, 35,* 1–8.

Ford, C. A., Millstein, S. G., Halpern-Felsher, B. L., & Irwin, C. E., Jr. (1997). Influence of physician confidentiality assurances on adolescents' willingness to disclose information and seek future health care: A randomized controlled trial. *JAMA, 278,* 1029–1034.

Gayes, L. A., & Steele, R. G. (2014). A meta-analysis of motivational interviewing interventions for pediatric health behavior change. *Journal of Consulting and Clinical Psychology, 82,* 521–535.

Ghitza, U. E., & Tai, B. (2014). Challenges and opportunities for integrating preventive substance-use-care services in primary care through the Affordable Care Act. *Journal of Health Care for the Poor and Underserved, 25,* 36–45.

Green-Hennessy, S. (2010). Children and adolescents. In B. L. Levin, K. D. Hennessy, & J. Petril (Eds.), *Mental health services: A public health perspective* (3rd ed., pp. 201–225). New York: Oxford University Press.

Gryczynski, J. (2015). *A randomized trial of SBIRT services in school-based health centers.* Baltimore: Friends Research Institute. Grantome. Retrieved from *http://grantome. com/grant/NIH/R01-DA036604-01.*

Harris, S. K., Csémy, L., Sherritt, L., Starostova, O., Van Hook, S., Johnson, J., et al. (2012). Computer-facilitated substance use screening and brief advice for teens in primary care: An international trial. *Pediatrics, 129,* 1072–1082.

Harris, S. K., Herr-Zaya, K., Weinstein, Z., Whelton, K., Perfas, F., Jr., Castro-Donlan, C., et al. (2012). Results of a statewide survey of adolescent substance use screening rates and practices in primary care. *Substance Abuse, 33,* 321–326.

Hibbard, J. H., Greene, J., & Overton, V. (2013). Patients with lower activation associated with higher costs: Delivery systems should know their patients' "scores." *Health Affairs, 32,* 216–222.

Hoagwood, K. E. (2010). Family support in children's mental health: A review and synthesis. *Clinical Child and Family Psychology Review, 13,* 1–45.

Institute of Medicine. (2001). *Crossing the quality chasm: A new health system for the 21st century.* Washington, DC: National Academy Press.

Institute of Medicine. (2006). *Improving the quality of care for mental and substance use conditions: Quality chasm series.* Washington, DC: National Academy Press.

Jones, D. J. (2014). Future directions in the design, development, and investigation of technology as a service delivery vehicle. *Journal of Clinical Child and Adolescent Psychology, 43,* 128–142.

Kadivar, H., Thompson, L., Wegman, M., Chisholm, T., Khan, M., Eddleton, K., et al. (2014). Adolescent views on comprehensive health risk assessment and counseling: Assessing gender differences. *Journal of Adolescent Health, 55,* 24–32.

Kazdin, A. E., & Rabbitt, S. M. (2013). Novel models for delivering mental health services and reducing the burdens of mental illness. *Clinical Psychological Science, 1,* 170–191.

Kemp, S. P., Marcenko, M. O., Lyons, S. J., & Kruzich, J. M. (2014). Strength-based practice and parental engagement in child welfare services: An empirical examination. *Children and Youth Services Review, 47,* 27–35.

Kumar, S., Nilsen, W. J., Abernethy, A., Atienza, A., Patrick, K., Pavel, M., et al. (2013). Mobile health technology evaluation: The mHealth evidence workshop. *American Journal of Preventive Medicine, 45,* 228–236.

Lenhart, A. (2015). Teens, social media and technology overview 2015. Pew Research

Center. Retrieved November 20, 2015, from *www.pewinternet.org/files/2015/04/ PI_TeensandTech_Update2015_0409151.pdf*.

Levy, S. J. L., & Kokotailo, P. K. (2011). Substance use screening, brief intervention, and referral to treatment for pediatricians. *Pediatrics, 128*(5), e1330–e1340.

Levy, S., Weiss, R., Sherritt, L., Ziemnik, R., Spalding, A., Van Hook, S., et al. (2014). An electronic screen for triaging adolescent substance use by risk levels. *JAMA Pediatrics, 168*(9), 822–828.

Liddle, H. A. (2002). *Multidimensional family therapy for adolescent cannabis users: Cannabis youth treatment series, Vol. 5* (DHHS Publication No. 02-3660). Rockville, MD: Center for Substance Abuse Treatment, Substance Abuse and Mental Health.

Logan, D. E., & King, C. A. (2001). Parental facilitation of adolescent mental health services utilization: A conceptual and empirical review. *Clinical Psychology: Science and Practice, 8*, 319–333.

Macfarlane, D. (2005). *Current state of collaborative mental health care.* Mississauga: Canadian Collaborative Mental Health Initiative. Retrieved December 3, 2015, from *www.ccmhi.ca/en/products/documents/12_OverviewPaper_EN.pdf*.

McGillicuddy, N. B., Rychtarik, R. G., Morsheimer, E. T., & Bruke-Storer, M. R. (2012). Agreement between parent and adolescent reports of adolescent substance use. *Journal of Child and Adolescent Substance Abuse, 16*, 59–78.

McLellan, A. T., & Meyers, K. (2004). Contemporary addiction treatment: A review of systems problems for adults and adolescents. *Biological Psychiatry, 56*(10), 764–770.

Mitchell, S. G., Gryczynski, J., O'Grady, K. E., & Schwartz, R. P. (2013). SBIRT for adolescent drug and alcohol use: Current status and future directions. *Journal of Substance Abuse Treatment, 44*, 463–472.

Mitchell, S. G., Schwartz, R. P., Kirk, A. S., Dusek, K., Oros, M., Hosler, C., et al. (2016). SBIRT implementation for adolescents in urban federally qualified health centers. *Journal of Substance Abuse Treatment, 60*, 81–90.

Moyer, V. A. (2013). Screening and behavioral counseling interventions in primary care to reduce alcohol misuse: U.S. Preventive Services Task Force recommendation statement. *Annals of Internal Medicine, 159*, 210–218.

National Drug Intelligence Center. (2011). *The economic impact of illicit drug use on American society.* Washington, DC: U.S. Department of Justice.

National Institute on Alcohol Abuse and Alcoholism. (2011). *Alcohol screening and brief intervention for youth: A practitioner's guide* (NIH Publication No. 11-7805). Bethesda, MD: Author.

Ozechowski, T. J., Becker, S. J., & Hogue, A. (2016). SBIRT-A: Adapting SBIRT to maximize developmental fit for adolescents in primary care. *Journal of Substance Abuse Treatment, 62*, 28–37.

Ozechowski, T. J., & Waldron, H. B. (2010). Assertive outreach strategies for narrowing the adolescent substance abuse treatment gap: Implications for research, practice, and policy. *Journal of Behavioral Health Services and Research, 37*, 40–63.

Pedersen, E. R., Grow, J., Duncan, S., Neighbors, C., & Larimer, M. E. (2012). Concurrent validity of an online version of the Timeline Followback assessment. *Psychology of Addictive Behaviors, 26*, 672.

President's New Freedom Commission on Mental Health. (2003). *Achieving the promise:*

Transforming mental health care in America (Final Report) (DHHS Publication No. SMA-03-3832). Rockville, MD: Substance Abuse and Mental Health Services Administration.

Roy-Byrne, P., Bumgardner, K., Krupski, A., Dunn, C., Ries, R., Donovan, D., et al. (2014). Brief intervention for problem drug use in safety-net primary care settings: A randomized clinical trial. *JAMA, 312,* 492–501.

Saitz, R., Palfai, T. P., Cheng, D. M., Alford, D. P., Bernstein, J. A., Lloyd-Travaglini, C. A., et al. (2014). Screening and brief intervention for drug use in primary care: The ASPIRE randomized clinical trial. *JAMA, 312,* 502–513.

Sanders, J., & Munford, R. (2014). Youth-centered practice: Positive youth development practices and pathways to better outcomes for vulnerable youth. *Children and Youth Services Review, 46,* 160–167.

Sterling, S., Kline-Simon, A. H., Wibbelsman, C., Wong, A., & Weisner, C. (2012). Screening for adolescent alcohol and drug use in pediatric health-care settings: Predictors and implications for practice and policy. *Addiction Science and Clinical Practice, 7,* 13.

Stiffman, A. R., Pescosolido, B., & Cabassa, L. J. (2004). Building a model to understand youth service access: The gateway provider model. *Mental Health Services Research, 6*(4), 189–198.

Stoner, S. A., Mikko, A. T., & Carpenter, K. M. (2014). Web-based training for primary care providers on screening, brief intervention, and referral to treatment (SBIRT) for alcohol, tobacco, and other drugs. *Journal of Substance Abuse Treatment, 47,* 362–370.

Stroul, B. A., & Blau, G. M. (2008). *The system of care handbook: Transforming mental health services for children, youth, and families.* Baltimore: Brookes.

Substance Abuse and Mental Health Services Administration. (2013). *Systems-level implementation of screening, brief intervention, and referral to treatment* (Technical Assistance Publication [TAP] Series 33; HHS Publication No. [SMA] 13-4741). Rockville, MD: Author.

Szapocznik, J., Zarate, M., Duff, J., & Muir, J. (2013). Brief strategic family therapy: Engaging drug using/problem behavior adolescents and their families in treatment. *Social Work in Public Health, 28,* 206–223.

Tanner-Smith, E. E., & Lipsey, M. W. (2015). Brief alcohol interventions for adolescents and young adults: A systematic review and meta-analysis. *Journal of Substance Abuse Treatment, 51,* 1–18.

Turner, S. D., Spithoff, S., & Kahan, M. (2014). Approach to cannabis use disorder in primary care: Focus on youth and other high-risk users. *Canadian Family Physician, 60,* 801–808.

U.S. Department of Health and Human Services. (1999). *Mental Health: A Report of the Surgeon General.* Rockville, MD: Substance Abuse and Mental Health Services Administration and National Institutes of Health, National Institute of Mental Health.

Walton, M. A., Bohnert, K., Resko, S., Barry, K. L., Chermack, S. T., Zucker, R. A., et al. (2013). Computer and therapist based brief interventions among cannabis-using adolescents presenting to primary care: One year outcomes. *Drug and Alcohol Dependence, 132,* 646–653.

Wandersman, A., Chien, V. H., & Katz, J. (2012). Toward an evidence-based system for innovation support for implementing innovations with quality: Tools, training, technical assistance, and quality assurance/quality improvement. *American Journal of Community Psychology, 50,* 445–459.

Winters, K. C., Fahnhorst, T., Botzet, A., Lee, S., & Lalone, B. (2012). Brief intervention for drug-abusing adolescents in a school setting: Outcomes and mediating factors. *Journal of Substance Abuse Treatment, 42,* 279–288.

Winters, K. C., Leitten, W., Wagner, E., & O'Leary Tevyaw, T. (2007). Use of brief interventions within a middle and high school setting. *Journal of School Health, 77,* 196–206.

Wissow, L. S., Brown, J., Fothergill, K. E., Gadomski, A., Hacker, K., Salmon, P., et al. (2013). Universal mental health screening in pediatric primary care: A systematic review. *Journal of the American Academy of Child and Adolescent Psychiatry, 52,* 1134–1147.

Yatchmenoff, D. K. (2005). Measuring client engagement from the client's perspective in nonvoluntary child protective services. *Research on Social Work Practice, 15,* 84–96.

Zarkin, G., Bray, J., Hinde, J., & Saitz, R. (2015). Costs of screening and brief intervention for illicit drug use in primary care settings. *Journal of Studies on Alcohol and Drugs, 76,* 222–228.

PART II

CLINICAL GUIDE

*Application of Brief Interventions
in Diverse Settings and Populations*

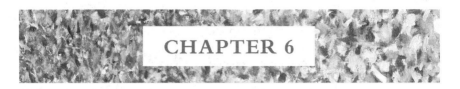

CHAPTER 6

Motivational Enhancement in Medical Settings for Adolescent Substance Use

Tracy O'Leary Tevyaw, Anthony Spirito,
Suzanne M. Colby, and Peter M. Monti

$\mathcal{A}$dolescent substance use and abuse is a significant public health concern due to its prevalence and associated negative consequences (see Schulenberg, Maslowsky, Maggs, & Zucker, Chapter 1, and Winters, Botzet, & Lee, Chapter 3, this volume). Two-thirds of 12th graders have tried alcohol in their lifetime (Johnston, O'Malley, Miech, Bachman, & Schulenberg, 2014). Using alcohol and other substances during adolescence is particularly concerning because early-onset substance use increases the risk of developing a substance use disorder (SUD; Flory, Lynam, Milich, Leukefeld, & Clayton, 2004; Winters & Lee, 2008). Moreover, regular alcohol use during adolescence is associated with myriad adverse outcomes, including co-occurring mental health problems, school dropout, delinquency, sexual risk behaviors, and related sexually transmitted infections (Armstrong & Costello, 2002; Barnes, Welte, & Hartman, 2002; Tubman, Gil, Wagner, & Artigues, 2003). Recent research strongly suggests that alcohol and substance use during this vulnerable period may result in irreversible damage to the developing brain (Brown et al., 2008; Spear, 2014; Lisdahl, Shollenbarger, Sagar, & Gruber, Chapter 2, this volume). Indeed, alcohol use plays a major role in the three leading causes of death among adolescents: unintentional injury (e.g., motor vehicle crashes, drowning), suicide, and homicide (Heron, 2013).

Because adolescents typically do not identify themselves as problem drinkers, an optimal approach includes proactive screening, assessment, and interventions in medical settings, where adolescents are likely to present. For instance, in 2010 there were approximately 189,000 emergency department (ED) visits for underage drinking (Substance Abuse and Mental Health Services Administration, Center for Behavioral Health Statistics and Quality, 2012). Rates of alcohol misuse in adolescents who present to the ED range from 4 to 10% (Fairlie, Sindelar, Eaton, & Spirito, 2006; Kelly, Donovan, Kinnane, & Taylor, 2002; Spirito et al., 2004). In one study of a Level I pediatric trauma center, 30% of adolescents admitted to the hospital following a trauma-related injury screened positive for alcohol misuse (Ehrlich et al., 2010). Rates of positive substance abuse screens among adolescents in primary care clinics approaches 15% (Knight et al., 2007).

Medical settings also provide an opportunity to reach adolescents who need intervention but who are not served by other services. In one retrospective study of a large health care plan that included privately insured adolescents and adolescents insured through government programs, close to 70% of adolescents received preventive medical care at least once annually (Nordin, Solberg, & Parker, 2010).

For the past two decades, our group has focused on detecting and screening for alcohol use in teens in the ED (Barnett et al., 1998; Chung et al., 2000; Colby et al., 1999, 2002). Our approach is consistent with the SBIRT model—Screening, Brief Interventions, and Referral to Treatment—a public health approach to early identification and intervention for at-risk alcohol and other substance use in targeted settings (see Mitchell, Gryczynski, O'Grady, & Schwartz, 2013, for a review of SBIRT for adolescents).

We have examined characteristics of and risk factors for alcohol use among adolescents in the ED setting (Barnett, Goldstein, Murphy, Colby, & Monti, 2006; Barnett et al., 2003; Monti, 1997; Spirito et al., 2001), and developed and tested brief interventions for adolescents in the ED (Monti et al., 2007; Spirito et al., 2004, 2011). Conducting a brief alcohol intervention in the ED also allows us to capitalize on a "teachable moment" or a "window of opportunity." For example, adolescents treated in an ED for an alcohol-related event (such as an alcohol overdose or an alcohol-related motor vehicle crash) may be especially receptive to an alcohol intervention due to the salience of the event and their negative emotional reaction to it. Furthermore, if they are frightened and upset when they arrive, it is likely that the confusion and often long wait in a busy ED will increase their discomfort. In our own work (Barnett et al., 2002), we have found that adolescents whose injuries were severe enough that they were later admitted to the hospital from the ED reported greater intent to change drinking than those not admitted. Clinicians can capitalize on these compelling factors to elicit ambivalence from teens about their alcohol use and promote interest in reducing dangerous drinking. A recent meta-analysis of six motivational interviewing (MI) trials delivered in ED settings to adolescents found that drinking frequency decreased significantly more among adolescents receiving MI versus a control condition, and drinking quantity decreased significantly more among adolescents receiving MI versus control (Kohler & Hofmann, 2015).

In this chapter we present our MI approach that we believe is particularly well suited for use in an ED. It combines a collaborative, nonjudgmental, empathic therapeutic style (Miller & Rollnick, 2012) with personalized feedback regarding drinking patterns and effects. The brevity of an MI makes it particularly suitable for use in an ED or other medical settings. This chapter outlines clinical research that has been conducted with adolescents who range from 13 to 19 years of age. All teens were treated individually with the same treatment approach, except that the parents of 13- to 17-year-olds were approached for informed consent and possible involvement in the treatment. Although our work has involved adolescents who volunteer to participate in our studies, this approach has wide applicability to treatment programs, to programs for adjudicated youths, and to a variety of prevention efforts.

In the following section, we first present detailed step-by-step coverage of our MI approach, illustrated with relevant clinical examples. Next, we present several topics that require special attention, including counselor training, other populations of interest, treatment modality issues, and dealing with other substances of abuse. Finally, we briefly present empirical results for our approach, conclusions, and some future directions for this line of research.

THE MI SESSION

The MI protocol we have developed for our research program focuses on alcohol consumption and risky behavior, with an emphasis on heavy drinking and driving after drinking. As is consistent with an MI approach, the intervention should be modified, as appropriate, to be meaningful for each teen and his or her level of interest in changing. The session description that follows is typically conducted in about 45 minutes. Because we are intervening with teens who have been treated in an ED for alcohol-related reasons (e.g., motor vehicle crash, assault, intoxication), we wait for their blood alcohol concentration (BAC) to decrease and administer a Mini-Mental State Exam to ensure that they are able to understand and provide informed consent to participate in the intervention.

Introduction and Engagement

The introduction can be made prior to the assessment (which may promote more honest responding to questions) or prior to the MI. The purpose of the introduction is to provide the teen with an idea of the content, style, and limitations of the time that will be spent with the counselor. We introduce the session as an opportunity for teens to talk about their thoughts and feelings regarding the event that brought them to the ED, to get some information about their pattern of drinking, the effects of alcohol on their behavior, and to spend some time, if they are interested, talking about ways to avoid similar things happening in the future. Counselors emphasize that they will not tell the teen what to do—rather, it is up to the teen to make decisions and choices about drinking and about things he or she does when drinking. The circumstances that precipitated the ED visit are then explored, including how much the teen had been drinking, with whom he or she was drinking, and any injuries sustained or consequences suffered. The use of open-ended questions in this part of the interview enhances rapport and helps the counselor rapidly develop an understanding of the teen's recent drinking patterns and associations. An open-ended question is a question that cannot be answered with one word or very brief responses. For example, asking "Tell me more about what happened around the time of the incident" is open-ended, whereas "Were you drinking at the time of the incident?" is not.

For sessions that are preventive in nature (i.e., not following an identifiable alcohol-related event), the purpose of the session can be articulated as an opportunity to talk about experiences with alcohol and to address any concerns or questions the teen might have. Whether or not there is a precipitating event, the counselor should overtly state his or her interest in getting the teen's perspective at the outset and demonstrate that interest throughout the session.

The introduction provides an opportunity to establish rapport and minimize defensiveness. The counselor should present an empathic, concerned, nonauthoritarian, and nonjudgmental style (Miller & Rollnick, 2012). It is important for teens to believe that the counselor respects their ideas, is interested in hearing about their experiences, and will not scold them or make disapproving statements about their behavior. This introduction is straightforward and can be used regardless of the nature of the referral (i.e., voluntary or involuntary).

The following introductory statements illustrate the manner in which we describe the MI session to teens. We discuss the structure, content, and aim of the session, with repeated emphasis on the teen's personal responsibility and choice regarding changing alcohol use. Notice the collaborative tenor of the introduction, in that the counselor is establishing that the two will work together to generate strategies to avoid similar situations in the future.

> "What I'd like to do now is explore with you your alcohol use. We're concerned about risky drinking and other risky behaviors that tend to go along with drinking, like driving. I can't tell you what to do; only you can decide what you'll do. Rather, I'd like to find out what you think about drinking after this experience and maybe see if together we can come up with some ways to avoid these kinds of situations in the future. You're the one who will decide what happens with your drinking. If you choose, you can make changes in

your drinking, but that's really up to you. How does that sound? Can we try this out?"

Many teens express concerns about divulging information about their alcohol use. The following illustrates how we broach the sensitive topic of confidentiality with teens in the ED. Brittany, a 17-year-old white female who arrived by ambulance at the ED after being involved in a motor vehicle crash in which she was the driver, shares her concerns with the counselor.

COUNSELOR: First, before we begin, I'd like to talk to you about the project and what we'll be doing. I'll ask you questions about your alcohol use and other substance use, ask you about the events that led up to the car crash, give you some information from the questionnaires you completed earlier if you're interested, and talk about some ways you may be able to avoid this kind of thing happening again. How does that sound?

BRITTANY: Well, I don't know. . . . I don't know how much I want to talk about what happened. I don't want this going on my permanent record. I really don't want anyone to know what happened, and besides, I was in a car accident. I probably shouldn't say anything at all.

COUNSELOR: I can understand how you might feel that way. Let me tell you about confidentiality and its limits. Everything you tell us is kept strictly confidential—that means that I will not share the information you give me nor anything you say during our discussion with anyone, including your parents or the staff here at the ED. The only times when I'm required by law to report information to the authorities are as follows: when a person says that they are going to hurt themselves or hurt others or when there's suspicion of child abuse or neglect or elder abuse or neglect.

At this point, the counselor would describe the limits to confidentiality specific to their local laws and jurisdiction. The clinician would also inform the adolescent that the contents of the clinical note entered into their medical record would be limited to a discussion with the adolescent about the car crash. Researchers working with adolescents in clinical trials can also secure a certificate of confidentiality from the National Institutes of Health (NIH), through the institution where the research is being conducted. A certificate of confidentiality serves to further protect the privacy of adolescents who participate in research considered sensitive, which includes research on substance use. The interested reader is directed to NIH's website *https://humansubjects.nih.gov/coc/background* for further information.

BRITTANY: Um, I don't want the police to know what I say.

COUNSELOR: We also protect your confidentiality outside of the ED setting. So, if the police, your school, or anyone else called and wanted information, we couldn't release anything to them. We also don't acknowledge that you even participated in the project. The only way they would know if you participated in this project would be if you told them.

BRITTANY: Oh, I see. Well, I guess that sounds OK. What if I decide that I don't want to do this anymore? Will you tell anyone then?

COUNSELOR: No. If you decided not to continue in the project, we wouldn't tell anyone about any of the information you gave us. We keep all of the information teenagers give us in a locked filing cabinet, and the only people who have access to it are those directly involved in the research project. Your name is not on any of the questionnaires you answer.

BRITTANY: OK, I feel a little better about it. You can go ahead with your questions.

COUNSELOR: Great. Let's get started.

Participant Assessment

In our program, assessment instruments serve a dual purpose. They are used as a measure of target behaviors at the initial session and at later assessments to detect any changes over time, and they are also used to provide personalized feedback to teens within the MI session. Assessments are administered after the basic structure of the program has been described. In our ED setting, measures are interviewer administered, but other facilities may prefer to have teens self-administer the questionnaires. Paper-and-pencil versions may be used, or measures can be computerized for ease of administration, data collection, and development of personalized feedback. The structure of the program and the resources available will determine the nature of the assessment. An important distinction when choosing assessments is to decide whether it is an objective of the program to provide teens with a perspective on how they compare with other teens of the same gender and age. In order to provide such "normative information," it is necessary to use measures that have age and gender norms available.

In an ED setting, our goal is to construct an assessment that is sufficiently comprehensive to obtain an accurate baseline evaluation, as well as feedback for the MI, yet brief enough to keep intervention in the ED feasible. Our assessment includes measures on alcohol frequency and quantity, alcohol tolerance and withdrawal (e.g., drinking to intoxication, needing to drink more to obtain the same effects, experiencing hangovers), drinking to cope with negative affect, negative consequences related to alcohol use, alcohol-related injuries, engagement in risky or hazardous behaviors and the degree to which alcohol was involved, and utilization of safe strategies to avoid drinking and driving. In other settings, more extensive assessment sessions at baseline may be desirable. (See National Institute on Alcohol Abuse and Alcoholism, 2003; Winters et al., Chapter 3, this volume, for information on instruments appropriate for use with adolescents.)

Exploring Motivation

Once the assessment is complete and teens have been oriented to the MI session, they are asked what they like and don't like about drinking. Open-ended
questions are used to encourage teens to generate all their likes and dislikes
about drinking and to talk about the effects that matter most to them. In our
program, teens are also asked why they might drive after drinking and what
they do not like about driving after drinking (including the worst thing they
could imagine happening). They are asked to elaborate on their parents' and
friends' attitudes toward drinking and toward drinking and driving and on how
those attitudes might affect their own drinking behaviors.

The counselor's goal in this section of the MI session is to gain an understanding of the teen's perceptions about his or her drinking. By discussing the
teen's perceived pros and cons of drinking, the counselor and teen can develop
a shared understanding of what aspects serve as reinforcers for drinking (which
could be potential barriers to change) and what elements (i.e., consequences
of drinking) might serve as reasons for reducing alcohol use. The counselor
can then tailor the MI to these personalized barriers and facilitators of change,
while keeping in mind the teen's interest in and readiness for changing drinking behavior. This discussion also assists the counselor in identifying influences
on the teen's behaviors in the form of peer and parental behavior and attitudes
and the importance of these influences, according to the teen.

Although it can be useful to elicit the pros as well as the cons of drinking, particularly among adolescents showing strong resistance to considering
making any changes, current research has shown that the emphasis of the MI
session should be on the cons of drinking and facilitating and promoting *change
talk* (self-expressed language that demonstrates movement toward change) versus *sustain talk* (self-expressed language against change; Apodaca et al., 2014,
2016; Baer et al., 2008; Gaume et al., 2016; Magill et al., 2016). Change talk
(Moyers & Martin, 2006) are in-session verbalizations that are more likely to
occur when therapists engage in MI-consistent behaviors (affirm strengths,
emphasize the individual's control over decision making, seek permission to
give feedback or advice) versus MI-inconsistent behaviors (give advice without
permission, confront individuals, provide unsolicited instructions on how to
change). Indeed, Baer and colleagues (2008) reported that among adolescents
who were not treatment seeking, change talk during MI sessions was associated
with significantly greater reductions in substance use at follow-up. In contrast,
sustain talk, specifically, adolescents' statements about not wanting, not needing, or not feeling able to change, was significantly associated with worse outcomes, *even when sustain talk was infrequently verbalized by the adolescent in session.* This illustrates how important it is for the counselor to guide discussions
to topics focused on reasons for change and to avoid discussions that promote
sustain talk. Moreover, in one of our studies of younger adults in the ED (average age = 28.6 years, SD = 9.2), we found that change talk was more likely to

occur in MI sessions when discussing (1) barriers to and facilitators of change (e.g., "What obstacles do you see getting in the way of making these changes?"; "What gives you hope that you can change your drinking?"), (2) the benefits of target behavior change (e.g., "What are some of the good things that will happen if you make these changes?"), and (3) change planning (e.g., "Where does this leave you in terms of making a change in your drinking?"; Kahler et al., 2016). However, there may be an important exception to this rule, as reviewed in the example below.

Jayden, a 19-year-old Latino male working full time after graduating from high school, was seen in the ED after suffering lacerations following a fight in a nightclub. The lack of perceived cons of drinking on Jayden's part, coupled with his statements regarding his alcohol use, indicate that he is not considering changing his drinking. He does not perceive himself to have any alcohol-related problems and has expressed no intentions to change his drinking in the near future. In working with adolescents like Jayden who express little to no ambivalence about their substance use, the counselor's aim is to develop rapport by understanding Jayden's perceived pros for drinking, and *then* to actively steer the discussion toward change talk topics, while affirming Jayden's autonomy and control in the decision-making process. Eliciting and listening to Jayden's perspectives first, without jumping in too early to discuss reasons to change, allows the counselor to set a more collaborative, less confrontational tone and decrease the likelihood of increasing resistance. Indeed, using reflective listening skills when reviewing perceived pros and cons with adolescents may serve to heighten ambivalence about use and to potentially increase opportunities for change talk (Feldstein Ewing, Apodaca, & Gaume, 2016). A recent meta-analysis of eight studies of brief alcohol interventions for adolescents showed significantly greater reductions in alcohol consumption levels when decisional balance (reviewing pros and cons of drinking) and goal-setting exercises were used (Tanner-Smith & Lipsey, 2015).

COUNSELOR: What do you like about your drinking?

JAYDEN: Hmm . . . I like how I feel when I drink.

COUNSELOR: In what way?

JAYDEN: Uh, well, drinking relaxes me. It's a social thing, a way to hang out with my boys at the club and have a good time.

COUNSELOR: You enjoy the chance to socialize with your friends. Anything else?

JAYDEN: I can forget about work. It's a way to celebrate the end of the week for me. I work 60 hours a week doing construction, man. It's hard work.

COUNSELOR: So, you like drinking because it makes you feel relaxed. It's a means for getting together with friends, and forgetting about work. Is that about right?

JAYDEN: Yeah, and I like the way it tastes, especially when I've been working outside.

COUNSELOR: How about the things you don't like as much about your drinking?

JAYDEN: Well, there's really nothing I don't like about it. I don't have any problems with drinking. Just because I got into a fight doesn't mean I have an alcohol problem.

COUNSELOR: You feel that drinking isn't an issue for you.

JAYDEN: Absolutely, and I won't listen to someone telling me that it is!

COUNSELOR: I hear a lot of irritation in your voice, and I wonder if there have been people in your life who have accused you of having an alcohol problem.

JAYDEN: Oh, yeah. My mother and my girlfriend. What do they know? They don't drink and they think it's OK to get on my back because I have a few beers on the weekend.

COUNSELOR: We both agree that it's not helpful to make judgments about others, and I'm not here to tell you what to do. We've just met, and I'd like to hear your own perspective and thoughts. What are some of the not-so-good things about drinking?

JAYDEN: Like I said, there's not really anything I don't like. Well, maybe the cost. I only like the good stuff, and after a while it can add up.

COUNSELOR: So, how much money you're spending is one thing you don't like about drinking. What else?

JAYDEN: That's it.

COUNSELOR: May I ask you about some things that others have said they don't like about drinking and hear your thoughts on them?

JAYDEN: Sure. Whatever.

COUNSELOR: Some people don't like how they feel the next day after drinking; they might get very sick, or hung over, or can't remember everything that happened the night before.

JAYDEN: Oh, I see what you mean. Of course, I don't enjoy getting hangovers. That doesn't happen too much, so it's not a problem for me.

COUNSELOR: So, let's see if I have it right. There are a few things you like about drinking, but there are several things you don't like about drinking—the amount of money you spend on alcohol, getting hangovers, and having to deal with your mother and your girlfriend getting on your case about drinking.

JAYDEN: You hit the nail on the head. That's about it.

COUNSELOR: "Where does this leave you now?"

It is important to note that development of the capacity for abstract reasoning, self-reflection, and other executive functions involved in self-regulation and the processing of ambivalence can vary among adolescents of the same age (Lyons & Zelazo, 2011). Arun, a 16-year-old Asian male, was admitted to the ED following injuries sustained in a bicycle accident where alcohol was involved. He perceived the pros of his alcohol use to far outweigh the cons; this was mainly due to his perceived lack of negative consequences from drinking, as well as the recent onset of his alcohol use (in the past 3 months). The following vignette illustrates how the counselor "tips the balance" to highlight the negative consequences of drinking and thereby increase discrepancy between Arun's drinking behaviors and his goals.

COUNSELOR: So, you mentioned earlier some of the things you like about your drinking. Tell me some of the things you don't like as much about your drinking.

ARUN: There's really nothing I don't like about drinking. It's not like I've been drinking a long time, you know.

COUNSELOR: You shared with me earlier that you fell off your bike while giving your friend a ride and that you and he had been drinking. How does alcohol fit into what happened to bring you to the emergency room tonight?

ARUN: Oh. I guess that's true, I was drinking before it happened, but only a little bit.

COUNSELOR: So, although you feel you weren't drinking that much tonight, you see that maybe there's a connection between drinking and falling.

ARUN: Yeah, I see what you mean. Not a big connection, though! If my friend knew how to balance on the back, it wouldn't have happened.

COUNSELOR: And what has it been like for you here in the ED?

ARUN: Well, it sucks. I have a broken arm, it hurts a lot, and the doctors make you wait forever before one of them even talks to you!

COUNSELOR: So, if I were to sum up, there are some things you like about alcohol. However, you see a link between drinking and having this broken arm and having to spend your evening stuck here in the hospital, which hasn't been pleasant for you at all! Do I have that about right?

ARUN: Yeah. This is the first time that I've had something like this happen to me.

COUNSELOR: And it sounds like you want it to be your last bad experience!

Enhancing Motivation

The purpose of this section of the MI is to increase teens' understanding of their patterns of alcohol use, to provide information about indicators of problem drinking, and to promote interest in making positive changes to hazardous drinking patterns. We do this in three ways. We provide personalized feedback from the assessment instruments, including a comparison of the teen's scores to age and gender norms. We also provide information about alcohol and its effects, for example, alcohol's effects on driving skills. Finally, we ask the teens to elaborate on what they imagine the future would be like if they were to change.

Personalized Feedback

Personalized feedback has been a key element of many effective brief interventions (Dotson, Dunn, & Bowers, 2015). Face-to-face feedback from a counselor appears to result in significantly better outcomes than computerized feedback without a counselor present (Barnett, Sussman, Smith, Rohrback, & Spruijt-Metz, 2012; Walton et al., 2010), and thus feedback from the counselor is a central feature of our intervention. The computer program we have developed generates a printed personalized feedback sheet that the counselor discusses and reviews with the teen that summarizes information gathered during the assessment. This feedback provides age- and gender-based normative information (i.e., percentile rank) on drinking frequency and quantity per drinking episode; frequency of drunkenness; and alcohol-related problems with family, friends, and school. Indices of physical and emotional dependence (including signs of tolerance and withdrawal) and risk taking related to alcohol use are also provided. In addition, we provide personalized feedback about the number of strategies the teen has used in the past to avoid driving or riding with a drinking driver. A computer program is not necessary in order to provide feedback; information from normative tables and levels of risk can be transcribed or hand calculated.

The counselor can give the assessment feedback to the teen all at once, reserving discussion for the very end, or discuss the separate sections as they are presented. Throughout, the counselor determines whether the teen understands the information and elicits reactions and questions. As in other parts of the interview, the counselor must make decisions about what aspects of the feedback to focus on or emphasize. For example, less severe scores on feedback sections might be highlighted as a sign of strength or potential for change, or, if the counselor is trying to elicit concern from the teen, might be de-emphasized. Once the feedback has been explained, it is useful to ask teens what aspects they were most surprised by and what was most disturbing to them. The counselor should help the teen interpret the meaning of the feedback. For example, teens who are discouraged by the results can be reminded that negative results can improve with behavior change.

In the interest of time, we present an abbreviated version of the feedback to the teen during the MI and provide a more detailed version to take home. Language is kept simple and to the point, with risks expressed in a concerned, but matter-of-fact, way. Including simple graphics to illustrate scores and statistics in the feedback helps to engage teens and can better facilitate work with those who do not read well. As with text, graphics should be explained. This section is designed to correct overestimations, common among adolescents, about the prevalence of alcohol and other substance use in their age group (i.e., the false consensus effect) and to provide an opportunity to discuss the increased problems that are associated with heavy alcohol and other substance use.

Ryan is a 15-year-old white male brought into the ED after becoming intoxicated at a school dance. He is not only surprised about his personalized assessment feedback but is also challenging the veracity of the information and the counselor's interpretation of the results. Rather than increasing resistance by telling Ryan that he's wrong, the counselor instead reflects Ryan's disbelief and uses it as a means of developing discrepancy between his alcohol use and his future goals, and heightening ambivalence about his alcohol use. The following clinical vignette illustrates the use of reflective listening and rolling with resistance.

COUNSELOR: What I'd like to do now is go over the results of some of the questionnaires you answered with me. How does that sound?

RYAN: OK, I guess.

COUNSELOR: There are a lot of numbers here, but I'll explain each one. Please ask questions or make comments as we go along. On this first section, we compared your drinking with the drinking of other teenage males your age. You drink more than 8 out of 10 of them.

RYAN: No way! That can't be right. I have friends who drink way more than I do.

COUNSELOR: So, you don't think these numbers are correct.

RYAN: Well, I didn't say that. I just don't drink that much compared to all my friends, that's all.

COUNSELOR: I can see how this might be confusing to you. You don't feel that you drink very much at all, compared to your friends, and yet your drinking rates turn out to be higher than most teenage males your age. It's hard to figure out.

RYAN: Definitely! Some of my friends can drink a six-pack no problem, and they're fine. Where did you get this from?

COUNSELOR: These figures are from a statewide survey of teenagers on alcohol use. I can see why you'd be surprised, because your friends drink more than you do and yet your levels are higher than most teenagers in our state. The reason for this is that the survey reflects a large number of teenagers. Some of them drink more than you do, some drink less, and still others don't drink alcohol at all. This feedback compares you to all of those teenagers.

RYAN: But what about my friends? I also know a lot of other guys who drink a lot more than I do. How do you explain that?

COUNSELOR: What happens is that we tend to hang out with people who are similar to ourselves and who like to do the same things. People who drink at higher levels usually have friends who drink at those same levels. So, it can seem like most guys your age drink the same as you do, because that's been your experience. In fact, more boys your age drink less than you do.

RYAN: Wow, that's really hard to believe. (*Looks surprised, becomes quiet.*)

COUNSELOR: This really doesn't fit with how you see yourself.

RYAN: Yeah. I don't know what to think about it. I honestly never thought I drank that much.

Information

When relevant, information about blood alcohol level and metabolization of alcohol, effects of alcohol on driving, and related topics can be discussed. In our program, teens are tested for their blood alcohol levels at the time they are treated at the hospital, which provides the basis for discussion. Teens are usually receptive to information about the effects of alcohol at different levels, including the fact that even very low levels of alcohol can impair driving. Information about estimated blood alcohol concentration (eBAC) may also be provided, given that individuals often have difficulty accurately assessing their own BAC level (see Grant, LaBrie, Hummer, & Lac, 2012; Quinn & Fromme, 2011). This can be particularly helpful feedback for those with low sensitivity to the effects of alcohol (i.e., less reported subjective perceptions of intoxication), which is a well-established risk factor for alcohol use disorder. For example, in one study of younger social drinkers, low alcohol sensitivity was associated with a pattern of drinking "too much, too fast" as seen by a steeper ascending eBAC trajectory (Trela, Piasecki, Bartholow, Heath, & Sher, 2016). The "too much, too fast" pattern is akin to binge drinking. For teens, discussion of this topic could include feedback about the benefits of being aware and mindful of the amount of alcohol consumed and the potential pitfalls of relying on how "buzzed" the teen feels when making decisions about drinking.

Envisioning the Future

Motivation can be further enhanced by asking teens to imagine the future if their drinking were to change. This approach is intended to introduce the idea of making a change that might have a positive outcome. If there is a discrepancy between a teen's current drinking pattern and his or her goals for the future, such a discrepancy may provide a motivating function and should be highlighted. For example, if a teen has future athletic aspirations, the counselor could highlight the discrepancy between the goal of highly skilled performance in his or her sport and the teen's current pattern of behavior. Some areas to introduce are the possible reactions of family and friends. An example of a prompt might be "If you decided to make a change, what do you think would become easier in your life?"

Establishing a Plan

Regardless of the setting in which the intervention is conducted or the focus or length of the MI, the counselor and adolescent should leave the session with an understanding of what the teen is willing to do next. For example, if the motivational session is used as a precursor to entering a treatment program, appropriate goals might be to engage in the treatment program by attending a specific number of sessions or contributing at least one comment in each group attended. For other adolescents, one session of MI can be conceptualized as a precursor to self-change. In either case, teens have a greater chance of being successful at changing if they establish a well-considered plan and make a commitment to it.

Prior to discussing a plan, it is helpful to reassess the teens' interest in changing. Good open-ended questions to use are "Where does this leave you now?" or "What would you like to change?" Clinical tools, such as the readiness ruler (Maisto et al., 2011a, 2011b), also can be used. The readiness ruler provides an easily understood basis for talking about the teen's interest in changing and has anchors ranging from 1 (not ready to change) to 10 (trying hard to change). The teen is asked, "On a scale from 1 to 10, how interested are you in _____?" Follow-up questions, such as "What do you think would have to happen to increase that number?" can be used (Rollnick, Mason, & Butler, 1999).

The requirements and/or limitations of any further treatment should be understood and discussed with the teen when creating the behavior change plan. For example, adolescents entering a hospital treatment program likely will be required to abstain from alcohol or drug use, and this may be the expectation as well when they leave the program. In other settings (e.g., college campuses), abstinence may not be a realistic expectation, and both the counselor and the adolescent may be more comfortable taking a moderation approach to reduction in the harmful consequences of drinking. Although having predetermined behavioral expectations, such as abstinence, may limit the degree to which the MI is experienced as client centered and runs the risk of eliciting counterproductive or resistant responses from the adolescent, it is not an impossible situation and has been successfully integrated into 12-step treatment models (see Kelly, Cristello, & Bergman, Chapter 15, this volume).

In the final phase, the adolescent and counselor develop a plan for the future that covers goals for behavior change, barriers to changes, and strategic advice. A "goals sheet," which contains a variety of alcohol/other substance use moderation and harm reduction goals, as well as blank spaces for filling in other goals, such as attending school, can be used. Adolescents are asked to select the goals that they would like to attempt and to generate other goals that they have. In the final phase, the adolescent and counselor develop a plan for the future that covers goals for behavior change, barriers to changes, and strategic advice. Having adolescents select their goals provides the opportunity for the counselor to support the adolescent's self-efficacy about making changes.

The following vignette describes the process by which a counselor helps a 14-year-old ED patient in developing a behavior change plan for refraining from alcohol use. Kimani, an African American female, was found unconscious in a park and was brought to the ED by some concerned neighbors. She reported to the counselor at the ED that she had consumed several shots of tequila with friends in the park, passed out, and woke up to find herself in the

ED. The counselor and Kimani have reviewed her perceived pros and cons of drinking and have covered the results of the assessment.

COUNSELOR: What I'd like to do is talk to you a bit about what you think will happen if you continue to drink the same way.

KIMANI: I dunno. . . . I'm not supposed to drink at all, not just because it's against the law, either. I live in a group home, and I could get kicked out for this whole thing. Then I won't have a place to live, and they'll send me back into foster care.

COUNSELOR: So, right now you're worried about what will happen at the group home and whether you'll be allowed to continue to live there.

KIMANI: Yeah. (*Looks away, bites nails.*)

COUNSELOR: Clearly, then, if you keep drinking the way you did today, you won't be allowed to live in the group home. There's a good chance that you might have to leave. What else will happen?

KIMANI: (*Shrugs shoulders.*) I don't know.

COUNSELOR: May I tell you some of my own concerns as well?

KIMANI: If you want, I guess. I don't care.

COUNSELOR: Well, one concern is that your drinking levels are high compared with other girls your age. We talked earlier about tolerance, dependence, and withdrawal, and all of those things could worsen if you continue to drink at the same levels. Another concern is what we call "self-medicating" with alcohol. Your answers indicated that a lot of your drinking has to do with trying to feel better and forget about problems in your life. Generally, if a person keeps drinking for these reasons, it's not uncommon for them to have to drink even more over time to experience the same effects. Drinking at higher and higher levels is also related to experiencing more problems in life, so it can turn out to be a vicious cycle of drinking at higher levels, having more problems, and in turn, drinking even more.

KIMANI: Hmm. . . .

COUNSELOR: What would be the good things that would happen if you stopped drinking?

KIMANI: Um, well, I would be able to keep living in the group home.

COUNSELOR: Yes! That seems important to you. What else?

KIMANI: I wouldn't, like, get sick or have any more hangovers.

COUNSELOR: So, physically you'd feel better. What else?

KIMANI: My social worker might stop asking me her stupid questions about, like, "substance use."

COUNSELOR: You'd look forward to the end of those questions, because you could tell her that you're no longer drinking. That would be a relief, huh?

KIMANI: Yeah.

COUNSELOR: You know, just from our talk, I could imagine one or two more—would you like to hear them?

KIMANI: Yeah, sure.

COUNSELOR: One other good thing about stopping drinking is that your need to drink to cope with your feelings might also decrease. In other words, by not drinking, you might find other ways of feeling emotionally better—healthier ways that wouldn't get you in trouble and wouldn't cause more problems down the road. I can talk to you later about some of those ways to feel better without drinking, if you're interested.

KIMANI: Oh, you mean, like, exercising, or yoga? My social worker wants me to do that.

COUNSELOR: That's definitely one way to feel better, and there are other ways, too. I'd be happy to go over those with you. Now, back to the good things about stopping drinking, from what you've told me it seems that you are not allowed to drink at all, so you feel that you have to stop drinking altogether.

KIMANI: I'm not allowed to use anything or drink while I live in the group home. I can't even smoke, it's so bad in there.

COUNSELOR: Let's see . . . what are some ways that you can successfully stop drinking? What would work for you?

KIMANI: I have to say that I hate to exercise! I don't want to do that.

COUNSELOR: OK, so you feel that wouldn't work for you. Like I said, there are lots of strategies that people use. Would you be interested in going over some of the ones that others have tried that work?

KIMANI: Um, all right.

COUNSELOR: (Shows list of strategies to patient, and emphasizes abstinence-based strategies.) We can use this checklist as a jumping-off point. What do you think about some of these?

KIMANI: Uh, well, I think the one about talking to or texting a friend about how I feel—that might be OK. I like to text, so I can try that out. Maybe this one, too, about reminding myself of all the reasons why I don't want to drink and why I can't drink—like because I'll get kicked out of the group home if I do.

COUNSELOR: OK, you seem to have a good sense of what you want to try. That sounds like a great plan. Now part of the reason you said you were drinking today was because you were hanging out with friends who like to drink. What kinds of things can you do to keep yourself from drinking when you're with these friends?

KIMANI: I can ask them not to drink around me, but I don't think that they should have to stop what they're doing just because of me.

COUNSELOR: What else could you do that would work?

KIMANI: Um . . . I'm not sure.

COUNSELOR: May I suggest a few things?

KIMANI: Sure.

COUNSELOR: Sometimes people will ask their friends to do fun things that don't involve alcohol or to go places where alcohol isn't allowed. Other people will spend more time with friends who don't drink and spend less time with friends who do drink, because it's such a tempting situation for them. Which of those ideas might work for you?

KIMANI: I could do both of those things. That might work.

COUNSELOR: What might get in the way of you making these changes?

KIMANI: Well, if I'm around my friends who drink, and they give me a drink. I can never say no to that!

COUNSELOR: What could you do to avoid drinking if you're offered one?

KIMANI: Maybe ask them not to give me anything before I even get there, or maybe leave when I know that they're going to start to drink.

COUNSELOR: Those are great strategies!

The counselor can assist the teen in developing short- and long-term goals that are specific, measurable, attainable, reasonable, and time limited. This should include generating strategies for reducing drinking and risky behavior, determining which methods are acceptable to the teen, and exploring how these can be accomplished. If the teen is able to generate appropriate ways to reduce drinking and related behaviors, the counselor's main task is to help the teen specify which strategies to try and when as well as to imagine how they might work. However, teenagers will often be vague or uncertain about what they would like to do differently, and counselors must help them develop a list of specific strategies. For example, a teenager might say, "I just won't drink as much." The counselor's task in this case would be to help the adolescent specify a reduction goal that would place the teen at lower risk. Open-ended explorations, such as "Tell me how you might do that," can be used. A more direct response would be "We know that if you were to have no more than one drink an hour, your blood alcohol level wouldn't get too high. What do you think about that for a goal?" Depending on the teen, other suggestions about moderate drinking approaches, such as refusal skills and alternative coping strategies, can be presented.

Developing a plan with teens who are clear about not being interested in making any changes to their drinking is more challenging. In most cases, there will be some things the teen would like to avoid, like getting hurt after drinking or getting into dangerous circumstances. In these cases, focusing on avoiding those harmful consequences rather than alcohol consumption per se can be effective. In other cases, teens may be interested in keeping track of their drinking, such as self-monitoring drinks, or calculating how much money they spend on alcohol over a period of time. The purpose of these strategies is to increase the teen's awareness of his or her drinking and possibly raise his or her level of concern. Suggestions for working with adolescents with different degrees of interest and ideas about changing are presented in Table 6.1.

Josh, an 18-year-old white college student, admitted himself to the ED after sustaining injuries from falling off a porch at a party. His blood alcohol level registered at 0.20, indicating heavy, recent alcohol consumption. During the assessment, Josh reported engaging in several high-risk behaviors while drinking, particularly unprotected sexual activity. Although Josh was receptive to the intervention, he was reluctant to change his alcohol use altogether. Below is a description of the counselor guiding Josh in developing a harm reduction plan.

COUNSELOR: So, we've covered a lot of material together. I'm wondering, where does this leave you?

JOSH: I have no idea. Like I said, I'm not trying to be difficult, but I don't have an "alcohol problem." I drink just like everyone else at college does. I just had some bad luck tonight, that's all. In the wrong place at the wrong time, you know?

COUNSELOR: OK, so it's clear that you feel that your drinking isn't the issue here but that having to come to the ED was a stroke of bad luck. Nevertheless, I wonder if there are some things that you could do to prevent something similar from happening again to you, so that you can avoid this unpleasant experience altogether.

JOSH: You know, the funny thing is that I really didn't have fun at the party. I don't know why I went, really. One of the guys we were with wanted to go there, the idiot. There was a ton of people there and it was way too crowded. That's how I fell off the porch and hurt my leg—someone knocked into me. Now I'll have a nice scar to remind me forever of this miserable night.

COUNSELOR: It sounds like you're saying that going to parties that are very crowded is not fun for you, and it seems like you're leaning toward avoiding those kinds of situations from now on.

JOSH: Yeah, I think so.

COUNSELOR: You also mentioned that you were concerned about sleeping with people when you had been drinking and without using protection. From what you said, it sounded like you tend to do this when you've been drinking more than your usual amount, and typically this happens at parties like the one tonight. Is that right?

JOSH: Yup.

COUNSELOR: In addition to avoiding crowded parties, what are some other ways to avoid these kinds of situations?

JOSH: I only do this when I'm really wrecked out of my mind. I probably should pay more attention to how much I'm drinking so that I don't get lit.

COUNSELOR: How would you be able to tell when you're starting to "get lit"?

TABLE 6.1. How to Respond to Adolescents at Different Levels of Interest in Changing

Adolescent presentation	Counselor's task
The adolescent is interested in changing and has ideas about things to try.	1. Help the adolescent be specific about ways to reduce drinking and risk-related behavior. 2. Identify things that might get in the way of changing and help problem-solve around barriers: "What might make it hard to cut down on your drinking when you are with your friends? What could you do to handle that?" 3. Assess and enhance self-efficacy: "You have a lot of good ideas about what might work for you. What is it about you that makes you feel you will be successful?" 4. Write down the goals and strategies for accomplishing the goals. Include target dates for attempting the goals. Give a copy of the plan to the teen.
The adolescent is interested in changing but has no ideas or only vague ideas about how to change.	1. Ask the teen's permission to give some examples of what other people have tried. If he or she is agreeable, provide a list of goals that vary in intensity. 2. Identify which goals the adolescent would like to try, and discuss how he or she imagines they would turn out. Identify what might get in the way of success and help problem-solve around barriers. 3. Assess and enhance self-efficacy. 4. Write down the goals and give a copy to the adolescent.
The adolescent is not interested in changing.	1. Establish whether the teen is willing to see a list of things that other people who were not interested in changing have tried: "I get it that you don't want to change anything right now. I wonder if you would be interested in seeing some ways to learn more about alcohol in general and your drinking in particular?" 2. Identify goals, such as observing other people's behavior when they are drinking, counting their drinks, reading informational materials. 3. Write down the goals and give a copy to the adolescent.

JOSH: Well, like, after about three or four beers I'll get a good buzz going, but then I keep drinking anyway, and after about seven beers I'm hammered.

COUNSELOR: So, it sounds like when you limit yourself to three beers, you're feeling more in control.

JOSH: Yeah, pretty much.

COUNSELOR: I think paying closer attention to the amount that you drink sounds good. That will also help in terms of your judgment and remembering to use protection when you have sex with someone.

JOSH: Oh, yeah, like I told you earlier, if I've been drinking, I don't think at all about condoms. So, I see what you're saying—I should drink less because it'll help me make better decisions about stuff like that.

COUNSELOR: That's one benefit. Also, sometimes when people drink, they do things that they normally wouldn't if they were sober, like sleep with people who they don't know well.

JOSH: I see. Yeah, I admit that happens. I'd like to stop that. In fact, a friend was telling me that some girl told him that she's pregnant and he's the father, and he, like, has no idea which party he met this girl at. Pretty scary. I'm in college, just trying to have a good time.

COUNSELOR: Yes, that would be a big deal. So, you think that you probably need to make some changes, given your own experience and that of your friend. You're really thinking about this.

JOSH: Yeah. I like drinking, but it's not worth getting hammered and having to deal with all this crap. I'm young, and I don't want to have to worry about getting someone pregnant, or getting a disease, or worse.

COUNSELOR: So, you're ready to take the steps necessary to change these things about your drinking and the things that have gone along with it, like having sex without condoms, so that you don't have to worry and can still have a good time with your friends.

One aid that can be used with teens at this point is a list of behavioral change strategies. Specific and clear strategies should be provided, such as "After having an alcoholic drink I will have a nonalcoholic drink," or "I won't 'chug' or 'shotgun' drinks." Such a list can be introduced as things that other people have successfully done and should include a variety of change strategies so that adolescents at any level of readiness to change could find something that they would be interested in trying. We believe that tailoring this kind of intervention (i.e., presenting goals and strategies that seem appropriate to the teen's level of drinking and readiness to change) is promising, but it may also be worthwhile to expose teens to strategies that are action oriented. In this way, the teen is exposed to an array of possibilities. For example, a teen who had initially been showing no interest in changing might select a more action-oriented strategy than might have been anticipated. Those who decide not to attempt behavior change are at least exposed to these ideas and may use them if they become more interested in changing once the session is over. Regardless of their level of interest in changing, teens should not have goals selected for them and should have a variety of options.

Goal setting is most successful when goals are personalized, specific, behavioral, simple but well elaborated, and include a timeline. In order to capitalize on any enhanced motivation as a result of the session, teens should be encouraged to specify a time within the next few days that they will attempt a goal. As with the feedback sheet, one copy of the list of goals and their target dates should be given to the teen, and one copy should be retained by the counselor as a reference for future sessions if applicable. In support of this approach, a recent meta-analysis of 138 studies examined the role of progress monitoring on goal attainment across a variety of behavioral change interventions (Harkin et al., 2016). Overall, results showed larger effect sizes on goal attainment when individuals make a public commitment to change (e.g., stating an intention to change during a treatment session with a counselor, or informing others of their goals) and when an individual's monitoring of behavior was physically recorded—when it was written down or reported to someone (Harkin et al., 2016). Additionally, interventions that included elements of goal setting, action planning, and immediate feedback on behavior, along with progress monitoring, had larger effects than interventions without these elements (Harkin et al., 2016). The authors propose that monitoring progress toward one's goals serves to highlight discrepancies between current behaviors and stated goals—a topic that MI-based interventions can handily address.

Anticipating Barriers

When developing the behavior-change plan, the counselor should help the teen imagine how his or her strategies will work and actively problem-solve around barriers that might get in the way of being successful at the plan. For example, the counselor could ask how the teen imagines his or her friends would react to his or her deciding to cut down on drinking. Asking the teen to anticipate and prepare for ways to handle challenging situations will serve to help the teen and the counselor to develop further needed details of the plan and to evaluate and enhance the teen's self-efficacy.

Providing Advice

Giving advice about limiting drinking (vs. recommending abstinence) may be controversial when working with minors. However, providing advice is warranted in some cases, including those in which adolescents are not able to generate ideas, in which they ask for advice, or in which they are not developing appropriate goals.

Madison, a 16-year-old white female, arrived by ambulance at the ED after sustaining a broken arm in a car accident in which she was a passenger. As it turned out, the driver of the car had a positive BAC, as did Madison. Here, the counselor reframes some misconceptions and misinformation that Madison has about the effects of alcohol and provides her with advice as to how to avoid similar situations in the future.

COUNSELOR: You seem really shaken and upset by this whole experience. How are you feeling about it?

MADISON: Oh, my God, I never want to go through this again. This was a terrible night. I'm just glad my friends are all OK.

COUNSELOR: What a relief that is.

MADISON: Yeah, thank God. Justin seemed OK at the time, you know, we had no idea that he was that drunk when we got in the car.

COUNSELOR: It's really not obvious, is it?

MADISON: No, it's not. At least, not with some guys. With girls, you can always tell if they've been drinking.

COUNSELOR: So, by looking at the way someone's acting, you can tell how much he or she has had to drink.

MADISON: Yeah, usually.

COUNSELOR: That's one way to judge, but sometimes it can be misleading. Some people get affected right away, and others take longer to show effects, depending on how much alcohol they've had and how quickly they drink it. It can be tough to tell just how much a person's had to drink, even for a professional. That's why a blood alcohol test is used here in the hospital—it gives the fastest and most reliable information about how much alcohol a person has had.

MADISON: Oh. What was my blood alcohol test?

COUNSELOR: Your reading was .034 when you arrived at the ED. Are you familiar with what that means?

MADISON: Um, well, I think that if it's .10, that means you're drunk, right? I know that you can get a DUI if your test is higher than that.

COUNSELOR: Actually, you're referring to the legal limit, which for adults in this state is .08 and for anyone under age 21 is .02. So, if you were driving and you got pulled over and your test was .02 or higher, you could be charged with a DUI.

MADISON: Oh, wow, I didn't know that. Why is it lower for kids?

COUNSELOR: Because this state has what's called a "zero-tolerance law" for underage drinking. For most people, having one standard drink of alcohol raises their blood alcohol level to .02. So, basically, the message is that the police will arrest you if you're driving and if you've had anything at all to drink, even if it's one beer.

MADISON: But that seems ridiculous. One or two beers doesn't do anything to you. I mean, like, I know lots of people who drive after drinking that amount.

COUNSELOR: I can see why this seems confusing, especially if you don't feel the effects of alcohol after one or two beers—why should such a small amount of alcohol be grounds for getting a DUI?

MADISON: Uh huh.

COUNSELOR: Would you be interested in hearing more information about this?

MADISON: Um, OK.

COUNSELOR: Well, alcohol affects motor coordination, such as reaction time, hand–eye coordination, and the ability to pay attention to two or more things at once. These are skills needed for driving. This effect can happen at blood alcohol levels starting as low as .02, which is about equivalent to one drink.

These effects tend to be more pronounced for younger, less experienced drivers.

MADISON: Oh.

COUNSELOR: Plus, it can be tough for someone to judge not only how much someone else has had to drink but also how intoxicated they themselves are. That's because of three factors. The first is that our judgment is impaired by alcohol. Second, our ability to estimate how intoxicated we are is less accurate when our blood alcohol levels are going down than when they are rising. For example, after you have a drink, your blood alcohol continues to rise for 20–30 minutes to its highest point and then begins to fall more gradually. When it begins to fall, people tend to think that they're less intoxicated than they actually are.

MADISON: So, like, you can judge better right away how buzzed you are, but it's harder after you've been drinking for a while.

COUNSELOR: Exactly! Finally, becoming tolerant to alcohol's effects makes us less able to judge how intoxicated we are. If you have a few drinks at a time on a regular basis, your body gets used to it in that you lose some of the ability to feel alcohol's effects. However, your ability to drive is still affected at the same number of drinks as before—you just can't feel it. You temporarily lose some of the "warning system" your body had before.

MADISON: I see. I didn't know that. So that's why my guy friends who drink a lot seem like they're not drunk, but maybe they are?

COUNSELOR: Yes. Would you be interested in hearing about some ways to avoid a situation like getting into a car with a driver who's been drinking or driving after drinking?

MADISON: Yeah, I guess.

COUNSELOR: Here's a list that we can go over together. Let's read off each of these and see which ones might work for you: sleep over, find someone who has not been drinking at all to drive you home, designate a driver beforehand who won't drink at all, call a taxi, take a bus, call a parent for a ride, call another adult for a ride, walk home, only go to places where no alcohol is available, don't drink, and don't go out with people who drink.

MADISON: Uh, let me think. . . . I could sleep over, call a taxi, call my cousin for a ride, um, I don't think I want to call my parents, though, because they'll just, like, freak about it if they know I'm at a party where there's alcohol, and, um, maybe designate a driver beforehand.

COUNSELOR: Terrific! How do you think those strategies will work?

MADISON: OK, I guess. I'd either just sleep over or call my cousin, probably. I don't like buses or taxis, and no way am I walking home late at night.

COUNSELOR: So, the strategies you've picked out should work well in helping you avoid a situation like this in the future.

MADISON: (*Nods head.*)

Enhancing Self-Efficacy

If the adolescent makes a plan to change, it is critical that he or she feels hopeful about and capable of implementing this plan. So, in addition to being willing to change, we also want the teen to feel confident that he or she can be successful. Therefore, one of the counselor's primary responsibilities is to enhance the teen's sense that he or she can effectively make changes. The counselor can do this by reinforcing promising but realistic ideas, by making supportive statements about the adolescent's strengths, and by being optimistic about his or her future once change is implemented. One of the more important actions a counselor can take is to affirm the teen's efforts and intentions, and to make statements about his or her own belief that the teen has the resources to be successful in carrying out the plan.

Planning Further Contact

Even minimal counselor contact outside of the treatment session has been shown to increase engagement in treatment and participation in ongoing treatment. Therefore, counselors should consider whether further contact is feasible. The purpose of further sessions would be to reinforce the process of motivation toward behavior change begun in the initial session. The counselor draws upon information from the initial session, including the teen's (1) interest in changing, (2) perceptions about his or her drinking and its effects, (3) concerns about changing, and (4) assessment feedback. Progress toward goals should be discussed, problems and barriers identified, and strategies reviewed. Suggestions for responding to different teen presentations are presented in Table 6.2.

OTHER CONSIDERATIONS

The preceding sections describe in some detail the basic elements of our brief MI approach with adolescents. To illustrate our approach, we have provided many examples from among the hundreds of adolescents with whom we have worked. In this section we discuss several additional considerations that can be best described as process/procedural issues.

Counselor Training Recommendations

As is true for all types of therapy, there is no substitute for a well-trained counselor. Because manualized behavioral treatment approaches are sometimes misunderstood as being applied in a "cookbook fashion"—that is, in the absence of careful consideration of the training of the counselor and the unique needs of each adolescent—it is of paramount importance that counselors have therapy

TABLE 6.2. Follow-Up Sessions: Three Possible Presentations and Suggested Responses

1. *The adolescent didn't try anything.* If the adolescent had at the initial meeting set some concrete goals but reports that none were attempted, open-ended questions and reflective listening should be used extensively to understand the teen's situation before continuing. Explore what the interim time period has been like for the teen. Some possibilities are that the goals were not appropriate, that the teen's interest in changing has declined, or that some unanticipated events occurred that made it difficult for the teen to attempt change. As rapport is built in the second session, further information about the teen's pattern of drinking, other behavior, or life circumstances may be revealed. The aim of the session should be maintaining the relationship with the teen, minimizing resistance and sustain talk, and establishing an appropriate course from this point. Motivational enhancement strategies that increase change talk (i.e., the discussion of barriers to change and facilitators of change, discussion of benefits of change) should be used to attempt to renew the adolescent's commitment to making a change.

2. *The adolescent attempted goals but was not successful.* If the adolescent reports having attempted some goals but had limited success, the strategies should be reviewed, as well as what difficulties the teen had in implementing them. It may be that he or she did not anticipate certain barriers and that the goals and strategies for addressing barriers to change should be discussed at length. The counselor should affirm and commend the adolescent for attempting his or her goals, and then assist the adolescent in problem solving around obstacles and barriers.

3. *The adolescent attempted change and experienced some success.* For teens who report having met some or all of the goals set at baseline, the counselor would first review this success, asking such questions as "What did you do?"; "How did that work?"; and "How do you feel about making this change?" This is a critical time for the counselor to affirm the teen, commend him or her for progress toward goals, and reinforce self-efficacy by making statements such as "I'm impressed with how you were able to make this change." After getting a good sense of the teen's experience, the counselor can help him or her determine whether further goals should be set ("What do you think needs to happen next?"). It is also important to pursue discussion of change planning—how to ensure that changes are maintained ("Where does this leave you now in terms of sticking to your goal in the future?").

experience and are well versed in behavioral principles (see Creed et al., 2016). Of equal importance, counselors must have good interpersonal skills that enable them to "connect" with adolescents and strong therapy skills in adhering to the spirit of MI (Feldstein Ewing et al., 2016; Miller & Moyers, 2015; Moyers & Miller, 2013).

A master's degree in a mental health discipline (e.g., child psychology, child development, clinical or counseling psychology) is considered "entry level" for counselors in our trials. We occasionally employ individuals with bachelor's degrees, particularly if they have adolescent-related clinical experiences. One year of clinical experience is the usual minimum required for our counselor training program. Training consists of several elements, including approximately 75 hours of one-on-one training and viewing videotaped clinical demonstrations, such as those produced by Miller, Moyers, and Rollnick (2013). An excellent resource is the Motivational Interviewing Network of Trainers (MINT; *www.motivationalinterviewing.org/category/resource-tag/dvd*), an international organization that promotes high-quality MI practice, fidelity to the spirit of MI, and training.

Our training also includes reading Miller and Rollnick (2013), listening to several hours of audiotaped MIs, extensive observed role plays, and ongoing weekly supervision as part of our training program. Ratings from our adolescents, counselors, and trained observers have provided us with evidence that our training has been successful in teaching counselors to consistently adhere to the stylistic and protocol-driven elements of the MI in the context of an empathic interaction with our teens (Monti et al., 2007).

As is the case in other clinical work, use of appropriate self-disclosure and humor can be helpful clinical tools, especially in dealing effectively with adolescents. One self-disclosure issue that occasionally comes up is the question regarding the drinking practices of the counselor. As a general guideline to our counselors, we emphasize that it is not so important whether the question gets answered as that the teen feels that he or she is being understood.

The issue of handling personal questions directed at the counselor during the MI can be thorny, particularly with questions having to do with the counselor's own experiences with alcohol. Below is a vignette illustrating how a counselor fielded such inquiries from Malik, an 18-year-old African American college male who was found intoxicated in his dormitory room and was brought to the ED by university emergency medical technicians (EMTs).

MALIK: So, you keep asking me all these questions about drinking. You must have gone to college to have your job—didn't you drink when you were in school?

COUNSELOR: It seems strange to you that I'd be asking you these questions about drinking, as if I didn't know firsthand what drinking was like.

MALIK: Yeah.

COUNSELOR: I can see why you'd wonder that. The reason I ask those questions is because people can have different reactions to drinking. I'm interested to hear about your perceptions and feelings and what you've personally experienced. Plus, I don't want to assume anything—I'd rather hear what you think and how you feel about drinking. You're the expert on you. Sometimes, people ask that question because they're concerned that if the other person has never been drunk or hasn't ever had alcohol, they might not be able to understand or help.

MALIK: Uh, well . . . yeah, I don't know how someone could be helpful if they've never had alcohol. Where I go to school, being hungover is pretty normal. Everyone has a wicked hangover on Sunday, that's just a fact.

COUNSELOR: I can see your point. What I'm here to do is to help people to avoid situations where they drink too much, like what happened to you this evening, or drink in situations that are risky or dangerous that increase their chances of getting hurt. So, I help people to take a look at their drinking and make changes in their drinking that are effective, if they're interested. I'm not here to pass judgment on what's normal or not normal, but rather, what you'd like to do about drinking. Again, that's your choice and completely up to you.

MALIK: All right. Fair enough.

Population and Modality

As was mentioned earlier in this chapter, adolescents with whom we have worked range from 13 to 19 years of age and have been enrolled because they are in the ED after having been involved in an alcohol-related incident, or else having screened positive for a recent history of harmful drinking. Thus, the population of teens with whom we have the most experience is fairly restricted and deserves comment. Perhaps the least restricted aspect of this population is the age range that it spans. Development matters and must be seriously considered in designing interventions (see Schulenberg et al., Chapter 1, this volume). Some issues that we have come to deal with on a routine basis include the different patterns of drinking and problems seen in younger adolescents versus young adults (i.e., younger adolescents may not have established a pattern of regular drinking, younger adolescents are more likely to be seen for intoxication), the necessity for parental involvement and perhaps even parental intervention with younger teens, issues of consent and confidentiality that emerge in dealing with parent–teen dyads, and the fact that younger teens may require a more structured approach than older teens. Each of these issues requires careful and considerable clinical judgment.

One issue is that feedback material must be presented in a format and modality that is sensitive to age and level of comprehension. Our counselors do not assume reading competence. Rather, the entire protocol is implemented in the context of a discussion between the counselor and the teen. Although multimodal presentation is generally preferable, it is especially appropriate when dealing with younger teens. Computerized interventions and interventions involving text messaging are appealing to youth and becoming increasingly more prevalent (e.g., Suffoletto, Calloway, Kristan, Monti, & Clark, 2013; Suffoletto et al., 2014).

Dealing with Other Drugs of Abuse

A recent review of 39 MI interventions for adolescent substance use found that 67% of studies showed statistically improved substance use outcomes (Barnett et al., 2012). Specific to marijuana, seven out of nine studies reported reductions in adolescent marijuana use following the delivery of MI targeting marijuana use (Barnett et al., 2012). Although we do not directly address other substances in the brief intervention illustrated in this chapter, we have found (Monti, 1999) that the effects of our brief alcohol intervention with older adolescents seemed to generalize to marijuana use at a 12-month follow-up; we found similar reductions in marijuana use in another brief alcohol intervention study described below (Spirito et al., 2011). This contrasts with a more recent meta-analytic review of 30 studies showing that while brief interventions for adolescents targeting both alcohol and other substances were effective in reducing alcohol and the other targeted substances, interventions that target only alcohol did not show carryover effects on reducing other substances (Tanner-Smith, Steinka-Fry, Hennessy, Lipsey, & Winters, 2016).

While conducting our alcohol-focused randomized control trials (RCTs) in the ED, we noted the higher than average prevalence of smoking among the adolescent ED patients, and considered whether the MI for alcohol might be adapted for smokers in the same setting. In the ED, the approach to MI was different for smoking than it had been for alcohol. The conversation about alcohol was set up well by the context for the ED visit: an alcohol-related event. In contrast, the smoking intervention was more opportunistic; adolescents came to the ED for treatment for any type of urgent care—usually unrelated to smoking. Our earliest pilot study provided initial support for the promise of this approach (Colby et al., 1998) and two subsequent RCTs, spanning a range of settings (ED, specialty clinics, primary care, schools), provided additional support for these brief, proactive interventions with adolescent smokers (Colby et al., 2005, 2012). However, overall, trials of MI for smoking had tended to be small and underpowered, making it challenging to detect the differences between MI and comparison treatments. More recently, a meta-analysis by Hettema and Hendricks (2010) and a pooled analysis by Heckman, Egleston, and Hofmann (2010) have provided more compelling support demonstrating the efficacy of MI for promoting smoking cessation generally and with adolescent smokers specifically. A detailed review of this literature and description of our MI protocol adapted for smoking interventions can be found in Colby (2015).

EMPIRICAL SUPPORT, CONCLUSIONS, AND FUTURE DIRECTIONS

Our first ED intervention trial (Monti et al., 1999), conducted with 94 adolescents ages 18–19 years, showed promising effects of MI compared to standard care, which consisted of assessment and informational handouts. Teens were interviewed 3 and 6 months following their ED visit, with follow-up rates averaging 91% across the two conditions. Regardless of group assignment, teens showed a reduction in overall drinking, with the greatest reduction occurring from baseline to 3-month follow-up. Alcohol use did not differ between the two treatment groups, and there may be several reasons for this. First, it is plausible that the experience of having an alcohol-related ED visit causes short-term reductions in alcohol use, regardless of intervention. It should also be noted that our control condition provided more than typical hospital care in that teens received detailed assessments about their alcohol use and its consequences, informational handouts, and follow-up assessments. Reactivity to assessment may account for the lack of group differences in alcohol use.

However, despite no group differences in alcohol use at follow-up, MI did result in greater reduction in *harm* associated with alcohol use. Specifically, compared with teens who received standard care, teens who received MI had fewer alcohol-related injuries, fewer social problems, were less likely to report drinking and driving at 6-month follow-up, and were significantly less likely to have a traffic violation within the follow-up period, as verified by Department of Motor Vehicle records. The clinical significance of these effects is of particular interest: 6 months after their ED visit, the MI group showed a 32% reduction in drinking and driving and had half the occurrence of alcohol-related injuries of the standard-care group. Thus, our brief MI had a meaningful effect on clinically significant sequelae of drinking behavior, with harm reduction effects maintained at 12 months following the alcohol-related event.

In a concurrent trial, we also examined MI compared to standard care on alcohol use and consequences in an ED sample of 13- to 17-year-olds. In this trial, we did not find a main effect of treatment condition on alcohol outcomes in the overall sample. This may have been due to the substantially lower overall rates of alcohol use and consequences at baseline in this younger group than in the older group. Indeed, it was sometimes the case that the incident leading to the ED visit had been the teen's first exposure to alcohol. Thus, there was less room to demonstrate differential improvement over time. When we identified those adolescents who screened positive for problematic alcohol use at the baseline assessment in the ED, and tested the effects of MI on this subset of patients, we found that those who received MI reported significantly greater reductions in drinking frequency and in frequency of high-volume drinking compared with teens in standard care (Spirito et al., 2004).

We have also evaluated a combination of two brief, evidence-based MI models, one for parents and one for teens. In a 2011 RCT, families of adolescents (ages 13–17) treated in an urban ED for an alcohol-related event were randomized to receive either an individual teen MI only or an individual teen MI plus a Family Check-Up (FCU; Dishion & Stormshak, 2007; Dishion, Stormshak, & Kavanaugh, 2011). Both conditions resulted in reduced alcohol and marijuana use over the 12-month follow-up, with the strongest effects at 3 and 6 months. Adding the FCU to MI was associated with fewer high-volume drinking days at 3 months. Even though treatment focused primarily on alcohol, the FCU + MI condition had lower average likelihood of marijuana use across the three follow-up time points (30.4%) than the MI-only condition (40.1%). For those with a history of problematic substance use at baseline, effect sizes of the FCU on marijuana use were especially strong at 3 months ($h = .61$) and medium effects remained at 6 months ($h = .46$), and 12 months ($h = .38$; Spirito et al., 2011).

Although our MI is a promising approach for ED settings, and perhaps other settings in which there is the potential for a teachable moment, older adolescents and young adults who are severe problem drinkers and/or drug users may not respond solely to a brief intervention. (See Esposito-Smythers, Rallis, Machell, Williams, & Fisher, Chapter 7, Dauria, McWilliams, & Tolou-Shams, Chapter 8, and Kelly et al., Chapter 15, this volume, for information on treating more severely impaired adolescents.) One possibility might be to use MI as a preparation for standard adolescent treatment programs (see Kelly et al., Chapter 15, this volume), to facilitate more intensive treatment options (see Dauria et al., Chapter 8, this volume), and to enhance medication compliance (see Miranda & Treloar, Chapter 13, this volume).

In summary, our work to date suggests that the brief MI outlined in this chapter, when introduced at a teachable moment during an ED visit, is particularly effective in reducing harmful behaviors, such as drinking and driving, alcohol-related injuries, alcohol-related problems, and traffic violations among older adolescents, and reducing drunkenness and driving after drinking among younger adolescents. Developmental differences and the broad range of adolescents we have treated are likely to account for the different patterns of results. The addition of follow-up contact using technology, such as text messaging (see Braciszewski & Havlicek, Chapter 9, this volume), more systematic study of developmental considerations and their interaction with MI treatment; possible matching, particularly with more severely impaired adolescents; and combining MI with other forms of compatible adolescent treatment are all possibilities for extending motivational enhancement effects with alcohol-involved adolescents.

REFERENCES

Apodaca, T. R., Borsari, B., Jackson, K. M., Magill, M., Longabaugh, R., Mastroleo, N. R., et al. (2014). Sustain talk predicts poorer outcomes among mandated college student drinkers receiving a brief motivational intervention. *Psychology of Addictive Behaviors, 28*, 631–638.

Apodaca, T. R., Jackson, K. M., Borsari, B., Magill, M., Longabaugh, R., Mastroleo, N. R., et al. (2016). Which individual therapist behaviors elicit client change talk and sustain talk in motivational interviewing? *Journal of Substance Abuse Treatment, 61*, 60–65.

Armstrong, T. D., & Costello, E. J. (2002). Community studies on adolescent substance use, abuse, or dependence and psychiatric comorbidity. *Journal of Consulting and Clinical Psychology, 70*, 1224–1239.

Baer, J. S., Beadnell, B., Garrett, S. B., Hartzler, B., Wells, E. A., & Peterson, P. L. (2008). Adolescent change language within a brief motivational intervention and substance use outcomes. *Psychology of Addictive Behaviors, 22*, 570–575.

Barnes, G. M., Welte, J. W., & Hoffman, J. H. (2002). Relationship of alcohol use to delinquency and illicit drug use in adolescents: Gender, age, and racial/ethnic differences. *Journal of Drug Issues, 32,* 153–178.

Barnett, E., Sussman, S., Smith, C., Rohrback, L. A., & Spruijt-Metz, D. (2012). Motivational interviewing for adolescent substance use: A review of the literature. *Addictive Behaviors, 37,* 1325–1334.

Barnett, N. P., Lebeau-Craven, R., O'Leary, T. A., Colby, S. M., Rohsenow, D. J., Monti, P. M., Woolard, R., & Spirito, A. (2002). Predictors of motivation to change after medical treatment for drinking-related events in adolescents. *Psychology of Addictive Behaviors, 16,* 106–112.

Barnett, N. P., Goldstein, A. L., Murphy J. G., Colby, S. M., & Monti, P. M. (2006). "I'll never drink like that again": Characteristics of alcohol-related incidents and predictors of motivation to change in college students. *Journal of Studies on Alcohol, 67,* 754–763.

Barnett, N. P., Monti, P. M., Spirito, A., Colby, S. M., Rohsenow, D. J., Ruffolo, L., et al. (2003). Alcohol use and related harm among older adolescents treated in an emergency department: The importance of alcohol status and college status. *Journal of Studies on Alcohol, 64,* 342–349.

Barnett, N. P., Spirito, A., Colby, S. M., Vallee, J. A., Woolard, R., Lewander, W., et al. (1998). Detection of alcohol use in adolescent patients in the emergency department. *Academic Emergency Medicine, 5*(6), 607–612.

Brown, S. A., McGue, M., Maggs, J., Schulenburg, J., Hingson, R., Swartzwelder, S., et al. (2008). A developmental perspective on alcohol and youths 16 to 20 years of age. *Pediatrics, 121,* S290–S310.

Chung, T., Colby, S. M., Barnett, N. P., Rohsenow, D. J., Monti, P. M., & Spirito, A. (2000). Screening adolescents for problem drinking: Performance of brief screens against DSM-IV alcohol diagnoses. *Journal of Studies on Alcohol, 61,* 579–587.

Colby, S. M. (2015). Motivational interviewing for smoking cessation with adolescents. In H. Arkowitz, W. R. Miller, & S. Rollnick (Eds.), *Motivational interviewing in the treatment of psychological problems* (2nd ed., pp. 296–319). New York: Guilford Press.

Colby, S. M., Barnett, N. P., Eaton, C. A., Spirito, A., Woolard, R., Lewander, W., et al. (2002). Potential biases in case detection of alcohol involvement among adolescents in an emergency department. *Pediatric Emergency Care, 18,* 350–354.

Colby, S. M., Monti, P. M., Barnett, N. P., Rohsenow, D. J., Weissman, K., Spirito, A., et al. (1998). Brief motivational interviewing in a hospital setting for adolescent smoking: A preliminary study. *Journal of Consulting and Clinical Psychology, 66,* 574–578.

Colby, S. M., Monti, P. M., Barnett, N. P., Spirito, A., Myers, M., Rohsenow, D. J., et al. (1999, June). Effects of a brief motivational interview on alcohol use and consequences: Predictors of response to intervention among 13- to 17-year-olds. In R. Longabaugh & P. Monti (Chairs), *Brief motivational interventions in the emergency department for adolescents and adults.* Symposium conducted at the annual meeting of the Research Society on Alcoholism, Santa Barbara, CA.

Colby, S. M., Monti, P. M., Tevyaw, T. O., Barnett, N. P., Spirito, A., Rohsenow, D. J., et al. (2005). Brief motivational intervention for adolescent smokers in a hospital setting. *Addictive Behaviors, 30,* 865–874.

Colby, S. M., Nargiso, J., Tevyaw, T., Barnett, N. P., Metrik, J., Woolard, R. H., et al. (2012). Enhanced motivational interviewing versus brief advice for adolescent smoking cessation: A randomized clinical trial. *Addictive Behaviors, 37,* 817–823.

Creed, A., Frankel, S. A., German, R. E., Green, K. L., Jager-Hyman, S., Taylor, K. P., et al. (2016). Implementation of transdiagnostic cognitive therapy in community behavioral health: The Beck Community Initiative. *Journal of Consulting and Clinical Psychology, 84*(12), 1116–1126.

Dishion, T. J., & Stormshak, E. (2007). *Intervening in children's lives: An ecological, family-centered approach to mental health care.* Washington, DC: American Psychological Association.

Dishion, T. J., Stormshak, E. A., & Kavanagh, K. (2011). *Everyday parenting: A professional's guide to building family management skills.* Champaign, IL: Research Press.

Dotson, K. B., Dunn, M. E., & Bowers, C. A. (2015). Stand-alone personalized normative feedback for college student drinkers: A meta-analytic review, 2004 to 2014. *PLOS ONE, 10*(10), e0139518.

Ehrlich, P. F., Maio, R., Drongowski, R., Wagaman, M., Cunningham, R., & Walton, M. A. (2010). Alcohol interventions for trauma patients are not just for adults: Justification for brief interventions for the injured adolescent at a pediatric trauma center. *Journal of Trauma: Injury, Infection, and Critical Care, 69,* 202–210.

Fairlie, A. M., Sindelar, H. A., Eaton, C. A., & Spirito, A. (2006). Utility of the AUDIT for screening adolescents for problematic alcohol use in the emergency department. *International Journal of Adolescent Medical Health, 18,* 115–122.

Feldstein Ewing, S. W., Apodaca, T. R., & Gaume, J. (2016). Ambivalence: Prerequisite for success in motivational interviewing with adolescents? *Addiction, 111*(11), 1900–1907.

Flory, K., Lynam, D., Milich, R., Leukefeld, C., & Clayton, R. (2004). Early adolescent through young adult alcohol and marijuana use trajectories: Early predictors, young adult outcomes, and predictive utility. *Development and Psychopathology, 16,* 193–213.

Gaume, J., Longabaugh, R., Magill, M., Bertholet, N., Gmel, G., & Daeppen, J. B. (2016). Under what conditions?: Therapist and client characteristics moderate the role of change talk in brief motivational intervention. *Journal of Consulting and Clinical Psychology, 84,* 211–220.

Grant, S., LaBrie, J. W., Hummer, J. F., & Lac, A. (2012). How drunk am I?: Misperceiving one's level of intoxication in the college drinking environment. *Psychology of Addictive Behaviors, 26,* 51–58.

Harkin, B. W., Thomas, L., Chang, B. P. I., Prestwich, A., Conner, M., Kellar, I., et al. (2016). Does monitoring goal progress promote goal attainment?: A meta-analysis of the experimental evidence. *Psychological Bulletin, 142,* 198–229.

Heckman, C. J., Egleston, B. L., & Hofmann, M. T. (2010). Efficacy of motivational interviewing for smoking cessation: A systematic review and meta-analysis. *Tobacco Control, 19,* 410–416.

Heron, M. (2013). Deaths: Leading causes for 2010. *National Vital Statistics Reports, 62*(6), 1–96. Retrieved from September 7, 2016, from *www.cdc.gov/nchs/data/nvsr/nvsr62/nvsr62_06.pdf.*

Hettema, J. E., & Hendricks, P. S. (2010). Motivational interviewing for smoking cessation: A meta-analytic review. *Journal of Consulting and Clinical Psychology, 78,* 868–884.

Johnston, L. D., O'Malley, P. M., Miech, R. A., Bachman, J. G., & Schulenberg, J. E. (2014). *Monitoring the Future national survey results on drug use: 1975–2013:*

Overview, key findings on adolescent drug use. Ann Arbor: Institute for Social Research, University of Michigan.

Kahler, C. W., Caswell, A. J., Laws, M. B., Walthers, J., Magill, M., Mastroleo, N. R., et al. (2016). Using topic coding to understand the nature of change language in a motivational intervention to reduce alcohol and sex risk behaviors in emergency department patients. *Patient Education and Counseling, 99,* 1595–1602.

Kelly, T. M., Donovan, J. E., Kinnane, J. M., & Taylor, D. M. (2002). A comparison of alcohol screening instruments among under-aged drinkers treated in the emergency department. *Alcohol and Alcoholism, 37,* 444–450.

Knight, J. R., Harris, S. K., Sherritt, L., Van Hook, S., Lawrence, N., Brooks, T., et al. (2007). Prevalence of positive substance abuse screen results among adolescent primary care patients. *Archives of Pediatric Adolescent Medicine, 161,* 1035–1041.

Kohler, S., & Hofmann, A. (2015). Can motivational interviewing in emergency care reduce alcohol consumption in young people?: A systematic review and meta-analysis. *Alcohol and Alcoholism, 50,* 107–117.

Lyons, K. E., & Zelazo, P. D. (2011). Monitoring, metacognition, and executive function: Elucidating the role of self-reflection in the development of self-regulation. In J. B. Benson (Ed.), *Advances in child development and behavior* (pp. 379–411). Burlington, VT: Academic Press.

Magill, M., Walthers, J., Mastroleo, N. R., Gaume, J., Longabaugh, R., & Apodaca, T. R. (2016). Therapist and client discussions of drinking and coping: A sequential analysis of therapy dialogues in three evidence-based alcohol use disorder treatments. *Addiction, 111,* 1011–1020.

Maisto, S. A., Krenek, M., Chung, T. A., Martin, C. S., Clark, D., & Cornelius, J. R. (2011a). Comparison of the concurrent and predictive validity of three measures of readiness to change marijuana use in a clinical sample of adolescents. *Journal of Studies on Alcohol and Drugs, 72,* 592–601.

Maisto, S. A., Krenek, M., Chung, T. A., Martin, C. S., Clark, D., & Cornelius, J. R. (2011b). A comparison of the concurrent and predictive validity of three measures of readiness to change alcohol use in a clinical sample of adolescents. *Psychological Assessment, 23,* 983–994.

Miller, W. R., & Moyers, T. B. (2015). The forest and the trees: Relational and specific factors in addiction treatment. *Addiction, 110,* 410–413.

Miller, W. R., Moyers, T. B., & Rollnick, S. (2013). *Motivational interviewing: Helping people change, based on the new motivational interviewing, third edition* [DVD or streaming online]. Carson City, NV: Change Companies. Retrieved from *www.changecompanies.net/products/motivational-interviewing.*

Miller, W. R., & Rollnick, S. (2012). *Motivational interviewing: Helping people change* (3rd ed.). New York: Guilford Press.

Mitchell, S. G., Gryczynski, J., O'Grady, K. I. E., & Schwartz, R. P. (2013). SBIRT for adolescent drug and alcohol use: Current status and future directions. *Journal of Substance Abuse Treatment, 44,* 463–472.

Monti, P. M. (1997, July). Motivational interviewing with alcohol-positive teens in an emergency department. In E. Wagner (Chair), *Innovations in adolescent substance abuse intervention.* Symposium conducted at the annual meeting of the Research Society on Alcoholism, San Francisco, CA.

Monti, P. M. (1999, June). Brief intervention for harm reduction with alcohol-positive older adolescents in a hospital emergency department. In R. Longabaugh & P. Monti (Chairs), *Brief motivational interventions in the emergency department for adolescents and adults.* Symposium conducted at the annual meeting of the Research Society on Alcoholism, Santa Barbara, CA.

Monti, P. M., Barnett, N. P., Colby, S. M., Gwaltney, C. J., Spirito, A., Rohsenow, D. J., & et al. (2007). Motivational interviewing versus feedback only in emergency care for young adult problem drinking. *Addiction, 102,* 1234–1243.

Monti, P. M., Colby, S. M., Barnett, N. P., Spirito, A., Rohsenow, D. J., Myers, M., et al. (1999). Brief intervention for harm reduction with alcohol-positive older adolescents in a hospital emergency department. *Journal of Consulting and Clinical Psychology, 67,* 989–994.

Moyers, T. B., & Martin, T. (2006). Therapist influence on client language during motivational interviewing sessions. *Journal of Substance Abuse Treatment, 30,* 245–251.

Moyers, T. N., & Miller, W. R. (2013). Is low therapist empathy toxic? *Psychology of Addictive Behaviors, 27,* 878–884.

National Institute on Alcohol Abuse and Alcoholism. (2003). *Assessing alcohol problems: A guide for clinicians and researchers* (2nd ed.; NIH Publication No. 03-3745). Bethesda, MD: U.S. Department of Health and Human Services.

Nordin, J. D., Solberg, L. I., & Parker, E. D. (2010). Adolescent primary care visit patterns. *Annals of Family Medicine, 8,* 511–516.

Quinn, P. D., & Fromme, K. (2011). Predictors and outcomes of variability in subjective alcohol intoxication among college students: An event-level analysis across 4 years. *Alcoholism: Clinical and Experimental Research, 25,* 484–495.

Rollnick, S., Mason, P., & Butler, C. (1999). *Health behaviour change: A guide for practitioners.* Edinburgh, UK: Churchill Livingstone.

Spear, L. P. (2014). Adolescents and alcohol: Acute sensitivities, enhanced intake, and later consequences. *Neurotoxicology and Teratology, 41,* 51–59.

Spirito, A., Barnett, N. P., Lewander, W., Colby, S. M., Rohsenow, D. J., Eaton, C. A., et al. (2001). Risks associated with alcohol-positive status among adolescents in the emergency department: A matched case-control study. *Journal of Pediatrics, 139,* 694–699.

Spirito, A., Monti, P. M., Barnett, N. P., Colby, S. M., Sindelar, H., Rohsenow, D. J., et al. (2004). A randomized clinical trial of a brief motivational intervention for alcohol-positive adolescents treated in an emergency department. *Journal of Pediatrics, 145,* 396–402.

Spirito, A., Sindelar-Manning, H., Colby, S. M., Barnett, N. P., Lewander, W., Rohsenow, D. J., et al. (2011). Individual and family motivational interventions for alcohol-positive adolescents treated in an emergency department: Results of a randomized clinical trial. *Archives of Pediatric Adolescent Medicine, 165,* 269–274.

Substance Abuse and Mental Health Services Administration, Center for Behavioral Health Statistics and Quality. (2012). *The DAWN Report: Highlights of the 2010 Drug Abuse Warning Network (DAWN) findings on drug-related emergency department visits.* Rockville, MD: Author.

Suffoletto, B., Calloway, C. B., Kristan, J., Monti, P. M., & Clark, D. B. (2013). Mobile phone text message intervention to reduce binge drinking among young adults: Study protocol for a randomized controlled trial. *Trials, 14,* 93.

Suffoletto, B., Kristan, J., Callaway, C., Kim, K., Chung, T., Monti, P. M., et al. (2014). A text-message alcohol intervention for young adult emergency department patients: A randomized clinical trial. *Annals of Emergency Medicine, 64,* 664–672.

Tanner-Smith, E. E., & Lipsey, M. W. (2015). Brief alcohol interventions for adolescents and young adults: A systematic review and meta-analysis. *Journal of Substance Abuse Treatment, 51,* 1–18.

Tanner-Smith, E. E., Steinka-Fry, K. T., Hennessy, E. A., Lipsey, M. W., & Winters K. C. (2016). Can brief alcohol interventions for youth also address concurrent illicit drug use?: Results from a meta-analysis. *Journal of Youth and Adolescence, 44,* 1011–1023.

Trela, C. J., Piasecki, T. M., Bartholow, B. D., Heath, A. C., & Sher, K. J. (2016). The natural expression of individual differences in self-reported level of response to alcohol during ecologically assessed drinking episodes. *Psychopharmacology, 233,* 2185–2195.

Tubman, J. G., Gil, A. G., Wagner, E. F., & Artigues, H. (2003). Patterns of sexual risk behaviors and psychiatric disorders in a community sample of young adults. *Journal of Behavioral Medicine, 26,* 473–500.

Walton, M. A., Chermack, S. T., Shope, J. T., Bingham, C. R., Zimmerman, M. A., Blow, F. C., et al. (2010). Effects of a brief intervention for reducing violence and alcohol misuse among adolescents: A randomized controlled trial. *JAMA, 304,* 527–535.

Winters, K. C., & Lee, C. Y. S. (2008). Likelihood of developing an alcohol and cannabis use disorder during youth: Association with recent use and age. *Drug and Alcohol Dependence, 92,* 239–247.

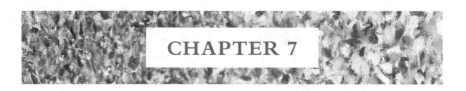

CHAPTER 7

Brief Interventions for Adolescents with Substance Abuse and Comorbid Psychiatric Problems

Christianne Esposito-Smythers, Bethany Rallis,
Kyla Machell, Caitlin Williams, and Sarah Fischer

*T*he presence of comorbid psychiatric disorders (CPDs) among adolescents with substance use disorders (SUDs) is the rule rather than the exception. Comorbidity is common among adolescents with SUDs found across community, treatment, and juvenile justice settings. Comorbidity rates range from an average of 60% in community-based settings to as high as 80% in inpatient treatment (Abrantes, Brown, & Tomlinson, 2003; Armstrong & Costello, 2002; Storr, Pacek, & Martins, 2012). Moreover, comorbidity rates increase with severity of SUDs (i.e., abuse vs. dependence; Roberts, Roberts, & Xing, 2007). Disruptive behavior disorders (oppositional defiant and conduct disorders) are most commonly diagnosed among adolescents with SUDs, followed by mood and anxiety disorders (Armstrong & Costello, 2002). Given the strong association between SUDs and psychiatric disorders, it is important to gain a thorough understanding of the nature of this relationship and the degree to which it impacts treatment of adolescent SUDs. The purpose of this chapter is to provide an overview of literature on the association between adolescent SUDs and CPDs in an effort to inform clinical practice and research. Below, we review the status of the field, including research on comorbidity rates across settings, gender and race/ethnic differences in comorbidity, comorbidity patterns across substances, the effect of order of onset of SUDs and psychiatric disorders on outcomes, and leading theories that help explain this association. Next, we review guidelines for assessing psychiatric comorbidity. We then present data on the effect of comorbidity on SUD treatment outcomes. Following this review, we discuss strategies for addressing comorbidity in the context of brief interventions. We conclude with a discussion of future clinical and research directions.

STATUS OF THE FIELD

Numerous studies have examined rates of CPDs among adolescents with SUDs across community, treatment (substance abuse outpatient and inpatient/residential), and juvenile justice settings. Full descriptions of the disorders included in these studies can be found in the fifth edition of the *Diagnostic and Statistical Manual of Mental Disorders* (DSM-5; American Psychiatric Association, 2013). Most studies have been conducted with community samples, with a comprehensive review suggesting that, on average, 60% of adolescents with an SUD have at least one CPD (Armstrong & Costello, 2002). Comorbidity rates are higher in clinical samples seeking treatment for SUDs. Rates of CPDs in adolescent outpatient treatment samples range from 62 to 88%, and upward of 80% in inpatient/residential samples. Rates of CPDs among adolescents with SUDs in juvenile justice settings are comparable to those found in clinical samples. See Table 7.1 for a representative review of studies that present rates of comorbid internalizing and externalizing disorders across settings.

Notably, many adolescents with SUDs have more than one comorbid disorder. For example, in community-based samples, Essau (2011) found that 37% of adolescents with an SUD had one CPD, 11.8% two disorders, and 3.9% three disorders. Roberts et al. (2007) found the mean number of CPDs to range from 1.7 to 2.8. In an outpatient substance abuse treatment setting, Rowe, Liddle, Greenbaum, and Henderson (2004) found that 20% of adolescents met criteria for only one psychiatric disorder, 24% for two, 17% for three, and 26% for four or more. When examined across subtypes, 35% of the sample had only a comorbid externalizing disorder, 5% only an internalizing disorder, and 48% both an internalizing and an externalizing disorder. In a sample of adolescents seeking inpatient treatment for an SUD, Stowell and Estroff (1992) found that 82% met criteria for a psychiatric disorder and 74% had two or more disorders (61% mood, 54% conduct, 43% anxiety). Thus, as discussed in further detail below, a comprehensive assessment for CPDs is warranted when working with adolescents with SUDs.

Gender and Race/Ethnic Differences

A review of community-based studies concluded that most fail to find gender differences in comorbidity rates among adolescents with SUDs, and among those that do, results are mixed (Armstrong & Costello, 2002). Studies

TABLE 7.1. Rates of Comorbid Externalizing and Internalizing Disorders by Study Sample

Authors	Disorder	Comorbidity rate	Type of study sample
	Externalizing disorders		
Armstrong & Costello (2002)	CD, ODD, ADHD	46% (median)	Community
Rowe, Liddle, Greenbaum, & Henderson (2004)	Externalizing disorders CD ADHD	35% 69% 28%	Outpatient treatment
Mason & Posner (2009)	ADHD	30%	Outpatient treatment
Dennis et al. (2004)	CD ADHD	53% 38%	Outpatient treatment
Stowell & Estroff (1992)	CD	54%	Inpatient treatment
Abrantes, Brown, & Tomlinson (2003)[a]	CD ODD ADHD	84% 61% 34%	Inpatient treatment
Tomlinson, Brown, & Abrantes (2004)[a]	CD or ODD ADHD	65% 29%	Inpatient treatment
Grella, Joshi, & Hser (2004)	CD ADHD	57% 13%	Substance abuse residential, inpatient, and outpatient treatment
Stahlberg, Anckarsater, & Nilsson (2010)	CD ADHD	84% 45%	Juvenile detention
Abram, Teplin, McClelland, & Dulcan (2003)	CD, ODD, and/or ADHD	62% male, 65% female	Juvenile detention
Sittner Hartshorn, Whitbeck, & Prentice (2015)	CD ADHD	75% 13%	Juvenile justice involvement (arrest in last year)
	Internalizing disorders		
Armstrong & Costello (2002)	Any depressive disorder[b] Any anxiety disorder	19% 16–18% (medians)	Community

(continued)

TABLE 7.1. (*continued*)

Authors	Disorder	Comorbidity rate	Type of study sample
Center for Behavioral Health Statistics & Quality (2015)	MDD	11%	Community
Essau (2011)	Any depressive disorder[b]	35%	Community
	Any anxiety disorder	22%	
Rowe et al. (2004)	Internalizing disorders	5%	Outpatient treatment
	Any depressive disorder[b]	30%	
	Any anxiety disorder	38%	
Mason & Posner (2009)	MDD	40%	Outpatient treatment
	GAD	13%	
	PTSD	13%	
Dennis et al. (2004)	MDD	18%	Outpatient treatment
	GAD	23%	
	PTSD or acute stress disorder	14%	
Stowell & Estroff (1992)	Any mood disorder[c]	61%	Inpatient treatment
	Any anxiety disorder	43%	
Abrantes et al. (2003)[a]	MDD	64%	Inpatient treatment
	Dysthymic disorder	40%	
	Social anxiety disorder	30%	
	Separation anxiety disorder	22%	
	Obsessive–compulsive disorder	21%	
	GAD	14%	
	Agoraphobia	10%	
	Panic	6%	
Tomlinson et al. (2004)[a]	Any mood disorder[c]	70%	Inpatient treatment
	Any anxiety disorder	57%	

(*continued*)

TABLE 7.1. (*continued*)

Authors	Disorder	Comorbidity rate	Type of study sample
Grella et al. (2004)	MDD	14%	Substance abuse residential, inpatient, and outpatient treatment
Stahlberg et al. (2010)	Any depressive disorder[b]	33%	Juvenile detention
	Any anxiety disorder	20%	
Sittner et al. (2015)	MDD	9%	Juvenile justice involvement (arrest in last year)
Abram et al. (2003)	Any mood disorder[c]	21% males, 26% females	Juvenile detention
	Any anxiety disorder	29% males, 34% females	

Note. CD, conduct disorder; ODD, oppositional defiant disorder; ADHD, attention-deficit/hyperactivity disorder; MDD, major depressive disorder; GAD, generalized anxiety disorder; PTSD, posttraumatic stress disorder; SUD, substance abuse disorder; CPD, comorbid psychiatric disorder.
[a]These studies included only adolescents with SUDs and CPDs in their samples.
[b]Depressive disorders = unipolar mood disorders (major depressive, dysthymia).
[c]Mood disorders = unipolar and/or bipolar (bipolar I and II, cyclothymia) mood disorders. Many authors did not specify the mood, depressive, or anxiety disorders assessed. Percentages are rounded to the whole number.

conducted with clinical samples also yield few differences. For example, in a clinical sample of alcohol-dependent adolescents, males had higher rates of attention-deficit/hyperactivity disorder (ADHD) than females. No difference in rates of *diagnosis* of comorbid major depression, oppositional defiant disorder, conduct disorder, or posttraumatic stress disorder (PTSD) were found. However, females reported more *symptoms* of major depression and PTSD, whereas males reported more *symptoms* of conduct disorder and ADHD (Clark et al., 1997). In a sample of Native American adolescents admitted to a residential substance abuse treatment facility, males reported higher rates of conduct disorder than females, but no differences were found in disruptive behavior, major depressive, or anxiety disorders (Novins, Fickensher, & Manson, 2006). In a sample of incarcerated adolescents with an SUD, no gender difference in rates of psychosis, mania, or major depression were found. Approximately one-third (31% males, 30% females) had comorbid disruptive behavior disorders, and half of these youth also had mood disorders, anxiety disorders, or both (Abram, Teplin, McClelland, & Dulcan, 2003).

Very few studies have examined race/ethnic differences in community or clinical settings, limiting conclusions that can be drawn (Armstrong & Costello, 2002; Storr et al., 2012). Chisolm, Mulatu, and Brown (2009) conducted one of the only comprehensive studies that examined race/ethnic differences. In a large sample of adolescents seeking outpatient or residential substance abuse treatment services ($n = 9{,}030$), African American, Hispanic, and mixed-race adolescents reported more co-occurring internalizing symptoms than white adolescents. Further, African American and Native American adolescents reported fewer externalizing and combined internalizing and externalizing symptoms than white adolescents.

Type of Substance and Pattern of Comorbidity

There is a paucity of research that examines whether type of comorbidity varies by type of SUD. Most studies suggest that alcohol and/or cannabis use disorders are associated with increased odds of comorbid disruptive behavior disorders (oppositional defiant or conduct disorders; Armstrong & Costello, 2002; Hollen & Ortiz, 2015; Roberts et al., 2007). Results of studies that examine differences in rates of mood and anxiety disorders are mixed. In a review of community-based studies, Armstrong and Costello (2002) found that adolescents with an alcohol or cannabis use disorder did not have increased odds of depressive or anxiety disorders. However, in a more recent epidemiological study, Roberts et al. (2007) found that an alcohol use disorder (AUD) was associated with increased odds of comorbid mood (major depressive, dysthymic, bipolar), but not anxiety (agoraphobia, generalized anxiety, panic, social phobia, posttraumatic stress) disorders or ADHD. Cannabis use disorder was not associated with increased risk for a mood or anxiety disorder. Interestingly, in a recent study conducted with a large sample of high school students, Essau (2011) found that the presence of an anxiety disorder (panic, agoraphobia, social, specific, generalized, obsessive–compulsive, posttraumatic, not otherwise specified) was more common among adolescents with cannabis relative to AUDs (23.1% vs. 18.6%), whereas depressive disorders (major depressive and dysthymia) were more frequent among youth with alcohol relative to cannabis use disorders (24.7% vs. 20.0%). Other illicit SUDs were not associated with increased odds of any particular CPD in community samples (Armstrong & Costello, 2002; Roberts et al., 2007) but were found to be related to conduct disorder in an inpatient sample (Hollen & Ortiz, 2015). Mixed study results may have resulted from the fact that the disorders included in mood and anxiety disorder composite variables differed across studies as did the nature of study samples. Further disorder-specific research is needed before conclusions can be drawn.

Temporal Order

The temporal order of onset of psychiatric disorder relative to SUDs is also important to consider. This information informs theory pertaining to the development of both types of disorders and holds treatment implications, as discussed in further detail below. Most literature that examines the temporal order of SUDs and CPDs suggests that disruptive behavior and anxiety disorders tend to precede or occur in close proximity to the onset of SUDs for most youth, whereas depression tends to precede and follow SUDs at equal rates (Storr et al., 2012). For example, in a large sample of high school students, Rohde, Lewinsohn, and Seeley (1996) found that comorbid anxiety (88%, average onset age 8) and disruptive behavior (80%, average onset age 12) disorders preceded the onset of AUD (average onset age 15) for most youth. For depression, just over half (58%) reported that depression preceded the onset of the AUD. In a clinical sample of alcohol-dependent adolescents, for most males and females, conduct disorder preceded the onset of AUD (63–65%), with fewer reporting onset in the same year (20–28%) or secondary (7–17%) onset. Though less consistency was evident across genders with regard to comorbid depression, most reported that major depression preceded (31% males, 50% females) or followed (59% males, 47% females) the onset of AUD. Few youth reported onset within the same year (10% males, 3% females; Clark et al., 1997). Deas-Nesmith, Brady, and Campbell (1998) found that anxiety disorders and PTSD preceded SUDs for all adolescents assessed, with an average of 2 years between the onset of anxiety symptoms and substance use, in an adolescent clinical sample. The most commonly diagnosed disorders were social phobia and PTSD. In a sample of incarcerated adolescents, Abram et al. (2003) found that most youth (63% females, 54.3% males) with comorbid SUD and psychiatric disorders reported onset in the same year. Fewer participants reported that the psychiatric disorder preceded the SUD (28% females, 25% males) or that the SUD preceded the psychiatric disorder (10% females, 21% males).

Theories Explaining Comorbidity

Why is psychiatric comorbidity so common among adolescents with SUDs? In addition to research suggesting shared genetic and environmental influences (Storr et al., 2012), there are at least two well-known theories about this association. The first is the self-medication hypothesis, which suggests that substances are used to reduce feelings of distress, depression, or anxiety (Khantzian, 1997). Adolescents who use substances for self-medication often hold positive substance use expectancies (e.g., drinking leads to relaxation/tension reduction) and coping motives (e.g., drinking will improve coping; Cooper, 2004) that drive their use. Expectancies are thought of as underlying beliefs about the effects of substance use or associations between past experiences and use, while motives represent an immediate urge to use.

Expectancies and motives are distinct but related risk factors for substance use (e.g., Agrawal et al., 2008; see Davis, Riley, & Smith, Chapter 4, this volume). Expectancies can be learned in a variety of contexts: in the home, via media, and through peers. For example, a person who grows up in a home in which parents drink at the end of each day may develop positive beliefs about the relaxing effects of alcohol (e.g., "Drinking alcohol is a good way to unwind"). This is, essentially, an " 'if–then" statement (e.g., "If I drink alcohol at the end of the day, then I will feel more relaxed"). Notably, expectancies may develop before any substance use has ever occurred—individuals can develop beliefs about substances simply through observation (Smith, Goldman, Greenbaum, & Christiansen, 1995). Motives, on the other hand, characterize the reason that an individual is using a substance *right now*. For example, an individual may hold many positive expectancies about drinking (e.g., "Drinking is a good way to relax"; "Drinking helps me socialize at parties") but is motivated to drink in a specific situation by a proximal urge (e.g., "I want to have more fun at this party tonight, so I'm having another drink").

A second leading theory is problem behavior theory, which suggests that substance use is one of many delinquent behaviors that form an underlying "syndrome" of problem behavior (Donovan & Jessor, 1985). Adolescents who engage in delinquent behaviors are more prone to engage in illicit activities and associate with delinquent peers who have similarly poor social and problem-solving skills, victimize other youth, and both use and distribute illicit drugs (Loeber et al., 2001). Specific temperamental and neurological factors increase risk for this wide variety of "problem behaviors." For example, poor planning, impulse control, and impaired executive functioning may underlie multiple diagnoses associated with delinquent behaviors and substance use, such as ADHD and conduct disorder (Clark, Parker, & Lynch, 1999; Tarter et al., 1999).

ASSESSMENT OF COMORBIDITY

As most adolescents with an SUD will have a CPD, it is important to conduct a comprehensive assessment of both disorders when developing treatment plans. A multimethod assessment approach that includes a diagnostic interview, broadband assessments, and briefer area-specific assessments is recommended when possible. Below is a review of some of the strengths and drawbacks of each type of assessment approach.

Diagnostic Interviews

Structured and semistructured diagnostic interviews are useful tools to help derive diagnoses. Use of interviews allows one to obtain a comprehensive assessment of psychiatric diagnoses, which is extremely helpful in developing an accurate case formulation (i.e., understanding of the development of presenting problems) and treatment plans. They also capture areas of difficulties not shared during a clinical history interview that may affect treatment approach and outcomes. For example, it is not uncommon for adolescents with oppositional behavior and substance abuse problems to have an underlying anxiety disorder that is not reported during unstructured clinical interviews, yet plays a large role in both behaviors and requires intervention. Some diagnostic interviews are also free of cost. Drawbacks of diagnostic interviews are that they require training and can be lengthy (e.g., 1–2 hours if both adolescent and parent interviews are conducted) depending on the number of diagnoses present and skill level of the interviewer.

There are four well-validated diagnostic interviews commonly used to assess psychiatric disorders and SUDs in adolescents, all of which include parent- and adolescent-report versions. The Schedule for Affective Disorders and Schizophrenia for School-Age Children—Present and Lifetime Version (K-SADS-PL; Kaufman et al., 1997) is a widely used, semistructured, clinician-administered interview that provides a reliable and valid measurement of DSM-IV disorders. A DSM-5 version is also now available. The NIMH Diagnostic Interview Schedule for Children Version IV (DISC-IV; Shaffer, Fisher, Lucas, Dulcan, & Schwab-Stone, 2000) is a computer-assisted structured interview that generates DSM-IV diagnoses. There are clinician-administered and voice-assisted versions. The Diagnostic Interview for Children and Adolescents (DICA; Reich, 2000) is semistructured and assesses for the full range of DSM-IV diagnoses, and is available in computer and paper-and-pencil versions. The Anxiety Disorders Interview Schedule for DSM-IV for Child and Parent (ADIS-IV; Silverman, Saavedra, & Pina, 2001) is semistructured and assesses mood, anxiety, and disruptive behavior disorders. There are also screens to assess for substance abuse, psychosis, and selective mutism, as well as eating, somatoform, and developmental and learning disorders. Development of the DSM-5 version is under way.

Broadband Assessment of Psychiatric Symptoms

Similar to diagnostic interviews, broadband instruments allow one to assess for adolescent psychiatric symptoms across multiple disorders, many of which may not have been reported during a standard clinical interview. This information can also be used to inform case formulation and treatment planning as well as to assess change over time if readministered during and/or at the end of treatment. Broadband assessments take less time to administer than diagnostic interviews and do not require training because they are self-report instruments completed by adolescents, parents, and teachers. Many also come with computerized scoring and generate a feedback report that summarizes findings, which increases ease of scoring and interpretation. This feedback report includes cutoff scores to denote clinically significant symptoms in a problem area and many also flag critical items (i.e., those that indicate risk of harm to self or others) in need of immediate attention. The drawbacks of broadband assessments are that most require at least 20 minutes to complete, can be costly to purchase, and though they provide evidence for diagnoses, cannot be used to make actual psychiatric diagnoses. See Table 7.2 for examples of commonly used broadband instruments and helpful details about each.

Area–Specific Assessments

Area-specific assessments can also be useful assessment tools. Similar to broadband assessments, they can be used to determine severity of psychiatric symptoms, track youth outcomes over time, and can be completed by multiple informants when parent and/or teacher versions are available. They are briefer than broadband assessments, typically only requiring 5–15 minutes to complete, tend to be more sensitive to change in symptoms over time, typically include cutoff scores to denote clinically significant symptoms, and are less costly than broadband assessments. They are ideal to use when tracking progress in one problem area over time, and can easily be administered at the start of every counseling session. The drawbacks of area-specific assessments are that they typically assess only one specific problem area, many come only in an adolescent self-report version, scoring has to be completed by hand, and they cannot be used to yield actual diagnoses. See Table 7.2 for examples of commonly used area-specific assessments and helpful details about each instrument.

EMPIRICAL DATA ON THE EFFECT OF COMORBIDITY ON SUD INTERVENTION OUTCOMES

CPDs among adolescents with SUDs have been shown to negatively impact treatment outcomes across outpatient (Rowe et al., 2004; Tomlinson, Brown, & Abrantes, 2004), intensive outpatient (White et al., 2004), and inpatient/residential (McCarthy, Tomlinson, Anderson, Marlatt, & Brown, 2005; Shane, Jasiukaitis, & Green 2003) SUD treatment. Generally, most research suggests that youth with internalizing *and* externalizing disorders, or more diagnoses in total, report worse outcomes (Rowe et al., 2004; Shane et al., 2003; Tomlinson et al., 2004). When the effect of comorbid internalizing and externalizing symptoms are compared, comorbid externalizing symptoms appear to be associated with worse outcomes (Tomlinson et al., 2004; Winters, Stinchfield, Latimer, & Stone, 2008). Interestingly, when comorbid internalizing disorders, or depression in particular, is examined in relation to SUD outcomes, results are quite mixed. In a review conducted by Hersh, Curry, and Kaminer (2014) that examined the effect of depression on adolescent SUD outcomes across multiple settings, depression was found to have a positive effect on outcomes in some studies and a negative or lack of effect in others. It has been suggested that depression may differentially affect youth. For some, depression may have a motivating effect on engagement. Depressed youth may be more likely to acknowledge that they have a problem, desire relief from their depression, and

TABLE 7.2. Examples of Broadband and Area-Specific Assessment Instruments for Adolescent Psychiatric Symptoms

Instrument	Type of assessment	Response format(s)	Items	Information yielded
Achenbach System of Empirically Based Assessment (Achenbach, 2009)	Broadband	Parent report (CBCL), youth self-report (YSR), and teacher report (TRF)	113	Composite scores for internalizing, externalizing, and total problems, as well as eight behavioral syndromes and six DSM-oriented scales. Many scales are DSM-5 compatible.
Behavior Assessment System for Children (Reynolds & Kamphaus, 2015)	Broadband	Adolescent self-report of personality (SRP), parent rating scale (PRS), and teacher rating scale (TRS)	175	DSM-5 symptoms. The PRS and TRS yield composite (Externalizing Problems, Internalizing Problems, Behavioral Symptoms Index, Adaptive Skills, Executive Functioning Index), clinical, and content (e.g., anger control, bullying) scores. The SRP yields clinical and adaptive scale scores across domains.
Youth's Inventory–4 (Gadow et al., 2002)	Broadband	Self-report	120	Symptoms of 18 DSM-IV disorders.
Child and Adolescent Symptom Inventory (Gadow & Sprafkin, 2015; Gadow et al., 2002)	Broadband	Parent report Teacher report	142 105	Symptoms of 18 DSM-IV disorders and DSM-5 items and scales.
Beck Youth Depression Inventory (Beck, Beck, Jolly, & Steer, 2005)	Specific (depression)	Self-report	20	Negative thoughts (about self, life, and the future), sadness and guilt, and sleep disturbance associated with depression.
Reynolds Adolescent Depression Scale–2 (Reynolds, 2002)	Specific (depression)	Self-report	30	Subscales (dysphoric mood, anhedonia/negative affect, negative evaluation, somatic complaints) and a total depressive score.

(*continued*)

TABLE 7.2. (*continued*)

Instrument	Type of assessment	Response format(s)	Items	Information yielded
Beck Youth Anxiety Inventory (Beck et al., 2005)	Specific (anxiety)	Self-report	20	Worries about school performance, the future, negative reactions, fears, and physiological symptoms associated with anxiety.
Screen for Child Anxiety Related Emotional Disorders (Birmaher et al., 1997)	Specific (anxiety)	Self-report and parent report	41	Five subscales (somatic/panic, generalized anxiety, separation anxiety, social phobia, school phobia) and a total anxiety scale.
Beck Disruptive Behavior Inventory for Youth (Beck et al., 2005)	Specific (disruptive behavior)	Self-report	20	Behaviors and attitudes associated with conduct disorder and oppositional defiant disorder.
Brown Attention-Deficit Disorder Scales (Brown, 2001)	Specific (disruptive behavior)	Self-report, parent report, and teacher report	40	Executive function impairments associated with ADHD.
Conners 3rd Edition (Conners, 2008)	Specific (disruptive behavior)	Self-report (SR), parent report (PR), and teacher report (TR)	41 SR, 41 TR, 45 PR; short form	DSM-5 criteria for ADHD, oppositional defiant disorder and conduct disorder; subscale scores for inattention, hyperactivity/impulsivity, learning problems, executive functioning, ADHD, oppositional defiant disorder, conduct disorder, defiance/aggression, peer/family relations, general psychopathology.

Note. ADHD, attention-deficit/hyperactivity disorder.

thus be more likely to engage in treatment (Pagnin, de Queiroz, & Saggese, 2005; Tapert et al., 2003). For others it may be a liability, impeding the ability to mobilize the resources needed to engage in treatment (Tapert et al., 2003).

Relative to more intensive treatment, very few studies have examined the effect of comorbidity on substance outcomes in the context of brief interventions for adolescents. Becker, Curry, and Yang (2011) conducted an open trial of motivational enhancement therapy (MET; two sessions) plus cognitive-behavioral therapy (CBT; three sessions) with 106 adolescents with an SUD (38% depressive, 10% anxiety, 27% posttraumatic, and 50% conduct disorders). Neither severity of depressive nor conduct symptoms predicted change in substance use *frequency* over 12 months. However, in a second study that used a subsample of 90 of these adolescents, lower baseline depressive symptoms predicted worse substance use *problems*. Further, more severe conduct symptoms predicted greater substance use *frequency*, but only among those with lower (vs. higher) depressive symptoms at 6 months (Hersh, Curry, & Becker, 2013).

Tapert et al. (2003) examined the effect of depressed mood on intervention outcomes among 268 adolescents treated for injury or alcohol intoxication in a hospital emergency department or self-reported alcohol use at time of the visit. Adolescents were randomized to brief motivational interviewing (MI) or standard care. At 6-month follow-up, higher depressed mood at baseline predicted less drinking for younger females, more drinking for younger males and older females, and had no effect on drinking outcomes for older males.

Stein et al. (2011) examined whether depressive symptoms moderated intervention effects in a sample of 162 incarcerated adolescents, most of whom met criteria for an SUD prior to incarceration (60% alcohol, 90% cannabis). Adolescents were randomly assigned to MI or relaxation training. At 3-months postrelease, MI was associated with lower rates of substance use (drinks per drinking day and days used marijuana) than relaxation training, but only among those with low levels of depression. Within the relaxation training condition, adolescents with higher versus lower depressive symptoms reported less substance use (days used marijuana and trend for drinks per drinking day) at follow-up. Depressive symptoms did not influence outcome within the MI condition.

As is evident, comorbidity does not appear to have a clear pattern of effects on brief interventions for SUDs. Rather, results appear to vary by age, gender, severity of symptoms, and brief intervention type. For younger adolescents (i.e., ages 12–14), particularly those recruited from community-based samples, depressive symptoms may be milder in nature and less stable, relative to older adolescents (i.e., ages 15–17), who may have a longer history of depression. Thus, their depressive symptoms may dissipate more quickly as might their ability to engage in alcohol-related activities if caught drinking by their parents (Tapert et al., 2003). As suggested by Tapert et al. (2003), this may be particularly true for young females who tend to be more closely monitored by their parents relative to males (Svensson, 2003). Depression may also have a greater impact on social drinking for younger adolescents because it requires a more proactive effort on their part relative to more autonomous older adolescents who can often drive (Tapert et al., 2003). Older adolescents, on the other hand, may have greater access to alcohol and thus use it more readily to address depressive symptoms. A more frequent drinking pattern, in turn, may cause or exacerbate their depressed mood (Tapert et al., 2003), thus strengthening the nature of this relationship.

Interestingly, the studies conducted by Becker et al. (2011) and Hersh et al. (2013) suggest that comorbid depressive symptoms either have no effect or a protective effect on frequency of substance use, particularly in the presence of conduct problems. Adolescents with more severe conduct problems, particularly those with deviant peer groups, may lack motivation to change their substance use. When comorbid depressive symptoms are present, it may provide some internal motivation to change due to associated negative feelings and affect. Depressive symptoms may also reflect that the adolescent feels guilt or remorse for deviant acts, which may also increase the likelihood of positive change.

The effect of depressive symptoms on brief interventions for substance use also appears to vary by type of intervention. Depressive symptoms may have a greater impact on brief MI, which focuses on improving motivation for change and increasing change talk. Adolescents with heightened depression may not be able to readily attend to MI or mobilize the resources needed to make changes, even if desired. On the other hand, brief interventions that include some active skill instruction, such as cognitive-behavioral skills (e.g., relaxation, problem solving), may have a direct positive effect on depressive symptoms and thus provide greater benefit to depressed youth. For example, according to Stein et al. (2011), the meditational and mindfulness components of relaxation may help youth with heightened depressive symptoms better manage their affect, which in turn may decrease their need to use substances for affect regulation purposes. Indeed, prior research suggests that adults with SUDs who are high in depressed mood fare better in a mindfulness treatment than usual care (Witkiewitz & Bowen, 2010). Further research in this area is needed before any definitive conclusions can be drawn about the effect of comorbidity on brief interventions for SUDs.

IMPLICATIONS FOR BRIEF SUBSTANCE ABUSE INTERVENTIONS

As described above, comorbid conditions may impact the efficacy of interventions for adolescent SUDs. Perhaps more importantly, it is highly likely that an adolescent who requires intervention for an SUD will experience comorbid psychopathology. Thus, it is imperative that comorbidity is assessed and discussed during brief interventions for SUDs.

How can a medical or mental health professional address comorbidity within brief MI for an adolescent SUD? The first step is to assess for symptoms of CPD. As described earlier, there are several assessment tools that can be used. Once this information is gathered, the clinician can provide feedback about these symptoms. This information can be integrated into feedback pertaining to the adolescent's level of current substance use. For example, in many brief interventions, a clinician will assess the adolescent's current level of substance use and associated problems, and then provide feedback regarding how much the adolescent is using substances compared with peers and the degree to which it has caused problems in his or her life. A similar process can be used to integrate feedback about CPDs. For example, when working with an adolescent with comorbid depression, a clinician might share that the adolescent reported clinically significant depressive symptoms, depression is a medical condition that commonly occurs among adolescents with SUDs, and that effective treatments are available. The clinician might also share that substance use can worsen depression, increase the length of depressive episodes, increase the risk of suicidal thoughts and behavior, decrease the effectiveness of psychiatric medications, and cause dangerous drug interactions if used with psychiatric medications. Such feedback can enhance understanding of the severity of problem substance use and distressing emotions, address misperceptions, and enhance motivation for treatment of both disorders.

Feedback of this type is very important given that adolescents tend to estimate that their peers use substances at much higher rates or in greater quantities than they actually do, and thus perceive that their own use is within normal limits (Buckner, Ecker, & Proctor, 2011). Adolescents also tend to underestimate the base rates of youth psychiatric symptoms, have social norms about the need for secrecy of psychiatric symptoms, and endorse perceived norms about the lack of availability of help (e.g., Wilson, Deane, Marshall, & Dalley, 2010). The implication of this research is that adolescents who use substances and have CPDs may be even less likely to seek help or express motivation for therapy than those without comorbidity. They may not perceive substance use as a problem because it is viewed as "normal," and at the same time, believe that their psychological difficulties are "abnormal." Their substance use may also facilitate connectedness and belonging to desired peer groups, whereas acknowledging and seeking help for psychological difficulties may make them feel different and isolated from peers. Thus, they may retain secrecy and avoid seeking professional help to maintain their relationships.

Other common components of brief MI involves asking adolescents to brainstorm the pros and cons of substance use and to envision the future if changes in substance use are made. With regard to the former, adolescents can be asked to think about how their substance use may impact their CPD when developing their pros and cons list. For pros, adolescents commonly share that substances help them temporarily forget about their depression or decrease their anxiety in social situations, consistent with the self-medication model. Adolescents should also be encouraged to think about the cons of using to manage depression (e.g., worsens depression, can increase suicidal thinking) and anxiety (e.g., effects are temporary, impairs judgment). A similar approach can be taken when asking adolescents about the not-so-good and good things that may happen in the future if changes in substance use are made.

Adolescents should be encouraged to think about how changes or lack thereof may affect their psychiatric condition. If the adolescent has difficulty, it can be helpful to share that psychiatric disorders tend to worsen when substances are used and when mental health treatment is not obtained. This can lead to the need for hospitalization or residential placement. If the teen has a history of suicidal behavior, a future suicide attempt and completion is also more likely.

Goal setting is another core component of brief interventions for adolescent SUDs. Adolescents with comorbid psychiatric conditions should be encouraged to set goals not only for their substance use but also their psychiatric disorder. It should be repeated that SUDs are often interconnected and that progress in one area will positively affect the other. Though there are several brief interventions that have an impact on adolescent substance use, the treatment of comorbid mood, anxiety, and disruptive behavior disorders are generally most effective when the adolescent can participate in multiple therapy sessions, which often include family work and consultation with schools and other medical and mental health professionals involved in their care (see David-Ferdon & Kaslow, 2008; Epstein et al., 2015; Evans, Owens, & Bunford, 2014, for reviews of evidence-based interventions). Thus, one goal for comorbid youth may be to seek an adjunctive intervention for CPDs. Other more immediate goals may involve attempting to use adaptive strategies to manage difficult emotions in place of substances (e.g., call a friend if sad, talk with best friend if nervous at a party).

After goals are selected, a discussion of barriers typically ensues. The adolescent should be asked to consider what could get in the way of both substance- and mental health-related goals, so that the clinician can assist the adolescent in problem solving around barriers. In instances where a goal is attending adjunctive mental health therapy, the clinician should be prepared to address misconceptions about therapy. The clinician might ask questions such as "What do you think happens in therapy?" and "How many sessions do you think it takes to get better?" to open the line of communication in this area. The clinician might also ask about things that will get in the way of therapy attendance. Common responses often include the belief that it means the teen is crazy, friends will make fun of the teen, parents are the problem, parents will get upset if family problems are discussed, the teen would rather do other things, transportation problems, and forgetting appointments. The clinician will need to help the adolescent process and/or problem-solve these obstacles. At the end of this discussion, the clinician should be sure to help the adolescent generate self-efficacy statements around goals for both substance use and CPDs. The clinician might ask questions such as "What personal strengths will help you to successfully meet your goals?" and "What strengths have family or friends noticed in you?" After strengths have been identified, the clinician can help the adolescent articulate how identified strengths can facilitate success toward goals. For example, the clinician might state "Your intelligence will clearly help you learn and use skills taught during therapy needed to feel better and avoid drinking." If psychoeducational handouts are sent home at the end of the intervention, the clinician may consider sending home materials pertaining to relevant CPDs (e.g., causes, symptoms, effective treatments) in addition to SUDs.

As adolescent attendance at adjunctive evidence-based mental health interventions often requires parental engagement (consent, transportation, payment) and involvement (parent and family sessions), it will be necessary to have a discussion with parents about their adolescent's psychiatric symptoms and need for mental health treatment. In some instances, the clinician may need to use psychoeducation and motivational techniques to enhance parental understanding and engagement in the adolescent's treatment goals. The clinician will also likely need to help parents problem-solve barriers to therapy attendance. To further improve the likelihood of adolescent attendance and optimal treatment outcomes, referrals for parental treatment (substance abuse, mental health, couple counseling, etc.) should be offered as needed, particularly if parental difficulties contribute to the adolescent's substance or mental health problems. The clinician may emphasize that parents may be best able to help their child if they are feeling well, and that their health is just as important as that of their child.

DETERMINING THE NEED FOR ADJUNCTIVE MENTAL HEALTH INTERVENTIONS

The need for an adjunctive mental health intervention as well as its optimal length and intensity may vary across adolescents with SUDs. To help inform this decision, it is important to determine both a timeline for the development of the SUD and CPDs as well as a thorough understanding of the sequencing of symptoms and use in daily life. SUDs may precede, follow, or develop simultaneously with CPDs. Temporal order may suggest different etiologies, which may require different approaches for optimal outcomes (Brook, Whiteman, Finch, & Cohen, 1995). For example, when internalizing disorders precede SUDs and substances are used to relieve or dampen distress, adequate treatment of the internalizing disorder may result in reductions in substance use. Under such conditions, only a brief adjunctive SUD intervention may be needed. In instances where the psychopharmacological effects of the substances result in or exacerbate internalizing disorders (e.g., via additional stress, withdrawal symptoms), adequate treatment of the SUD may result in reductions in comorbid symptoms. There does exist some evidence to suggest that outpatient treatment of SUDs alone is associated with reductions in comorbid internalizing symptoms (Horigian et al., 2013). When an SUD and CPDs onset simultaneously, consistent with a reciprocal causation model (Johnson & Kaplan, 1990), it is possible that concurrent or integrated treatment may be needed for optimal outcomes. Indeed, comorbid symptoms directly associated with substance use will likely have a different effect on outcomes relative to symptoms resulting from an organic disorder (Hersh et al., 2014). For example, depressed mood resulting from substance withdrawal may remit upon completion of successful SUD treatment, whereas depressed mood associated with comorbid major depressive disorder may require an evidence-based intervention that directly targets depressive symptoms. Understanding the temporal precedence of SUDs and CPDs can offer valuable information to help inform treatment planning (Brook et al., 1995).

Though temporal precedence is informative, an understanding of the sequencing of symptoms and substance abuse *in daily life* may lead to a more precise understanding of the SUD–comorbidity relationship and how to approach treatment. This requires the use of a functional analysis, which is a step-by-step examination of the environmental events, cognitions, emotions, physical sensations, and behaviors in the hours leading up to an episode of substance use, as well as immediate reinforcers of use. Functional analysis is essential in order for clinicians to understand when (e.g., alone, with friends, weekends), why (e.g., self-medicinal purposes, peers using substances), and under what conditions (mood states, etc.) substances are used. This information can aid in an overarching conceptualization of the interrelationship of substances and psychiatric symptoms to guide treatment planning. Figure 7.1 includes examples of therapist questions that are asked to help prepare a depressed client for a functional analysis of marijuana use as well as sample client responses. Notably, the therapist included "depression" as a factor that increased the client's vulnerability to a lapse in abstinence. Figure 7.2 includes an example of a functional analysis of events that led up to the depressed client's marijuana use and lapse in abstinence. Also of note is that some of the client's negative thoughts are reflective of black-and-white thinking common to depression (i.e., "Nothing I do is right") as are identified behaviors (i.e., social isolation) associated with the client's marijuana use.

CONCLUSIONS AND FUTURE DIRECTIONS

CPDs occur at high rates among adolescents with SUDs. Moreover, various patterns of comorbidity have differential effects on treatment outcome. Research is sorely needed to examine the processes through which comorbidity affects SUD outcomes, conditions under which adolescents who are comorbid are most likely to relapse, and conditions that yield the most optimal treatment outcomes (Tomlinson et al., 2004). It is imperative to assess for and measure the effect of comorbid conditions on outcomes for SUDs. These data will add to the dearth of literature in this area and inform future thinking about how to best meet the needs of this complex population. To our knowledge, brief interventions simultaneously targeting adolescent SUDs (alcohol; cannabis; other hard, illicit drugs) and comorbid conditions have not been tested. This

What is the behavior I am working on?	What trigger started the chain to my behavior?	What things in myself and my environment made me vulnerable?
Marijuana use	Being picked on at school	1. My depression 2. Isolating myself 3. Not sleeping enough 4. Fight with my mom

FIGURE 7.1. Preparatory therapist questions and sample client responses that aid in preparation for a functional analysis of substance use.

may stem from the fact that evidence-based interventions for psychiatric disorders tend to include a long course of treatment, and comorbid youth tend to have more severe symptoms than noncomorbid youth. However, not all youth with SUDs and comorbid psychiatric symptoms seen in the context of brief interventions may require a full course of adjunctive mental health treatment. Treatment models that incorporate the great heterogeneity of substance-abusing youth are essential.

There are a few potential approaches to addressing comorbid substance use and psychiatric comorbidity in brief interventions that may benefit from examination. First, as discussed earlier, it is indeed possible to integrate comorbidity-related feedback, exercises, goals, and recommendations into standard brief MI protocols for SUDs. While this approach may not remediate psychiatric symptoms in those with full-blown and/or severe psychiatric disorders, it can be used to engage adolescents in adjunctive treatment. If comorbid psychiatric symptoms are not severe or are due to the direct effect of substances (e.g., withdrawal symptoms), the integration of a behavior functional analysis and a few selected transdiagnostic CBT sessions could lead to reductions in comorbid psychiatric symptoms.

Transdiagnostic skills are techniques that help remediate multiple types of mental health and substance use problems (e.g., problem solving, cognitive restructuring). Parents could simultaneously receive a few transdiagnostic parent-training sessions (e.g., problem solving, communication, monitoring, behavioral contracting). Indeed, the Family Check-Up (Stormshak & Dishion, 2009), a well-known brief substance abuse preventive intervention, incorporates parent training to enhance skills in areas known to protect against SUDs and externalizing problems. For example, if an adolescent presented with alcohol abuse and depressive symptoms, the therapist could teach problem solving to work on both problems. The therapist would begin by identifying common triggers for both urges to use alcohol and depressive symptoms (e.g., conflict with parents, bullying). If the primary trigger identified was conflict with a parent, the problem could be defined as "how to decrease conflict with my parent."

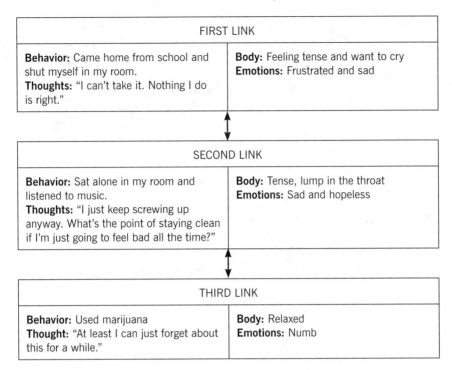

FIGURE 7.2. Example of a functional analysis of events that led up to using marijuana and a lapse in abstinence.

The therapist and adolescent would then work collaboratively to brainstorm potential options, such as asking for time to cool down, use a calm voice, come home on time, and drink to numb out. They would then evaluate each of these options, rating whether each would likely lead to a positive and/or negative outcome. Based on these ratings, the option(s) associated with the most positive outcomes would be selected and the adolescent would be asked to try to implement these options at home. The adolescent's parents could be taught the same problem-solving skill to help decrease conflict with their adolescent. However, they would be asked to generate options that they could implement to help decrease conflict (e.g., not engage in discussions when angry, take time to cool down when getting upset, work in therapy to create a behavioral contract with rewards and consequences for specified adolescent behaviors). They, too, would evaluate and then select the most optimal potential solutions to implement at home. Discussion would also be devoted to how to carry out solutions (e.g., where to go to cool down and things that can be done to self-soothe) as well as how to work through potential obstacles to implementation. The therapist would then meet with the adolescent and parent together to discuss their respective plans to decrease conflict at home.

Another novel approach may be to use a stepped-care model to address variability in SUD treatment response and the effect of comorbidity on outcomes. In a stepped-care model, adolescents would enter the lowest level of care and transition to more intensive treatment only if they exhibit poor treatment outcomes at that level (Kaminer & Godley, 2010). Treatment algorithms are created, with accompanying decision rules, to guide treatment decisions based on progress in target symptoms (e.g., substance use, depressive symptoms, conduct problems). For example, adolescents may enter a brief intervention for substance use. If they do not show an adequate reduction in substance or comorbid symptoms (e.g., depression, anxiety, conduct problems), they could be "stepped up" to more intensive intervention in the area of need. In this fashion, adolescents receive needed targeted treatment only in select areas, which improves cost effectiveness, feasibility, and utility of the intervention (Hersh et al., 2014). If we are to move science forward and adequately address comorbidity among youth with SUDs, it is imperative to develop and test novel and hopefully effective approaches to this often very complex condition.

ACKNOWLEDGMENTS

This research was supported by two National Institutes of Health grants (R01MH087520 and R01MH097703) awarded to Christianne Esposito-Smythers and colleagues.

REFERENCES

Abram, K. M., Teplin, L. A., McClelland, G. M., & Dulcan, M. K. (2003). Comorbid psychiatric disorders in youth in juvenile detention. *Archives of General Psychiatry, 60,* 1097–1108.

Abrantes, A. M., Brown, S. A., & Tomlinson, K. L. (2003). Psychiatric comorbidity among inpatient substance abusing adolescents. *Journal of Child and Adolescent Substance Abuse, 13,* 83–101.

Achenbach, T. M. (2009). *The Achenbach System of Empirically Based Assessment (ASEBA): Development, findings, theory, and applications.* Burlington: University of Vermont Research Center for Children, Youth, and Families.

Agrawal, A., Dick, D. M., Bucholz, K. K., Madden, P. A., Cooper, M. L., Sher, K. J., et al. (2008). Drinking expectancies and motives: A genetic study of young adult women. *Addiction, 103,* 194–204.

American Psychiatric Association. (2013). *Diagnostic and statistical manual of mental disorders* (5th ed.). Arlington, VA: Author.

Armstrong, T. D., & Costello, E. J. (2002). Community studies on adolescent substance use, abuse, or dependence and psychiatric comorbidity. *Journal of Consulting and Clinical Psychology, 70,* 1224–1239.

Beck, J. S., Beck, A. T., Jolly, J. B., & Steer, R. A. (2005). *Beck Youth Inventories: For children and adolescents.* San Antonio, TX: Psychological Corporation.

Becker, S. J., Curry, J. F., & Yang, C. (2011). Factors that influence trajectories of change in frequency of substance use and quality of life among adolescents receiving a brief intervention. *Journal of Substance Abuse Treatment, 41*, 294–304.

Birmaher, B., Khetpal, S., Brent, D., Cully, M., Balach, L., Kaufman, J., et al. (1997). The Screen for Child Anxiety Related Emotional Disorders (SCARED): Scale construction and psychometric characteristics. *Journal of the American Academy of Child and Adolescent Psychiatry, 36*, 545–553.

Brook, J. S., Whiteman, M., Finch, S. J., & Cohen, P. (1995). Aggression, intra-psychic distress and drug use: Antecedent and intervening processes. *Journal of the American Academy of Child and Adolescent Psychiatry, 34*, 1076–1083.

Brown, T. E. (2001). *Brown Attention-Deficit Disorder Scales® for Children and Adolescents.* San Antonio, TX: Psychological Corporation.

Buckner, J. D., Ecker, A. H., & Proctor, S. L. (2011). Social anxiety and alcohol problems: The roles of perceived descriptive and injunctive peer norms. *Journal of Anxiety Disorders, 25*, 631–638.

Center for Behavioral Health Statistics and Quality. (2015). Behavioral health trends in the United States: Results from the 2014 National Survey on Drug Use and Health (HHS Publication No. SMA 15-4927, NSDUH Series H-50). Retrieved from www.samhsa.gov/data.

Chisolm, D. J., Mulatu, M. S., & Brown, J. R. (2009). Racial/ethnic disparities in the patterns of co-occurring mental health problems in adolescents in substance abuse treatment. *Journal of Substance Abuse Treatment, 37*, 203–210.

Clark, D., Parker, A., & Lynch, K. (1999). Psychopathology and substance-related problems during early adolescence: A survival analysis. *Journal of Clinical Child Psychology, 28*, 333–341.

Clark, D. B., Pollock, N., Bukstein, O. G., Mezzich, A. C., Bromberger, J. T., & Donovan, J. E. (1997). Gender and comorbid psychopathology in adolescents with alcohol dependence. *Journal of the American Academy of Child and Adolescent Psychiatry, 36*, 1195–1203.

Conners, C. K. (2008). *The Conners 3rd Edition* (Conners 3). North Tonawanda, NJ: Multi Health System.

Cooper, M. L. (1994). Motivations for alcohol use among adolescents: Development and validation of a four-factor model. *Psychological Assessment, 6*, 117.

David-Ferdon, C., & Kaslow, N. J. (2008). Evidence-based psychosocial treatments for child and adolescent depression. *Journal of Clinical Child and Adolescent Psychology, 37*, 62–104.

Deas-Nesmith, D., Campbell, S., & Brady, K. (1998). Substance use disorders in an adolescent inpatient psychiatric population. *Journal of the National Medical Association, 90*, 233–238.

Dennis, M., Godley, S. H., Diamond, G., Tims, F. M., Babor, T., Donaldson, J., et al. (2004). The Cannabis Youth Treatment (CYT) Study: Main findings from two randomized trials. *Journal of Substance Abuse Treatment, 27*, 197–213.

Donovan, J. E., & Jessor, R. (1985). Structure of problem behavior in adolescence and young adulthood. *Journal of Consulting and Clinical Psychology, 53*, 890–904.

Epstein, R., Fonnesbeck, C., Williamson, E., Kuhn, T., Lindegren, M. L., Rizzone, K., et al., (2015). Psychosocial and pharmacologic interventions for disruptive behavior in children and adolescents (Comparative Effectiveness Review No. 154, pp. ES1–ES21; AHRQ Publication No. 15(16)-EHC019-EF). Rockville, MD: Agency for

Healthcare Research and Quality. Retrieved from *www.effectivehealthcare.ahrq.gov/reports/final.cfm.*

Essau, C. A. (2011). Comorbidity of substance use disorders among community based and high-risk adolescents. *Psychiatry Research, 185,* 176–184.

Evans, S. W., Owens, J. S., & Bunford, N. (2014). Evidence-based psychosocial treatments for children and adolescents with attention-deficit/hyperactivity disorder. *Journal of Clinical Child and Adolescent Psychology, 43,* 527–551.

Gadow, K. D., & Sprafkin, J. (2015). *The Symptom Inventories: An annotated bibliography.* Stony Brook, NY: Checkmate Plus.

Gadow, K. D., Sprafkin, J., Carlson, G. A., Schneider, J., Nolan, E. E., Mattison. R. E., et al. (2002). A DSM-IV-referenced, Adolescent Self-Report Rating Scale. *Journal of the American Academy of Child and Adolescent Psychiatry, 41,* 671–679.

Grella, C. E., Joshi, V., & Hser, Y. I. (2004). Effects of comorbidity on treatment processes and outcomes among adolescents in drug treatment programs. *Journal of Child and Adolescent Substance Abuse, 14,* 13–31.

Hersh, J., Curry, J. F., & Becker, S. J. (2013). The influence of comorbid depression and conduct disorder on MET/CBT treatment outcome for adolescent substance use disorders. *International Journal of Cognitive Therapy, 6,* 325–341.

Hersh, J., Curry, J. F., & Kaminer, Y. (2014). What is the impact of comorbid depression on adolescent substance abuse treatment? *Substance Abuse, 35,* 364–375.

Hollen, V., & Ortiz, G. (2015). Mental health and substance use comorbidity among adolescents in psychiatric inpatient hospitals: Prevalence and covariates. *Journal of Child and Adolescent Substance Abuse, 24,* 102–112.

Horigian, V. E., Weems, C. F., Robbins, M. S., Feaster, D. J., Ucha, J., Miller, M., et al. (2013). Reductions in anxiety and depression symptoms in youth receiving substance use treatment. *American Journal of Addiction, 22,* 329–337.

Johnson, R. J., & Kaplan, H. B. (1990). Stability of psychological symptoms: Drug use consequences and intervening processes. *Journal of Health and Social Behavior, 31,* 277–291.

Kaminer, Y., & Godley, M. (2010). From assessment reactivity to aftercare for adolescent substance abuse: Are we there yet? *Child and Adolescent Psychiatric Clinics of North America, 19,* 577–590.

Kaufman, J., Birmaher, B., Brent, D., Rao, U. M. A., Flynn, C., Moreci, P., et al. (1997). Schedule for Affective Disorders and Schizophrenia for School-Age Children—Present and Lifetime Version (K-SADS-PL): Initial reliability and validity data. *Journal of the American Academy of Child and Adolescent Psychiatry, 36,* 980–988.

Khantzian, E. J. (1997). The self-medication hypothesis of substance use disorders: A reconsideration and recent applications. *Harvard Review of Psychiatry, 4,* 231–244.

Loeber, R., Farrington, D. P., Stouthamer-Loeber, M., Moffitt, T. E., Caspi, A., & Lynam, D. (2001). Male mental health problems, psychopathy, and personality traits: Key findings from the first 14 years of the Pittsburgh Youth Study. *Clinical Child and Family Psychology Review, 4,* 273–297.

Mason, M. J., & Posner, M. A. (2009). Brief substance abuse treatment with urban adolescents: A translational research study. *Journal of Child and Adolescent Substance Abuse, 18,* 193–206.

McCarthy, D. M., Tomlinson, K. L., Anderson, K. G., Marlatt, G. A., & Brown, S. A. (2005). Relapse in alcohol and drug disordered adolescents with comorbid psychopathology: Changes in psychiatric symptoms. *Psychology of Addictive Behaviors, 19,* 28–34.

Novins, D. K., Fickensher, A., & Manson, S. M. (2006). American Indian adolescents in substance abuse treatment: Diagnostic status. *Journal of Substance Abuse Treatment, 30,* 275–284.

Pagnin, D., de Queiroz, V., & Saggese, E. G. (2005). Predictors of attrition from day treatment of adolescents with substance-related disorders. *Addictive Behaviors, 30*(5), 1065–1069.

Reich, W. (2000). Diagnostic Interview for Children and Adolescents (DICA). *Journal of the American Academy of Child and Adolescent Psychiatry, 39,* 59–66.

Reynolds, W. M. (2002). *Reynolds Adolescent Depression Scale* (2nd ed.). Lutz, FL: Psychological Assessment Resources.

Reynolds, W. M., & Kamphaus, R. W. (2015). *Behavioral Assessment Scale for Children* (3rd ed.). Circle Pines, MN: American Guidance Service.

Roberts, R. E., Roberts, C. R., & Xing, Y. (2007). Comorbidity of substance use disorders and other psychiatric disorders among adolescents: Evidence from an epidemiological survey. *Drug and Alcohol Dependence, 88S,* S4–S13.

Rohde, P., Lewinsohn, P. M., & Seeley, J. R. (1996). Psychiatric comorbidity with problematic alcohol use in high school students. *Journal of the American Academy of Child and Adolescent Psychiatry, 35*(1), 101–109.

Rowe, C. L., Liddle, H. A., Greenbaum, P. E., & Henderson, C. E. (2004). Impact of psychiatric comorbidity on treatment of adolescent drug abusers. *Journal of Substance Abuse Treatment, 26,* 129–140.

Shaffer, D., Fisher, P., Lucas, C. P., Dulcan, M. K., & Schwab-Stone, M. E. (2000). NIMH Diagnostic Interview Schedule for Children Version IV (NIMH DISC-IV): Description, differences from previous versions, and reliability of some common diagnoses. *Journal of the American Academy of Child and Adolescent Psychiatry, 39,* 28–38.

Shane, P. A., Jasiukaitis, P., & Green, R. S. (2003). Treatment outcomes among adolescents with substance abuse problems: The relationship between comorbidities and post-treatment substance involvement. *Evaluation and Program Planning, 26,* 393–402.

Silverman, W. K., Saavedra, L. M., & Pina, A. A. (2001). Test–retest reliability of anxiety symptoms and diagnoses with the Anxiety Disorders Interview Schedule for DSM-IV: Child and Parent Versions. *Journal of the American Academy of Child and Adolescent Psychiatry, 40,* 937–944.

Sittner Hartshorn, K., Witbeck, L., & Prentice, P. (2015). Substance use disorders, comorbidity, and arrest among indigenous adolescents. *Crime and Delinquency, 61,* 1311–1332.

Smith, G. T., Goldman, M. S., Greenbaum, P. E., & Christiansen, B. A. (1995). Expectancy for social facilitation from drinking: The divergent paths of high-expectancy and low-expectancy adolescents. *Journal of Abnormal Psychology, 104,* 32–40.

Stahlberg, O., Anckarsater, H., & Nilsson, T. (2010). Mental health problems in youths committed to juvenile institutions: Prevalences and treatment needs. *European Child and Adolescent Psychiatry, 19,* 893–903.

Stein, L. A. R., Colby, S. M., Barnett, N. P., Lebeau, R., Monti, P. M., & Golembeske, C. (2011). Motivational interviewing for incarcerated adolescents: Effects of depressive symptoms on reducing alcohol and marijuana use after release. *Journal of Studies on Alcohol and Drugs, 72,* 497–506.

Stormshak, E. A., & Dishion, T. J. (2009). A school-based, family-centered intervention to prevent substance use: The Family Check-Up. *American Journal of Drug and Alcohol Abuse, 35,* 227–232.

Storr, C. L., Pacek, L. R., & Martins, S. S. (2012). Substance use disorders and adolescent psychopathology. *Public Health Reviews, 34*(2). Retrieved from *www.publichealthreviews.eu/upload/pdf_files/12/00_Storr.pdf.*

Stowell, R. J. A., & Estroff, T. W. (1992). Psychiatric disorders in substance-abusing adolescent inpatients: A pilot study. *Journal of the American Academy of Child and Adolescent Psychiatry, 31,* 1036–1040.

Svensson, R. (2003). Gender differences in adolescent drug use: The impact of parental monitoring and peer deviance. *Youth and Society, 34,* 300–329.

Tapert, S. F., Colby, S. M., Barnett, N. P., Spirito, A., Rohsenow, D. J., Myers, M. G., et al. (2003). Depressed mood, gender, and problem drinking in youth. *Journal of Child and Adolescent Substance Abuse, 12,* 55–68.

Tarter, R., Vanyukov, M., Giancola, P., Dawes, M., Blackson, T., Mezzich, A., et al.,(1999). Etiology of early age onset substance use disorder: A maturational perspective. *Developmental Psychopathology, 11,* 657–683.

Tomlinson, K. L., Brown, S. A., & Abrantes, A. (2004). Psychiatric comorbidity and substance use treatment outcomes of adolescents. *Psychology of Addictive Behaviors, 18,* 160–169.

White, A. M., Jordan, J. D., Schroeder, K. M., Acheson, S. K., Georgi, B. D., Sauls, G., et al. (2004). Predictors of relapse during treatment and treatment completion among marijuana dependent adolescents in an intensive outpatient substance abuse program. *Substance Abuse, 25,* 53–59.

Wilson, C. J., Deane, F. P., Marshall, K. L., & Dalley, A. (2010). Adolescents' suicidal thinking and reluctance to consult general medical practitioners. *Journal of Youth and Adolescence, 39,* 343–356.

Winters, K. C., Stinchfield, R. D., Latimer, W. W., & Stone, A. (2008). Internalizing and externalizing behaviors and their association with the treatment of adolescents with substance use disorder. *Journal of Substance Abuse Treatment, 35,* 269–278.

Witkiewitz, K., & Bowen, S. (2010). Depression, craving, and substance use following a randomized trial of mindfulness-based relapse prevention. *Journal of Consulting and Clinical Psychology, 78,* 362–374.

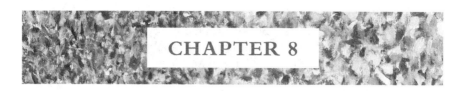

CHAPTER 8

Substance Use Prevention and Treatment Interventions for Court-Involved, Non-Incarcerated Youth

Emily F. Dauria, Melissa A. McWilliams,
and Marina Tolou-Shams

*I*n the United States, there are 31 million adolescents involved in the juvenile justice system. Each year, another 1.4 million adolescents are arrested (Hockenberry & Puzzanchera, 2014). In 2013, 62% of juveniles in the justice system identified as European American and 38% identified as racial or ethnic minority (with 92% of those minority youth identifying as African American, representing 35% of youth overall; Sickmund, Sladky, & Kang, 2015). In this same year, girls accounted for more than one-quarter of all juvenile arrests and roughly half of all juveniles involved in the system were under the age of 16 (Sickmund et al., 2015).

Adolescents involved in the justice system are convicted of committing many different types of crimes—the most common are labeled as "property offenses" (e.g., car theft, vandalism, stolen property; Furdella & Puzzanchera, 2015). Youth are least likely to commit crimes labeled as "crimes against the person," which involve the use of force against another individual and include assault, forcible rape, and kidnapping (Furdella & Puzzanchera, 2015).

Over the past few years, there has been a focus on diverting, or redirecting, youth away from processing in the juvenile justice system. To date, 80% of arrested youth are not detained or incarcerated (Puzzanchera, 2013). Programs designed to divert youth from detention or incarceration are implemented at various points throughout the juvenile's contact with the justice system. For example, diversion programs can be initiated at early stages of justice involvement (e.g., at the point of contact with law enforcement) or at later stages of justice involvement (e.g., through juvenile specialty court processing, such as juvenile drug courts [JDCs]). Throughout this chapter, we refer to the population of youth encountered in the diversion stage as court-involved, non-incarcerated (CINI) youth. Substance use assessment and treatment studies for juvenile justice youth have defined their samples in multiple different ways, often referring to youth as "juvenile offenders" or "justice-involved youth." Fewer studies focus only on CINI or diverted youth, and research has yet to fully determine how CINI youth's substance use treatment needs may be similar to or different from the needs of detained or incarcerated youth. Thus, we draw upon the overarching body of juvenile justice substance use literature to guide our review of interventions, both brief and intensive. We highlight throughout which studies and available treatment options include CINI youth to inform recommendations for future intervention development and testing.

STATUS OF THE FIELD: SUBSTANCE USE AMONG JUSTICE-INVOLVED YOUTH

To frame our discussion regarding substance use interventions for CINI youth, we use Munetz and Griffin's (2006) sequential intercept model (SIM; see Figure 8.1). The SIM emphasizes a series of "points of intercepts" where various interventions (including those targeting substance use) can be delivered to prevent the further entrenchment of juveniles in the justice system. The five intercepts identified by Munetz and Griffin (2006) represent the flow of individuals throughout the justice system. Unless otherwise noted, the substance use interventions described throughout the chapter focus on Intercept 2 of the SIM. This intercept represents the initial court hearing stage (i.e., after a youth has been arrested but before he or she has a trial) and includes screening, pretrial diversion, and service linkage activities. Brief intervention models for substance use may be ideal for development and testing at Intercept 2 because it is possible that a youth's substance use is less severe and his or her contact with the court is briefer than those youth involved at Intercepts 3–5.

Substance Use, Mental and Physical Health, and Delinquency

Youth involved in the justice system have higher rates of substance use and substance use disorders than juveniles not involved in the justice system (Domalanta, Risser, Roberts, & Risser, 2003; Grisso, 2004; Johnson et al., 2004; Mauricio et al., 2009; Otto-Salaj, Gore-Felton, McGarvey, & Canterbury,

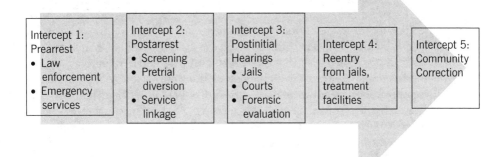

| Intercept 1:
Prearrest
• Law
  enforcement
• Emergency
  services | Intercept 2:
Postarrest
• Screening
• Pretrial
  diversion
• Service
  linkage | Intercept 3:
Postinitial
Hearings
• Jails
• Courts
• Forensic
  evaluation | Intercept 4:
Reentry
from jails,
treatment
facilities | Intercept 5:
Community
Correction |

FIGURE 8.1. The sequential intercept model. From Munetz and Griffin (2006). Reproduced by permission.

2002; Ryan & Redding, 2004). The substances used most often by adolescents are alcohol and marijuana (Johnston, O'Malley, Bachman, & Schulenberg, 2012). Depending on which research study and which juvenile justice population studied, the rates of DSM-5 substance use disorder diagnosis range from 25 to 87% (Chesney-Lind, 2001; Johnson et al., 2004; Prescott, 1997; Teplin, Abram, McClelland, Dulcan, & Mericle, 2002). Research suggests that there are notable racial/ethnic differences in substance use among justice-involved adolescents (Braithwaite, Conerly, Robillard, Woodring, & Stephens, 2003; Feldstein Ewing, Venner, Mead, & Bryan, 2011). For example, European American justice-involved adolescents have the greatest rates of substance use across a number of categories (e.g., frequency of marijuana use, age of first marijuana use), whereas African American adolescents have the lowest rates of use (Braithwaite et al., 2003; Feldstein Ewing et al., 2011). Due to differences in patterns of substance use by race and ethnicity, as well as continued disproportionate representation of racial/ethnic-minority youth entering the juvenile justice system, culturally responsive and tailored substance use treatment programs are sorely needed. Examples of such interventions are presented later in this chapter.

Substance use can impair judgment and can be associated with aggression and violence, which can then result in youth contact with police (law enforcement) and/or the courts (Dishion & Andrews, 1995; Mauricio et al., 2009; Thornberry, Krohn, Lizzotte, & Chard-Wierschem, 1993). Youth with substance use disorders often have repeat contact with the justice system (Belenko & Sprott, 2002; National Center on Addiction and Substance Abuse at Columbia University, 2004; Hussong, Curran, Moffit, Caspi, & Carrig,

2004), which has been referred to as a "drug-crime cycle" (Chassin, Knight, Vargas-Chanes, Losoya, & Naranjo, 2009). Indeed, CINI youth diagnosed with both a psychiatric disorder (e.g., depression, anxiety, conduct disorder [CD]) and a substance use disorder (referred to as "dually diagnosed") are at increased risk for future detention in a juvenile facility relative to those who are not diagnosed with a co-occurring substance use disorder (Tolou-Shams et al., 2014). Treating substance use that co-occurs with psychiatric symptoms and/ or diagnosis presents with unique challenges (Bukstein, Glancy, & Kaminer, 1992; Dembo, Pacheco, Schmeidler, Fisher, & Cooper, 1997; Goldstein et al., 2003; Rowe, Liddle, Greenbaum, & Henderson, 2004). Among the general adolescent population, substance abusers with co-occurring psychiatric disorders present for treatment with more frequent substance use, have more parental psychopathology, and poorer family relationships (Riggs, Baker, Mikulich, Young, & Crowley, 1995) than nondually diagnosed youth. They are also at high risk to drop out of treatment (Wise, Cuffe, & Fischer, 2001) and have poor long-term treatment outcomes (Crowley, Mikulich, MacDonald, Young, & Zerbe, 1998) than those without a co-occurring psychiatric disorder. Coordinated treatment efforts are therefore needed in order to prevent adolescent offenders most at risk (i.e., adolescents with comorbid psychiatric symptoms) from further entrenchment in the justice system—yet, there are very few evidence-based "dual diagnosis" interventions for juvenile justice youth (Belendiuk & Riggs, 2014).

Substance use also has implications for adolescents' physical health and development (e.g., impaired neurological development, cognitive deficiencies; Harrison, 2001). Research suggests that young offenders who use substances also engage in high-risk sexual activity, including having a high number of sexual partners (Canterbury et al., 1995) and using condoms less frequently (Kingree & Betz, 2003; Morris, Baker, Valentine, & Pennisi, 1998). These risk behaviors place substance-using juvenile offenders at high risk for sexually transmitted infections, including HIV, as well as unwanted pregnancies (Castrucci & Martin, 2002; Kingree & Betz, 2003; Morris et al., 1998; Teplin, Mericle, McClelland, & Abram, 2003). These sexual and substance use risk behaviors are as prevalent among CINI youth as they are among detained or incarcerated youth (Dembo, Belenko, Childs, Greenbaum, & Wareham, 2010; Dembo, Belenko, Childs, & Wareham, 2009; Tolou-Shams, Brown, Gordon, & Fernandez, 2007; Tolou-Shams, Brown, Houck, Lescano, & Project SHIELD Study Group, 2008)—however, it is important to note the methodological limitation that none of these studies have directly compared rates of substance use between CINI and detained youth. Due to the high prevalence of co-occurring substance use and sexual risk behaviors among youth involved in the justice system across a number of intercepts, it is important to develop and deliver public health interventions as early as possible in the juvenile justice continuum.

Access to Treatment and JDCs

Juvenile justice settings provide an opportunity to link adolescents with substance use disorders to treatment and care. In fact, the juvenile justice system is the major referral source for adolescent substance users (Office of Applied Studies, 2000). However, despite these youth's clear need for substance use treatment, access to appropriate substance use screening, referral, and treatment services is often fragmented and not effective (Young, Dembo, & Henderson, 2007), and few empirically supported interventions exist (Braukman et al., 1985; Friedman, Terras, & Glassman, 2002; Henggeler, Pickrel, & Brondino, 1999; Smith, Chamberlain, & Eddy, 2010)—this makes it challenging for juvenile justice systems to refer these youth for effective substance use treatment whether brief or intensive.

JDCs were developed with the aim of improving access to substance use treatment and thereby reductions in use for CINI youth to prevent recidivism. Drug courts (for adults) were developed in the late 1980s as an alternative to incarceration, with the goal of providing intensive treatment services that are more appropriate to address the complex needs of substance-using individuals (Bureau of Justice Assistance, 2003). The first JDC began in 1995 (Sloan & Smykla, 2003)—as of 2014, there were 433 JDCs operating in the United States (National Institute of Justice, 2014). JDCs have five primary goals: (1) provide immediate intervention treatment, (2) improve CINI juveniles' functionality in their current living environment, (3) provide CINI juveniles with skills to lead substance- and crime-free lives, (4) strengthen the families of substance-using CINI juveniles, and (5) promote accountability for CINI juveniles and their service providers (National Institute of Justice, 2014). Judges provide close oversight of each JDC case, and treatment service teams typically include representatives from social and mental health services, law enforcement, school and vocational training programs, and probation (Bureau of Justice Assistance, 2003).

Although JDCs have been operating nationally for over two decades, a relatively small number of studies have evaluated how effective they are in reducing CINI juveniles' recidivism and substance use. The existing literature provides conflicting results. Some studies provide encouraging support for the efficacy of JDCs in reducing substance use and delinquency (Henggeler et al., 2008; Latessa, Sullivan, Blair, Sullivan, & Smith, 2013; Rodriguez & Webb, 2004; Shaffer, Listwan, Latessa, & Lowenkamp, 2008), while others fail to find any impact at all (Wright & Clymer, 2001). One evaluation of nine JDCs found that juveniles who completed JDC recidivated at significantly higher rates than their counterparts who completed formal court hearings (Latessa et al., 2013). Although overall findings may appear discouraging, some of these programs produced significant positive outcomes and have several commonalities worth noting. First, research suggests that when parents and guardians attend hearings, juveniles are less likely to be late or absent from treatment or school, provide a positive drug test, or receive sanctions for behavioral issues occurring in the program (Salvatore, Henderson, Hiller, White, & Samuelson, 2010). It is recommended that JDC hearings serve as a time to teach caregivers how to interact and deliver appropriate consequences for their youth's behavior (Salvatore et al., 2010). Next, having judges (as opposed to community panels) oversee JDCs is critical to consider. A multisite study of JDCs in Iowa found that over a 4-year period, there were no differences in rearrest rates for JDC completers versus noncompleters, suggesting that JDCs are ineffective in reducing recidivism—however, 62% of these JDC youth were not overseen by a judge, which suggests that judicial monitoring of youth's progress might be essential to their outcomes (Cook, Watson, & Stageberg, 2009). Additional factors that are thought to improve the results of JDCs include reducing JDC-participating youth's involvement with substance-using and delinquent peers, not relying on detention as a sanction or punishment, and modeling reliable disciplinary practices (Marlowe, 2010).

EMPIRICAL EVIDENCE FOR SUBSTANCE USE INTERVENTIONS FOR JUVENILE JUSTICE POPULATIONS

An emerging area of research shows that interventions can reduce substance use among youth involved in the juvenile justice system (Braukman et al., 1985; Dennis et al., 2004; Friedman et al., 2002; Henggeler et al., 1999; Randall & Cunningham, 2003; Smith et al., 2010). This body of work suggests that interventions may reduce substance use in the short term and be particularly successful in reducing alcohol and marijuana use (Dennis et al., 2004; Gil, Wagner, & Tubman, 2004; Tripodi & Bender, 2011). However, to date, researchers have found that no single treatment produces the best substance use reduction outcomes and *very few are brief interventions* (Baldwin, Christian, Berkeljon, & Shadish, 2012; Catalano, Hawkins, Wells, Miller, & Brewer, 1990; Chassin, 2008; Williams & Chang, 2000). In Table 8.1, we present brief descriptions of treatments that have some demonstrated success in reducing substance use among juvenile justice populations, including CINI youth. Of these, four—the Family Check-Up, five -session motivational enhancement therapy + cognitive-behavioral therapy, brief strategic family therapy, and ATTAIN—may be considered "brief" interventions, in that the intervention can be delivered in anywhere from one to eight sessions (e.g., Dennis et al., 2004; Dishion, Nelson, & Kavanagh, 2003; Godley, Godley, Dennis, Funk, & Passetti, 2006; Stormshak, Fosco, & Dishion, 2010). These brief interventions have demonstrated reductions in substance use and/or improved legal outcomes (e.g., preventing future arrests) with samples of youth that have included CINI youth (five-session motivational enhancement therapy

+ cognitive-behavioral therapy, ATTAIN), or youth at high risk for court/ legal involvement (brief strategic family therapy), or detained/incarcerated youth (the Family Check-Up, five-session motivational enhancement therapy + cognitive-behavioral therapy). In addition, the brief intervention model Screening, Brief Intervention, and Referral to Treatment (SBIRT; Substance Abuse and Mental Health Services Administration, 2015) is described in Table 8.1. Although not yet a published evidence-based practice with juvenile justice youth, SBIRT is currently being delivered in juvenile justice settings as part of a larger implementation project and represents a promising brief intervention for substance-using CINI youth (see National Center for Mental Health and Juvenile Justice; *www.ncmhjj.com/projects/sbirt-in-jj*).

Brief Interventions

Motivational Enhancement Therapy + Cognitive-Behavioral Therapy and the Cannabis Youth Treatment Study

The motivational enhancement therapy + cognitive-behavioral therapy (MET-CBT) model incorporates a combination of individual motivational interviewing sessions and group CBT and can be delivered in five- or 12-session formats (indicated by MET-CBT 5 and MET-CBT 12, respectively). The "brief" format of MET-CBT, MET-CBT 5, consists of two 60-minute individual MET sessions followed by three 75-minute group CBT sessions. MET-CBT addresses teens' and young adults' motivation to change and helps to develop skills to increase social support, how to engage in non-drug-related activities, and develop avoidance and coping mechanisms to deal with relapse issues (National Council of Juvenile and Family Court Judges, 2015).

In 2004, the Cannabis Youth Treatment (CYT) study conducted two randomized trials with 600 marijuana users (the majority of whom were under the supervision of the criminal justice system including CINI youth), and evaluated the effectiveness of short-term (90 days or less) outpatient interventions for adolescents with cannabis use disorders (Dennis et al., 2004). Study interventions included MET-CBT 5 and MET-CBT 12 and multidimensional family therapy (MDFT). MDFT is an intensive (i.e., nonbrief) family-based intervention widely used in the juvenile justice field and is described in greater detail below (see the "Intensive Interventions" section). CYT study participants were predominantly white males, ages 15–16 years, the majority of whom reported no previous substance abuse or mental health treatment. The authors found that both MET-CBT and MDFT interventions demonstrated a significant effect on pre–post treatment on the two marijuana outcomes of interest (i.e., days of abstinence and the percentage of adolescents in recovery). Clinical outcomes were similar across sites and conditions and, in line with previous research (Tripodi & Bender, 2011), the treatment effect sizes were generally small.

TABLE 8.1. Evidence-Based Brief and Intensive Interventions to Reduce Substance Use among Juvenile Justice Youth

Intervention	Target population	Typical length	Brief description
Screening, Brief Intervention, and Referral to Treatment (SBIRT)*	Adolescents with substance use disorders or those at risk of developing these disorders	N/A	Aims to identify, reduce, and prevent problematic substance use; includes substance use assessment, brief intervention to increase insight regarding substance use, and referral to more extensive treatment when needed
Family Check-Up (FCU)*	Severe substance-using, antisocial youth	Up to three sessions	Incorporates motivational interviewing techniques to engage family, improve parenting practices, and reduce youth's risk behavior and family conflict
Motivational enhancement therapy + cognitive-behavioral therapy (MET-CBT)*	Juvenile justice youth ages 12–18 with problematic marijuana use; not suitable for those with severe conduct disorder	Five to seven sessions	Incorporates combination of individual MET sessions and group CBT; primary goal is to enhance motivation to change marijuana use and develop skills needed to gain control over use and achieve abstinence
Alcohol treatment targeting adolescents in need (ATTAIN)*	Alcohol- and marijuana-using adolescents	Seven sessions	Motivational, cognitive-behavioral intervention that seeks to reduce alcohol and marijuana use; individually tailored to youth's cultural, etiologic, and risk factors
Brief strategic family therapy (BSFT)*	CINI youth	Eight to 24 sessions	Culturally sensitive family intervention to reduce delinquency and drug use and strengthen family unit; uses a structured, problem-focused, and practical approach; focuses on improving parent–child interactions, developing conflict resolution, and parenting and communication skills
Adolescent contingency management (Adol CM)	Adolescents with alcohol and/or drug addictions	Three or more months, often in conjunction with other treatments	Uses reward system to reinforce certain behaviors, such as abstaining from drugs or attending therapy sessions; reinforcements are introduced when treatment goals are met and withheld (or, alternatively, given punishment) when adolescent exhibits undesirable behavior

TABLE 8.1. (continued)

Intervention	Target population	Typical length	Brief description
Familias Unidas	Hispanic youth whose families immigrated to the United States	Three to 5 months, two sessions per week	Family-centered, group-based approach aimed at promoting positive school, family, behavioral, legal, and health outcomes, and decreasing substance use, sexual risk behaviors, and antisocial behavior; includes parent–child interaction observations
Multidimensional family therapy (MDFT)	Substance-abusing or dependent adolescents	Three to 6 months, one to three sessions per week	Individual and family therapy sessions; comprehensive team works to provide services to youth and family of origin; foster family implements behavior management techniques; clinicians teach youth interpersonal skills and work with family of origin in family therapy
Multidimensional treatment foster care (MTFC)	Adolescent offenders ages 12–17	Six to 9 months in therapeutic foster home	Includes parent training and support for foster parents, family therapy for biological parents, skills training and supportive therapy for youth, school-based interventions and academic support, and psychiatric consultation and medication management when needed
Multisystemic therapy (MST)	Youth ages 11–18 and their families	Clinicians available 24 hours per day, 7 days per week	Home-based, goal-oriented approach that focuses on home, school, peer groups, and community systems; seeks to improve parenting practices, engage youth in prosocial peer groups and away from delinquent peers, and reduce youth's favorable attitudes toward drug use

Note. The table outlines information regarding each treatment's target population, typical length of service delivery, and a brief description of its major components. These treatments will be explained in greater detail throughout the following sections. Asterisks (*) represent brief interventions.

Brief Strategic Family Therapy

Brief strategic family therapy (BSFT; Szapocznik, Schwartz, Muir, & Brown, 2012) is a family-based intervention relevant for CINI youth that may be considered "brief" if successfully implemented within eight sessions. BSFT aims to treat adolescent drug use and co-occurring problem behaviors, is implemented within eight to 24 sessions, and has demonstrated long-term effects (into young adulthood) in reducing arrests, incarcerations, and other externalizing behaviors (Horigian et al., 2015). Thus, while this intervention has not necessarily been directly tested with a sample of all CINI youth, it has relevance to the CINI youth population in that the study population focus is adolescent substance abusers with co-occurring conduct problems (and likely many with some level of police or court contact at time of BSFT intervention).

The Family Check-Up

The Family Check-Up (FCU) is another empirically validated, individually tailored, brief (up to three-session) intervention that seeks to address some of the key issues related to engaging families in treatment (Stormshak et al., 2010). Based on motivational interviewing (Miller & Rollnick, 2002), the FCU is designed to enhance parental recognition of the adolescent's risk behaviors, provide support for reducing these behaviors, help parents reflect on their parenting practices, and promote motivation to change maladaptive parenting (Chiapa et al., 2015; Connell, Dishion, & Klostermann, 2012; Dishion et al., 2003; Slavet et al., 2005; Stormshak & Dishion, 2009). The three-session intervention includes family-based assessment, interview, and feedback sessions that include videotaping of parent–child interaction, and feedback based on that videotaped assessment. The FCU has improved family engagement in treatment and has been associated with declines in youth-reported antisocial behavior and total number of arrests during adolescence (Connell et al., 2012); enhancing treatment at juvenile justice facilities, improving engagement in postrelease discharge services, and generating greater postrelease family functioning (Slavet et al., 2005); and enhancing parenting skills, improving parent monitoring, reducing family conflict, and reducing adolescent substance use (Dishion et al., 2003; Stormshak & Dishion, 2009).

Alcohol Treatment Targeting Adolescents in Need

Gil et al. (2004) developed this alcohol treatment targeting adolescents in need (ATTAIN) intervention, a brief (seven-session) motivational, cognitive-behavioral intervention incorporating guided self-change, and tested its effectiveness across different racial and ethnic groups. The ATTAIN intervention was designed to address cultural-specific factors while simultaneously addressing common etiologic and risk factors for substance use.

Ninety-seven Hispanic and African American juvenile offenders completed treatment at the time of study publication. Researchers observed significant reductions in alcohol and marijuana for both ethnic groups from baseline to postintervention. Additional findings suggest that cultural factors can both positively and negatively influence treatment outcomes. Notably, adolescents with greater mistrust of other racial/ethnic groups demonstrated less response to treatment, and adolescents with greater ethnic pride and "Hispanic" orientation demonstrated better response to treatment. Findings support the notion that culturally tailored interventions may be effective in reducing substance use among racial- and ethnic-minority CINI youth (or those who are presenting with conduct problems) but suggest the need for future research on culturally tailored substance use interventions.

Screening, Brief Intervention, and Referral to Treatment

SBIRT is an evidence-based practice developed to identify, reduce, and prevent alcohol or illicit substance misuse and dependency (Becker, Ozechowski, & Hogue, Chapter 5, this volume). There are three main components of SBIRT practices: (1) *screening,* when a health care professional assesses an individual for risky substance use behaviors; (2) *brief intervention,* in which the health care professional engages an individual with risky substance use behaviors in a short conversation providing advice and guidance to reduce risk; and (3) *referral to treatment,* where an individual identified to be in need of additional services is referred to brief therapy or treatment (Substance Abuse and Mental Health Services Administration, 2015).

Intensive Interventions

By way of comparison, Table 8.1 includes examples of intensive interventions that have produced favorable outcomes for substance-abusing or -dependent adolescents such as home-based interventions and those that address known determinants of clinical difficulties (e.g., individual, family, school) in the environments where problems occur (Randall & Cunningham, 2003). These interventions work across multiple domains or environments of the participant's life, and sessions occur frequently over a period of at least several months (Liddle, Dakof, Parker, Diamond, & Barrett, 2001; Liddle, Rowe, Dakof, Henderson, & Greenbaum, 2009). Familias Unidas is an empirically supported intensive family-based intervention that was developed specifically with and for Hispanic immigrant families in the United States and has demonstrated efficacy in reducing substance use (along with improving safer sex practices) among Latinx youth (Pantin et al., 2003). Gender-specific programs and services have been identified as a priority for juvenile justice populations (Office of Juvenile Justice and Delinquency Prevention, 2015) because girls have different, unique pathways into the juvenile justice system than boys that warrant separate, focused attention to address their behavioral and emotional presentations and risk for recidivism. Yet to date there have been no large-scale brief or intervention trial results published of gender-responsive substance use interventions for adolescent female offenders (whether CINI or incarcerated girls).

Other Integrated Treatment Interventions

Given the disproportionate rate of psychiatric symptoms and HIV/sexually transmitted infection (STI) risk behaviors among substance-abusing juvenile offenders (Elkington et al., 2008; Teplin et al., 2005), researchers are beginning to develop and test integrated interventions (i.e., those addressing substance use and mental health outcomes and/or HIV/STI risk behaviors) with juvenile justice populations (Marvel, Rowe, Colon-Perez, DiClemente, & Liddle, 2009; Mouttapa et al., 2009; Roberts-Lewis, Welch-Brewer, Jackson, Martin Pharr, & Parker, 2010). Thus far, there is limited empirical evaluation of these integrated substance use interventions on substance use outcomes. Further, the majority of these interventions would not be considered "brief" and most have been tested with detained and not CINI youth populations (see Marvel et al., 2009, and Tolou-Shams et al., 2017, as exceptions). However, findings suggest that integrated treatment may be effective at improving psychosocial functioning (e.g., mental health, family relations, peer relations) and improving HIV/STI- and substance use-related behaviors (e.g., increasing ease in carrying and using condoms, improving self-efficacy in avoiding substance use; Mouttapa et al., 2009). Research is still needed to test and evaluate integrated treatment interventions with substance-using CINI populations.

"Best Practices" in Juvenile Justice Substance Use Treatment

In an effort to further guide the development and implementation of substance use treatment, several governing bodies have identified a set of common characteristics that constitute "best practices" for substance use services for justice-involved youth (Bukstein, 2005; Henderson, Taxman, & Young, 2008; National Institutes of Drug Abuse, 2006). The components of these identified "best practices" include a comprehensive, integrated treatment approach; family involvement; gender and cultural competence; continuity of care; assessment and treatment of co-occurring disorders; and a length of at least 90 days. Many of these characteristics are included in the interventions presented in Table 8.1 (with the exception of the length of treatment for brief interventions).

Despite these specific recommendations, however, research suggests that providing juvenile offenders with *any type* (e.g., individual, family based) of substance use intervention may positively impact their substance use behaviors. For example, Chassin et al. (2009) studied a sample of 420 young males found guilty of a serious offense and surveyed them every 6 months (up to 12 months posttreatment) to examine their participation in substance use treatment and self-reported substance abuse. Of those who were surveyed, 34% reported receiving any form of substance abuse treatment (e.g., participation in court-ordered substance abuse sessions with a psychologist or social worker). The authors found that participation in some form of substance abuse treatment reduced alcohol use in both the short- and long term. Furthermore, receiving treatment for more than 90 days was associated with significant reductions in marijuana and alcohol use, which may suggest why the field has tended toward "nonbrief" or more intensive interventions.

In a systematic literature review published in 2011, Tripodi and Bender examined how effective substance abuse treatment interventions are in reducing young offenders' alcohol and marijuana use (Braukman et al., 1985; Friedman et al., 2002; Godley et al., 2006; Henggeler et al., 1999; Smith et al., 2010). Interventions represented a variety of individual and family-based modalities (i.e., multisystemic therapy [MST], multidimensional treatment foster care, assertive continuing care, and triple-modality social learning), ranging in length from 12 to 90 weeks, and were conducted in a number of settings (e.g., clinics, homes, aftercare services). Their findings suggest that this series of rigorously tested substance use (intensive or nonbrief) interventions for juvenile offenders have small to moderate effects on reducing alcohol and marijuana use. When examining commonalities of the successful substance use interventions the authors note that, for most interventions, the role of family (both families of origin and therapeutic families) appeared to play an important role in changing substance use behaviors.

Summary of "Best Practices"

The majority of interventions tested and found to be effective in reducing juvenile offenders' alcohol and drug use to date have been intensive and have incorporated family-based approaches along with various combinations of other characteristics noted above to be important (Chassin et al., 2009; Sickmund & Puzzanchera, 2014; Williams & Chang, 2000). However, there have been a few brief interventions tested with some success in improving substance use outcomes, of which some have included CINI youth. Commonalities among these brief interventions include extraindividual approaches (group, family); a focus on culture, race, and ethnicity; and flexible delivery within the juvenile justice system.

Limitations on "Best Practices" for CINI Youth

There are several limitations to underscore in these findings as they relate to CINI youth. While family-based interventions have demonstrated success in reducing substance use, they have primarily been tested and used with heavier-using subpopulations in the juvenile justice system (e.g., violent offenders, severe substance-using youth, antisocial youth; Borduin, Mann, Cone, & Henggeler, 1995; Henggeler, Melton, Brondino, Scherer, & Hanley, 1997; Randall & Cunningham, 2003)—therefore, these intensive substance abuse interventions may be less appropriate and effectual in meeting the needs of substance-using youth at their first point of criminal justice involvement. Furthermore, despite their demonstrated effectiveness, substance use treatment programs that incorporate family therapy or counseling are the least likely substance abuse services provided in juvenile justice settings (Sickmund & Puzzanchera, 2014), particularly those in brief detention or postadjudicated incarcerated settings. Given that there is often still family involvement at the postarrest, pretrial intercept of the SIM and that youth are not intentionally separated from their families (as they are when detained or put in residential out-of-home juvenile justice placement), family-based approaches to substance use treatment may be more easily implemented or considered at this stage (e.g., in juvenile court settings or community-based diversion programs).

Another limitation to the current state of successful substance use interventions is their length or intensity. As noted above, existing literature primarily supports interventions that last 3 months or longer to efficaciously treat substance use in juvenile justice populations (Chassin et al., 2009; Sickmund & Puzzanchera, 2014; Williams & Chang, 2000). Such intensive interventions may not be suitable for CINI youth who are coming into contact with the justice system for the first time—however, this remains a hypothesis to be tested. Brief intervention models noted in Table 8.1, such as SBIRT, that appear promising for reducing substance use in general-population adolescent samples are only just being implemented and tested with juvenile justice youth (National Center for Mental Health and Juvenile Justice; *https://www.ncmhjj.com/projects/sbirt-in-jj/*). Greater emphasis on development and testing of brief interventions for the CINI youth population is needed and warranted.

A third limitation is that the most effective, research-based treatments are challenging to implement in real-world settings—they do not afford the same ability to be strictly controlled or manipulated as the tightly controlled efficacy trials (Chassin, 2008; Chassin et al., 2009). Moreover, the treatments are often not delivered as intended. Recent research has shown that "the most common treatments that are actually received by adolescent offenders are not research therapies, but rather community therapies, which are delivered under non-standardized conditions by leaders who may not be highly trained (and perhaps themselves in recovery from drug abuse)" (Chassin et al., 2009, p. 184). These implementation discrepancies can result in greatly reduced treatment effects compared with the research trials (Chassin et al., 2009; Curtis, Ronan, & Borduin, 2004). Thus, further research on the efficacy of brief interventions conducted in real-world settings is strongly needed.

CLINICAL APPLICATIONS:
SUBSTANCE-USING CINI YOUTH

In order to understand how a clinician might apply the intervention informa-tion presented throughout this chapter thus far, we present two clinical case studies of substance-using CINI youth followed by discussion of (1) the type of intervention that might be most appropriate to address the youth's substance use and, as relevant, co-occurring psychiatric needs; and (2) challenges to treatment delivery. This is followed by a more general discussion of challenges to treatment engagement for this youth population and contextual factors (e.g., culture, motivation, family involvement) critical to consider when implement-ing substance use intervention with CINI youth.

Case Example 1: Robert

Robert is a 16-year-old European American male who has spent the last 7 years moving between multiple foster home placements. He has been in his current foster home for the past 2 years with two younger siblings and the family would like to move toward adoption. His biological father has been incarcerated since Robert was a young child. At 9 years old, Robert was removed from his biologi-cal mother's care by the state child welfare agency due to her excessive drug use and substantiated neglect of Robert. For the past 3 years, Robert has openly identified as a gang member and routinely carries a knife on his person (per Robert for self-protection against rival gang members). According to Robert's record, he has a history of oppositional, delinquent, and antisocial behaviors in school and in the community (e.g., defiance, destruction of property, dis-respect toward others, dishonesty, and physical violence). He was diagnosed with CD at the age of 13 but has never completed interventions due to his lack of stable family involvement. Robert was recently charged with assault with a deadly weapon during a gang fight and is now in detention. Upon admission to detention, Robert was mandated to complete a breathalyzer and urine drug toxicology screen for which the results indicated recent high levels of alcohol and marijuana use. However, when questioned about his substance use, Robert denied using any substances in the past month.

Type of Intervention

CD is a psychiatric disorder occurring in childhood and adolescence that is marked by a long-standing pattern of aggression, theft, vandalism, violation of rules, defiance, lying, and/or other antisocial behaviors. Like substance use disorders, CD responds best to family-based therapies. Although Robert's bio-logical parents are not involved in his life, he has been living with his foster family consistently for the past 2 years and may soon be adopted by them.

Involving his new family in family-based therapy could beneficially target his CD and substance use problems, while simultaneously cultivating new family relationships. MST, an intensive and integrated family-based treatment that emphasizes functioning within a series of interconnected contexts (e.g., home, school, neighborhood), reduces substance use and antisocial behaviors among children and adolescents with CD. This treatment would be valuable for Robert and his family. Additionally, Robert's foster parents could benefit from CD psychoeducation and parent management training (PMT) focused on enhancing various parenting skills (e.g., reinforcing positive behaviors, parent monitoring, limit setting) that are important in establishing a healthy and consistent home environment for youth with CD.

Challenges to Delivering Treatment

Engaging juvenile offenders in substance use and mental health treatment can be a difficult process, especially when they present with disruptive behavioral disorders. As Robert presents with co-occurring substance use disorder and CD, his therapist may have difficulty initially building rapport and trust, engaging Robert in treatment, and overcoming treatment resistance. One strategy to help address these obstacles to treatment is to employ MET, an adaptation of motivational interviewing. MET is a brief, nonconfrontational client-feedback intervention geared toward establishing a working alliance, helping clients explore and resolve ambivalence, and promoting readiness to change. As it is typically limited to a single session (with more if needed), MET may help Robert and his therapist collaborate to quickly and effectively overcome his initial resistance to treatment.

Robert's detention status presents additional treatment barriers for him and his foster family. As MST is a family-based intervention, the foster family must be able to attend the therapy sessions. Factors such as schedule coordination, travel distance, and transportation contingencies (including financial and time burden associated with travel) need to be considered and addressed during his detention interval. Telepsychiatry (the delivery of psychiatric assessment and care through telecommunications technology, usually videoconferencing) is a promising solution to circumvent these potential barriers to family-based intervention within the juvenile justice system. Several states have put telepsychiatry infrastructure in place in order to provide timely, cost-effective, and appropriate health care, as well as a means for implementing family therapy and visitation for juveniles who are not geographically close to their families or community support system (Fox, Somes, & Waters, 2007; Kaliebe, Heneghan, & Kim, 2011). Upon Robert's release, the telepsychiatrist can continue working with Robert until the juvenile justice system organizes aftercare services for him and his foster family to ensure the continuing care necessary for Robert to feel adequately supported and prepared for community reentry.

Case Example 2: Gabriela

Gabriela (Gabi) is a 15-year-old Hispanic female who currently resides with her biological mother, older brother, one younger sister, and maternal grandmother. Gabi and her siblings were all born in the United States and are the only first-generation Americans in the family. Gabi's biological father was recently deported to their native home of Guatemala and Gabi is very nervous that her mother and grandmother may also be required to leave the United States given their undocumented status.

Gabi rarely attended school over the past year and was recently charged with disorderly conduct and possession of alcohol. As these were her first offenses (truancy, disorderly conduct, alcohol possession), she was diverted from detention and referred to a diversion program that requires 10 hours of community service and attendance at an alcohol education program. Gabi's mother desires to be actively involved in her daughter's legal proceedings and treatment but is nervous of others learning of their undocumented status and thus does not want to take Gabi to a therapist. Gabi's mother expressed a number of worries to the juvenile court staff (that is monitoring Gabi's diversion program compliance) that may be negatively impacting Gabi's ability to function successfully in both her school and community. According to her mother, Gabi has had difficulty relating to her peers, is currently failing her classes, and does not seem to enjoy school at all. She reported that Gabi has always had a hard time focusing and paying attention, does not seem to listen when spoken to, is often forgetful, and can be impulsive. She admits that needing to repeatedly ask Gabi to do something at home in order to get it done is frustrating. A review of school records (provided by Gabi's mother) indicates that testing done within the past year suggested that Gabi meets DSM-5 criteria for attention-deficit/hyperactivity disorder (ADHD)—predominantly inattentive presentation.

Having adopted the SBIRT model approach to alcohol and drug use treatment, the court staff globally screened and interviewed Gabi to gain information about her substance use. Gabi tested positive for marijuana and admitted that she occasionally drinks alcohol but that she prefers marijuana. She smokes marijuana daily but does not feel she has a problem with substance use or that it is related to her current legal involvement.

Type of Intervention

Gabi presents with daily marijuana use, occasional alcohol use, and symptoms of ADHD—predominantly inattentive presentation, a psychological disorder that is marked by a persistent pattern of inattention (usually without hyperactivity and impulsivity features) that interferes with an individual's functioning and development. While still at court, Gabi might benefit from brief motivational interviewing to enhance her insight into her substance use and motivate her to consider reducing or abstaining from substance use (the "BI" of SBIRT).

Additionally, it is recommended that the court clinician, Gabi, and Gabi's mother collaborate to develop a parent-implemented contingency management contract. The contingency management approach seeks to encourage and reinforce changes in behavior by rewarding adolescents for objective evidence of change in the target behavior (Stanger & Budney, 2010; Winters, Botzet, & Fahnhorst, 2011). During this process, the clinician, Gabi, and Gabi's mother would agree on the target behavior(s) and the reward-and-consequence system. Gabi's mother would be provided with and trained on any related contingency management materials she would need in order to successfully implement the contingency management contract at home.

When developing ideas for appropriate community referrals for Gabi's needs (the "RT" of SBIRT), the court staff must consider factors other than her co-occurring substance use and ADHD symptoms—namely, her gender, her Hispanic culture, and her family's trepidation in disclosing too much information to others (and not knowing whom to trust) given their undocumented status. It is important for court staff to consider these contextual factors with Gabi and her mother in order to assist Gabi in getting the type of care she needs. A resource that could be beneficial for Gabi and her family is a program like Familias Unidas, if it is available in their community. This community, family-based program could help Gabi's mother (and grandmother) develop and maintain positive parenting practices and family support and improve parent–child communication with Gabi. Additionally, it could provide Gabi's mother with an important parent social support network within the Hispanic community. If this program is not available in their community or they do not have access to the Internet version, other culturally sensitive, family-based intervention programs that Gabi and her family may benefit from include ATTAIN, MST, and BSFT.

In addition to substance use treatment, Gabi and her family could benefit from individual behavioral interventions and behavioral parenting training focused on her ADHD symptoms. Behavioral therapy could help Gabi develop problem-solving skills and learn to become more organized, avoid distractions, and cope with her symptoms. Parent training could enhance Gabi's mother's parenting practices to create an environment conducive to ADHD success, such as developing a consistent family routine, modifying her communication with Gabi (e.g., using clear, brief directions/explanations rather than long-winded directions/explanations), effectively limiting Gabi's choices, and employing alternate methods of discipline. If the situation is unresponsive to behavioral interventions, stimulant medications could be carefully considered—with acknowledgment of Gabi's active substance use. For instance, prescribing stimulant medications in a long-acting form and in a controlled manner could help to minimize the risk for becoming physically dependent on, misusing, and diverting (e.g., trading or selling) them (Harstad, Levy, & Committee on Substance Abuse, 2014). If there is abundant concern about dependency, misuse, and diversion, nonstimulant medications can be considered for treatment despite being less effective than stimulants (Harstad et al., 2014). Regardless of the physician's ultimate prescription choice, it will be important to carefully monitor medication adherence.

Challenges to Delivering Treatment

Gabi's case presents a variety of treatment challenges, including Gabi's limited insight into the adverse consequences of her substance use—especially as it relates to her delinquent behavior and current legal difficulties. Brief motivational interviewing techniques might help establish greater patient engagement, rapport, and working alliance that would then open the door to discussing her substance use more openly—all of which could improve treatment outcomes. A second consideration is that the court staff and any providers be mindful of Gabi's cultural and family history and immigration status and how this cultural and family context is critical to consider through substance use assessment, referral, and treatment procedures.

WAYS TO ENHANCE TREATMENT ENGAGEMENT

Providing brief interventions to the juvenile justice population has several inherent challenges that mental health providers must consider in order for treatment to be most effective. Adolescents can present unique, developmentally relevant barriers to engaging in treatment. Systems routinely mandate interventions based on the expectation that the weight of the court encourages compliance. Experience does not always support that assumption, as adolescents who are ordered into treatment by a judge can be highly resistant to the process. There is no guarantee that mandated individuals will be engaged in or even complete the treatment process. The following domains are important for therapists and researchers alike to consider in order to enhance our understanding of what constitutes effective treatment for juveniles and how to provide the care they need to support them in achieving positive life outcomes into adulthood.

Motivation

"Motivation is an important factor in seeking, engaging, and remaining in treatment, and in achieving positive posttreatment outcomes" (Battjes, Gordon, O'Grady, & Carswell, 2003, p. 222). However, adolescents rarely perceive a need for treatment and tend to enter it as a result of external influences such as legal or family pressure rather than internal motivation (Battjes et al., 2003; Chassin, 2008). Furthermore, youth who have had previous contact with the juvenile justice system may harbor cynicism and skepticism about the potential of receiving any professional help that would be beneficial to them (Nissen,

2006), making it extremely difficult to engage and retain juveniles in treatment. Incorporating brief motivational interventions into their treatment plan can help mental health professionals overcome some of these barriers in engaging juveniles. By incorporating motivational techniques, adolescents should not only feel empowered during the treatment process to provide ideas and make decisions on how to improve their own lives but also feel like their experiences are acknowledged and validated rather than minimized (Nissen, 2006). Moreover, it can help juveniles in recognizing the consequences of their substance use (e.g., problems with interpersonal relationships, employment, health and legal status, collateral harm to their families), exploring and resolving ambivalence regarding change, actively engaging in and completing their treatment, and enrolling in aftercare services (Battjes et al., 2003; Chassin, 2008).

Cultural Differences

For decades, there has been a disproportionate overrepresentation of youth of color in the juvenile justice system (Nissen, 2006; Watson, Bisesi, Tanamly, & Mai, 2003). Therefore, infusing culturally relevant best practices into substance use treatment programs is essential in providing effective services to these diverse juveniles and their families. Effective interventions should embrace culture by carefully and thoroughly considering the cultural perspectives of youth and their families and how these perspectives relate to the treatment process (Watson et al., 2003). Cultural competency can build mental health professionals' capacity to properly address the common factors that influence amenability to treatment such as perceived discrimination, cultural mistrust, and acculturation (Gil et al., 2004; Nissen, 2006). This involves understanding the overt and subtle cultural variables that affect the development and maintenance of substance use and mental health problems as well as understanding the cultural perceptions of seeking and engaging in treatment (Watson et al., 2003). Watson and his colleagues (2003) offer the following practical advice for providing culturally sensitive treatment for juveniles:

> (a) address the needs of juveniles of various cultures in a way that elevates and does not denigrate their culture, (b) provide access to staff and/or posi-tive role models that represent the juvenile's cultural background, (c) [pro-vide services that] are language-appropriate, (d) recognize varying degrees of acculturation and cultural conflict within the family and understand that perceptions of the majority cultures and minority cultures may differ con-siderably about treatment, and (e) incorporate a variety of strategies that build on cultural strengths to engage and retain the juvenile in treatment. (p. 396)

By following these guidelines, mental health professionals can develop better treatment plans that honor a given culture's values and experiences and enhances the cultural pride of the juvenile and his or her family (Watson et al., 2003). Acknowledging and embracing cultural differences can break down the barriers of perceived discrimination and mistrust and improve the working alliance between the therapist and client. In fact, "minority parents [often] report less satisfaction with treatment when they perceive that providers have not considered their cultural values" (Algeria, Carson, Goncalves, & Keefe, 2011, p. 26; Walker, 2001).

Lack of language concordance between the mental health provider and the adolescent and his or her family is another cultural barrier that can impact adherence to treatment, retention, and overall quality of treatment (Algeria et al., 2011). Therefore, employing evidence-based intervention programs in clients' primary language that considers relevant cultural factors helps to overcome some of the key obstacles to treating adolescents and their families who are English language learners or have English as their second language.

Linking and Engagement in Care

Approximately two-thirds of youth will be rearrested and up to one-third of youth will be reincarcerated within a few years after their release (Mears & Travis, 2004). Challenges in linking youth to mental health and substance abuse treatment to counteract this trajectory are the result of (1) insufficient and fragmented services by an overburdened juvenile justice system, and (2) personal challenges within their family and community that affect their ability to successfully comply with treatment and avoid substance abuse (Sung, Mahoney, & Mellow, 2011; Watson, 2004). Systemic difficulties include a lack of coordination, integration, and communication among service systems (i.e., juvenile justice and mental health systems); difficulty accessing services; a lack of uniformity of standards, procedures, and practices among the thousands of U.S. juvenile justice jurisdictions; and high caseloads and staff turnover among service agencies (Kapp, Petr, Robbins, & Choi, 2013; Maschi, Hatcher, Schwalbe, & Rosato, 2008; Watson, 2004). Personal difficulties include lack of transportation to or availability of treatment services; strained family ties; and living in communities wrought with concentrated disadvantage, where exposure to violence and crime is widespread, opportunities for employment and education are limited, and quality of public services is suboptimal (Mears & Travis, 2004; Weaver & Campbell, 2015). A focus on community- and home-based brief interventions may therefore be more realistic and appropriate to implement given these real-life system barriers to successfully providing more intensive evidence-based treatments.

IMPLICATIONS AND NEXT STEPS FOR BRIEF TREATMENT DEVELOPMENT WITH CINI YOUTH

Brief interventions for substance use treatment are largely untested with CINI youth, which is a significant gap given that 80% of all arrested youth never reach detention or incarceration and many CINI youth and families do not have the time or resources to participate in intensive, longer-term intervention. Court and diversion settings therefore give a true window of opportunity to provide brief substance use intervention for CINI youth. More widely known brief interventions, such as SBIRT, are just being implemented and tested at the juvenile diversion level—thus, it remains to be seen what the outcomes of these will be for CINI youth.

Some key elements of empirically supported substance use interventions for juvenile justice youth include motivational enhancement techniques, family involvement, cultural consideration, and concurrent treatment of co-occurring psychiatric disorders/symptoms. Among more severely substance-using justice-involved youth, longer, more intensive, family-based interventions have demonstrated positive effects in reducing substance use and reoffending. Several of these interventions have already been widely disseminated in the juvenile justice system and community. Brief interventions, however, might have a role to play in treatment engagement and helping to address the real-world barriers to engaging in treatments that are common to many justice-involved youth and their families. Among CINI youth in particular, brief intervention may be appropriate as a first option for youth with less frequent or severe substance use and/or psychiatric symptoms. Brief interventions might also be appropriate when all that is feasible is a brief treatment due to lesser time in contact with the system. Brief interventions might also assist with engagement and linkages to community-based treatment that can then be more intensive, as needed, depending on the youth's behaviors and clinical symptoms. In sum, there is a great need—in partnership with the justice system, youth, families, and their communities—to develop an evidence base that supports the efficacy and implementation of brief interventions to reduce substance use among CINI youth.

REFERENCES

Algeria, M., Carson, N. J., Goncalves, M., & Keefe, K. (2011). Disparities in treatment for substance use disorders and co-occurring disorders for ethnic/racial minority youth. *Journal of the American Academy of Child and Adolescent Psychiatry, 50*(1), 22–31.

Baldwin, S., Christian, S., Berkeljon, A., & Shadish, W. (2012). The effects of family therapies for adolescent delinquency and substance abuse: A meta-analysis. *Journal of Marital and Family Therapy, 38*(1), 281–304.

Battjes, R. J., Gordon, M. S., O'Grady, K., & Carswell, M. A. (2003). Factors that predict adolescent motivation for substance abuse treatment. *Journal of Substance Abuse Treatment, 24*(3), 221–232.

Belendiuk, K. A., & Riggs, P. (2014). Treatment of adolescent substance use disorders. *Current Treatment Options in Psychiatry, 1*(2), 175–188.

Belenko, S., & Sprott, J. B. (2002). *Comparative recidivism rates of drug and nondrug juvenile offenders: Results from three jurisdictions.* Paper presented at the Academy of Criminal Justice Sciences annual conference, Anaheim, CA.

Borduin, C., Mann, B., Cone, L., & Henggeler, S. (1995). Multisystemic treatment of serious juvenile offenders: Long-term prevention of criminality and violence. *Journal of Consulting and Clinical Psychology, 63*(4), 569–578.

Braithwaite, R. L., Conerly, R. C., Robillard, A. G., Woodring, T., & Stephens, T. T. (2003). Alcohol and other drug use among adolescent detainees. *Journal of Substance Use, 8*(2), 126–131.

Braukman, C. J., Bedlington, M. M., Belden, B. D., Braukmann, P. D., Husted, J. J., & Ramp, K. K. (1985). Effects of community-based group-home treatment programs on male juvenile offenders use and abuse of drugs and alcohol. *American Journal of Drug and Alcohol Abuse, 11*(3–4), 249–278.

Bukstein, O. (2005). Practice parameter for the assessment and treatment of children and adolescents with substance use disorders. *Journal of the American Academy of Child and Adolescent Psychiatry, 44*(6), 609–621.

Bukstein, O. G., Glancy, L. J., & Kaminer, Y. (1992). Patterns of affective comorbidity in a clinical population of dually diagnosed adolescent substance abusers. *Journal of the American Academy of Child and Adolescent Psychiatry, 31*(6), 1041–1045.

Bureau of Justice Assistance. (2003). Juvenile drug courts: Strategies in practice. Retrieved from *www.ncjrs.gov/pdffiles1/bja/197866.pdf.*

Canterbury, R. J., McGarvey, E. L., Sheldon-Keller, A. E., Waite, D., Reams, P., & Koopman, C. (1995). Prevalence of HIV-related risk behaviors and STDs among incarcerated adolescents. *Journal of Adolescent Health, 17*(3), 173–177.

Castrucci, B. C., & Martin, S. L. (2002). The association between substance use and risky sexual behaviors among incarcerated adolescents. *Maternal and Child Health Journal, 6*(1), 43–47.

Catalano, R. F., Hawkins, J. D., Wells, E. A., Miller, J., & Brewer, D. (1990). Evaluation of the effectiveness of adolescent drug abuse treatment, assessment of risks for relapse, and promising approaches for relapse prevention. *International Journal of Addiction, 25*(9A–10A), 1085–1140.

Chassin, L. (2008). Juvenile justice and substance use. *Future of Children, 18*(2), 165–183.

Chassin, L., Knight, G., Vargas-Chanes, D., Losoya, S. H., & Naranjo, D. (2009). Substance use treatment outcomes in a sample of male serious juvenile offenders. *Journal of Substance Abuse Treatment, 36*(2), 183–194.

Chesney-Lind, M. (2001). What about the girls?: Delinquency programming as if gender mattered. *Corrections Today, 63*(1), 38.

Chiapa, A., Smith, J. D., Kim, H., Dishion, T. J., Shaw, D. S., & Wilson, M. N. (2015). The trajectory of fidelity in a multiyear trial of the Family Check-Up predicts change in child problem behavior. *Journal of Consulting and Clinical Psychology, 83*(5), 1006–1011.

Connell, A. M., Dishion, T. J., & Klostermann, S. (2012). Family Check-Up effects on adolescent arrest trajectories: Variation by developmental subtype. *Journal of Research on Adolescence, 22*(2), 367–380.

Cook, M., Watson, L., & Stageberg, P. (2009). *Statewide process and comparative outcomes study of 2003 Iowa adult and juvenile drug courts.* Des Moines: Division of Criminal and Juvenile Justice Planning, Statistical Analysis Center, Iowa Department of Human Rights.

Crowley, T. J., Mikulich, S. K., MacDonald, M., Young, S. E., & Zerbe, G. O. (1998).

Substance-dependent, conduct-disordered adolescent males: Severity of diagnosis predicts 2-year outcome. *Drug and Alcohol Dependence, 49*(3), 225–237.

Curtis, N., Ronan, K., & Borduin, C. (2004). Multisystemic treatment: A meta-analysis of outcome studies. *Journal of Family Psychology, 18*(3), 411–419.

Dembo, R., Belenko, S., Childs, K., Greenbaum, P., & Wareham, J. (2010). Gender differences in drug use, sexually transmitted diseases, and risky sexual behavior among arrested youths. *Journal of Child and Adolescent Substance Abuse, 19*(5), 424–446.

Dembo, R., Belenko, S., Childs, K., & Wareham, J. (2009). Drug use and sexually transmitted diseases among female and male arrested youths. *Journal of Behavioral Medicine, 32*(2), 129–141.

Dembo, R., Pacheco, K., Schmeidler, J., Fisher, L., & Cooper, S. (1997). Drug use and delinquent behavior among high risk youths. *Journal of Child and Adolescent Substance Abuse, 6*(2), 1–25.

Dennis, M., Godley, S. H., Diamond, G., Tims, F. M., Babor, T., Donaldson, J., et al. (2004). The Cannabis Youth Treatment (CYT) Study: Main findings from two randomized trials. *Journal of Substance Abuse Treatment, 27*(3), 197–213.

Dishion, T., & Andrews, D. (1995). Preventing escalation in problem behaviors with high-risk young adolescents: Immediate and 1-year outcomes. *Journal of Consulting and Clinical Psychology, 63*(4), 538–548.

Dishion, T. J., Nelson, S. E., & Kavanagh, K. (2003). The Family Check-Up with high-risk young adolescents: Preventing early-onset substance use by parent monitoring. *Behavior Therapy, 34*(4), 553–571.

Domalanta, D. D., Risser, W. L., Roberts, R. E., & Risser, J. M. (2003). Prevalence of depression and other psychiatric disorders among incarcerated youth. *Journal of the American Academy of Child and Adolescent Psychiatry, 42*(4), 477–484.

Elkington, K., Teplin, L., Mericle, A., Welty, L., Romero, E., & Abram, K. (2008). HIV/sexually transmitted infection risk behaviors in delinquent youth with psychiatric disorders: A longitudinal study. *Journal of the American Academy of Child and Adolescent Psychiatry, 47*(8), 901–911.

Feldstein Ewing, S. W. F., Venner, K. L., Mead, H. K., & Bryan, A. D. (2011). Exploring racial/ethnic differences in substance use: A preliminary theory-based investigation with juvenile justice-involved youth. *BMC Pediatrics, 11*(71), 71–80.

Fox, K. C., Somes, G. W., & Waters, T. M. (2007). Timeliness and access to healthcare services via telemedicine for adolescents in state correctional facilities. *Journal of Adolescent Health, 41*(2), 161–167.

Friedman, A. S., Terras, A., & Glassman, K. (2002). Multimodel substance use intervention program for male delinquents. *Journal of Child and Adolescent Substance Abuse, 11*(4), 43–64.

Furdella, J., & Puzzanchera, C. (2015). *Delinquency cases in juvenile court, 2013* (NCJ 248899). Washington, DC: Office of Juvenile Justice and Delinquency Prevention.

Gil, A. G., Wagner, E. F., & Tubman, J. G. (2004). Culturally sensitive substance abuse intervention for Hispanic and African American adolescents: Empirical examples from the Alcohol Treatment Targeting Adolescents in Need (ATTAIN) Project. *Addiction, 99*(S2), 140–150.

Godley, M. D., Godley, S. H., Dennis, M. L., Funk, R., & Passetti, L. L. (2006). Preliminary outcomes from the assertive continuing care experiment for adolescents discharged from residential treatment. *Journal of Substance Abuse Treatment, 23*(1), 21–32.

Goldstein, N. E., Arnold, D. H., Weil, J., Mesiarik, C. M., Peuschold, D., Grisso, T., et al. (2003). Comorbid symptom patterns in female juvenile offenders. *International Journal of Law and Psychiatry, 26*(5), 565–582.

Grisso, T. (2004). Reasons for concern about mental disorders of adolescent offenders. In *Double jeopardy: Adolescent offenders with mental disorders* (pp. 3–26). Chicago: University of Chicago Press.

Harrison, L. D. (2001). The revolving prison door for drug-involved offenders: Challenges and opportunities. *Crime and Delinquency, 47*(3), 462–484.

Harstad, E., Levy, S., & Committee on Substance Abuse. (2014). Attention-deficit/hyperactivity disorder and substance abuse. *Pediatrics, 134*(1), 293–301.

Henderson, C., Taxman, F., & Young, D. (2008). A Rasch model analysis of evidence-based treatment practices used in the criminal justice system. *Drug and Alcohol Dependence, 93*(1–2), 163–175.

Henggeler, S. W., Chapman, J. E., Rowland, M. D., Halliday-Boykins, C. A., Randall, J., Shackelford, J., et al. (2008). Statewide adoption and initial implementation of contingency management for substance abusing adolescents. *Journal of Consulting and Clinical Psychology, 76*(4), 556–567.

Henggeler, S., Melton, G., Brondino, M., Scherer, D., & Hanley, J. (1997). Multisystemic therapy with violent and chronic juvenile offenders and their families: The role of treatment fidelity in successful dissemination. *Journal of Consulting and Clinical Psychology, 65*(5), 821–833.

Henggeler, S. W., Pickrel, S. G., & Brondino, M. J. (1999). Multisystemic treatment of substance abusing and dependent delinquents: Outcomes, treatment fidelity, and transportability. *Mental Health Services Research, 1*(3), 171–184.

Hockenberry, S., & Puzzanchera, C. (2014). Juvenile and court statistics 2011. Retrieved from *www.ncjj.org/pdf/jcsreports/jcs2011.pdf.*

Horigian, V. E., Feaster, D. J., Brincks, A., Robbins, M. S., Perez, M. A., & Szapocznik, J. (2015). The effects of brief strategic family therapy (BSFT) on parent substance use and the association between parent and adolescent substance use. *Addictive Behaviors, 42*, 44–50.

Hussong, A. M., Curran, P. J., Moffitt, T. E., Caspi, A., & Carrig, M. M. (2004). Substance abuse hinders desistance in young adults' antisocial behavior. *Developmental Psychopathology, 16*(4), 1029–1046. Retrieved from *www.ncbi.nlm.nih.gov/pubmed/15704826.*

Johnson, T. P., Cho, Y. I., Fendrich, M., Graf, I., Kelly-Wilson, K., & Pickup, L. (2004). Treatment need and utilization among youth entering the juvenile corrections system. *Journal of Substance Abuse Treatment, 26*(2), 117–128.

Johnston, L. D., O'Malley, P. M., Bachman, J. G., & Schulenberg, J. E. (2012). *Monitoring the Future national results on adolescent drug use: Overview of key findings, 2011.* Ann Arbor: Institute for Social Research, University of Michigan.

Kaliebe, K. E., Heneghan, J., & Kim, T. J. (2011). Telepsychiatry in juvenile justice settings. *Child and Adolescent Psychiatric Clinics of North America, 20*(1), 113–123.

Kapp, S. A., Petr, C. G., Robbins, M. L., & Choi, J. J. (2013). Collaboration between community mental health and juvenile justice systems: Barriers and facilitators. *Child and Adolescent Social Work Journal, 30*(6), 505–517.

Kingree, J. B., & Betz, H. (2003). Risky sexual behavior in relation to marijuana and alcohol use among African-American, male adolescent detainees and their female partners. *Drug and Alcohol Dependence, 72*(2), 197–203.

Latessa, E. J., Sullivan, C., Blair, L., Sullivan, C. J., & Smith, P. (2013). Final report: Outcome and process evaluation of juvenile drug courts. Retrieved from *www.ncjrs.gov/pdffiles1/ojjdp/grants/241643.pdf*.

Liddle, H., Dakof, G., Parker, K., Diamond, G., & Barrett, K. (2001). Multidimensional family therapy for adolescent drug abuse: Results of a randomized clinical trial. *American Journal of Drug and Alcohol Abuse, 27*(4), 651–688.

Liddle, H., Rowe, C., Dakof, G., Henderson, C., & Greenbaum, P. (2009). Multidimensional family therapy for young adolescent substance abuse: Twelve-month outcomes of a randomized controlled trial. *Journal of Consulting and Clinical Psychology, 77*(1), 12–25.

Marlowe, D. (2010). Research update on juvenile drug treatment courts. Retrieved from *www.ndci.org/research*.

Marvel, F., Rowe, C., Colon-Perez, L., DiClemente, R., & Liddle, H. (2009). Multidimensional family therapy HIV/STD risk reduction intervention: An integrative family-based model for drug involved juvenile offenders. *Family Process, 48*(1), 69–83.

Maschi, T., Hatcher, S. S., Schwalbe, C. S., & Rosato, N. S. (2008). Mapping the social service pathways of youth to and through the juvenile justice system: A comprehensive review. *Children and Youth Services Review, 30*(12), 1376–1385.

Mauricio, A., Little, M., Chassin, L., Knight, G., Piquero, A., Losoya, S., et al. (2009). Juvenile offenders' alcohol and marijuana trajectories: Risk and protective factor effects in the context of time in a supervised facility. *Journal of Youth and Adolescence, 38*(3), 440–453.

Mears, D. P., & Travis, J. (2004). Youth development and reentry. *Youth Violence and Juvenile Justice, 2*(1), 3–20.

Miller, W. R., & Rollnick, S. (2002). *Motivational interviewing: Preparing people for change* (2nd ed.). New York: Guilford Press.

Morris, R., Baker, C., Valentine, M., & Pennisi, A. (1998). Variations in HIV risk behaviors of incarcerated juveniles during a four-year period: 1989–1992. *Journal of Adolescent Health, 23*(1), 39–48.

Mouttapa, M., Watson, D., McCuller, W., Reiber, C., Tsai, W., & Plug, M. (2009). HIV prevention among incarcerated male adolescents in an alternative school setting. *Journal of Correctional Health Care, 16*(1), 27–38.

Munetz, M. R., & Griffin, P. A. (2006). Use of the sequential intercept model as an approach to decriminalization of people with serious mental illness. *Psychiatric Services, 57*(4), 544–549.

National Center on Addiction and Substance Abuse at Columbia University. (2004). *Criminal neglect: Substance abuse, juvenile justice and the children left behind.* New York: Author.

National Council of Juvenile and Family Court Judges. (2015). Motivational enhancement therapy and cognitive-behavioral therapy (MET/CBT 5 or 12 sessions). Retrieved from *www.ncjfcj.org/motivational-enhancement-therapy-cognitive-behavioral-therapy-metcbt-5-or-12-sessions*.

National Institute of Justice. (2014). Number and types of drug courts (as of June 2014). Retrieved from *www.nij.gov/topics/courts/drug-courts/pages/welcome.aspx*.

National Institutes on Drug Abuse. (2006). Principles of drug abuse treatment for criminal justice populations: A research-based guide (06–5316). Retrieved from *www.drugabuse.gov/sites/default/files/txcriminaljustice_0.pdf.*

Nissen, L. B. (2006). Effective adolescent substance abuse treatment in juvenile justice settings: Practice and policy recommendations. *Child and Adolescent Social Work Journal, 23*(3), 298–314.

Office of Applied Studies. (2000). Substance abuse treatment in adult and juvenile correctional facilities: Findings from the Uniform Facility Data Set 1997 Survey of Correctional Facilities. Retrieved from *https://web.archive.org/web/20150421110525/ http://files.eric.ed.gov/fulltext/ED449405.pdf.*

Office of Juvenile Justice and Delinquency Prevention. (2015). Girls and the juvenile justice system. Retrieved from *www.ojjdp.gov/policyguidance/girls-juvenile-justice-system.*

Otto-Salaj, L., Gore-Felton, C., McGarvey, E., & Canterbury, R. (2002). Psychiatric functioning and substance use: Factors associated with HIV risk among incarcerated adolescents. *Child Psychiatry and Human Development, 33*(2), 91–106.

Pantin, H., Coatsworth, J., Feaster, D., Newman, F., Briones, E., Prado, G., et al. (2003). Familias unidas: The efficacy of an intervention to promote parental investment in Hispanic immigrant families. *Prevention Science, 4*(3), 189–201.

Prescott, L. (1997). Adolescent girls with co-occurring disorders in the juvenile justice system. Retrieved from *www.addictioncounselorce.com/articles/101360/GAINS_ Adol_girls.pdf.*

Puzzanchera, C. (2013). Juvenile arrests 2011. Retrieved from *www.ojjdp.gov/ pubs/244476.pdf.*

Randall, J., & Cunningham, P. (2003). Multisystemic therapy: A treatment for violent, substance-abusing and substance-dependent juvenile offenders. *Addictive Behaviors, 28*(9), 1731–1739.

Riggs, P. D., Baker, S., Mikulich, S. K., Young, S. E., & Crowley, T. J. (1995). Depression in substance-dependent delinquents. *Journal of the American Academy of Child and Adolescent Psychiatry, 34*(6), 764–771.

Roberts-Lewis, A. C., Welch-Brewer, C. L., Jackson, M. S., Martin Pharr, O., & Parker, S. (2010). Female juvenile offenders with HEART: Preliminary findings of an intervention model for female juvenile offenders with substance use problems. *Journal of Drug Issues, 40*(3), 611–626.

Rodriguez, N., & Webb, V. J. (2004). Multiple measures of juvenile drug court effectiveness: Results of a quasi-experimental design. *Crime and Delinquency, 50*(2), 292–314.

Rowe, C. L., Liddle, H. A., Greenbaum, P. E., & Henderson, C. E. (2004). Impact of psychiatric comorbidity on treatment of adolescent drug abusers. *Journal of Substance Abuse Treatment, 26*(2), 129–140.

Ryan, E., & Redding, R. (2004). A review of mood disorders among juvenile offenders. *Psychiatric Services, 55*(12), 1397–1407.

Salvatore, C., Henderson, J. S., Hiller, M. L., White, E., & Samuelson, B. (2010). Inside the "black box" of the prehearing team conference and status review hearing of a juvenile drug court. *Drug Court Review, 7,* 95–124.

Shaffer, D. K., Listwan, S. J., Latessa, E. J., & Lowenkamp, C. T. (2008). Examining the differential impact of drug court services by court type: Findings from Ohio. *Drug Court Review, 6,* 33–66.

Sickmund, M., & Puzzanchera, C. (Eds.). (2014). Juvenile offenders and victims: 1999 national report. Washington, DC: National Center for Juvenile Justice. Retrieved from *www.ojjdp.gov/ojstatbb/nr2014/downloads/NR2014.pdf*.

Sickmund, M., Sladky, A., & Kang, W. (2015). Easy access to juvenile court statistics: 1985–2013. Retrieved from *www.ojjdp.gov/ojstatbb/ezajcs/asp/demo.asp*.

Slavet, J. D., Stein, L. A. R., Klein, J. L., Colby, S. M., Barnett, N. P., & Monti, P. M. (2005). Piloting the Family Check-Up with incarcerated adolescents and their parents. *Psychological Services, 2*(2), 123–132.

Sloan, J. J., & Smykla, J. O. (2003). Juvenile drug courts: Understanding the importance of dimensional variability. *Criminal Justice Policy Review, 14*(3), 339–360.

Smith, D., Chamberlain, P., & Eddy, J. (2010). Preliminary support for multidimensional treatment foster care in reducing substance use in delinquent boys. *Journal of Child and Adolescent Substance Abuse, 19*(4), 343–358.

Stanger, C., & Budney, A. J. (2010). Contingency management approaches for adolescent substance use disorders. *Child and Adolescent Psychiatric Clinics of North America, 19*(3), 547–562.

Stormshak, E. A., & Dishion, T. J. (2009). A school-based, family-centered intervention to prevent substance use: The Family Check-Up. *American Journal of Drug and Alcohol Abuse, 35*(4), 227–232.

Stormshak, E. A., Fosco, G., & Dishion, T. (2010). Implementing interventions with families in schools to increase youth school engagement: The Family Check-Up model. *School Mental Health, 2*(2), 82–92.

Substance Abuse and Mental Health Services Administration. (2015). Screening, Brief Intervention, and Referral to Treatment (SBIRT). Retrieved from *www.samhsa.gov/sbirt*.

Sung, H. E., Mahoney, A. M., & Mellow, J. (2011). Substance abuse treatment gap among adult parolees: Prevalence, correlates, and barriers. *Criminal Justice Review, 36*(1), 40–57.

Szapocznik, J., Schwartz, S., Muir, J., & Brown, C. (2012). Brief strategic family therapy: An intervention to reduce adolescent risk behavior. *Couple and Family Psychology: Research and Practice, 1*(2), 134–145.

Teplin, L. A., Abram, K. M., McClelland, G. M., Dulcan, M. K., & Mericle, A. A. (2002). Psychiatric disorders in youth in juvenile detention. *Archives of General Psychiatry, 59*(12), 1133–1143.

Teplin, L. A., Elkington, K., McClelland, G., Abram, K., Mericle, A., & Washburn, J. (2005). Major mental disorders, substance use disorders, comorbidity, and HIV-AIDS risk behaviors in juvenile detainees. *Psychiatric Services, 56*(7), 823–828.

Teplin, L. A., Mericle, A. A., McClelland, G. M., & Abram, K. M. (2003). HIV and AIDS risk behaviors in juvenile detainees: Implications for public health policy. *American Journal of Public Health, 93*(6), 906–912.

Thornberry, T. P., Krohn, M. D., Lizotte, A. J., & Chard-Wierschem, D. (1993). The role of juvenile gangs in facilitating delinquent behaivor. *Journal of Research in Crime and Delinquency, 30*(1), 55–87.

Tolou-Shams, M., Brown, L. K., Gordon, G., & Fernandez, I. (2007). Arrest history as an indicator of adolescent/young adult substance use and HIV risk. *Drug and Alcohol Dependence, 88*(1), 87–90.

Tolou-Shams, M., Brown, L. K., Houck, C., Lescano, C. M., & Project SHIELD Study Group. (2008). The association between depressive symptoms, substance abuse and HIV risk among youth with an arrest history. *Journal of Studies on Alcohol and Drugs, 69*(1), 58–64.

Tolou-Shams, M., Dauria, E., Conrad, S., Kemp, K., Johnson, S., & Brown, L. K. (2017). Outcomes of a family-based HIV prevention intervention for substance using juvenile offenders. *Journal of Substance Abuse Treatment, 77,* 115–125.

Tolou-Shams, M., Rizzo, C. J., Conrad, S. M., Johnson, S., Oliveira, C., & Brown, L. K. (2014). Predictors of detention among juveniles referred for a court clinic forensic evaluation. *Journal of the American Academy of Psychiatry and the Law, 42*(1), 56–65.

Tripodi, S. J., & Bender, K. (2011). Substance use treatment for juvenile offenders: A review of quasi-experimental and experimental research. *Journal of Criminal Justice, 39*(3), 246–252.

Walker, J. S. (2001). Caregivers' views on the cultural appropriateness of services for children with emotional or behavioral disorders. *Journal of Child and Family Studies, 10*(3), 315–331.

Watson, D. (2004). Juvenile offender comprehensive reentry substance abuse treatment. *Journal of Correctional Education, 55*(3), 211–224.

Watson, D. W., Bisesi, L., Tanamly, S., & Mai, N. (2003). Comprehensive residential education, arts, and substance abuse treatment (CREASAT): A model treatment program for juvenile offenders. *Youth Violence and Juvenile Justice, 1*(1), 388–401.

Weaver R. D., & Campbell, D. (2015). Fresh start: A meta-analysis of aftercare programs for juvenile offenders. *Research on Social Work Practice, 25*(2), 201–212.

Williams, R., & Chang, S. (2000). A comprehensive and comparative review of adolescent substance abuse treatment outcome. *Clinical Psychology: Science and Practice, 7*(2), 138–166.

Winters, K. C., Botzet, A. M., & Fahnhorst, T. (2011). Advances in adolescent substance abuse treatment. *Current Psychiatry Reports, 13*(5), 416–421.

Wise, B. K., Cuffe, S. P., & Fischer, T. (2001). Dual diagnosis and successful participation of adolescents in substance abuse treatment. *Journal of Substance Abuse Treatment, 21*(3), 161–165.

Wright, D., & Clymer, B. (2001). Beckham County Juvenile Drug Court: Phase II analysis and evaluation. *Oklahoma Criminal Justice Resource Center.*

Young, D., Dembo, R., & Henderson, C. (2007). A national survey of substance abuse treatment for juvenile offenders. *Journal of Substance Abuse Treatment, 32*(3), 255–266.

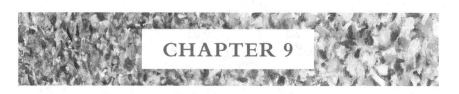

CHAPTER 9

Engaging Adolescents in Unstable Environments

Interventions with Foster Youth

Jordan M. Braciszewski and Judy Havlicek

*P*ublic health officials have asserted that child maltreatment warrants as much research attention as other concerns affecting young people, such as HIV/AIDS, smoking, and obesity (World Health Organization, 2006). While related to a host of negative outcomes, maltreatment and other adverse childhood experiences are particularly associated with increased alcohol and drug use (Dube et al., 2003, 2006). Indeed, a strong, graded relationship exists between accumulated experiences of these events (e.g., abuse, neglect, household dysfunction) and substance use severity, particularly at younger ages (Dube et al., 2003).

Youth receiving foster care services—a population nearing half a million in the United States each year—are exposed to such adverse events at alarming rates. Recent epidemiological data indicate that, compared to young people living in two-parent homes, youth residing in foster care report over 50 times the rate of being exposed to four or more adverse childhood experiences (0.9% vs. 48.3%, respectively; Bramlett & Radel, 2014). Not surprisingly, while rates of alcohol and marijuana use among foster youth are relatively similar to that of the general population of young people, use of other "hard" drugs are much higher for this vulnerable group (see Braciszewski & Stout, 2012, for a review).

Foster youth may also engage in substance use earlier than their general population peers (Braciszewski & Stout, 2012), findings that coincide with the strong link between early experience of adverse experiences during childhood

242

and substance use severity. Early initiation could lead to a greater propensity for both "hard" drug use (i.e., drugs other than alcohol and marijuana) and a higher level of substance use problems (i.e., diagnoses). Indeed, alcohol use disorders were found to occur up to four times more often among a sample of adolescents (ages 12–17) with a history of foster care (Pilowsky & Wu, 2006). Lifetime rates of substance (i.e., nonalcohol) use disorders for older adolescents in foster care have reached as high as 14%—two to three times higher than that of older adolescent norms (Keller, Salazar, & Courtney, 2010). As youth exit the system, diagnostic rates escalate rapidly. Longitudinal data indicate an increase of 11% and 13% for alcohol and substance use disorders, respectively, within 1 year of emancipation (Courtney et al., 2005). Comparatively, these rates among general population emerging adults are approximately 1–2% (Substance Abuse and Mental Health Services Administration, 2009). Interventions are clearly needed to reduce high levels of substance use within foster care, as well as curb the major spike in problematic alcohol and drug use postemancipation.

STATUS OF THE FIELD

Availability and utilization of substance use services are critical during young adulthood, a time where important milestones and tasks are negotiated. Despite this necessity, adolescents and young adults who demonstrate the need for substance use services are unlikely to receive them (Substance Abuse and Mental Health Services Administration, 2010). For youth in foster care, this gap between need and availability or access is even wider, despite Medicaid eligibility (Casanueva, Stambaugh, Urato, Fraser, & Williams, 2011). While entry into the child welfare system would be an optimal environment in which to systematically address health needs, few states are engaged in a comprehensive effort to assess and treat mental health and substance use conditions. For example, in a national review of child welfare systems, results indicated that few states require screening or assessment of mental health and substance use upon entry into foster care (McCarthy, Van Buren, & Irvine, 2007), striking given that a substantial proportion of youth report having a caregiver with alcohol and/or drug problems (Courtney, Terao, & Bost, 2004).

For state agencies where mental health and substance use screening or assessment *does* take place, substance use was identified as an area in which these efforts are not sufficiently comprehensive (McCarthy et al., 2007). In addition to the absence of public policy requirements for screening/assessment, the predominant focus in child protection on (1) *parental* substance use and (2) *infants* affected by substance use may contribute to a lack of emphasis on or quality assessment of problematic alcohol and drug use by young people in foster care (Casanueva et al., 2011). Indeed, the primary function of child welfare systems is to promote the safety, permanence, and well-being of children, though many would agree that well-being has received the least attention (Wulczyn, Barth, Yuan, Harden, & Landsverk, 2005). Finally, when the results of an assessment indicate a need for substance use services, availability and access to quality care are low. Among a host of possible services including trauma treatment; placement resources; culturally relevant services; crisis services; and services for lesbian, gay, bisexual, and transgender (LGBT) youth, substance use services ranked highest in terms of insufficiency (McCarthy et al., 2007).

Barriers that are also found among general population youth contribute to this disconnect between need for and access to treatment. Many youth do not perceive the need for substance use services, despite meeting criteria for alcohol and substance use diagnoses (Wu & Ringwalt, 2006), believing that such behavior is normative, given their developmental stage. Additionally, however, many population-specific roadblocks have been identified for foster youth. Such obstacles include a fear of consequences (e.g., being removed from a program) upon acknowledgment of substance use; reluctance to bond with a provider given difficult experiences with previous close relationships or individuals in authority; general mistrust of service systems; and lack of delivery, coordination, or continuity of care, given housing instability or overburdened case managers (Braciszewski, Moore, & Stout, 2014; Schneiderman, 2004; Simms, Dubowitz, & Szilagyi, 2000). Youth in foster care are also more likely to live in low-income homes compared to nonfoster youth (O'Hare, 2008), further limiting access to reliable health care. Consequently, foster youth often rely upon acute health services and emergency clinics, doing so at rates far greater than other low-income, Medicaid-eligible adolescents (Rubin, Alessandrini, Feudtner, Localio, & Hadley, 2004).

As indicated above, substance use continues to escalate as youth exit the foster care system. Simultaneously, however, access to substance use services becomes more difficult. Using data from a nationally representative study of youth in child welfare, for example, Casanueva et al. (2011) found that while use of illicit substances predicted receipt of substance use services while in the child welfare system, this relationship disappeared postexit, as substance use increased and receipt of both outpatient and inpatient substance use services diminished. Thus, despite having access to Medicaid or other public health resources, linkages between the child and adult service systems may break down as youth exit care.

In summary, foster youth represent a unique, at-risk population, in that they have diminished access to substance use treatment and other services while under the umbrella of the foster care system—a system purported to provide such services. Upon release from state and foster custody, access diminishes precipitously concurrent with a severe escalation of risk. Of the issues most salient to foster youth, substance use is among the more serious—however, to date, little attention has been paid to screening, assessment, prevention, or treatment of these problems. Combined with population-specific barriers to intervention availability, access, and acceptability, innovative solutions should be a priority for youth aging out of foster care.

GUIDELINES FOR DELIVERING
BRIEF INTERVENTIONS

As we have described, there is no established, systematic method for delivering substance use interventions, brief or otherwise, to youth in foster care. However, a review of the literature suggests that brief interventions may provide an excellent fit for this population. In the rest of this chapter, we focus attention on one particular method that is currently being tested and describe how it might be implemented throughout the foster care and child welfare systems.

Screening, Brief Intervention, and Referral to Treatment

Briefly, Screening, Brief Intervention, and Referral to Treatment (SBIRT) involves routine screening of alcohol and drug use, often within a primary care setting, the results of which help identify substance use severity and appropriate intervention level (Becker, Ozechowski, & Hogue, Chapter 5, this volume). Brief interventions are offered to those of moderate severity, while patients requiring more extensive interventions are referred to treatment. Given this approach, SBIRT has strong potential to address the health service disparity experienced by foster youth. SBIRT has been endorsed for use in a variety of service systems (Bernstein, Bernstein, Stein, & Saitz, 2009) and has shown success in emergency departments (Spirito et al., 2004), pediatric clinics (D'Amico, Miles, Stern, & Meredith, 2008), and schools (Mitchell et al., 2012). For the past 12 years, the Center for Substance Abuse Treatment (CSAT) at the Substance Abuse and Mental Health Services Administration has aided in the implementation of SBIRT in a number of settings. Three primary delivery systems have emerged from this endeavor, all of which could be implemented in foster care systems.

First, state and/or private agency case managers have the most face-to-face contact with foster youth, meeting regularly to check on safety issues, manage behavior, and advocate for services and legal rights. Given consistent contact with youth, case managers could both conduct an SBIRT-based intervention and provide follow-up contacts (i.e., boosters). Second, counselors, psychologists, and other mental health professionals who are already embedded in child welfare systems would be excellent candidates to provide SBIRT in foster care. Although training and support in administering SBIRT would be required for each group given the subtleties involved in delivering interventions for risky behavior, SBIRT is relatively straightforward to administer. Youth may also view mental health professionals as a group that does not make decisions about, for instance, placements or access to programs, increasing comfort with disclosing information about substance use. Finally, hiring a trained SBIRT professional would likely serve as the most optimal method. Such an individual would be "outside" of the child welfare system and, therefore, perceived as the least likely to impede access to other services, advocacy, or placements. Although contracted professionals would require training about the population, implementation would likely be fastest and most efficient. Indeed, of the CSAT-funded organizations that have incorporated SBIRT, the majority eventually adopted this model of hiring an external SBIRT professional (Bernstein et al., 2009).

If an SBIRT model were implemented in foster care, screening would best be completed upon entry into the foster care system or in early adolescence for youth who are already residing in foster care. Regardless of the delivery system chosen for a particular state, booster sessions are recommended. Previous studies conducted in emergency departments have noted that the chaos of the setting may mitigate the effectiveness of a brief intervention (Bernstein & Bernstein, 2008). Similarly, entry into the foster care system could be a confusing and difficult time for a young person, limiting initial intervention impact.

ISSUES IN ENGAGEMENT

Development of a working alliance with a young person in foster care involves not only considerations that would cut across all adolescents but also myriad, population-specific issues. While the list contained here is not exhaustive, we believe these are the most salient factors for implementation of a brief intervention with youth in foster care.

Development and Disability

Over two decades of research indicates that young people with disabilities are much more likely to experience maltreatment and neglect compared to their peers without disabilities (American Academy of Pediatrics, 2001). For example, recent data suggest that children with disabilities are 3.4 times more likely to be victims of abuse (Sullivan & Knutson, 2000). These young people are also more likely to be placed in out-of-home care, stay longer in foster care, and have a decreased likelihood of reunification (Lightfoot, Hill, & LaLiberte, 2011).

Developmental delays, in particular, are highly prevalent among youth in out-of-home care, with estimates ranging from 23 to 61% (Leslie, Gordon, Ganger, & Gist, 2002). Thus, factors such as reading level, comprehension, general cognitive ability, and mental health have strong potential to slow the process of alliance development. Brief interventions should, therefore, be delivered in a developmentally appropriate manner. Such accommodations could include adapting written materials to an appropriate reading level; having key informants (e.g., foster parents, teachers) be active collaborators in the treatment planning and execution process; and holding more frequent, closely spaced booster sessions.

Trauma

Growing evidence suggests that the maltreatment histories of foster youth prior to and during foster care are often extensive (Courtney & Heuring, 2005). An examination of administrative records by one of us (J. H.) indicated a lag time of 3 years between maltreatment investigation and foster care entry (Havlicek, 2014), suggesting elongated stays in highly challenging circumstances at young ages. Indeed, the largest subgroup (37%) of these young people faced five or more types of maltreatment, which persisted across three or more developmental periods and was perpetrated by three or more individuals. Another large group (26%) was characterized by a high probability of physical and sexual abuse. Although child welfare systems are designed to protect children from harm, as many as 11% of this sample also had a substantiated allegation of maltreatment by a foster care provider.

These chronic and high-impact forms of child victimization may ultimately result in a greater risk of developing trauma-related symptoms or posttraumatic stress disorder (PTSD), a diagnosis strongly linked to substance use (Giaconia et al., 2000). Across studies using standardized clinical assessments, the prevalence rate of lifetime PTSD among older foster youth ranges from 14 to 16% (Courtney et al., 2004; Keller et al., 2010; McMillen et al., 2005), a rate that is twice as high as the general population of young people (Merikangas et al., 2010), and also represents the most frequent mental health diagnosis among adolescents in foster care (Keller et al., 2010). While the extent to which foster youth receive treatment for PTSD remains unclear, untreated PTSD may ultimately heighten the risk for substance use in adolescence and adulthood. To date, brief interventions for trauma have been limited to veteran populations with small sample sizes (e.g., Steenkamp et al., 2011). However, these studies have been successful in reducing PTSD symptoms and could inform the development of trauma-related components within a brief substance use intervention.

Trust

By definition, youth in foster care have had at least one, if not multiple, experiences of abusive, neglectful, and/or transient experiences with adults. Given that attachment serves as the foundation for trust and forming healthy relationships (Bowlby, 1969), many youth in foster care may struggle to develop alliances with health professionals or other authority figures. Indeed, young people who have experienced maltreatment are more likely to have a disorganized attachment with their caretakers (Van IJzendoorn, Schuengel, & Bakermans-Kranenburg, 1999) and can sometimes misread neutral or ambiguous social interactions as negative or threatening (Luecken, Roubinov, & Tanaka, 2013). Cyclic patterns of relationships throughout the foster care experience (e.g., school mobility, multiple placements) can perpetuate these challenges. For example, a study of case manager turnover indicated that young people can develop strong attachments to these providers, only to lose that relationship and disrupt the development of a nurturing bond (Strolin-Goltzman, Kollar, & Trinkle, 2010), furthering youth skepticism about the perceived costs and benefits involved in relationship building. This may extend to difficulties in forming doctor–patient trust (DiGiuseppe & Christakis, 2003). As such, in a recent focus group study conducted by one of us (J. M. B.), foster care staff, administrators, and parents expressed strong concern about brief interventions in particular (Braciszewski, Moore, et al., 2014). Participants informed us that developing a trusting relationship quickly would be unlikely. Furthermore, if such a relationship were to develop, respondents strongly feared that this would not be in the youth's best interest, given previous experiences with starting and stopping relationships. Development of a trusting relationship within a short time frame may present the most significant challenge for the implementation of face-to-face brief interventions within the foster care system.

Social Support

Social support—specifically, support for abstinence from alcohol and drugs—is among the most robust predictors of sustained abstinence (Kelly, Hoeppner, Stout, & Pagano, 2012). However, young people who have been exposed to adverse events in childhood have been shown to have smaller social networks (Ford, Clark, & Stansfeld, 2011). Potential intervention content related to accessing such support has been rated negatively by foster youth (Braciszewski, Tran, et al., 2017). Participants remarked that encouragement to use support networks reminded them that few or sometimes no people existed on whom they could rely, which in turn increased their desire to use alcohol or drugs. Additional qualitative research with foster youth is needed to best understand how to leverage this important mechanism of behavior change.

Continuation of Care

Another challenge for engaging foster youth is the tendency for these young people to have less continuity of health care (i.e., a reliable link from screening to intervention). Without systematic screening of health needs, case managers may often rely upon foster parents or group home leaders to identify health care needs (Simms et al., 2000). However, these individuals may not have the legal power to provide treatment consent—rather, biological parents can sometimes remain in charge of consent, causing a delay in service access. If consent is granted, the complexity of these cases (e.g., legal involvement, multiple health issues, obtaining health histories), paired with low insurance reimbursement relative to time invested, can serve as a deterrent to receipt of care (Simms et al., 2000).

Foster youth often experience significant residential mobility, circulating between foster homes, group homes, homelessness, biological parents' home, and kinship foster care. Former foster youth participating in studies with one of us (J. M. B.) have indicated 1.5 placements per year; other researchers have reported even greater frequency of mobility (Newton, Litrownik, & Landsverk, 2000). These moves can lead to changes in health providers, further delaying timely assessment or treatment. Even if providers remain the same over time, housing disruptions can negatively impact consistent health monitoring. Results from an analysis of Medicaid claims data suggested that foster care status was associated with decreased continuity of care when compared with similarly insured, but non-foster care youth (DiGiuseppe & Christakis, 2003). Finally, for older adolescents in foster care, maintenance of health coverage can present challenges. Among a sample of 206 young people who had left the foster care system, two out of three lost insurance coverage within 3 months—those who were able to regain their coverage did so only after a period of 8 months on average (Raghavan, Shi, Aarons, Roesch, & McMillen, 2009). Implementation of brief interventions will require understanding of the health care systems involved and work within their associated complexity.

Staff Knowledge

An additional challenge for treatment engagement is the extent to which important stakeholders (e.g., case managers, foster parents, group home providers) receive training and support to identify and address substance use. In a national survey of licensed foster parents, 40% said they had fostered a child with a substance use disorder—however, less than two-thirds of those parents (61%) reported receiving any type of training specific to parenting a child with such an issue (Meyers, Kaynak, Clements, Bresani, & White, 2013). Support for foster parents with substance-using youth was not universal, as 28% of parents indicated that their agency was not helpful when they were experiencing problems with their substance-using foster child, which could reflect a lack of training on the part of case managers and other child welfare agency workers. Indeed, substance use training in social work education and content within child welfare curricula have frequently been absent (Schroeder, Lemieux, & Pogue, 2008), despite the strong presence of substance use among child welfare families. In addition, lack of case worker knowledge about community-based resources and treatment programs have been cited as barriers to service provision for both parents and youth (American Academy of Pediatrics, 2002). We strongly recommend continuing education courses and training on substance use for child welfare case managers. Indeed, when case managers receive such education/training, they reduce their negative attitudes toward substance use and increase their willingness to add substance-using young people to their caseloads (Amodeo, 2000; Amodeo & Fassler, 2000). Training should also focus on improving linkages to community-based substance use service agencies.

Family Dynamics

Parental substance use is often a driving contributor to a child's involvement in child protective service and placement in out-of-home care. Prevalence rates of substance use among child welfare-involved parents range from 40% in all cases involving unsubstantiated reports to 75% in out-of-home placement cases (Young, Gardner, & Dennis, 1998). In addition to being a precipitating factor in removal of a child from the home, parental substance use is also associated with delays in reunification (Brook, McDonald, Gregoire, Press, & Hindman, 2010) and reentry into foster care (Brook & McDonald, 2009). Given that parent involvement has the potential to augment brief intervention outcomes for adolescents (Spirito et al., 2011; Winters & Leitten, 2007), brief interventions for foster youth may require unique innovation around family dynamics. For example, engaging youth in conversations about parental substance abuse histories may ultimately help identify their own risks for substance dependence and future goals as adults. Given that many foster youth seek out their parents following emancipation, engaging youth in conversations about familial patterns of substance use may also help youth to navigate complex issues following exit from care. Finally, involvement of foster parents may serve as a helpful proxy for an adult collaborator within a brief intervention.

SUPPORT FOR BRIEF INTERVENTIONS

iHeLP: Interactive Technology to Prevent Substance Use

Over the past 3 years, one of us (J. M. B.) and his team have been working to develop the first brief substance use intervention specifically for youth in foster care (Braciszewski et al., 2016). Interactive Healthy Lifestyle Preparation (iHeLP) initially involves a computerized screening and brief intervention (SBI) to target substance use reduction in foster youth. The SBI utilizes computerized intervention authoring software (CIAS; Ondersma, Chase, Svikis, & Schuster, 2005), a sophisticated intervention development tool that allows for the modification and delivery of screening, assessment, and intervention, personalized for individual participants.

CIAS has often been used with other populations for whom disclosure of risky behavior presents additional challenges. Initial studies focused on perinatal drug use (Ondersma et al., 2005), and then expanded to postpartum, substance-using women (Ondersma, Svikis, & Schuster, 2007), pregnant alcohol and drug users (Ondersma, Winhusen, Erickson, Stine, & Wang, 2009; Tzilos, Sokol, & Ondersma, 2011), drug-using women who were also victims of intimate partner violence (Choo et al., 2016), and young people with HIV

(Naar-King et al., 2013). CIAS is unique in that it utilizes an animated narrator to deliver intervention content. The narrator, named Peedy the Parrot, can talk, move, gesture, display emotional reactions, and make empathic reflections that parallel those seen in a person-to-person interaction. Use of headphones and narration by Peedy allows access at any literacy level and provides a confidential setting regardless of location. While other characters and voices are available within CIAS, previous studies (Ondersma et al., 2005) and our own work have indicated a preference for Peedy.

The SBI addresses alcohol and illicit drug use by using an approach consistent with motivational interviewing (MI; Miller & Rollnick, 2012) and following the FRAMES (Miller & Sanchez, 1994) approach to brief interventions. FRAMES involves six major elements found in effective, brief clinical trials: (1) constructive, nonconfrontational Feedback, tailored to the individual; (2) emphasizing personal control and Responsibility; (3) provision of nonjudgmental Advice through educational information or suggestions; (4) offering a Menu of options or strategies; (5) displaying Empathy; and (6) promoting feelings of Self-efficacy.

To illustrate, after completing a brief assessment battery, Peedy orients participants to the intervention process, first by indicating his approach.

> "Now we are moving into the next part of this study, which will have fewer questions and will feel more like a real conversation between you, and a handsome green bird . . . that would be me! I'm going to ask you a few more questions, and I'm going to use your answers to give you some information that is designed just for you. Remember that I never lecture or judge people. Basically, I just want to help you think about whether or not you want to make any changes right now. If you want to change something, I can help you with that."

After asking for an initial Readiness Ruler score, Peedy presents facts about the participant's drug of choice, always emphasizing autonomy. Subject matter changes relative to the drug of choice and includes five to six topics such as mental health, sexual health, preventing injury, and, as presented below, brain development, and success at work/school.

> "Drinking while you are getting out on your own has the potential to get in the way of your long-term goals and your ability to become successfully independent. Remember, change can be different for everyone . . . some people may drink less often . . . others may have fewer drinks when they drink . . . and some people may quit drinking altogether. While the choice is yours, getting out on your own with a completely clear vision can be helpful. Let me share with you why. First, research shows that people who cut down their drinking in young adulthood are much less likely to develop alcohol problems later on. Your brain is still developing until roughly age 25, so people who cut down their drinking are likely to have better memory, attention,

and decision-making skills. Second, you will improve the likelihood of being successful at school or work since alcohol use can cause people to miss school, or work, and to fall behind."

Participants are then asked whether they are interested in making a change. In one scenario, Frank chooses to stay the same.

Peedy says, "So, it looks like you plan to keep drinking alcohol, at least for now. I'm sure that you have your reasons for this. I definitely don't judge you for it, and I won't try to force you to change. I'm just a fat green parrot anyway. But if it's OK, I'd like to talk with you just a little bit about what you're thinking right now. No pressure or anything, I just want to help you think about what, if anything, you want to change."

Frank is then asked to select the biggest reason he continues to drink, from a list of options. After his choice is reflected back to him and normalized (e.g., "This is pretty common"), he is asked to choose up to three "less good sides to drinking," which are also reflected back to him. Finally, Frank is asked to indicate the best thing about changing, which includes an option to write in a custom answer.

Peedy then summarizes Frank's responses: "Thanks for helping me understand your take on this. It looks like you don't like that alcohol is hurting your health and that it costs a lot of money. Overall, you think that drinking alcohol has had a kind of bad effect on your life. You also think that, if you were to cut down, or quit drinking, your relationships would improve."

In the next section, Frank is provided with feedback about his alcohol use, relative to both the general population of young adults and youth exiting foster care. We have found that using the foster care community as a comparison has more impact than the general population of young people. After asking for Frank's feedback about that section, he is asked whether he wants to quit, cut down, or stay the same; being unsure is also an option.

If he wants to stay the same, Peedy responds in a nonjudgmental manner: "Well, you've clearly thought about all of this information and right now you don't think that you want to change anything about your drinking. But, it also sounds like you would know when it would be time to think about making a change, if you needed to."

If Frank is unsure, Peedy inquires why he isn't ready, what makes him think he might want to change, and how he'll know whether it's time. The choices to cut down or quit are very similar, with only slight changes in wording. Peedy first reflects Frank's "not so good things" about drinking and his "best thing about changing." He then offers brief information about the change process. Finally, he offers Frank the option of discussing a change plan. If Frank says yes, Peedy gives three short tips about risky situations and then asks Frank about his own toughest situations, how to deal with them, and how Frank will know whether he needs a different plan.

Maria provides an example of someone who says yes to the first change question. In response, Peedy says, "First, I just want to say that you seem to know yourself well. You've made a decision on your own, and you have the strength to see it through. By deciding to cut down, or quit, you are taking steps towards a healthy transition out of DCYF [Department of Children, Youth and Families] care and improving your chances of short- and long-term health."

Peedy then asks Maria her three biggest reasons to change, how she wants to do it, and how others could help her, each from multiple-choice lists with options to write in answers. Peedy then takes Maria through the same change plan process as Frank, orienting her to the change process, how to deal with difficult situations, including social pressure, and developing her own plan to cope with these situations.

Peedy then summarizes Maria's answers: "Let me see if I have this right. You want to cut down, or quit drinking. I admire your commitment to this goal. You want to do this because you want to get someone off your back, you're trying to get back in school, and you want to be safer when you party. To do this, you want to tell your friends that you're cutting down and get away from a certain person. You think that cutting down, or quitting will be pretty hard."

At this point, both Frank and Maria would respond to one final Readiness Ruler question, which would trigger the second component of iHeLP: short message service (SMS) text messaging. Participants receive daily text messages for a period of 3 months, followed by an additional 3 months of messages sent every other day. Message content is theoretically grounded in MI and the transtheoretical model (TTM; Prochaska & DiClemente, 1992). The TTM posits that behavior change occurs in increments along stages: not being interested (precontemplation), considering change (contemplation), getting ready (preparation), starting to make changes (action), and maintaining those changes (maintenance). MI and TTM are complementary, as MI is a method of conversation that is particularly effective at the beginning TTM stages of readiness for change (DiClemente & Velasquez, 2002). Individual scores on the Readiness Ruler are anchored by stages analogous with the TTM and are highly predictive of drinking outcomes in adolescents (Maisto et al., 2011). To take advantage of this synchrony, messages are tailored to each participant's level of motivation to reduce his or her substance use by using content appropriate for that person's current stage of change, as measured by the post-SBI Readiness Ruler.

Motivation for behavior change, however, often fluctuates over time and should be considered when designing motivation-based interventions (Resnicow & Page, 2008). As such, individuals' motivational levels are likely to fluctuate over the course of the intervention. To account for these changes, iHeLP utilizes weekly "poll questions," sent via text message, to assess major outcomes and readiness to change. Answers to these questions are used by algorithms to determine the tailored messages each participant receives, allowing for fluid change in the intervention—that is, when participants respond with a Readiness Ruler score that alters their stage of change (e.g., moving from precontemplation to contemplation or from preparation to contemplation), the content of their messages reflects that change. This design allows for more up-to-the-minute tailoring of message content, rather than relying solely on baseline or follow-up data collected months after the initial interview.

iHeLP Development and Outcomes

One major goal of iHeLP development was to incorporate the preferences and voices of youth exiting foster care in a collaborative, participatory manner. This began by using the same inclusion criteria for all three phases of development (focus groups, open trial, pilot randomized controlled trial). In this way, feedback would always be provided by the same target population. During the focus group phase, participants were invited to posit their own intervention, given the concerns about elevated substance use postexit. Participants highlighted the need for a nonjudgmental stance, caution about working with service providers, preference for some type of interaction, and respect for autonomy and individuality (Braciszewski, Tran, Tzilos, & Moore, 2014). Youth were also heavily involved in providing direct feedback on text message content (Braciszewski et al., 2017), as well as writing messages that were incorporated into the larger study text bank. Altogether, focus group participants played a critical role in the design, content, and implementation of iHeLP for delivery in the open trial.

We then conducted an open trial where 17 participants completed iHeLP and provided feedback on their experiences. Results supported acceptability and feasibility (Braciszewski, Tzilos, Moore, & Stout, 2015). Specifically, all participants rated the computer as easy to work with and Peedy as nonjudgmental. Three times per week, text messages were followed with a question about the relevance/likability of that day's message—results indicated a 92% approval rating for the messages. The weekly poll question response rate was 87%, which is high, given the duration of the intervention (i.e., 6 months). Exit interviews indicated exceedingly positive reviews with many participants noting advantages over more traditional means of intervention, particularly those involving face-to-face contact with a physician, nurse, counselor, or case manager. In addition to high acceptability, implementation of iHeLP was shown to be feasible. Across the two phases, 45% of screened participants were eligible and only one participant directly refused participation. Target sample sizes were also achieved in less time than proposed.

Open-trial participant feedback has been incorporated into a final version of iHeLP, currently being tested in a small randomized trial. The two biggest additions were (1) weekly positive feedback if participants met their goal of cutting down/quitting that week, and (2) biweekly reminders of their reasons for change that they told Peedy. Thirty-three youth who are exiting care were assigned to either iHeLP or a control group focusing on diet, exercise, and general motivation. We will follow these young people for 1 year to track long-term intervention effects.

IMPLICATIONS FOR TREATMENT

Brief interventions hold a great deal of promise for the initial engagement of foster youth into a substance use intervention, as well as potential to reduce or eliminate alcohol and drug use. As we have described, however, youth in foster care often have complicated histories where substance use is only one of several health concerns. Trauma, family conflict, homelessness, low educational attainment, unemployment, tobacco use, physical illness, and risky sexual behavior are all, on average, higher among foster youth and foster care alumni than the general population (Auslander et al., 2002; Braciszewski & Colby, 2015; Courtney & Dworsky, 2006; Pecora et al., 2006). While brief interventions have the capacity to address more than one problem behavior simultaneously (e.g., Walton et al., 2010), many foster youth may require a higher level of care that can attend to the multidirectional relationships among these issues. Thus, brief intervention may serve an integral role in expediting enrollment in more intensive substance use and/or multidimensional treatment. Given the dearth of screening and assessment procedures in child welfare, this goal requires improved coordination among stakeholders and systems of care.

FUTURE DIRECTIONS

Addressing substance use among foster youth first requires acknowledgment of this important issue and subsequent improvement in the identification of alcohol and drug use. Given the barriers outlined above, leveraging technology is likely the most efficient and efficacious way to complete screening and assessment. Computers, mobile phones, and other means of electronic communication are increasingly being used to tackle a number of health issues. In addition to their ability to deliver evidence-based intervention content effectively, computer- and mobile phone-based interventions can address many of the barriers to foster youth receiving substance use services. First, the absence of screening and assessment is often an issue of finances (Casanueva et al., 2011). Utilization of new technologies can dramatically reduce such costs (Newman, Szkodny, Llera, & Przeworski, 2011), as the majority of funds are invested in intervention development while costs of delivery are relatively limited. Second, use of computers and mobile phones increases the likelihood of honest reporting through privacy and confidentiality (Turner et al., 1998), which may mitigate concerns among foster youth about negative consequences for reporting alcohol or drug use. Third, building therapeutic alliances within a maltreated population can present unique challenges. Technology-driven interventions not only circumnavigate this barrier, but could also increase the chances of future work with a counselor. Such low-intensity, high-frequency approaches could facilitate self-reflection and insight that more intensive services are needed. Likewise, technology could serve as a continued adjunct to formal treatment once it begins. Fourth, the frequent housing instability often experienced by foster youth can disrupt the continuity of a traditional model of care. Computers and mobile phones can be used across many environments, and text-based interventions, specifically, can be available 24 hours per day. Fifth, an intervention utilizing mobile technology can reach individuals unlikely to access traditional systems of care. Last, foster care staff and state social workers are often overburdened with large caseloads of youth and families experiencing considerable challenges. Using computers and mobile phones to address a significant health issue allows providers more flexibility with their time and efforts. Taken together, these advantages promote engagement, client satisfaction, and increased self-disclosure, all of which can potentially improve intervention response.

Technology-based brief interventions are not a panacea for foster youth. Issues of trauma, social support, family dynamics, and the negative attitudes of agency staff toward substance use remain essential issues for this population. Future research should examine the feasibility of incorporating trauma-based content, as well as adding family members or other important contacts as partners in behavior change. Training and education of social workers and other child welfare staff on substance use etiology, assessment, and intervention is also necessary. Finally, it is important for clinicians and researchers to understand that the culture of adolescents is significantly different from that of adults— thus, application of youth culture into intervention content and program development is needed. Indeed, programs that are developed with youth input are more likely to appeal to diverse groups of young people (D'Amico & Edelen, 2007). Creating culturally consistent interventions, making use of the population's vernacular, and reflecting the values and beliefs of group members can enhance service acceptability and efficacy (Nastasi et al., 2000), which ultimately should improve intervention effectiveness.

REFERENCES

American Academy of Pediatrics. (2001). Assessment of maltreatment of children with disabilities. *Pediatrics, 108*(2), 508–512.
American Academy of Pediatrics. (2002). Health care of young children in foster care. *Pediatrics, 109*(3), 536.
Amodeo, M. (2000). The therapeutic attitudes and behavior of social work clinicians with and without substance abuse training. *Substance Use and Misuse, 35*(11), 1507–1536.
Amodeo, M., & Fassler, I. (2000). Social workers and substance-abusing clients: Caseload composition and competency self-ratings. *American Journal of Drug and Alcohol Abuse, 26*(4), 629–641.
Auslander, W. F., McMillen, J. C., Elze, D., Thompson, R., Jonson-Reid, M., & Stiffman, A. (2002). Mental health problems and sexual abuse among adolescents in foster care: Relationship to HIV risk behaviors and intentions. *AIDS and Behavior, 6*(4), 351–359.

Bernstein, E., & Bernstein, J. (2008). Effectiveness of alcohol screening and brief motivational intervention in the emergency department setting. *Annals of Emergency Medicine, 51*(6), 751–754.

Bernstein, E., Bernstein, J. A., Stein, J. B., & Saitz, R. (2009). SBIRT in emergency care settings: Are we ready to take it to scale? *Academic Emergency Medicine, 16*(11), 1072–1077.

Bowlby, J. (1969). *Attachment.* London: Penguin.

Braciszewski, J. M., & Colby, S. M. (2015). Tobacco use among foster youth: Evidence of health disparities. *Children and Youth Services Review, 58,* 142–145.

Braciszewski, J. M., Moore, R. S., & Stout, R. L. (2014). Rationale for a new direction in foster youth substance use disorder prevention. *Journal of Substance Use, 19*(1–2), 108–111.

Braciszewski, J. M., & Stout, R. L. (2012). Substance use among current and former foster youth: A systematic review. *Children and Youth Services Review, 34*(12), 2337–2344.

Braciszewski, J. M., Stout, R. L., Tzilos, G. K., Moore, R. S., Bock, B. C., & Chamberlain, P. (2016). Testing a dynamic automated intervention model for emerging adults. *Journal of Child and Adolescent Substance Abuse, 25*(3), 181–187.

Braciszewski, J. M., Tran, T. B., Moore, R. S., Bock, B. C., Tzilos, G. K., Chamberlain, P., et al. (2017). Developing a tailored texting intervention: A card sort methodology. *Journal of Applied Biobehavioral Research, 22*(2), e12060.

Braciszewski, J. M., Tran, T. B., Tzilos, G. K., & Moore, R. S. (2014, March). *iHeLP: Improving substance use outcomes for foster youth.* Poster presented at the Society for Research on Adolescence, Austin, TX.

Braciszewski, J. M., Tzilos, G. K., Moore, R. S., & Stout, R. L. (2015, June). *iHeLP: A collaborative approach to substance use prevention for foster youth.* Paper presented at the Society for Community Research and Action, Lowell, MA.

Bramlett, M. D., & Radel, L. F. (2014). *Adverse family experiences among children in nonparental care, 2011–2012* (National Health Statistics Reports, Vol. 74). Hyattsville, MD: National Center for Health Statistics.

Brook, J., & McDonald, T. (2009). The impact of parental substance abuse on the stability of family reunifications from foster care. *Children and Youth Services Review, 31*(2), 193–198.

Brook, J., McDonald, T. P., Gregoire, T., Press, A., & Hindman, B. (2010). Parental substance abuse and family reunification. *Journal of Social Work Practice in the Addictions, 10*(4), 393–412.

Casanueva, C., Stambaugh, L., Urato, M., Fraser, J. G., & Williams, J. (2011). Lost in transition: Illicit substance use and services receipt among at-risk youth in the child welfare system. *Children and Youth Services Review, 33*(10), 1939–1949.

Choo, E. K., Zlotnick, C., Strong, D. R., Squires, D. D., Tapé, C., & Mello, M. J. (2016). BSAFER: A web-based intervention for drug use and intimate partner violence demonstrates feasibility and acceptability among women in the emergency department. *Substance Abuse, 37*(3), 441–449.

Courtney, M. E., & Dworsky, A. (2006). Early outcomes for young adults transitioning from out-of-home care in the USA. *Child and Family Social Work, 11*(3), 209–219.

Courtney, M. E., Dworsky, A., Ruth, G., Keller, T., Havlicek, J., & Bost, N. (2005). *Midwest evaluation of the adult functioning of former foster youth: Outcomes at age 19.* Chicago: Chapin Hall Center for Children, University of Chicago.

Courtney, M. E., & Heuring, D. H. (2005). The transition to adulthood for youth "aging out" of the foster care system. In D. W. Osgood, E. M. Foster, C. Flanagan, & G. Ruth (Eds.), *On your own without a net: The transition to adulthood for vulnerable populations* (pp. 27–67). Chicago: University of Chicago Press.

Courtney, M. E., Terao, S., & Bost, N. (2004) *Midwest evaluation of the adult functioning of former foster youth: Conditions of youth preparing to leave state care.* Chicago: Chapin Hall Center for Children, University of Chicago.

D'Amico, E. J., & Edelen, M. O. (2007). Pilot test of Project CHOICE: A voluntary afterschool intervention for middle school youth. *Psychology of Addictive Behaviors, 21*(4), 592.

D'Amico, E. J., Miles, J. N., Stern, S. A., & Meredith, L. S. (2008). Brief motivational interviewing for teens at risk of substance use consequences: A randomized pilot study in a primary care clinic. *Journal of Substance Abuse Treatment, 35*(1), 53–61.

DiClemente, C. C., & Velasquez, M. M. (2002). Motivational interviewing and the stages of change. In W. R. Miller & S. Rollnick (Eds.), *Motivational interviewing: Preparing people for change* (2nd ed., pp. 201–216). New York: Guilford Press.

DiGiuseppe, D. L., & Christakis, D. A. (2003). Continuity of care for children in foster care. *Pediatrics, 111*(3), e208–e213.

Dube, S. R., Felitti, V. J., Dong, M., Chapman, D. P., Giles, W. H., & Anda, R. F. (2003). Childhood abuse, neglect, and household dysfunction and the risk of illicit drug use: The Adverse Childhood Experiences Study. *Pediatrics, 111*(3), 564–572.

Dube, S. R., Miller, J. W., Brown, D. W., Giles, W. H., Felitti, V. J., Dong, M., et al. (2006). Adverse childhood experiences and the association with ever using alcohol and initiating alcohol use during adolescence. *Journal of Adolescent Health, 38*(4), 444.e1–444.e10.

Ford, E., Clark, C., & Stansfeld, S. A. (2011). The influence of childhood adversity on social relations and mental health at mid-life. *Journal of Affective Disorders, 133*(1), 320–327.

Giaconia, R. M., Reinherz, H. Z., Hauf, A. C., Paradis, A. D., Wasserman, M. S., & Langhammer, D. M. (2000). Comorbidity of substance use and post-traumatic stress disorders in a community sample of adolescents. *American Journal of Orthopsychiatry, 70*(2), 253.

Havlicek, J. (2014). Maltreatment histories of foster youth exiting out-of-home care through emancipation: A latent class analysis. *Child Maltreatment, 19*(3–4), 199–208.

Keller, T. E., Salazar, A. M., & Courtney, M. E. (2010). Prevalence and timing of diagnosable mental health, alcohol, and substance use problems among older adolescents in the child welfare system. *Children and Youth Services Review, 32*(4), 626–634.

Kelly, J. F., Hoeppner, B., Stout, R. L., & Pagano, M. E. (2012). Determining the relative importance of the mechanisms of behavior change within Alcoholics Anonymous: A multiple mediator analysis. *Addiction, 107*(2), 289–299.

Leslie, L. K., Gordon, J. N., Ganger, W., & Gist, K. (2002). Developmental delay in young children in child welfare by initial placement type. *Infant Mental Health Journal, 23*(5), 496–516.

Lightfoot, E., Hill, K., & LaLiberte, T. (2011). Prevalence of children with disabilities in the child welfare system and out of home placement: An examination of administrative records. *Children and Youth Services Review, 33*, 2069–2075.

Luecken, L. J., Roubinov, D. S., & Tanaka, R. (2013). Childhood family environment, social competence, and health across the lifespan. *Journal of Social and Personal Relationships, 30*(2), 171–178.

Maisto, S. A., Krenek, M., Chung, T., Martin, C. S., Clark, D., & Cornelius, J. (2011). A comparison of the concurrent and predictive validity of three measures of readiness to change alcohol use in a clinical sample of adolescents. *Psychological Assessment, 23*(4), 983–994.

McCarthy, J., Van Buren, E., & Irvine, M. (2007). Child and family services reviews, 2001–2004: A mental health analysis. Retrieved January 18, 2012, from *http://guc-chd.georgetown.edu/files/products_publications/TACenter/cfsr_analysis.pdf*.

McMillen, J. C., Zima, B. T., Scott, L. D., Auslander, W. F., Munson, M. R., Ollie, M. T., et al. (2005). Prevalence of psychiatric disorders among older youths in the foster care system. *Journal of the American Academy of Child and Adolescent Psychiatry, 44*(1), 88–95.

Merikangas, K. R., He, J.-P., Burstein, M., Swanson, S. A., Avenevoli, S., Cui, L., et al. (2010). Lifetime prevalence of mental disorders in US adolescents: Results from the National Comorbidity Survey Replication—Adolescent Supplement (NCS-A). *Journal of the American Academy of Child and Adolescent Psychiatry, 49*(10), 980–989.

Meyers, K., Kaynak, Ö., Clements, I., Bresani, E., & White, T. (2013). Underserved parents, underserved youth: Considering foster parent willingness to foster substance-using adolescents. *Children and Youth Services Review, 35*(9), 1650–1655.

Miller, W. R., & Rollnick, S. (2012). *Motivational interviewing: Helping people change* (3rd ed.). New York: Guilford Press.

Miller, W. R., & Sanchez, V. C. (1994). Motivating young adults for treatment and lifestyle change. In G. S. Howard & P. E. Nathan (Eds.), *Alcohol use and misuse by young adults* (pp. 55–81). Notre Dame, IN: University of Notre Dame Press.

Mitchell, S. G., Gryczynski, J., Gonzales, A., Moseley, A., Peterson, T., O'Grady, K. E., et al. (2012). Screening, Brief Intervention, and Referral to Treatment (SBIRT) for substance use in a school-based program: Services and outcomes. *American Journal on Addictions, 21*(Suppl. 1), S5–S13.

Naar-King, S., Outlaw, A. Y., Sarr, M., Parsons, J. T., Belzer, M., MacDonell, K., et al. (2013). Motivational enhancement system for adherence (MESA): Pilot randomized trial of a brief computer-delivered prevention intervention for youth initiating antiretroviral treatment. *Journal of Pediatric Psychology, 38*(6), 638–648.

Nastasi, B. K., Varjas, K., Schensul, S. L., Silva, K. T., Schensul, J. J., & Ratnayake, P. (2000). The participatory intervention model: A framework for conceptualizing and promoting intervention acceptability. *School Psychology Quarterly, 15*(2), 207–232.

Newman, M. G., Szkodny, L. E., Llera, S. J., & Przeworski, A. (2011). A review of technology-assisted self-help and minimal contact therapies for anxiety and depression: Is human contact necessary for therapeutic efficacy? *Clinical Psychology Review, 31*(1), 89–103.

Newton, R. R., Litrownik, A. J., & Landsverk, J. A. (2000). Children and youth in foster care: Disentangling the relationship between problem behaviors and number of placements. *Child Abuse and Neglect, 24*(10), 1363–1374.

O'Hare, W. P. (2008). *Data on children in foster care from the Census Bureau*. Baltimore: Annie E. Casey Foundation, Kids Count.

Ondersma, S. J., Chase, S. K., Svikis, D. S., & Schuster, C. R. (2005). Computer-based brief motivational intervention for perinatal drug use. *Journal of Substance Abuse Treatment, 28*(4), 305–312.

Ondersma, S. J., Svikis, D. S., & Schuster, C. R. (2007). Computer-based brief intervention: A randomized trial with postpartum women. *American Journal of Preventive Medicine, 32*(3), 231–238.

Ondersma, S. J., Winhusen, T., Erickson, S. J., Stine, S. M., & Wang, Y. (2009). Motivation enhancement therapy with pregnant substance-abusing women: Does baseline motivation moderate efficacy? *Drug and Alcohol Dependence, 101*(1), 74–79.

Pecora, P. J., Kessler, R. C., O'Brien, K., White, C. R., Williams, J., Hiripi, E., et al. (2006). Educational and employment outcomes of adults formerly placed in foster care: Results from the Northwest Foster Care Alumni Study. *Children and Youth Services Review, 28*(12), 1459–1481.

Pilowsky, D. J., & Wu, L. T. (2006). Psychiatric symptoms and substance use disorders in a nationally representative sample of American adolescents involved with foster care. *Journal of Adolescent Health, 38*(4), 351–358.

Prochaska, J. O., & DiClemente, C. C. (1992). Stages of change in the modification of problem behaviors. In M. Hersen, R. M. Eisler, & P. M. Miller (Eds.), *Progress in behavior modification* (Vol. 28, pp. 183–218). Sycamore, IL: Sycamore Press.

Raghavan, R., Shi, P., Aarons, G. A., Roesch, S. C., & McMillen, J. C. (2009). Health insurance discontinuities among adolescents leaving foster care. *Journal of Adolescent Health, 44*(1), 41–47.

Resnicow, K., & Page, S. E. (2008). Embracing chaos and complexity: A quantum change for public health. *American Journal of Public Health, 98*(8), 1382–1389.

Rubin, D. M., Alessandrini, E. A., Feudtner, C., Localio, A. R., & Hadley, T. (2004). Placement changes and emergency department visits in the first year of foster care. *Pediatrics, 114*(3), e354–e360.

Schneiderman, J. U. (2004). The health of children in foster care. *Journal of School Nursing, 20*(6), 343–351.

Schroeder, J., Lemieux, C., & Pogue, R. (2008). The collision of the Adoption and Safe Families Act and substance abuse: Research-based education and training priorities for child welfare professionals. *Journal of Teaching in Social Work, 28*(1–2), 227–246.

Simms, M. D., Dubowitz, H., & Szilagyi, M. A. (2000). Health care needs of children in the foster care system. *Pediatrics, 106*(4), 909–918.

Spirito, A., Monti, P. M., Barnett, N. P., Colby, S. M., Sindelar, H., Rohsenow, D. J., et al. (2004). A randomized clinical trial of a brief motivational intervention for alcohol-positive adolescents treated in an emergency department. *Journal of Pediatrics, 145*(3), 396–402.

Spirito, A., Sindelar-Manning, H., Colby, S. M., Barnett, N. P., Lewander, W., Rohsenow, D. J., et al. (2011). Individual and family motivational interventions for alcohol-positive adolescents treated in an emergency department: Results of a randomized clinical trial. *Archives of Pediatrics and Adolescent Medicine, 165*(3), 269–274.

Steenkamp, M. M., Litz, B. T., Gray, M. J., Lebowitz, L., Nash, W., Conoscenti, L., et al. (2011). A brief exposure-based intervention for service members with PTSD. *Cognitive and Behavioral Practice, 18*(1), 98–107.

Strolin-Goltzman, J., Kollar, S., & Trinkle, J. (2010). Listening to the voices of children in foster care: Youths speak out about child welfare workforce turnover and selection. *Social Work, 55*(1), 47–53.

Substance Abuse and Mental Health Services Administration. (2009). *Results from the 2008 National Survey on Drug Use and Health: National findings* (Office of Applied Studies, NSDUH Series H-36, HHS Publication No. SMA 09-4434). Rockville, MD: Author.

Substance Abuse and Mental Health Services Administration. (2010). *Results from the 2009 National Survey on Drug Use and Health: Vol. I. Summary of national findings* (Office of Applied Studies, NSDUH Series H-38A, HHS Publication No. SMA 10-4586 Findings). Rockville, MD: Author.

Sullivan, P., & Knutson, J. (2000). Maltreatment and disabilities: A population-based epidemiological study. *Child Abuse and Neglect, 24*(100), 1257–1273.

Turner, C. F., Forsyth, B. H., O'Reilly, J. M., Cooley, P. C., Smith, T. K., Rogers, S. M., et al. (1998). Automated self-interviewing and the survey measurement of sensitive behaviors. In M. P. Couper, R. P. Baler, J. Bethlehem, C. Z. Clark, J. Martin, W. Nicholls II, et al. (Eds.), *Computer-assisted survey information collection* (pp. 455–473). New York: Wiley.

Tzilos, G. K., Sokol, R. J., & Ondersma, S. J. (2011). A randomized phase I trial of a brief computer-delivered intervention for alcohol use during pregnancy. *Journal of Womens Health, 20*(10), 1517–1524.

Van IJzendoorn, M. H., Schuengel, C., & Bakermans-Kranenburg, M. J. (1999). Disorganized attachment in early childhood: Meta-analysis of precursors, concomitants, and sequelae. *Development and Psychopathology, 11*(2), 225–250.

Walton, M. A., Chermack, S. T., Shope, J. T., Bingham, C. R., Zimmerman, M. A., Blow, F. C., et al. (2010). Effects of a brief intervention for reducing violence and alcohol misuse among adolescents: A randomized controlled trial. *JAMA, 304*(5), 527–535.

Winters, K. C., & Leitten, W. (2007). Brief intervention for drug-abusing adolescents in a school setting. *Psychology of Addictive Behaviors, 21*(2), 249.

World Health Organization. (2006). *Preventing child maltreatment: A guide to taking action and generating evidence.* Geneva, Switzerland: Author.

Wu, L.-T., & Ringwalt, C. L. (2006). Use of alcohol treatment and mental health services among adolescents with alcohol use disorders. *Psychiatric Services, 57*(1), 84–92.

Wulczyn, F., Barth, R. P., Yuan, Y.-Y. T., Harden, B. J., & Landsverk, J. A. (2005). *Beyond common sense: Child welfare, child well-being, and the evidence for policy reform.* Piscataway, NJ: Aldine Transaction.

Young, N. K., Gardner, S., & Dennis, K. (1998). *Responding to alcohol and other drug problems in child welfare: Weaving together policy and practice.* Washington, DC: CWLA Press.

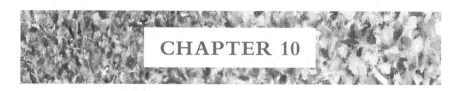

CHAPTER 10

Latino Youth, Acculturation, and Parenting

Lynn Hernandez and Oswaldo Moreno

*L*atinos represent the fastest-growing and youngest ethnic/racial-minority group in the United States, with 24.4% under the age of 18 (Colby & Ortman, 2015). It is, therefore, of concern that Latino young adolescents report more alcohol, cigarette, and illicit drug use, with the exception of amphetamines, than their non-Latino white and African American counterparts (Miech, Johnston, O'Malley, Bachman, & Schulenberg, 2015). Results from the Monitoring the Future study (Miech et al., 2015) demonstrate that while Latino adolescents have the highest rate of early alcohol and drug use initiation, by the time they reach the 12th grade, non-Latino white adolescents' use of both alcohol and drugs is higher, with the exception of marijuana use, which continues to increase for Latinos. Miech et al. (2015) note that although white non-Latino 12th graders tended to have higher rates of use for most drugs, Latino 12th graders had the highest usage rate for the most dangerous drugs (e.g., cocaine, crack, crystal methamphetamine). These researchers concluded that the decline of overall drug use among 12th-grade Latinos may be due to the fact that Latino students have the highest rate of high school dropout (Kena et al., 2014) and are therefore not included in the 12th-grade statistics. This may explain why, despite having lower alcohol and drug use rates in the 12th grade, as adults, Latinos have increased rates of alcohol use disorder (Mulia, Ye, Greenfield, & Zemore, 2009; Rios-Bedoya & Freile-Salinas, 2014), suffer from greater alcohol-related health problems (Yoon, Yi, & Thomson, 2011), and have higher death rates from alcohol-related motor vehicle accidents than their non-Latino white counterparts (West, Naumann, & Centers for Disease Control and Prevention, 2011). Further, findings indicate that the younger the age of substance use initiation, the higher the likelihood of developing a substance use disorder (Dawson, Goldstein, Chou, Ruan, & Grant, 2008; DeWit, Adlaf, Offord, & Ogborne, 2000; Guttmannova et al., 2011; Hingson, Heeren, & Winter, 2006).

Taken together, these results suggest that Latino adolescents are particularly vulnerable to progressing from use to problem use or dependence. This progression may be the result of unmet needs for early intervention for alcohol and other drug (AOD) use geared toward the specific needs of Latino youth. For this reason, understanding the role that particular factors play in Latino adolescents' AOD use trajectories as well as their treatment-seeking behaviors is crucial so that appropriate prevention and intervention programs are developed and implemented.

This chapter focuses on the influential role ethnocultural variables such as acculturation and *familismo* (familism) play in Latino adolescents' AOD use behaviors, and highlights the importance of addressing familial factors among acculturating Latino youth when intervening on their AOD use. We also discuss ways in which brief interventions may be one potential solution for increasing treatment access among this population. We begin our discussion by defining acculturation and familismo and reviewing empirical literature demonstrating the role they play in the etiology of AOD use behaviors among Latino youth. The goal of this chapter is to highlight the importance of addressing these two culturally relevant variables when delivering brief AOD interventions to Latino adolescents.

ETIOLOGY OF AOD USE BEHAVIORS AMONG LATINO ADOLESCENTS: THE ROLE OF ACCULTURATION AND FAMILY

There are a number of risk and protective factors that influence AOD use behaviors among adolescents in general, and Latino adolescents in particular. Pantin, Prado, Schwartz, and Sullivan (2005) categorize these factors into two domains: (1) intrapersonal factors (i.e., social cognitive attitudes, expectancies, and intentions regarding AOD use and perceived self-efficacy) and (2) contextual factors (i.e., family functioning, parent–adolescent communication about AOD use, and parental monitoring and supervision). In addition, cultural factors should be considered when developing, adapting, and implementing AOD use interventions. While Latinos are a heterogeneous group, and variations in AOD use exist within different Latino subgroups, specific processes inherent to this cultural group play a role in Latino adolescents' AOD behaviors. These cultural factors are discussed below.

Acculturation to the United States

There is a large body of literature demonstrating the role acculturation plays in the etiology and maintenance of AOD use behaviors among Latino adolescents immigrating and living in the United States (Ebin et al., 2001; Gil, Wagner, & Vega, 2000; Marsiglia & Waller, 2002; Nielsen & Ford, 2001; Ramirez et al., 2004; Unger et al., 2000). Acculturation is the developmental process by which an individual adopts the practices, values, and beliefs of the dominant culture while either retaining or abandoning the practices (e.g., language, food preferences, choice of peers, media), values (e.g., familismo, collectivism), and beliefs of their culture of origin. Acculturation is defined and measured inconsistently across studies with Latino adolescents, making it difficult to draw conclusions on its role in health-related outcomes. For instance, much of the earlier literature on acculturation examined the process on a spectrum where the two cultures of the individual—the new and native cultures—are on opposite ends of this spectrum. This unidimensional model classifies adolescents in the United States as "more acculturated" if they adopt the practices, values, and identity of the U.S. culture while abandoning the practices, values, and identity of the culture of origin. Alternatively, adolescents are classified as "less acculturated" if they retain the practices, values, and identity of their culture of origin and abandon the practices, values, and identity of the U.S. culture. Studies using this unidimensional scale demonstrate that Latinos classified as "more acculturated" have higher rates of AOD use than their "less acculturated" counterparts (Caetano & Raspberry, 2000; Caetano, Schafer, Clark, Cunradi, & Raspberry, 2000). Such findings have been consistently documented across a variety of Latino samples including migrant farmworkers in California (Lovato et al., 1994), Mexican American women (Gilbert, 1987), adolescents in New York City (Epstein, Botvin, Dusenbury, Diaz, & Kerner, 1996), and school-age children (Zapata & Katims, 1994).

The main problem with this unidimensional approach is that it prohibits an adolescent from being acculturated to both the U.S. culture and the culture of origin simultaneously, or being bicultural. According to Berry (1980), adoption of a new culture and retention of the culture of origin represent separate processes. Within this framework, acculturation is presented and measured as a bidimensional process—that is, Latino immigrant adolescents are faced with four options when arriving to the United States: (1) *assimilation*—identify with U.S. culture, (2) *separation*—retain and identify with the culture of origin, (3) *biculturalism*—identify with both cultures, or (4) *marginalization*—identify with neither culture. Therefore, within this framework, acculturation is defined as a bidimensional process whereby adolescents acquire the practices, values, and identity associated with the U.S. culture while also having the option to maintain the practices, values, and identity associated with the culture of origin (Schwartz et al., 2010). When acculturation is measured on a bidimensional scale, results demonstrate that retaining the practices, values, and identity of the culture of origin is associated with decreased risk for AOD use (De La Rosa, 2002; McQueen, Getz, & Bray, 2003; Schwartz et al., 2011). And while the effects of adopting the practices, values, and identity of the U.S. culture are less understood, studies demonstrate that bicultural adolescents—those who retain and identify with their culture of origin while also adopting and identifying with the U.S. culture—tend to be the least at risk for AOD use (Carvajal, Hanson, Romero, & Coyle, 2002; Nguyen & Benet-Martinez, 2013).

Despite these definitional challenges on acculturation, the literature on Latino youth suggests that increased acculturation to U.S. culture is associated with worsening behavior across a wide range of risk behaviors including AOD use. For instance, increased acculturation has been positively associated with AOD use when measured by English-language preference (Epstein et al., 1996; Nielsen & Ford, 2001; Zayas, Rojas, & Malgady, 1998), generational status (Ebin et al., 2001; Gil et al., 2000), and American-preferred media (Ramirez et al., 2004). For example, in studies where acculturation has been measured by language preferences when speaking with family and friends, Latino adolescents who primarily prefer speaking English are more likely to use AOD, while those who primarily speak Spanish are less likely to use (Epstein et al., 1996; Zayas et al., 1998). These studies highlight the protective role that maintaining an orientation toward Latino culture has on Latino adolescents' AOD use.

One model explaining the association between AOD use and acculturation was proposed by Szapocznik, Kurtines, and Hanna (1979). In their model, they identify acculturation gaps between adolescents and their parents as the primary pathways by which acculturation affects adolescents' AOD involvement. For example, by attending school in the United States, Latino adolescents are more readily exposed to U.S. culture and are given opportunities to learn the English language and associate with peers who may expose them to U.S. media, behaviors, and ways of identifying themselves. Conversely, Latino parents may choose to live in ethnic enclaves that may facilitate the use of the Spanish language as well as allow them to maintain behaviors and ways of identifying themselves that are consistent with their culture of origin. As a result, parents may become dependent on their adolescents to help them communicate in English-speaking situations and help them navigate U.S. culture, thus disrupting traditional hierarchical patterns in Latino families (Driscoll, Briggs, Brindis, & Yankah, 2001). Consequently, acculturation gaps emerge between parents and adolescents (Szapocznik, Scopetta, Kurtines, & Amalde, 1978). These acculturation gaps have a negative impact on communication and monitoring, two variables known to be protective against adolescent AOD use (Barnes & Farrell, 1992; Chilcoat & Anthony, 1996; Crosby & Miller, 2002; Ellickson & Morton, 1999; Peterson, Hawkins, Abbott, & Catalano, 1994; Small & Luster, 1994). Further, these acculturation gaps between parents and adolescents tend to undermine the influence of culture-specific protective factors such as *respeto,* the need to maintain respectful hierarchical relationships in Latino families (Raffaelli & Ontai, 2001), and familismo, the emphasis on the family as the primary source of one's social support and identity. These findings point to the important role that family plays in both protecting adolescents from AOD use as well as in buffering the harmful effects acculturation may have on adolescents' initiation of AOD use behaviors.

Familismo

In Latino cultures, familismo has been identified as a uniquely defining trait (Chandler, Tsai, & Wharton, 1999; Warner et al., 2006) and as a protective cultural value for Latinos (German, Gonzales, & Dumka, 2009; Romero & Ruiz, 2007). Familismo is a multidimensional construct that includes attitudinal components that reflect values and expectations for family relationships as well as behavioral components that reflect actual patterns of family interaction and resource exchange (Lugo Steidel & Contreras, 2003). These values and behaviors include the propensity to live in close proximity to the family (Romero & Ruiz, 2007), the use of family networks as sources of emotional and instrumental social support (German et al., 2009; Lugo Steidel & Contreras, 2003), positive interpersonal relationships within the family, high family unity and contact, and interdependence among nuclear and extended family members, as well as submission to a familial collective form of decision making (German et al., 2009; Gil et al., 2000; Romero & Ruiz, 2007; Smith-Morris, Morales-Campos, Alvarez, & Turner, 2013). Even though scholars may argue that the importance of family can be seen in many cultures (e.g., Schwartz, 2007), familismo in the Latino culture is particularly distinct as it encompasses having very close relations with family members throughout one's lifespan, which includes loyalty and solidarity (Marin & Gamba, 2003; Ramirez et al., 2004). Finch and Vega (2003) also note that for many Latinos, family is recognized primarily as a source of inspiration, strength, and support against threats that jeopardize health, status, and honor for the family.

In studies of culturally specific risk and protective factors, familismo and greater respeto (youth respect for their parents and elders) have been found to predict a lower disposition toward deviance and alcohol use in Latino adolescents living in the United States (Gil et al., 2000). Familismo has been associated with better health and fewer externalizing behavioral problems (e.g., lower rates of drug use, risky sexual behaviors, and delinquency) in Latino youth (Guilamo-Ramos, Bouris, Jaccard, Lesesne, & Ballan, 2009; Guilamo-Ramos, Bouris, Jaccard, Lesesne, Gonzalez, et al., 2009; Romero & Ruiz, 2007), as well as has been identified as a core protective factor that buffers against the effects of acculturation stress (Marsiglia, Kulis, Rodriguez, Becerra, & Castillo, 2009). Given these findings, it is not surprising that AOD use increases when acculturation erodes traditional family values, including respeto, family support, and family pride (Vega & Gil, 1999).

The central and protective role that the family plays among Latinos indicates that familismo is an important construct that must be considered when developing interventions for Latino adolescents. The knowledge base on familismo indicates that families are the ideal unit of intervention for Latinos. In situations in which acculturation gaps exist between parents and their acculturating adolescents, it is important that interventions address these gaps by fostering improved communication. Further, given that as adolescents acculturate, they adopt a new language and new ways of defining themselves, as well as new peers and new behaviors, it is important that parents are educated on the various cultural perspectives that may evolve within the adolescents. To date, only a few AOD use interventions addressing acculturation and including family components have been designed or adapted specifically for Latino adolescents. Building on our brief etiologic overview and discussion of acculturation and familismo, we next review the empirical literature on AOD use intervention development and treatment outcomes among Latino adolescents.

AOD USE INTERVENTIONS
FOR LATINO ADOLESCENTS

Several researchers have noted that treatment and intervention research falls behind in developing, adapting, and testing novel approaches with diverse populations (Bernal, 2006; Institute of Medicine, 2006; Vega et al., 2007). This is particularly true for AOD use treatment for Latino youth. Although extensive evidence documents the efficacy of interventions for children and adolescents, few clinical trials have included sufficient numbers of ethnic/racial-minority children to permit generalization across cultures (Chambless et al., 1996; Miranda, 1996; Miranda, Azocar, Organista, Munoz, & Lieberman, 1996). For instance, Szapocznik, Lopez, Prado, Schwartz, and Pantin (2006) conducted a review of empirically supported behavioral and pharmacological treatments for substance use between the years of 1972 and 2005 that contained a sample where at least 15% of the adolescents were Latino. In their review, six treatment studies were identified, but only three reported efficacy results specifically on Latino youth. Further, only one of these substance use treatments was specifically developed for Latino adolescents—brief strategic family therapy (BSFT; Szapocznik & Williams, 2000)—which is discussed below.

In a more recent review, Bandy and Moore (2011) evaluated findings from 33 randomized clinical trials that specifically targeted Latino youth or that contained a significant proportion of Latino youth in their sample. Overall, nine of the 33 programs reviewed targeted substance use among Latino youth. Of these nine, six had positive outcomes on at least one indicator of substance use at follow-up, while the remaining three had either mixed findings or produced no positive outcomes. Of the programs with positive outcomes, two were AOD use *intervention* programs, and the others were *prevention* programs designed for younger adolescents. Overall, programs that were culturally congruent with the target population, targeted the family, and included Spanish-speaking facilitators had the greatest effect on Latino adolescents' health outcomes (Bandy & Moore, 2011).

One intervention developed to align with Latinos' cultural value of family centrality is BSFT. BSFT was originally developed to address acculturation gaps between Cuban adolescents and their parents living in Miami (Szapocznik, Scopetta, & King, 1978) by restoring parents' leadership roles and improving the quality and effectiveness of parenting, improving family conflict resolution skills, and correcting parental over- and underinvolvement with the adolescent in 12–15 sessions (Szapocznik et al., 2006). In a clinical trial comparing BSFT with a group control condition, Latino adolescents in the BSFT condition demonstrated significant reductions in marijuana use and other conduct problems (Santisteban et al., 2003). Further, baseline family functioning moderated these treatment outcomes, such that those randomized to BSFT and with healthy family functioning at baseline maintained their healthy family functioning, and those with poor family functioning significantly improved their family functioning at follow-up. Realizing that they were unable to engage some families in treatment, Szapocznik, Kurtines, Foote, Perez-Vidal, and Hervis (1983, 1986) developed a one-on-one adaptation of BSFT. Although only the adolescent participates in this intervention, sessions focused on the family system and on the adolescent's role in this system. This one-person version of BSFT proved to be as efficacious as the standard conjoint BSFT, as adolescents in each condition demonstrated reductions in behavior problems and drug use (Szapocznik et al., 1983, 1986). This finding demonstrates that interventions that address family communication, even if done individually with the adolescent, can also be beneficial.

Although originally developed for Latinos, BSFT also has been applied to African American and non-Latino white adolescents (Robbins et al., 2011). However, outcomes seemed to be reached through different mediational pathways for different ethnic groups. Whereas BSFT seems to work by reducing associations with antisocial peers among African Americans, its success with Latinos may be more due to improving family functioning. These findings once again highlight the importance of addressing family factors among Latinos.

More recently, Burrow-Sanchez, Minami, and Hops (2015) compared a culturally accommodated group-based cognitive-behavioral therapy (CBT) intervention for substance use to its standard nonaccommodated CBT counterpart in 70 Latino juvenile justice-involved youth who met criteria for alcohol or drug abuse or dependence. The culturally accommodated CBT protocol addressed adolescents' ethnic identity as well as acculturation and acculturative stress. This protocol was also modified to include a preintervention *family introduction meeting* as well as regular phone and e-mail communication between the therapist and parents. Results demonstrated that Latino adolescents responded positively to both a standard and culturally accommodated CBT protocol by demonstrating decreases in number of use days at post and 3-month follow-ups regardless of treatment condition.

However, examination of cultural moderators of treatment outcomes showed that Latino adolescents with low commitment and exploration of their ethnic identity responded best to the standard condition, whereas Latino adolescents with higher commitment and exploration of their ethnic identity responded best to the accommodated condition. Similarly, adolescents whose parents indicated lower familismo responded best to the standard condition, whereas those whose parents indicated higher familismo responded best to the accommodated condition. Burrow-Sanchez et al. (2015) concluded that subgroups of Latino adolescents may experience better outcomes when interventions are congruent with their cultural values. They recommend the inclusion of measures of cultural characteristics, such as ethnic identity, acculturation, and individualistic versus collectivistic orientation in baseline assessments to be considered during treatment.

Taken together, these results highlight the positive effects interventions can have on Latino youth's AOD use outcomes when interventions are congruent with their cultural values and beliefs. However, the small number of interventions reviewed also highlights that this area of research is still in its infancy and that the pace of intervention research has not kept up with the rapid growth of the Latino population in the United States (Szapocznik et al., 2006). Findings from the studies reviewed along with the conceptual models and empirical evidence demonstrating the importance of family within Latino culture indicate that the family should be an important target for intervention-related change. However, this discussion also highlights the heterogeneity that exists within Latino subgroups and underscores the importance of assessing for important cultural characteristics that can be addressed during intervention delivery (Burrow-Sanchez et al., 2015). Indeed, it may be beneficial to assess the level of acculturation of adolescents and their parents as well as their orientation toward traditional Latino values such as familismo and respeto to provide therapists with guidance on personalized approaches to use during intervention sessions. However, developing AOD interventions and treatments that work is necessary but not sufficient, particularly if treatments are not made readily accessible to Latino communities. Given that Latinos tend to underutilize treatment services and experience multiple barriers to accessing such services, effective treatment protocols that also identify and address practical and attitudinal barriers to treatment services need to be developed.

MEETING THE SUBSTANCE USE TREATMENT NEEDS OF LATINO YOUTH THROUGH BRIEF INTERVENTIONS

Ethnic and racial disparities in the utilization of treatment services have been consistently documented (Delgado, Alegria, & Canive, 2006; Institute of Medicine, 2006; Marin, Escobar, & Vega, 2006; U.S. Department of

Health and Human Services, 2001). Inability to meet the needs of Latinos and the cultural incongruency between Latinos and available treatments may be contributing to the underutilization of such services and to the high dropout rates that exist. The surgeon general noted, "The culture of racial and ethnic minorities alter the types of mental health services they need. Clinical environments that do not respect, or are incompatible with the cultures of the people they serve, may deter minorities from using services and receiving appropriate care" (U.S. Department of Health Services, 2001, p. 8). Latino youth are much less likely to receive mental health services than white youth, despite rates of mental health problems being as high as or higher than other ethnic groups (Kataoka, Zhang, & Wells, 2002; McCabe et al., 1999; U.S. Department of Health and Human Services, 2001). For instance, combined data from 2003 to 2011 from the National Survey on Drug Use and Health (Substance Abuse and Mental Health Services Administration, 2013) indicate that Latinos were more likely than non-Latinos to have needed treatment for illicit drug or alcohol use in the past year. Further, among those who were ages 12 and older and in need of treatment, Latinos were less likely to have received substance use treatment. Other studies indicate that when Latino families do enter therapy, they are more likely to drop out of therapy prematurely than families from other ethnic groups (Huey, 1998). Studies have shown that multiple factors may be contributing to this underutilization of mental health services, but they also suggest the need for these services to be modified to be more culturally responsive to Latino youth and their families (Miranda, 1996; Vega et al., 2007).

Practical and Attitudinal Barriers

Underutilization of mental health services may be in part due to the multiple barriers to treatment services that Latinos tend to experience. For instance, a large number of Latino clients have limited English proficiency, and there is a lack of providers who have appropriate language skills. In fact, 30% of Latinos nationally report difficulty in communicating with their health care providers (Vega et al., 2007). Additional practical barriers include lack of transportation, child care, cultural differences between health care staff and the family, and lengthy waiting times (Flores, Abreu, Olivar, & Kastner, 1998). Given these barriers, some have recommended that programs designed for Latino populations contain explicit protocols for identifying and addressing these practical barriers that may discourage individuals from participating and engaging in programs (McCabe et al., 1999).

Research also clearly demonstrates that cultural and attitudinal barriers play a role in treatment underutilization. In a qualitative study, McCabe (2002) asked Latino families why they were less likely to bring their children in for therapy than other racial/ethnic groups. Parents reported the strong stigma associated with mental health treatments, lack of knowledge about where to find treatment, lack of information about what treatments are and how they work, tendency to "keep problems within the family," and embarrassment as reasons for not seeking treatment. In another study with 372 Latino families, 64% of families reported not seeking treatment because of concerns about what might happen in treatment and 45% reported concerns about the effectiveness of the services or about the characteristics of the providers not meeting their needs (Yeh, McCabe, Hough, Dupuis, & Hazen, 2003).

For substance abuse treatments to be successful, researchers and clinicians need to be cognizant of both the practical and attitudinal barriers experienced by Latinos. Procedures, techniques, and methods used during recruitment as well as the treatment process need to align with Latino cultural values. Further, protocols that specifically (1) address language barriers by not only hiring Spanish-speaking facilitators but also ensuring that all materials are carefully translated into Spanish, (2) take transportation and access barriers into consideration by taking interventions into the communities of the people they serve, and (3) provide regular cultural competency training and supervision for staff, have the potential to increase accessibility for Latino youth in need of AOD use intervention. Further, explicit protocols are also needed to assess individuals' attitudes toward treatment so that misconceptions can be addressed at the outset of treatment. Spending time with adolescents and their parents to address culturally based stigmas regarding substance treatment; to answer any questions, doubts, or misconceptions they may have; and to educate them on the process of therapy prior to commencing an intervention may be beneficial. Further, given the collectivistic values often seen in Latino families, it would be beneficial for therapists to foster strong interpersonal connections with their Latino clients (Szapocznik, Schwartz, Muir, & Brown, 2012).

Addressing Barriers through Brief Interventions

Brief interventions can be described as targeted, time-limited, and low-threshold services that aim to reduce substance use and its associated risks, as well as prevent progression to more severe levels of use (Babor et al., 2007). Brief interventions may be particularly suitable for Latino populations given their high rates of treatment underutilization, their high dropout rates, and the multiple practical and cultural barriers they experience when accessing substance use services. Further, engaging parents in programs targeting substance use remains a significant obstacle to the implementation of successful intervention programs (Spoth, Kavanagh, & Dishion, 2002). Research has shown that parent treatment groups usually suffer from low attendance rates and low participant retention rates (Goodman, 2002). In addition to the practical and attitudinal barriers already mentioned, low attendance rates can also be the result of parents' busy work schedules, their adolescents' extracurricular activity schedules, and can be related to lack of motivation from both the parents and adolescents. For families whose teens are in earlier stages of substance use and perhaps not seeking intensive treatment programs, brief interventions may not only be most appropriate but also more likely to engage families experiencing multiple barriers to treatment seeking.

While the literature on brief interventions with AOD-using Latino adolescents is quite scarce, brief motivational interventions have proven to be efficacious with ethnic/racial-minority populations (Hettema, Steele, & Miller, 2005; Lee et al., 2013), including Latino adolescents (Clair et al., 2013). Motivational interventions may be suitable for ethnic/racial-minority adolescents for several reasons. First, the idiographic perspective in motivational interventions offers individualized plans that are sensitive to what the adolescent defines as his or her culture and considers the adolescent's personal experience. Second, adolescents who may perceive discrimination from others and experience cultural mistrust may respond well to the self-guided techniques used in motivational interventions rather than directed interventions. Third, motivational interventions' emphasis on a collaborative relationship may help Latino teens think of counseling as more of a collaborative work experience that further alleviates the stigma attached to counseling and decreases reluctance to engage in counseling by reducing adolescents' views of counselors as authority figures.

One such intervention is guided self-change (GSC; Sobell & Sobell, 1998), a brief, behaviorally oriented motivational intervention designed for use with individuals with AOD problems. Over the last decade, GSC treatments underwent several modifications to make them both developmentally and culturally appropriate for work with adolescents of diverse backgrounds, and to generalize its behavioral and motivational strategies to co-occurring problem behaviors, such as AOD use, interpersonal violence, and HIV risk behaviors (Tubman, Wagner, Gil, & Pate, 2002). One study examining the efficacy of GSC among African American and Latino juvenile offenders modified treatment materials to be available in both English and Spanish as well as hired program staff that was multiethnic, multilingual, and representative of the adolescent population participating in the program (Gil, Wagner, & Tubman, 2004). Additionally, the program established clinics in specific neighborhoods to address practical barriers to treatment as well as allowed the inclusion of family members and used a "flexible" definition of family, so that extended family members would also be welcomed and included. Results demonstrated that adolescents reporting greater cultural mistrust (mistrust of others from a different ethnic/racial background) at baseline responded the least to the GSC intervention with lower reductions in alcohol and marijuana use days at follow-up, while those with greater Latino ethnic pride and ethnic orientation responded the best to the GSC intervention by demonstrating greater reductions in alcohol and marijuana use at follow-up (Gil et al., 2004). Another study (Wagner, Hospital, Graziano, Morris, & Gil, 2015) examined the efficacy of a school-based GSC protocol with a predominately Latino sample of 514 high school students. When compared with a standard care condition, GSC participants demonstrated significant reductions in total number of alcohol and drug use days at post and 3-month follow-ups.

Both of the studies reviewed above delivered a brief motivational intervention within community settings. When brief interventions are delivered within the communities of the populations they target, they offer greater access to care and greater ecological validity than more traditional approaches (Evans, 1999; Wagner, Tubman, & Gil, 2004; Waxman, Weist, & Benson, 1999). It is therefore important to provide services that are easily accessible for youth, especially when one considers the practical and cultural barriers Latino youth and their families experience in accessing substance use services. Community-based intervention models offer the advantage of delivering treatment directly to those who need it (Cowen, 1978), and circumvent many of the barriers to service access (Wagner et al., 2004). For Latino adolescents specifically, school-based models may be developmentally and culturally appropriate given that services are being provided in a high-impact social environment for shaping the development and adaptation of youth (Cowen, 1978), and represent one of the main social contexts contributing to the acculturation process (Nieri, 2012). Therefore, the development and implementation of community-based brief interventions is one potential approach for bridging the gaps that exist between Latino adolescents in need of substance use treatment and the actual treatment services.

CASE EXAMPLE

Below we present a case example that highlights the benefit of including assessments of cultural characteristics—such as ethnic identity, acculturation, and familismo—when tailoring an intervention to the specific needs and cultural background of a family. Attention to adolescent and family responses on such cultural measures will provide the counselor with information on what topics may be most beneficial to focus on while providing a culturally specific intervention.

The Martinez family is referred for counseling after their 15-year-old son, Jorge, is caught by school personnel smoking marijuana on school premises. At the first session, the counselor provides a brief introduction and focuses on building rapport with the family. This includes addressing cultural stigmas associated with counseling by exploring and discussing their personal attitudes and expectations regarding counseling, explaining the process and rationale for counseling, and making sure the family understands their collaborative role during the counseling process. Following this introduction, the counselor administers an assessment for the adolescent and parents to complete that contains measures of cultural factors (e.g., acculturation conflict and stress, ethnic identity) as well as measures of parenting practices (e.g., communication, supervision and monitoring, relationship quality) and adolescent factors (e.g., use patterns, peers).

While preparing for their second visit, the counselor notices that Jorge reports recently having started experimenting with marijuana. He also reports that his parents have never spoken to him about drugs. Seeing that Jorge and his parents have never had a discussion on drugs, the counselor looks at Jorge's and his parents' results on the acculturation measures and notices a discrepancy. The counselor also recalls Jorge speaking in English during their first session despite his parents only speaking Spanish. Jorge also reports experiencing conflict and frustration because his parents don't understand the "American" way of doing things. Despite this, he notes that Jorge ranked his family as being of utmost importance when asked about the things he values.

Based on this information, the counselor considers that the lack of substance-related communication may be due in part to an acculturation gap between Jorge and his parents. The counselor decides to have an individual session with Jorge's parents and focuses this session on psychoeducation. He believes that Jorge's parents may not have initiated a conversation with Jorge regarding drugs because they are not knowledgeable on the topic and feel that Jorge might know more about the topic than they do. Therefore, the counselor prepares information on alcohol and drugs, particularly within the context of the United States (terms used to refer to specific drugs, ways drugs are used, how they are accessed, etc.) to discuss with Jorge's parents and prepares to engage them in role-playing sessions focused on communicating drug-related expectations and limits. He also plans to address specific parenting practices, including family communication and supervision and monitoring. Given that Jorge's parents demonstrated strengths in their current parenting practices, the counselor considers that Jorge's parents may feel like they have less control over Jorge's life since arriving in the United States. Therefore, the counselor decides to focus on improving their parenting self-efficacy while capitalizing on their already strong parenting practices.

Given the acculturation gap between Jorge and his parents, the counselor decides to initiate his work with Jorge via an individual brief motivational intervention. However, given that Jorge endorsed a strong familisitic orientation during his assessment, the counselor enhances the family components in each of the motivational intervention exercises. For instance, during the decisional balance exercise, he probes Jorge on specific family situations (e.g., cons to using drugs: I will let my family down, I will cause shame to my family, I cannot fulfill my family responsibilities). He also engages Jorge in a discussion on ethnic identity, after noting that Jorge demonstrated cultural pride particularly as it pertains to foods, music, and sports specific to his cultural background. He engages Jorge in a discussion on how drug use fits within his self-definition as a bicultural individual. Finally, in a future goals exercise, the counselor asks Jorge to consider the role drug use may play in achieving his goals, particularly those pertaining to his family (e.g., being the first in his family to obtain a college education, supporting and providing for his family).

Through the use of cultural measures as well as general parenting measures, the counselor was able to obtain information that allowed him to tailor his intervention approach to the culturally specific needs of the Martinez family. Given that familismo is an integral part of the Latino culture, the counselor chose a family-based approach as his primary counseling intervention. Further, he recognized current strengths within the family and focused on improving parenting self-efficacy, which may be particularly useful for immigrant families, where parents may feel they have less control over the lives of their adolescents since arriving in the United States. Finally, it is important to note that literature demonstrates that some Latino parents do not engage in active communication about health-related behaviors with their adolescents due to a lack of knowledge regarding the specific health behavior as well as a lack of self-efficacy in discussing such topics with their adolescents (Mena, Dillon, Mason, & Santisteban, 2008; Umpierre et al., 2015). Therefore, combining this knowledge with information derived from the cultural assessments, the counselor was able to provide helpful psychoeducational information/feedback to Jorge's parents and develop a culturally specific treatment plan to address Jorge's marijuana use.

CONCLUSIONS AND IMPLICATIONS
FOR CLINICAL RESEARCH AND PRACTICE

The high prevalence of AOD use among Latino youth is of particular concern given recent demographic trends. Despite these high prevalence rates, AOD use treatment development and research lags behind. Knowledge on whether empirically supported treatments are effective in reducing AOD use in Latino youth or whether they need to be adapted is lacking given the low ethnic/racial-minority representation in randomized clinical trial studies. Even when studies do include a reasonable number of Latinos in their sample allowing for examination of differential response, outcome data are not provided separately for this group. Further, cultural factors such as acculturation, acculturation gaps, familismo, and respeto play a significant role in Latino youth's substance use. Including these factors in interventions targeted for Latinos may increase cultural sensitivity of existing treatments as well as treatment efficacy. Because Latinos tend to underutilize treatment services and experience multiple barriers to such services, protocols that identify and address practical and attitudinal barriers to treatment services must be developed.

The literature reviewed on existing AOD use interventions, while sparse, highlights the potential benefits of interventions that are both culturally responsive *and* engage the participation of family members in addressing AOD use and related negative consequences in young Latinos. Specifically, interventions are more likely to address the specific needs of Latino youth by:

1. Assessing acculturation, potential acculturation gaps between parents and adolescents, and cultural orientation to capture the heterogeneity among Latino subgroups and generate information that may offer guidance on what therapeutic approaches may offer the best "fit" for any given family.
2. Working with parents and adolescents to restore the protective factors of familismo and respeto by improving communication, particularly in situations where acculturation gaps exist.
3. Strengthening parenting practices (increasing monitoring and supervision) and parenting self-efficacy among Latino parents, who may feel they have lost control over the lives of their adolescents since arriving in the United States.
4. Educating parents on the various cultural perspectives their adolescents may be identifying with so that they understand and offer their adolescents culture-specific guidance.
5. Increasing access for Latino families by taking linguistically competent interventions out into the communities where they live or socialize in.
6. Including explicit protocols for addressing culturally based attitudinal stigmas and misconceptions regarding the therapy and the treatment process.
7. Stressing the importance of interpersonal connections with families, not only during the treatment process but also during recruitment and follow-up methods.

Finally, given the heterogeneity among Latino subgroups, it is important that counselors working with Latino families adopt a flexible approach that can be adjusted to meet the specific needs of any given client. Further, it is equally as important to keep in mind that Latino families bring with them significant strengths when coping with problems in the family, such as adolescent AOD abuse and related consequences. Therefore, when looking at the differences between values and attitudes of the Latino culture and the culture of the United States, it is important not to evaluate these differences as deficits within the Latino family. In fact, the literature reviewed in this chapter highlights protective factors that cultural values such as familismo and respeto play in adolescents' AOD use trajectories. Careful examination of the specific strengths any given Latino family may possess and developing treatment plans and interventions capitalizing on these specific strengths offers the opportunity for clinical research and practice to develop interventions that are both culturally sensitive and promote healthy development in Latino youth.

REFERENCES

Babor, T. F., McRee, B. G., Kassebaum, P. A., Grimaldi, P. L., Ahmed, K., & Bray, J. (2007). Screening, Brief Intervention, and Referral to Treatment (SBIRT): Toward a public health approach to the management of substance abuse. *Substance Abuse* 28(3), 7–30.

Bandy, T., & Moore, K. A. (2011). What works for Latino/Hispanic children and adolescents: Lessons from experimental evaluations of programs and interventions. ChildTrends Fact Sheet. Retrieved from *www.childtrends.org.*

Barnes, G. M., & Farrell, M. P. (1992). Parental support and control as predictors of adolescent drinking, delinquency, and related problem behaviors. *Journal of Marriage and the Family, 54*(4), 763–776.

Bernal, G. (2006). Intervention development and cultural adaptation research with diverse families. *Family Process, 45,* 143–151.

Berry, J. W. (1980). Acculturation as varieties of adaptation. In A. Padilla (Ed.), *Acculturation: Theory, models and findings* (pp. 9–25). Boulder, CO: Westview.

Burrow-Sanchez, J. J., Minami, T., & Hops, H. (2015). Cultural accommodation of group substance abuse treatment for Latino adolescents: Results of an RCT. *Cultural Diversity and Ethnic Minority Psychology, 21*(4), 571–583.

Caetano, R., & Raspberry, K. (2000). Drinking and DSM-IV alcohol and drug dependence among white and Mexican-American DUI offenders. *Journal of Studies on Alcohol, 61*(3), 420–426.

Caetano, R., Schafer, J., Clark, C. L., Cunradi, C. B., & Raspberry, K. (2000). Intimate partner violence, acculturation and alcohol consumption among Hispanic couples in the United States. *Journal of Interpersonal Violence, 15*(1), 30–45.

Carvajal, S. C., Hanson, C. E., Romero, A. J., & Coyle, K. K. (2002). Behavioural risk factors and protective factors in adolescents: A comparison of Latinos and non-Latino whites. *Ethnicity and Health, 7,* 181–193.

Chambless, D. L., Sanderson, W. C., Shoham, V., Johnson, S. B., Pope, K. S., & Crits-Christoph, P. (1996). An update on empirically validated therapies. *Clinical Psychologist, 49,* 5–18.

Chandler, C. R., Tsai, Y. M., & Wharton, R. (1999). Twenty years after: Replicating a study of Anglo- and Mexican-American cultural values. *Social Science Journal, 36*(2), 353–367.

Chilcoat, H. D., & Anthony, J. C. (1996). Impact of parent monitoring on initiation of drug use through late childhood. *Journal of the American Academy of Child and Adolescent Psychiatry, 35*(1), 91–100.

Clair, M., Stein, L. A., Soenksen, S., Martin, R. A., Lebeau, R., & Golembeske, C. (2013). Ethnicity as a moderator of motivational interviewing for incarcerated adolescents after release. *Journal of Substance Abuse Treatment, 45*(4), 370–375.

Colby, S. L., & Ortman, J. M. (2015). Projections of the size and composition of the U.S. population: 2014 to 2060, Current Population Reports. Retrieved from *www.census.gov/content/dam/Census/library/publications/2015/demo/p25-1143.pdf?.*

Cowen, E. L. (1978). Some problems in community program evaluation research. *Journal of Consulting and Clinical Psychology, 46*(4), 792–805.

Crosby, R. A., & Miller, K. S. (2002). Family influences on adolescent females' sexual health. In G. M. Wingood & R. J. DiClemente (Eds.), *Handbook of women's sexual and reproductive health* (pp. 113–127). New York: Kluwer Academic/Plenum.

Dawson, D. A., Goldstein, R. B., Chou, S. P., Ruan, W. J., & Grant, B. F. (2008). Age at first drink and the first incidence of adult-onset DSM-IV alcohol use disorders. *Alcoholism: Clinical and Experimental Research, 32*(12), 2149–2160.

De La Rosa, M. (2002). Acculturation and Latino adolescents' substance use: A research agenda for the future. *Substance Use and Misuse, 37*(4), 429–456.

Delgado, P., Alegria, M., & Canive, J. (2006). Depression and access to treatment among US Hispanics: A review of the literature and policy recommendations for future research. *Focus, 4*, 38–47.

DeWit, D. J., Adlaf, E. M., Offord, D. R., & Ogborne, A. C. (2000). Age at first alcohol use: A risk factor for the development of alcohol disorders. *American Journal of Psychiatry, 157*(5), 745–750.

Driscoll, A. K., Briggs, M. A., Brindis, C. D., & Yankah, E. (2001). Adolescent Latino reproductive health: A review of the literature. *Hispanic Journal of Behavioral Sciences, 23*(3), 255–326.

Ebin, V. J., Sneed, C. D., Morisky, D. E., Rotheram-Borus, M. J., Magnusson, A. M., & Malotte, C. K. (2001). Acculturation and interrelationships between problem and health-promoting behaviors among Latino adolescents. *Journal of Adolescent Health, 28*(1), 62–72.

Ellickson, P. L., & Morton, S. C. (1999). Identifying adolescents at risk for hard drug use: Racial/ethnic variations. *Journal of Adolescent Health, 25*(6), 382–395.

Epstein, J. A., Botvin, G. J., Dusenbury, L., Diaz, T., & Kerner, J. (1996). Validation of an acculturation measure for Hispanic adolescents. *Psychological Reports, 79*(3), 1075–1079.

Evans, S. W. (1999). Mental health services in schools: Utilization, effectiveness, and consent. *Clinical Psychology Review, 19*(2), 165–178.

Finch, B. K., & Vega, W. A. (2003). Acculturation stress, social support, and self-rated health among Latinos in California. *Journal of Immigrant Health, 5*(3), 109–117.

Flores, G., Abreu, M., Olivar, M. A., & Kastner, B. (1998). Access barriers to health care for Latino children. *Archives of Pediatric Adolescent Medicine, 152*(11), 1119–1125.

German, M., Gonzales, N. A., & Dumka, L. (2009). Familism values as a protective factor for Mexican-origin adolescents exposed to deviant peers. *Journal of Early Adolescence, 29*(1), 16–42.

Gil, A. G., Wagner, E. F., & Tubman, J. G. (2004). Culturally sensitive substance abuse intervention for Hispanic and African American adolescents: Empirical examples from the Alcohol Treatment Targeting Adolescents in Need (ATTAIN) project. *Addiction, 99*(Suppl. 2), 140–150.

Gil, A. G., Wagner, E. F., & Vega, W. A. (2000). Acculturation familism, and alcohol use among Latino adolescent males: Longitudinal relations. *Journal of Community Psychology, 28*(4), 443–458.

Gilbert, M. J. (1987). Alcohol consumption patterns in immigrant and later generation Mexican American women. *Hispanic Journal of Behavioral Sciences, 9*, 299–313.

Goodman, M. R. (2002). If we build it will parents come?: Parent participation in preventative parenting groups. Retrieved from *http://search.ebscohost.com/login. aspx?direct=true&db=psyh&AN=2002–95023–061&site=ehost-live Available from EBSCOhost psyh database.*

Guilamo-Ramos, V., Bouris, A., Jaccard, J., Lesesne, C., & Ballan, M. (2009). Familial and cultural influences on sexual risk behaviors among Mexican, Puerto Rican, and Dominican youth. *AIDS Education and Prevention, 21*(5), 61–79.

Guilamo-Ramos, V., Bouris, A., Jaccard, J., Lesesne, C. A., Gonzalez, B., & Kalogerogiannis, K. (2009). Family mediators of acculturation and adolescent sexual behavior among Latino youth. *Journal of Primary Prevention, 30*(3–4), 395–419.

Guttmannova, K., Bailey, J. A., Hill, K. G., Lee, J. O., Hawkins, J. D., Woods, M. L., et al. (2011). Sensitive periods for adolescent alcohol use initiation: Predicting the lifetime occurrence and chronicity of alcohol problems in adulthood. *Journal of Studies on Alcohol and Drugs, 72*(2), 221–231.

Hettema, J., Steele, J., & Miller, W. R. (2005). Motivational interviewing. *Annual Review of Clinical Psychology, 1,* 91–111.

Hingson, R. W., Heeren, T., & Winter, M. R. (2006). Age at drinking onset and alcohol dependence: Age at onset, duration, and severity. *Archives of Pediatric Adolescent Medicine, 160*(7), 739–746.

Huey, S. J. (1998). *Therapy termination among Black, Caucasian, and Latino children referred to community mental health clinics.* Unpublished dcotoral disertation, University of California, Los Angeles, CA.

Institute of Medicine. (2006). *Improving the quality of health care for mental and substance use conditions.* Washington, DC: National Academic Press.

Kataoka, S. H., Zhang, L., & Wells, K. B. (2002). Unmet need for mental health care among U.S. children: Variation by ethnicity and insurance status. *American Journal of Psychiatry, 159*(9), 1548–1555.

Kena, G., Aud, S., Johnson, F., Wang, X., Zhang, J., Rathbun, A., et al. (2014). The condition of education 2014. Retrieved from *http://nces.ed.gov/pubs2014/2014083.pdf.*

Lee, C. S., Lopez, S. R., Colby, S. M., Rohsenow, D., Hernandez, L., Borrelli, B., et al. (2013). Culturally adapted motivational interviewing for Latino heavy drinkers: Results from a randomized clinical trial. *Journal of Ethnicity in Substance Abuse, 12*(4), 356–373.

Lovato, C. Y., Litrownik, A. J., Elder, J., Nuñez-Liriano, A., Suarez, D., & Talavera, G. A. (1994). Cigarette and alcohol use among migrant Hispanic adolescents. *Family and Communication Health, 16,* 18–31.

Lugo Steidel, A. G., & Contreras, J. M. (2003). A new familism scale for use with Latino populations. *Hispanic Journal of Behavioral Sciences, 25,* 312–330.

Marin, G., Escobar, J., & Vega, W. A. (2006). Mental illness in American Hispanics: A review of the literature. *Focus, 4,* 23–37.

Marin, G., & Gamba, R. J. (2003). Acculturation and changes in cultural values. In K. M. Chun, P. B. Organista, & G. Marin (Eds.), *Acculturation: Advances in theory, measurement, and applied research* (pp. 83–93). Washington, DC: American Psychological Association.

Marsiglia, F. F., Kulis, S., Rodriguez, G. M., Becerra, D., & Castillo, J. (2009). Culturally specific youth substance abuse resistance skills: Applicability across the U.S.-Mexico border. *Reseach on Social Work Practice, 19*(2), 152–164.

Marsiglia, F. F., & Waller, M. (2002). Language preference and drug use among Southwestern Mexican American middle school students. *Child Schools, 25,* 145–158.

McCabe, K. M. (2002). Factors that predict premature termination among Mexican-American children in outpatient psychotherapy. *Journal of Child and Family Studies, 11,* 347–359.

McCabe, K. M., Yeh, M., Hough, R., Landsverk, J., Hurlburt, M., Culver, S., et al. (1999). Racial/ethnic representation across five public sectors of care for youth. *Journal of Emotional and Behavioral Disorders, 7,* 72–82.

McQueen, A., Getz, J. G., & Bray, J. H. (2003). Acculturation, substance use, and deviant behavior: Examining separation and family conflict as mediators. *Child Development, 74*(6), 1737–1750.

Mena, M. P., Dillon, F. R., Mason, C. A., & Santisteban, D. A. (2008). Communication about sexually-related topics among Hispanic substance-abusing adolescents and their parents. *Journal of Drug Issues, 38*(1), 215–234.

Miech, R. A., Johnston, L. D., O'Malley, P. M., Bachman, J. G., & Schulenberg, J. (2015). Monitoring the Future National Survey results on drug use, 1975–2014: Vol. I. Secondary school students. Retrieved from *http://monitoringthefuture.org/pubs.html-monographs.*

Miranda, J. (1996). Introduction to the special section on recruiting and retaining minorities in psychotherapy research. *Journal of Consulting and Clinical Psychology, 64*(5), 848–850.

Miranda, J., Azocar, F., Organista, K. C., Munoz, R. F., & Lieberman, A. (1996). Recruiting and retaining low-income Latinos in psychotherapy research. *Journal of Consulting and Clinical Psychology, 64*(5), 868–874.

Mulia, N., Ye, Y., Greenfield, T. K., & Zemore, S. E. (2009). Disparities in alcohol-related problems among white, black, and Hispanic Americans. *Alcoholism: Clinical and Experimental Research, 33*(4), 654–662.

Nguyen, A. M. D., & Benet-Martinez, V. (2013). Biculturalism and adjustment: A meta-analysis. *Journal of Cross-Cultural Psychology, 44,* 122–159.

Nielsen, A. L., & Ford, J. A. (2001). Drinking patterns among Hispanic adolescents: Results from a national household survey. *Journal of Studies on Alcohol, 62*(4), 448–456.

Nieri, T. (2012). School context and individual acculturation: How school composition affects Latino students' acculturation. *Sociological Inquiry, 82*(3), 460–484.

Pantin, H., Prado, G., Schwartz, S. J., & Sullivan, S. (2005). Methodological challenges in designing efficacious drug abuse and HIV preventive interventions for Hispanic adolescent subgroups. *Journal of Urban Health, 82*(2), 92–102.

Peterson, P. L., Hawkins, J. D., Abbott, R. D., & Catalano, R. F. (1994). Disentangling the effects of parental drinking, family management, and parental alcohol norms on current drinking by black and white adolescents. *Journal of Research on Adolescence, 4,* 203–227.

Raffaelli, M., & Ontai, L. L. (2001). She's 16 years old and there's boys calling over to the house: An exploratory study of sexual socialization in Latino families. *Culture, Health, and Sexuality, 3*(3), 295–310.

Ramirez, J. R., Crano, W. D., Quist, R., Burgoon, M., Alvaro, E. M., & Grandpre, J. (2004). Acculturation, familism, parental monitoring, and knowledge as predictors of marijuana and inhalant use in adolescents. *Psychology of Addictive Behavior, 18*(1), 3–11.

Rios-Bedoya, C. F., & Freile-Salinas, D. (2014). Incidence of alcohol use disorders among Hispanic subgrounds in the USA. *Alcohol and Alcoholism, 49,* 549–556.

Robbins, M. S., Feaster, D. J., Horigian, V. E., Rohrbaugh, M., Shoham, V., Bachrach, K., et al. (2011). Brief strategic family therapy versus treatment as usual: Results of a multisite randomized trial for substance using adolescents. *Journal of Consulting and Clinical Psychology, 79*(6), 713–727.

Romero, A. J., & Ruiz, M. (2007). Does familism lead to increased parental monitoring?: Protective factors for coping with risky behaviors. *Journal of Child and Family Studies, 16,* 143–154.

Santisteban, D. A., Coatsworth, J. D., Perez-Vidal, A., Kurtines, W. M., Schwartz, S. J., LaPerriere, A., et al. (2003). Efficacy of brief strategic family therapy in modifying Hispanic adolescent behavior problems and substance use. *Journal of Family Psychology, 17*(1), 121–133.

Schwartz, S. J. (2007). The applicability of familism to diverse ethnic groups: A preliminary study. *Journal of Social Psychology, 147*(2), 101–118.

Schwartz, S. J., Weisskirch, R. S., Zamboanga, B. L., Castillo, L. G., Ham, L. S., Huynh, Q. L., et al. (2011). Dimensions of acculturation: Assocations with health risk behaviors among college students from immigrant families. *Journal of Counseling Psychology, 58,* 27–41.

Small, S. A., & Luster, T. (1994). Adolescent sexual-activity: An ecological, risk-factor approach. *Journal of Marriage and the Family, 56*(1), 181–192.

Smith-Morris, C., Morales-Campos, D., Alvarez, A. C., & Turner, M. (2013). An anthropology of familismo: On narratives and description of Mexican immigrants. *Hispanic Journal of Behavioral Sciences, 35*(1), 35–60.

Sobell, M. B., & Sobell, L. C. (1998). Guided self-change treatment. In W. R. Miller & N. Heather (Eds.), *Treating addictive behaviors: Process of change.* New York: Plenum Press.

Spoth, R., Kavanagh, K., & Dishion, T. (2002). Family-centered preventive intervention science: Toward benefits to larger populations of children, youth, and families. *Prevention Science, 3*(3), 145–152.

Substance Abuse and Mental Health Services Administration. (2013). Results from the 2012 National Survey on Drug Use and Health: Summary of national findings. Retrieved from *www.samhsa.gov/data/sites/default/files/NSDUHmhfr2012/NSDUHmhfr2012.pdf.*

Szapocznik, J., Kurtines, W., & Hanna, N. (1979). Comparison of Cuban and Anglo-American cultural values in a clinical population. *Journal of Consulting and Clinical Psychology, 47*(3), 623–624.

Szapocznik, J., Kurtines, W. M., Foote, F. H., Perez-Vidal, A., & Hervis, O. (1983). Conjoint versus one-person family therapy: Some evidence for the effectiveness of conducting family therapy through one person. *Journal of Consulting and Clinical Psychology, 51*(6), 889–899.

Szapocznik, J., Kurtines, W. M., Foote, F., Perez-Vidal, A., & Hervis, O. (1986). Conjoint versus one-person family therapy: Further evidence for the effectiveness of conducting family therapy through one person with drug-abusing adolescents. *Journal of Consulting and Clinical Psychology, 54*(3), 395–397.

Szapocznik, J., Lopez, B., Prado, G., Schwartz, S. J., & Pantin, H. (2006). Outpatient drug abuse treatment for Hispanic adolescents. *Drug and Alcohol Dependence, 84*(1), S54–S63.

Szapocznik, J., Schwartz, S. J., Muir, J. A., & Brown, C. H. (2012). Brief strategic family therapy: An intervention to reduce adolescent risk behavior. *Couple and Family Psychology, 1*(2), 134–145.

Szapocznik, J., Scopetta, M. A., & King, O. E. (1978). Theory and practice in matching treatment to the special characteristics and problems of Cuban immigrants. *Journal of Community Psychology, 6*(2), 112–122.

Szapocznik, J., Scopetta, M. A., Kurtines, W., & Amalde, M. A. (1978). Theory and measurement of acculturation. *Interamerican Journal of Psychology, 12,* 113–130.

Szapocznik, J., & Williams, R. A. (2000). Brief strategic family therapy: Twenty-five years of interplay among theory, research and practice in adolescent behavior problems and drug abuse. *Clinical Child and Family Psychology Review, 3*(2), 117–134.

Tubman, J. G., Wagner, E. F., Gil, A. G., & Pate, K. N. (2002). Brief motivational intervention for substance-abusing delinquent adolescents: Guided self-change as a social work practice innovation. *Health and Social Work, 27*(3), 208–212.

Umpierre, M., Meyers, L. V., Ortiz, A., Paulino, A., Rodriguez, A. R., Miranda, A., et al. (2015). Understanding Latino parents' child mental health literacy: Todos a bordo/all aboard. *Research on Social Work Practice, 25*(5), 607–618.

Unger, J. B., Cruz, T. B., Rohrbach, L. A., Ribisl, K. M., Baezconde-Garbanati, L., Chen, X., et al. (2000). English language use as a risk factor for smoking initiation among Hispanic and Asian American adolescents: Evidence for mediation by tobacco-related beliefs and social norms. *Health Psychology, 19*(5), 403–410.

U.S. Department of Health and Human Services. (2001). *Mental health: Culture, race, and ethnicity—a supplement to mental health: A report of the surgeon general.* Rockville, MD: U.S. Department of Health and Human Services, Substance Abuse and Mental Health Services Administration, Center for Mental Health Services.

Vega, W. A., & Gil, A. (1999). A model for explaining drug use behavior among Hispanic adolescents. *Drugs and Society, 14,* 57–74.

Vega, W. A., Karno, M., Alegria, M., Alvidrez, J., Bernal, G., Escamilla, M., et al. (2007). Research issues for improving treatment of U.S. Hispanics with persistent mental disorders. *Psychiatric Services, 58*(3), 385–394.

Wagner, E. F., Hospital, M. M., Graziano, J. N., Morris, S. L., & Gil, A. (2015). A randomized controlled trial of guided self-change with minority adolescents. *Journal of Consulting and Clinical Psychology, 82*(6), 1128–1139.

Wagner, E. F., Tubman, J. G., & Gil, A. G. (2004). Implementing school-based substance abuse interventions: Methodological dilemmas and recommended solutions. *Addiction, 99*(2), 106–119.

Warner, L. A., Valdez, A., Vega, W. A., De La Rosa, M., Turner, R. J., & Canino, G. (2006). Hispanic drug abuse in an evolving cultural context: An agenda for research. *Drug and Alcohol Dependence, 84,* S8–S16.

Waxman, R. P., Weist, M. D., & Benson, D. M. (1999). Toward collaboration in the growing education-mental health interface. *Clinical Psychology Review, 19*(2), 239–253.

West, B. A., Naumann, R. B., & Centers for Disease Control and Prevention. (2011). Motor vehicle-related deaths: United States, 2003–2007. *MMWR Surveillance Summary, 60*(Suppl.), 52–55.

Yeh, M., McCabe, K., Hough, R. L., Dupuis, D., & Hazen, A. (2003). Racial/ethnic differences in parental endorsement of barriers to mental health services for youth. *Mental Health Services Research, 5*(2), 65–77.

Yoon, Y. H., Yi, H. Y., & Thomson, P. C. (2011). Alcohol-related and viral hepatitis C-related cirrhosis mortality among Hispanic subgroups in the United States, 2000–2004. *Alcohol Clinical and Experimental Research, 35*(2), 240–249.

Zapata, J. T., & Katims, D. S. (1994). Antecedents of substance use among Mexican American school-age children. *Journal of Drug Education, 24*(3), 233–251.

Zayas, L. H., Rojas, M., & Malgady, R. G. (1998). Alcohol and drug use, and depression among Hispanic men in early adulthood. *American Journal of Community Psychology, 26*(3), 425–438.

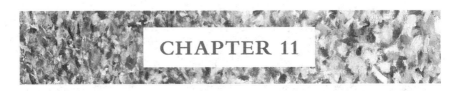

CHAPTER 11

Cultural Considerations and Recommendations for Implementing Brief Interventions with American Indian Adolescents

Nichea S. Spillane and Kamilla Venner

American Indians/Alaska Natives (AI/ANs) were the first inhabitants of North America. According to the last U.S. Census, there are approximately 2.9 million Americans who identified as solely AI/AN and another 2.3 million as both AI/AN and at least one other race that accounts for 1.7% of the U.S. population (Humes, Jones, & Ramirez, 2011). While the numbers of AI/ANs represent a small portion of the U.S. population, there is a tremendous amount of diversity within the AI/AN group. There are more than 560 AI/AN tribes and communities that are federally recognized (Humes et al., 2011). Twenty-two percent live on reservation lands or other trust lands and 60% of AI/ANs live in metropolitan areas, which is the lowest rate of metropolitan residence of any racial group (Humes et al., 2011).

Despite the large number of AI/ANs who abstain from alcohol and other drugs, negative consequences from substance use are among the most prevalent health concerns facing many AI communities today (Beauvais, 1996; Hawkins, Cummins, & Marlatt, 2004). Indeed, although alcohol use was not historically a part of the traditional AI way of life, alcohol and substance misuse now pose a significant public health problem (Spillane, Greenfield, Venner, & Kahler, 2015). AI/ANs face substance-related health disparities, including higher age-adjusted mortality rates attributable to alcohol use, chronic liver disease and cirrhosis, drug use, and lung cancer, compared with the United States "All Races" (U.S. Department of Health and Human Services, 2001). Alcohol is the leading contributor to increased mortality rates among AI/ANs compared to the U.S. population as a whole (U.S. Department of Health and Human Services, 2001). Rates of fetal alcohol syndrome (FAS) have been found to be as high as 9.0 per 1,000 live births in some AI communities in the Northern Plains, compared to a rate of 0.3 per 1,000 live births reported in a large multistate study (May & Gossage, 2001).

Among youth in 8th, 10th, and 12th grades, analyses comparing national data from the Monitoring the Future (MTF) study with data from a large sample of AI youth living on or near reservations found that the prevalence of alcohol and other drug use is higher among AI youth for nearly all substances studied (Stanley, Harness, Swaim, & Beauvais, 2014). For example, prevalence of youth who reported that they had gotten drunk in the past year in the 8th grade was 36.7% for AIs versus 14.8% for youth in the MTF sample. Prevalence of past-year drunkenness among 10th graders was 50.7% for AIs versus 37.2% for MTF youth, and among 12th graders was 52.9% for AIs versus 53.8% for MTF youth (Stanley et al., 2014). Prevalence estimates for marijuana use are 56.2% for AI youth versus 16.4% of MTF youth in the 8th grade, 61.4% for AI youth versus 33.4% of MTF youth in the 10th grade, and 67.9% for AI youth versus 43.8% of MTF youth in the 12th grade (Stanley et al., 2014).

Research conducted specifically with AI youth living on reservations has found that substance use during adolescence is associated with other risks such as early sex (Kaufman et al., 2007) and suicidal ideation (Yoder, Whitbeck, Hoyt, & LaFromboise, 2006), and predicts substance use in young adulthood (Mitchell, Beals, & Whitesell, 2008). Given that, compared with white youth, AI youth tend to initiate substance use at earlier ages (Beauvais, Jumper-Thurman, Helm, Plested, & Burnside, 2004; Spear, Longshore, McCaffrey, & Ellickson, 2005; Wallace et al., 2002), have higher rates of substance use (Stanley et al., 2014), and experience many health disparities related to substance use (Sarche & Spicer, 2008)—intervening on AI substance use at a young age is important.

The purpose of this chapter is to provide an overview of the literature on prevention and intervention efforts related to AI adolescent substance use. We begin with a review of the current status of the field. Next, we review guidelines for implementing brief interventions with indigenous youth. We then discuss implications for implementing brief interventions. We conclude with a discussion of future clinical and research directions.

STATUS OF THE FIELD

The research literature on prevalence rates of substance use and the high rates of negative consequences experienced as the result of problematic substance use highlight the need for substance use preventive interventions for AI youth. There is a strong need for programs that are culturally appropriate and that take into account their unique cultural identity, which can be influenced by historical, relational, and contextual factors (Harris, Carlson, & Poata-Smith, 2013). Developing and implementing culturally tailored programs is important not only for increasing program effectiveness but also for increasing acceptance in AI communities (Betancourt, Green, Carrillo, & Ananeh-Firempong, 2003; Whaley & Davis, 2007).

Epidemiological data clearly highlight the need for substance use and mental health services in AI country (Manson, 2000; Sarche & Spicer, 2008). However, it is unclear whether services exist but are not utilized, or whether there is a lack of services. One study examined treatment utilization in 109 youth in a Northern Plains reservation community and found that 21% were diagnosed as having a mental health or substance use disorder, or both, in the prior 6 months. Of those, 23% reported using services for symptoms of mental or substance use disorders during their lifetime, with most of the services being delivered in the school setting (Novins, Beals, Sack, & Manson, 2000). These studies point to a clear need for treatment services and indicate that substance-using individuals want to make a change. Making treatment more accessible to youth in a variety of settings (i.e., beyond the school setting) may be one way to increase utilization of treatment services.

In addition, intervening early in the trajectory of substance use may be particularly important for AI youth, and may help to prevent the many health disparities that are related to substance use. Prevention programs are grouped into three categories, including primary, secondary, and tertiary levels of prevention. Primary prevention programs focus on preventing youth from engaging in substance use (Lindsey, 2003), and are intended to be delivered prior to youth initiating any substance use. Secondary and tertiary prevention programs focus on youth who have begun using at different levels (Lindsey, 2003). Secondary prevention programs target youth who have begun experimenting or who have initiated substance use, but have not become dependent or experienced negative consequences. Tertiary programs are for youth who have already starting using substances and who are experiencing negative consequences related to their use. There are very few primary prevention programs for AI youth that have been the focus of research (Walsh & Baldwin, 2015). Most programs that have been evaluated in AI youth are secondary prevention programs, and there are even tertiary prevention programs.

While there are studies under way evaluating prevention programs for AI youth, these results are still pending. Many of the programs that have been tested are adaptations or modifications of mainstream programs. Among the very few exceptions, the Canoe Journey (Donovan et al., 2015) was developed within the Native culture. The Healing of the Canoe project is an excellent example of how university partners can collaborate with local tribes and work as coresearchers in addressing problems, identifying strengths, and even interpreting data (Donovan et al., 2015). The team, which included tribal members and university researchers, worked together to blend cognitive-behavioral life skills with culturally grounded, tribal-specific teachings, practices, and values that targeted both the prevention of substance use along with the promotion of cultural affiliation. The research development and planning phase took 3 years to complete. During this phase, community-based participatory research (CBPR) methods were employed to establish a working partnership with a focus on community engagement, conduct a community needs and resources assessment, identify and prioritize health disparities, specify a disorder to address through CBPR development of appropriate interventions, and develop community-based interventions. Preliminary findings evaluating this project showed reductions in substance use and increases in hope, optimism, and self-efficacy (Donovan et al., 2015). The mainstream programs that have been adapted and tested in AIs include Life Skills (Schinke, Tepavac, & Cole, 2000) and Drug Refusal Skills (Jumper-Reeves, Dustman, Harthun, Kulis, & Brown, 2014), which is an adaptation of the Keepin' It REAL program (Gosin, Marsiglia, & Hecht, 2003). Both of these programs utilize school-based curricula and are fairly long in duration. Living in Two Worlds, based on the Keepin' It REAL program, consists of 12 lessons delivered over 5 months (Kulis, Dustman, Brown, & Martinez, 2013). Life Skills contains 25–60 individual lessons that students participate in two to three times per week over 20–30 weeks (Schinke et al., 2000). Having prevention programs in the schools is important, but in high-risk populations, there is an opportunity to have culturally adapted programs outside of the school community. Programs that are shorter in duration may be more feasible in the community.

Although there are several, mostly secondary and tertiary prevention programs that have been implemented in indigenous communities, the continued disproportionally high rates of substance use among AI youth suggest that more work needs to be done. One approach that may offer promise is Screening, Brief Intervention, and Referral to Treatment (SBIRT; Becker, Ozechowski, & Hogue, Chapter 5, this volume; Parker-Langley, 2002). SBIRT is a comprehensive, integrated, public health approach to the delivery of early intervention and treatment services for persons with substance use disorders, as well as those who are at risk of developing these disorders. In an SBIRT session, clinicians within various treatment settings assess the severity of a client's substance use and potential need for treatment. Patients are then provided with a brief intervention, or referral to more intense treatment. Currently there are no studies examining SBIRT in AI adolescents. This is a missed opportunity, as SBIRT could be offered at primary care centers, hospital emergency rooms, trauma centers, and other community settings, providing opportunities for early intervention with at-risk substance-using youth before more severe consequences occur.

AI CULTURAL CONSIDERATIONS

As stated earlier, currently there are no publications on outcomes on screening and brief interventions with AI adolescents (or AI adults for that matter). In this section, we first provide a rationale for culturally adapting brief interventions for AI youth. Next, we discuss cultural considerations when adapting, and guidance for practitioners wishing to engage and intervene with AI adolescents. If AI adolescents are a new population for a practitioner, ethical guidelines encourage seeking appropriate supervision and consultation with a practitioner who has expertise and experience working with AI adolescents.

Reasons to Culturally Adapt

Cultural adaptations of evidence-based treatments (EBTs) is a burgeoning line of research in substance use disorder (SUD) treatment. Burlew, Copeland, Ahuama-Jonas, and Calsyn (2013) argue there are several reasons to consider culturally adapting an EBT: (1) the EBT is less (or not) effective with the subgroup; (2) the EBT is harmful for the subgroup; (3) the EBT is unacceptable to the subgroup; (4) an adaptation would increase attractiveness, engagement, retention, and outcomes; (5) cultural traditions influence behavior; and/or (6) it is more respectful to the ethnic cultural group's knowledge and worldview. Given that EBTs are rarely tested with sufficiently large samples of diverse racial and ethnic groups, the extent to which outcomes are similar or different across groups is often unknown, thus raising concerns about the validity of existing EBTs for racial/ethnic minorities (Bernal & Scharron-del-Rio, 2001).

The literature provides support for the value of culturally adapting EBTs for ethnic-minority groups. For example, there are empirical examples of unadapted EBTs that are less effective with an ethnic-minority group, such as an HIV risk-reduction intervention that was less effective for black men than for white men with substance abuse problems (Calsyn et al., 2012), whereas culturally adapted EBTs have been found to improve outcomes for ethnic minorities (Calsyn et al., 2012, 2013). It is thought that unadapted EBTs may be particularly unacceptable to AI/ANs based on clashes in worldview: (1) EBTs are secular and AI/AN traditional healing is spiritual; (2) EBTs take place in dyads or with one family and AI/AN traditional healing may involve the community; (3) SUD treatment often carries stigma, whereas AI/AN traditional healing is valued; and (4) EBTs do not explicitly include AI/AN worldviews, while AI/AN traditional healing promotes cultural identity and cultural preservation (e.g., Calabrese, 2008; Gone, 2007). Culturally adapting EBTs would serve to honor the effect of AI/AN culture on health risk and protective behaviors (Calabrese, 2008). Adding an explicit focus on AI culture, such as traditional spirituality and ceremonies and Native language, is a way to honor AI culture and contribute to its maintenance and strength.

Adapting EBTs while preserving the core components represents a pathway to dissemination and diffusion among AI/ANs (Venner & Bogenschutz, 2008; Venner, Feldstein, & Tafoya, 2008). Combining EBTs with indigenous knowledge, via cultural adaptations that are appropriate for AI/ANs with varying levels of acculturation, represents a compromise of strictly adhering to fidelity without cultural adaptations and culturally adapting EBTs without attention to fidelity (Castro, Barrera, & Holleran Steiker, 2010; Castro, Barrera, & Martinez, 2004). Culturally adapted EBTs should be empirically tested for efficacy and effectiveness as well as examining potential mediators and moderators to promote best practices for AI/ANs with SUD.

General Cultural Considerations

In this section, we discuss topics that are relevant to cultural adaptations, such as cultural identity, acculturation, spirituality, the role of extended family and nonsanguine (not biological) familial relationships, collectivism, and discrimination (Venner, Feldstein, & Tafoya, 2007).

Cultural Identity and Acculturation

Cultural identity can be defined as one's social identity in relation to one's group memberships, which may include ethnicity, gender, religion, class, nationality, and so on (Friedman, 1994). The stronger the client's cultural identity, the more likely culture will be important in considering conceptions of alcohol and addiction, motivations to use or change, goals and values, and social influences on drinking, such as social drinking norms and attitudes toward alcohol. It is helpful to inquire about the client's level of cultural salience—how important is the adolescent's AI identity to how the youth sees him- or herself and his or her worldview? High AI salience suggests more integration of AI culture within the brief intervention delivered. In contrast, in situations of higher client acculturation, or greater alignment with U.S. mainstream culture, it may be less important or even iatrogenic to explicitly include cultural adaptations. For example, Burrow-Sanchez, Minami, and Hops (2015) found that more acculturated adolescent Latino youth had poorer substance use outcomes if they were randomized to receive substance abuse treatment that had been culturally adapted for Latino youth than if they were randomized to unadapted treatment. For adolescents who are highly acculturated to U.S. mainstream culture, the provider might inquire about the youth's interest in learning more about AI culture and focusing on AI strengths in conversations about perceptions of substance use and motivations to change.

AI youth's level of cultural identity will influence how they introduce themselves in relation to their AI heritage, tribal enrollment, and clans. It is best to rely on a youth's self-identification of AI rather than asking about percentage of AI heritage. Asking specific questions about tribal enrollment may be a sensitive issue if the tribe does not have federal recognition or if the youth has heritage from multiple tribes and various other races/ethnicities. Finally, an AI youth may choose to share his or her clan membership. A clan refers to a group of people who may share descent or kinship. A person's clan will usually be the same as the mother's clan but may include aspects from both the mother and father or, less often, only the father. In sharing one's clan, people from within the same tribe will know how they are related, what their relationships ought to be, responsibilities to one another in difficult times, and they may proceed to call each other by their clan relationship (e.g., my daughter). For instance, when a close family member dies, people from a related clan will be responsible to do certain tasks such as serve as pallbearers. In some tribes, an AI provider may refer to the client by his or her clan relationship, which is viewed as a close connection and may help reduce the client's feelings of stigma and power differentials.

Religiosity and Spirituality

Religiosity and spirituality have important relationships to addiction and resolving addiction problems in the U.S. population and in AI communities. In the general U.S. population, almost 90% endorse a belief in God (Newport, 2016), and spirituality has consistently been demonstrated to be protective against the development of alcohol use disorders (AUDs; e.g., Miller, 2013). In AI communities, participation in traditional AI activities and spirituality have been helpful for AI adults in alcohol cessation (Stone, Whitbeck, Chen, Johnson, & Olson, 2006) and among AI adults ages 45 and older who are cutting down or quitting drinking, according to an epidemiological survey of Northern Plains and Southwestern tribes (Bezdek, Croy, Spicer, & Team, 2004). In a treatment study, AI adults exhibited increases in spirituality from baseline to follow-up (Greenfield et al., 2015). For AIs, spirituality may include traditional AI spirituality, Christianity, a blend of these, or something else (e.g., Garroutte et al., 2009). One should be cautious about asking about traditional AI spirituality due to its sacred and often secret nature, based on past historical oppression and outlawing of AI spirituality (Stannard, 1992). Rather than directly ask for specific information about traditional AI spirituality, religion, or the meaning of actions, dances, regalia, and other religious acts or pieces, providers might instead obtain such information by researching about a specific tribe, and seeking out a cultural broker who is knowledgeable about the tribe. Such an approach will help a provider to avoid serious breaches in the therapeutic alliance.

Collectivism and Conceptions of Family

Parental monitoring and supervision have been demonstrated to be critical for drug abuse prevention (National Institute on Drug Abuse, 2003). In non-AI populations, parental monitoring has been shown to be strongly protective against substance use in youth (Clark, Shamblen, Ringwalt, & Hanley, 2012; Kiesner, Poulin, & Dishion, 2010; Wang, Deveaux, Li, Marshall, Chen, & Stanton, 2014). Traditional parental monitoring consists of rule setting, monitoring youth activities, praise for appropriate behavior, and moderate, consistent discipline that enforces defined family rules (Kosterman, Hawkins, Haggerty, Spoth, & Redmond, 2001). However, traditional Western views of parenting are different from AI ways of parenting, which are more likely to involve family networks that often include grandparents, aunts, uncles, and sometimes fictive kin (not based on blood or marital relationships; Whitbeck, Sittner Hartshorn, & Walls, 2014). Therefore, "parenting" responsibilities may be spread throughout this extended network. Consistent with this more inclusive view of parenting, research with AI youth has found that the *number* of people monitoring an adolescent may be more strongly associated with reduced risk for substance use than parental monitoring when measured using a more mainstream, Western approach (Whitbeck, Sittner Hartshorn, Crawford, et al., 2014). Following from this, it may be important to include multiple family network members in prevention efforts, but to do so in a culturally consistent way. For example, discussions about family rules and values, family monitoring, and praise for appropriate behaviors should be encouraged in a way that is consistent with an AI approach to parenting. Few published studies have examined the influence of *family* monitoring. Whitbeck, Sittner Hartshorn, Crawford, and colleagues (2014) conducted a longitudinal study of North American indigenous youth and found that family monitoring served as a protective factor reducing the odds of smoking by 24%, but with no significant effect on marijuana or alcohol use. The role of family monitoring may be particularly salient for those residing in AI communities (e.g., reservations), where there are many family members living in close proximity and sharing parenting responsibilities.

Discrimination

The connection between discrimination and negative physical health effects is well documented, and the negative influence of discrimination on mental health is also gaining empirical support (e.g., Ngamake, Walch, & Raveepatarakul, 2016). Higher levels of perceived discrimination have been shown to be related to increased frequency of drinking and alcohol-related consequences among AI youth (Cheadle & Whitbeck, 2011; Whitbeck, Chen, Hoyt, & Adams, 2004). In a longitudinal study of AI youth, perceived discrimination predicted risk of developing an AUD (Armenta, Sittner, & Whitbeck, 2016). Drinking and other drug use are often considered maladaptive coping responses to discrimination in ethnic-minority and other oppressed groups (Gerrard et al., 2012; Wei, Alvarez, Ku, Russell, & Bonett, 2010).

Fortunately, research on the links between discrimination, alcohol and substance use, and mental health outcomes can provide some guidance to providers in helping young people choose positive coping skills to respond to stigma and discrimination. For example, researchers found that maladaptive (avoidant) coping strategies such as use of drugs and alcohol mediated the relationship between discrimination and depression, anxiety, and stress in a sample of sexual minority adults (Ngamake et al., 2016). Furthermore, internalization (i.e., blaming oneself for the discriminatory behavior) mediated the relationship between discrimination and anxiety, suggesting that internalization is one mechanism by which discrimination led to anxiety. Internalization also served to moderate the relationship between discrimination and depression and anxiety, such that those who rarely internalize showed increasing depression and anxiety as perceived discrimination increased. But for those high in internalization, their depression and anxiety were high no matter the level of perceived discrimination. Thus, it may be helpful to assist AI youth in identifying discrimination when it occurs and avoiding both internalization and use of maladaptive coping strategies such as alcohol and drug use in order to safeguard their mental health.

Microaggressions

Microaggressions are everyday interpersonal exchanges conveying negative messages about a person's group membership that vary from slights to blatant efforts to inflict harm—whether intentional or inadvertent, they have been related to psychological distress in the person experiencing the microaggressions (Sue & Sue, 2013). Examples include denial of racism, saying the person is being oversensitive (to discrimination); denial of importance of cultural heritage, beliefs, or practices; and even categorically romanticizing AI/ ANs. We are all exposed to many of the same socializing forces in the United States, such as media portrayals of AIs as either all wearing headdresses, romanticized, or depicted only in a negative light such as having severe drinking problems or being homeless. In addition, the U.S. power structure is evident in characteristics of people in power, such as presidents of companies, institutions, and of the United States in terms of nearly all being non-Hispanic white and male. Thus, we learn many stereotypes that may lead us to inadvertently commit microaggressions with our clients, or to resist further exploration of client experiences of microaggressions, in favor of questioning whether the client was being too sensitive or perhaps misread the person's intentions.

Well-intentioned people, including providers, may inadvertently commit a microaggression with a client (Owen, Tao, Imel, Wampold, & Rodolfa, 2014; Sue & Sue, 2013). Therapeutic microaggressions include messages minimizing or negating the client's culture, experiences of discrimination, and culturally inappropriate interventions (Burkard & Knox, 2004). A large online study of racial/ethnic-minority adults found 81% reported at least one microaggression during counseling (Hook et al., 2016). Another study at a university counseling center found that 53% of racial/ethnic-minority clients reported experiencing a microaggression by their therapist and such experiences were negatively related to working alliance (Owen et al., 2014). When the microaggression was not discussed in therapy (76%), working alliance was lower compared to when it was discussed (Owen et al., 2014). An important approach to maintaining the therapeutic alliance is to recognize one's own microaggression right away, have an open discussion about the microaggression, and apologize and work to repair therapeutic alliance. It is also crucial to respond as nondefensively as possible when a client brings it to our attention rather than first denying any malintent (see Balsam, Molina, Beadnell, Simoni, & Walters, 2011, for more information on microaggressions). AI-specific microaggressions to avoid include "You are so lucky to be Native American," and "My great-grandmother was a Cherokee princess" (Chae & Walters, 2009). Such statements may impact AI/AN youth negatively in thinking the provider puts all AI/ANs into one category or overly romanticizes being AI/AN or is making a claim to be AI when there were no AI/AN "princesses" in the past.

AI Stereotypes

We recommend that providers be aware of negative AI stereotypes. Often, AIs have internalized negative stereotypes (May & Smith, 1988) that have been refuted or not supported by research. AIs may internalize the stereotype that all AIs drink alcohol, when in actuality AIs have higher rates of abstinence than all races except Asian Americans (Grant et al., 2015; Spicer et al., 2003). Another widely held stereotype is that AIs have a slower rate of alcohol metabolism than non-AIs, however that is unlikely to be true (Garcia-Andrade, Wall, & Ehlers, 1997; Schaefer, 1981). A related harmful stereotypic belief is that AIs have a genetic predisposition to AUDs (Ehlers et al., 2004). Such stereotypes may contribute to drinking problems and interfere with efforts to reduce alcohol use or to abstain. Providers' awareness of these erroneous stereotypes will help reduce the likelihood of inadvertently perpetuating them.

CULTURALLY ADAPTED
BRIEF INTERVENTION GUIDELINES

The following section is based on research by one of us (K. V.) that is designed to culturally adapt motivational interviewing (MI). This line of research has used focus groups consisting of people from several tribes (Venner et al., 2007) and subsequent work involving another Southwestern pueblo (R01 DA021672) to adapt MI in partnership with tribal people (Venner, Greenfield, et al., 2016) and conduct a randomized controlled trial to compare the adapted MI to treatment as usual at the local SUD treatment agency.

Making Introductions

Culturally appropriate introductions may improve rapport building and provide role modeling with AI adolescent clients. Using MI as a foundation, we recommend introducing yourself, mentioning AI tribes or culture, providing structure for your time together, and emphasizing client autonomy (Miller & Rollnick, 2012). If you are an AI provider, we suggest sharing your tribal affiliation/membership and clans, if you feel comfortable doing so. For instance, one of us (K. V.) may share that she is from an Alaska Native tribe called Athabascan, and is part of the Caribou (udzih) clan. Sharing one's tribe and clan(s) accomplishes bringing AI culture to the forefront as well as modeling aspects of a proper AI introduction. If you are not AI, we suggest sharing your own heritage and bringing up AI culture as a way of priming culture (i.e., eliciting thoughts about culture and cultural influences) and as an invitation for the client to discuss culture during the session. One way to do this is to share your level of involvement with AI culture. This may include (1) how much interaction you have had with AI clients, (2) how long you have worked with a particular tribe, or (3) respect for AI focus on holistic conceptions of health and well-being. For example, a provider may say, "I have English and German heritage and my family has been in the U.S. for many generations. I am new to this area and am interested in how things are done around here and what is important to people in this area and to you. If your AI heritage is important to you and how you see your substance use, I would like to hear about any strengths you may find in your culture as well as any difficulties." At some point, it may be helpful to let the client know it is OK to talk about the therapeutic relationship and how he or she feels about working with a non-Native practitioner. For example, "How is it for you to work with someone who is not American Indian?" Even if you have very little knowledge and exposure to AI people, you might say that you are aware that AIs have many cultural strengths, such as some of the highest rates of alcohol abstinence (Spicer et al., 2003). For instance, "While I am new to this reservation, I am aware of some little-known AI strengths, such as very high rates of abstinence from alcohol." A strength-based focus may reassure an AI adolescent that you do not believe many negative stereotypes about AIs. It is also important to ask the adolescent whether it would be helpful to have a parent(s) or other family members present. Finally, you may simply say that you would like to know how much AI culture is important to that individual in general. Then, if it is important, you may explore how the client believes AI culture/community views well-being, or drinking and/or using substances.

Screening AI Youth for Risky Alcohol/Substance Use

Although screening may entail brief evidence-based measures such as the Alcohol Use Disorders Identification Test (AUDIT: Saunders, Aasland, Babor, de la Fuente, & Grant, 1993) and AUDIT-C (Garcia Carretero, Novalbos Ruiz,

Martinez Delgado, & O'Ferrall Gonzalez, 2016), here we focus on the provider–client interaction related to screening. In an effort to ease into the topic of alcohol or other drug (AOD) use and avoid triggering possible defensiveness about drinking/substance use and negative alcohol-related stereotypes of AIs, we suggest providing a rationale for asking about AOD consumption, and connecting how alcohol may impact people's health and well-being in ways that they might not have considered. For example, an AI psychiatrist recommended the following (paraphrased) wording during a qualitative interview (Sussman et al., 2015): "We are interested in your well-being and ask all of our patients questions about alcohol use. You may or may not have thought about how alcohol use may impact your health and well-being. I'd like to offer these questions for your consideration." Emphasizing a focus on health and well-being may convey more caring and emphasize a holistic view of the individual, and therefore may be more acceptable to AI youth as well as to youth of all cultural backgrounds.

Providing Information

In MI, feedback may include screening results, information, advice, and concerns (Miller & Rollnick, 2012). In general, providing information includes asking the client permission to discuss topics, asking for the client's knowledge on the topic, providing the information in a neutral manner, and asking for the client's thoughts and reactions to the information. The idea is to invite the client to consider your information, though he or she has the autonomy to disagree with or reject it. A common example is providing information about the definition of moderate drinking levels. Cultural adaptations for AIs may include information on the following topics: (1) high abstinence rates among AIs, (2) AI adaptations of 12-step programs (Coyhis, 2010a, 2010b), and (3) knowledge of negative stereotypes of the "drunken Indian" or differences in alcohol metabolism and sensitivity (e.g., Garcia-Andrade et al., 1997). As stated above, it is important for providers to be aware that these stereotypes exist, that the client may have internalized them, and that there is research evidence to document high AI abstinence rates, similar rates of alcohol metabolism among AIs compared with the general U.S. population, and no unique genetic predisposition among AIs to developing an AUD. If a provider wanted to highlight the AI abstinence rates, he or she might begin by asking what the AI youth already knows about AIs who do not drink alcohol. If the youth is not aware or is misinformed, then the provider would provide the information. For example, "Research has shown repeatedly that AIs have very high rates of abstaining from drinking alcohol, such that 63% have not drank alcohol in the past year compared to 42% of non-Hispanic whites. This is similar to Asian American abstinence rates of 67% (Substance Abuse and Mental Health Services Administration, 2014). What do you think about this information?" In this way, the provider may introduce ethnicity-specific information that highlights strengths associated with abstinence. This may help to correct erroneous descriptive norms about AI drinking and also may help counteract any internalized stereotypes about AIs and drinking.

Inviting Change Talk

Clients benefit when providers invite them to share their own arguments for change or "change talk." Change talk refers to client statements that favor making a change in substance use behavior (Miller & Rollnick, 2012). Evidence is building that the amount of change talk during sessions is related to treatment outcomes (Amrhein, Miller, Yahne, Palmer, & Fulcher, 2003) and is a mechanism of change for MI (D'Amico & Feldstein Ewing, Chapter 14, this volume; Moyers, Martin, Houck, Christopher, & Tonigan, 2009). Miller and Rollnick (2013) offer several ways to invite change talk, including (1) asking evocative questions, (2) using importance and confidence rulers, (3) querying extremes, and (4) exploring goals and values.

Including Culture When Inviting Change Talk

Although the sole use of these techniques may elicit cultural aspects of change talk, it may be necessary to explicitly include references to culture in your reflections or evocative questions. Relevant cultural topics may include cultural identity, acculturation, spirituality, extended family and nonsanguine familial relationships, collectivism, and discrimination (Venner et al., 2007). One way to enhance client motivation to change is to develop discrepancy between substance use and other aspects of the client, such as identity and values. Thus, a provider may ask how the client's tribal community or family views drinking. The provider may also ask, in a neutral manner, how drinking fits in with the client's traditional spirituality or ceremonies. The resulting dialogue may lead to opportunities to enhance motivation or to provide corrective information about AIs and drinking using an MI-consistent manner of providing information.

CULTURALLY ADAPTING RULERS

In MI, the rulers used to assess readiness to change or importance of change are presented as linear measuring tools, similar to actual rulers that measure inches or centimeters. However, in AI culture, conceptualizations and thinking often follow more circular than linear patterns. Based on responses from focus groups with AIs who varied by tribes, cultural identity, gender, and educational attainment, we (Venner et al., 2007) reported options for culturally adapting rulers. For instance, the Diné lifespan is represented by a circle that begins at zero and ends at 104 years of age, so some AI youth may relate to a circular representation of increasing numbers representing intensity of motivation for change. One may change the linear rulers to a circle and ask the AI youth to rate how important it is to make a change in his or her alcohol use from not at all to extremely important. Another option is to use words describing various anchors for levels of importance or competence, which may be combined with visual representations of growth or the development of animals, plants, or projects. For instance, using Native plants, such as corn, the lowest level of readiness or confidence could be that the ground is not ready for planting, whereas the highest level could be that the corn is ready for harvest.

Exploring Goals and Values

Exploring goals and values is helpful in eliciting change talk because alcohol and other substance use are usually not in alignment with those goals. When there is a mismatch between one's goals and behaviors, discomfort often arises as theoretically explained by either cognitive dissonance (e.g., Festinger, 1962) or a two-stage model of self-control (Myrseth, Fishbach, & Trope, 2009) whereby one recognizes the discrepancy and then resolves it by either changing the goal/value or by changing behavior (e.g., drinking less or quitting). One cultural adaptation to consider is, if an adolescent's cultural identity is high, yet the adolescent has not mentioned spirituality, to query gently about how spirituality may fit in with drinking. As mentioned above, one should exercise caution in asking about traditional AI spirituality due to its sacred and often secret nature based on past historical oppression and outlawing of AI spirituality (Stannard, 1992). One suggestion is to clarify that you do not want to ask about secret or sacred spiritual beliefs or practices, but are wondering whether spirituality might be related to his or her drinking or to a path whereby his or her alcohol problems may be resolved. For example, a provider might say, "I am hearing that you do not drink while participating in traditional ceremonies. Without going into any secret or sacred details, how have you been able to avoid drinking during those times?" Another possibility: "I can tell that your traditional spirituality has been important in your life. I am wondering how your drinking fits in with your spiritual beliefs?" In this way, one may respectfully mine for change talk while including cultural values and beliefs.

FUTURE DIRECTIONS AND NEXT STEPS

The literature on prevention/intervention in AI adolescents (and adults) is nascent and in desperate need of research funding and attention. Despite this, there are some important findings in the AI literature, such as work in spirituality, that can generalize to and enrich research conducted in other populations. The U.S. population is becoming more and more diverse—it will be important for all clinicians and researchers to understand the effects of stereotypes, discrimination, and poverty and how these relate to substance use and treatment outcomes. Research with AIs has established the importance of including spirituality in research (Graham, 2002; Greenfield et al., 2015). This finding can extend beyond AIs, since 89% of the population believes in God or another higher power (Lipka, 2015). Besides the twelve-step facilitation approach (Nowinski, Baker, & Carroll, 1999), EBTs have yet to include spirituality in an explicit and meaningful way, but will likely benefit from its inclusion by tapping into positive aspects of coping and associations with prevention and cessation of substance use.

Future AI addiction research needs to focus on increasing scientific rigor as well as incorporating cultural strengths and traditional healing into interventions where appropriate. Current efforts to increase AI scientific rigor that we are a part of include working with the National Institutes of Health to evaluate the state of the prevention and intervention literatures in addiction. In addition, delivering AI youth-focused prevention/interventions in a short amount of time, and including the use of technology, may increase the reach of our prevention and intervention programs and will likely appeal to youth, thereby increasing engagement. Finally, technology-based interventions such as telehealth interventions can ensure fidelity to EBT, in settings where EBT training is difficult or too costly or provider turnover is high.

We have provided some cultural considerations when working with AI clients and some guidance on how brief interventions might be culturally adapted. One of us (K. V.) has conducted work to adapt MI (Venner et al., 2007) and a combined MI and community reinforcement approach (MICRA) and found improved SUD outcomes for adult AIs (Venner, Greenfield, et al., 2016). The results of the randomized controlled trial comparing MICRA to treatment as usual revealed improvements in both groups but no significant differences between the two (Venner, Tonigan, et al., 2016). Working with Latino youth, Burrow-Sanchez et al. (2015) found that traditional youth had better outcomes in a culturally adapted CBT but that acculturated youth did better with unadapted EBT than with the culturally adapted EBT. Therefore, it is important to consider the acculturation status of clients prior to providing an adapted EBT. Future research should examine both how to effectively culturally adapt EBTs and for which youth adaptations are more effective. Finally, research regarding how to generalize findings from one tribe to another will facilitate dissemination.

Although AIs have among the highest rates of abstinence of all racial groups in the United States, those AIs who do engage in substance use experience a disproportionate amount of health disparities related to their use. It is important that research be supported that can find the most effective interventions for AI youth to address these alarming health disparities and strengthen protective factors such as high abstinence rates, spirituality, extended family, and collectivism.

REFERENCES

Amrhein, P. C., Miller, W. R., Yahne, C. E., Palmer, M., & Fulcher, L. (2003). Client commitment language during motivational interviewing predicts drug use outcomes. *Journal of Consulting and Clinical Psychology, 71*(5), 862–878.

Armenta, B. E., Sittner, K. J., & Whitbeck, L. B. (2016). Predicting the onset of alcohol use and the development of alcohol use disorder among indigenous adolescents. *Child Development, 87*(3), 870–882.

Balsam, K. F., Molina, Y., Beadnell, B., Simoni, J., & Walters, K. (2011). Measuring multiple minority stress: The LGBT People of Color Microaggressions Scale. *Cultural Diversity and Ethnic Minority Psychology, 17*(2), 163–174.

Beauvais, F., Jumper-Thurman, P., Helm, H., Plested, B., & Burnside, M. (2004). Surveillance of drug use among American Indian adolescents: Patterns over 25 years. *Journal of Adolescent Health, 34*(6), 493–500.

Bernal, G., & Scharron-del-Rio, M. R. (2001). Are empirically supported treatments valid for ethnic minorities?: Toward an alternative approach for treatment research. *Cultural Diversity and Ethnic Minority Psychology, 7*(4), 328–342.

Betancourt, J. R., Green, A. R., Carrillo, J. E., & Ananeh-Firempong, O., 2nd. (2003). Defining cultural competence: A practical framework for addressing racial/ethnic disparities in health and health care. *Public Health Reports, 118*(4), 293–302.

Bezdek, M., Croy, C., Spicer, P., & Team, A.-S. (2004). Documenting natural recovery in American-Indian drinking behavior: A coding scheme. *Journal of Studies on Alcohol and Drugs, 65*(4), 428–433.

Burkard, A. W., & Knox, S. (2004). Effect of therapist color-blindness on empathy and attributions in cross-cultural counseling. *Journal of Counseling Psychology, 51*(4), 387–397.

Burlew, A. K., Copeland, V. C., Ahuama-Jonas, C., & Calsyn, D. A. (2013). Does cultural adaptation have a role in substance abuse treatment? *Social Work in Public Health, 28*(3–4), 440–460.

Burrow-Sanchez, J. J., Minami, T., & Hops, H. (2015). Cultural accommodation of group substance abuse treatment for Latino adolescents: Results of an RCT. *Cultural Diversity and Ethnic Minority Psychology, 21*(4), 571–583.

Calabrese, J. D. (2008). Clinical paradigm clashes: Ethnocentric and political barriers to Native American efforts at self-healing. *Ethos, 36*(3), 334–353.

Calsyn, D. A., Burlew, A. K., Hatch-Maillette, M. A., Beadnell, B., Wright, L., & Wilson, J. (2013). An HIV prevention intervention for ethnically diverse men in substance abuse treatment: Pilot study findings. *American Journal of Public Health, 103*(5), 896–902.

Calsyn, D. A., Burlew, A. K., Hatch-Maillette, M. A., Wilson, J., Beadnell, B., & Wright, L. (2012). Real men are safe-culturally adapted: Utilizing the Delphi process to revise real men are safe for an ethnically diverse group of men in substance abuse treatment. *AIDS Education and Prevention, 24*(2), 117–131.

Castro, F. G., Barrera, M., Jr., & Holleran Steiker, L. K. (2010). Issues and challenges in the design of culturally adapted evidence-based interventions. *Annual Review of Clinical Psychology, 6*, 213–239.

Castro, F. G., Barrera, M., Jr., & Martinez, C. R., Jr. (2004). The cultural adaptation of prevention interventions: Resolving tensions between fidelity and fit. *Prevention Science, 5*(1), 41–45.

Chae, D. H., & Walters, K. L. (2009). Racial discrimination and racial identity attitudes in relation to self-rated health and physical pain and impairment among two-spirit American Indians/Alaska Natives. *American Journal of Public Health*, 99(Suppl. 1), S144–S151.

Cheadle, J. E., & Whitbeck, L. B. (2011). Alcohol use trajectories and problem drinking over the course of adolescence: A study of North American indigenous youth and their caretakers. *Journal of Health and Social Behavior*, 52(2), 228–245.

Clark, H. K., Shamblen, S. R., Ringwalt, C. L., & Hanley, S. (2012). Predicting high risk adolescents' substance use over time: The role of parental monitoring. *Journal of Primary Prevention*, 33(2–3), 67–77.

Coyhis, D. (2010a). *The medicine wheel and 12 steps for men workbook*. Colorado Springs, CO: Coyhis.

Coyhis, D. (2010b). *The medicine wheel and 12 steps for women workbook*. Colorado Springs, CO: Coyhis.

Donovan, D. M., Thomas, L. R., Sigo, R. L., Price, L., Lonczak, H., Lawrence, N., et al. (2015). Healing of the Canoe: Preliminary results of a culturally tailored intervention to prevent substance abuse and promote tribal identity for Native youth in two Pacific Northwest tribes. *American Indian and Alaska Native Mental Health Research*, 22(1), 42–76.

Ehlers, C. L., Gilder, D. A., Wall, T. L., Phillips, E., Feiler, H., & Wilhelmsen, K. C. (2004). Genomic screen for loci associated with alcohol dependence in Mission Indians. *American Journal of Medical Genetics Part B: Neuropsychiatric Genetics*, 129B(1), 110–115.

Festinger, L. (1962). Cognitive dissonance. *Scientific American*, 207, 93–102.

Friedman, J. (1994). *Cultural identity and global process*. London: SAGE.

Garcia-Andrade, C., Wall, T. L., & Ehlers, C. L. (1997). The firewater myth and response to alcohol in Mission Indians. *American Journal of Psychiatry*, 154(7), 983–988.

Garcia Carretero, M. A., Novalbos Ruiz, J. P., Martinez Delgado, J. M., & O'Ferrall Gonzalez, C. (2016). Validation of the Alcohol Use Disorders Identification Test in university students: AUDIT and AUDIT-C. *Adicciones*, 775.

Garroutte, E. M., Beals, J., Keane, E. M., Kaufman, C., Spicer, P., Henderson, J., et al. (2009). Religiosity and spiritual engagement in two American Indian populations. *Journal for the Scientific Study of Religion*, 48(3), 480–500.

Gerrard, M., Stock, M. L., Roberts, M. E., Gibbons, F. X., O'Hara, R. E., Weng, C. Y., et al. (2012). Coping with racial discrimination: The role of substance use. *Psychology of Addictive Behaviors*, 26(3), 550–560.

Gone, J. P. (2007). "We never was happy living like a Whiteman": Mental health disparities and the postcolonial predicament in American Indian communities. *American Journal of Community Psychology*, 40(3–4), 290–300.

Gosin, M., Marsiglia, F. F., & Hecht, M. L. (2003). Keepin' it R.E.A.L.: A drug resistance curriculum tailored to the strengths and needs of pre-adolescents of the southwest. *Journal of Drug Education*, 33(2), 119–142.

Graham, T. L. C. (2002). Using reasons for living to connect to American Indian healing traditions. *Journal of Sociology and Social Welfare*, 29(1), 55–75.

Grant, B. F., Goldstein, R. B., Saha, T. D., Chou, S. P., Jung, J., Zhang, H., et al. (2015). Epidemiology of DSM-5 alcohol use disorder: Results from the National Epidemiologic Survey on Alcohol and Related Conditions III. *JAMA Psychiatry*, 72(8), 757–766.

Greenfield, B. L., Hallgren, K. A., Venner, K. L., Hagler, K. J., Simmons, J. D., Sheche, J. N., et al. (2015). Cultural adaptation, psychometric properties, and outcomes of the Native American Spirituality Scale. *Psychological Services, 12*(2), 123–133.

Harris, M., Carlson, B., & Poata-Smith, E. S. (2013). *Indiengeous identitiies and the politics of authenticity.* Sydney, Australia: University of Technology Sydney E-Press.

Hawkins, E. H., Cummins, L. H., & Marlatt, G. A. (2004). Preventing substance abuse in American Indian and Alaska Native youth: Promising strategies for healthier communities. *Psychological Bulletin, 130*(2), 304–323.

Hook, J. N., Farrell, J. E., Davis, D. E., DeBlaere, C., Van Tongeren, D. R., & Utsey, S. O. (2016). Cultural humility and racial microaggressions in counseling. *Journal of Counseling Psychology, 63*(3), 269–277.

Humes, K. R., Jones, N. A., & Ramirez, R. R. (2011). *Overview of race and Hispanic origin: 2010.* Washington, DC: U.S. Census Bureau.

Jumper-Reeves, L., Dustman, P. A., Harthun, M. L., Kulis, S., & Brown, E. F. (2014). American Indian cultures: How CBPR illuminated intertribal cultural elements fundamental to an adaptation effort. *Prevention Science, 15*(4), 547–556.

Kaufman, C. E., Desserich, J., Big Crow, C. K., Holy Rock, B., Keane, E., & Mitchell, C. M. (2007). Culture, context, and sexual risk among Northern Plains American Indian youth. *Social Science and Medicine, 64*(10), 2152–2164.

Kiesner, J., Poulin, F., & Dishion, T. J. (2010). Adolescent substance use with friends: Moderating and mediating effects of parental monitoring and peer activity contexts. *Merrill–Palmer Quarterly, 56*(4), 529–556.

Kosterman, R., Hawkins, J. D., Haggerty, K. P., Spoth, R., & Redmond, C. (2001). Preparing for the drug free years: Session-specific effects of a universal parent-training intervention with rural families. *Journal of Drug Education, 31*(1), 47–68.

Kulis, S., Dustman, P. A., Brown, E. F., & Martinez, M. (2013). Expanding urban American Indian youths' repertoire of drug resistance skills: Pilot results from a culturally adapted prevention program. *American Indian and Alaska Native Mental Health Research, 20*(1), 35–54.

Lindsey, V. V. (2003). Primary, secondary, tertiary prevention programs. *Journal of Addictive Disorders.* Retrieved from *www.breining.edu.*

Lipka, M. (2015, November 4). Americans' faith in God may be eroding. Retrieved August 30, 2016, from *www.pewresearch.org/fact-tank/2015/11/04/americans-faith-in-god-may-be-eroding.*

Manson, S. M. (2000). Mental health services for American Indians and Alaska Natives: Need, use, and barriers to effective care. *Canadian Journal of Psychiatry, 45*(7), 617–626.

May, P. A., & Gossage, J. P. (2001). Estimating the prevalence of fetal alcohol syndrome: A summary. *Alcohol Research and Health, 25*(3), 159–167.

May, P. A., & Smith, M. B. (1988). Some Navajo Indian opinions about alcohol abuse and prohibition: A survey and recommendations for policy. *Journal of Studies on Alcohol and Drugs, 49*(4), 324–334.

Miller, W. R. (2013). Addiction and spirituality. *Substance Use and Misuse, 48*(12), 1258–1259.

Miller, W. R., & Rollnick, S. (2012). *Motivational interviewing: Helping people change* (3rd ed.). New York: Guilford Press.

Mitchell, C. M., Beals, J., & Whitesell, N. R. (2008). Alcohol use among American

Indian high school youths from adolescence and young adulthood: A latent Markov model. *Journal of Studies on Alcohol and Drugs, 69*(5), 666–675.

Moyers, T. B., Martin, T., Houck, J. M., Christopher, P. J., & Tonigan, J. S. (2009). From in-session behaviors to drinking outcomes: A causal chain for motivational interviewing. *Journal of Consulting and Clinical Psychology, 77*(6), 1113–1124.

Myrseth, K. O., Fishbach, A., & Trope, Y. (2009). Counteractive self-control. *Psychological Science, 20*(2), 159–163.

National Institute on Drug Abuse. (2003). Preventing drug use among children and adolescents: A research-based guide for parents, educators, and community leaders. Retrieved from *www.drugabuse.gov/sites/default/files/preventingdruguse_2.pdf*.

Newport, F. (2016, June). Most Americans still believe in God. *Social Issues*. Retrieved from *news.gallup.com/poll/193271/americans-believe-god.aspx*.

Ngamake, S. T., Walch, S. E., & Raveepatarakul, J. (2016). Discrimination and sexual minority mental health: Mediation and moderation effects of coping. *Psychology of Sexual Orientation and Gender Diversity, 3*(2), 213–226.

Novins, D. K., Beals, J., Sack, W. H., & Manson, S. M. (2000). Unmet needs for substance abuse and mental health services among Northern Plains American Indian adolescents. *Psychological Services, 51*(8), 1045–1047.

Nowinski, J., Baker, S., & Carroll, K. (1992). *Twelve-step facilitation therapy manual: A clinical research guide for therapists treating individuals with alcohol abuse and dependence* (NIAAA Project MATCH Monograph Series. Vol. 1. [DHHS Publication No. ADM 92-1893]). Washington, DC: U.S. Government Printing Office.

Owen, J., Tao, K. W., Imel, Z. E., Wampold, B. E., & Rodolfa, E. (2014). Addressing racial and ethnic microaggressions in therapy. *Professional Psychology: Research and Practice, 45*(4), 283–290.

Parker-Langley, L. (2002). *Alcohol prevention programs among American Indians: Research findings and issues* (Vol. 37). Washington, DC: Department of Health and Human Services.

Sarche, M., & Spicer, P. (2008). Poverty and health disparities for American Indian and Alaska Native children: Current knowledge and future prospects. *Annals of the New York Academy of Sciences, 1136*, 126–136.

Saunders, J. B., Aasland, O. G., Babor, T. F., de la Fuente, J. R., & Grant, M. (1993). Development of the Alcohol Use Disorders Identification Test (AUDIT): WHO collaborative project on early detection of persons with harmful alcohol consumption–II. *Addiction, 88*(6), 791–804.

Schaefer, J. M. (1981). Firewater myths revisited: Review of findings and some new directions. *Journal of Studies on Alcohol and Drugs, 9*, 99–117.

Schinke, S. P., Tepavac, L., & Cole, K. C. (2000). Preventing substance use among Native American youth: Three-year results. *Addictive Behaviors, 25*(3), 387–397.

Spear, S., Longshore, D., McCaffrey, D., & Ellickson, P. (2005). Prevalence of substance use among white and American Indian young adolescents in a Northern Plains state. *Journal of Psychoactive Drugs, 37*(1), 1–6.

Spicer, P., Beals, J., Croy, C. D., Mitchell, C. M., Novins, D. K., Moore, L., et al. (2003). The prevalence of DSM-III-R alcohol dependence in two American Indian populations. *Alcoholism: Clinical and Experimental Research, 27*(11), 1785–1797.

Spillane, N. S., Greenfield, B., Venner, K., & Kahler, C. W. (2015). Alcohol use among reserve-dwelling adult First Nation members: Use, problems, and intention to change drinking behavior. *Addictive Behaviors, 41*, 232–237.

Stanley, L. R., Harness, S. D., Swaim, R. C., & Beauvais, F. (2014). Rates of substance use of American Indian students in 8th, 10th, and 12th grades living on or near reservations: Update, 2009–2012. *Public Health Reports, 129*(2), 156–163.

Stannard, D. E. (1992). *American holocaust: The conquest of the New World*. New York: Oxford University Press.

Stone, R. A., Whitbeck, L. B., Chen, X., Johnson, K., & Olson, D. M. (2006). Traditional practices, traditional spirituality, and alcohol cessation among American Indians. *Journal of Studies on Alcohol and Drugs, 67*(2), 236–244.

Substance Abuse and Mental Health Services Administration. (2014). *Results from the 2013 National Survey on Drug Use and Health: Summary of national findings* (NSDUH Series H-48, HHS Publication No. SMA 14–4863). Rockville, MD: Author.

Sue, D. W., & Sue, D. (2013). *Counseling the culturally diverse: Theory and practice* (6th ed.). Hoboken, NJ: Wiley.

Sussman, A. L., Venner, K. L., Sanchez, V., Williamson, R. L., Getrich, C., Root, M., et al. (2015). *Developing culturally appropriate screening and treatment strategies for alcohol and opiate use and primary care settings*. Paper presented at the New Mexico Public Health Association Conferences, Albuquerque, NM.

U.S. Department of Health and Human Services. (2001). *Mental health, culture, race, and ethnicity—a supplement to mental health: A report of the Surgeon General*. Rockville, MD: Author.

Venner, K. L., & Bogenschutz, M. P. (2008). *Cultural and spiritual dimensions of addictions treatment*. Center City, MI: Hazelden.

Venner, K. L., Feldstein, S. W., & Tafoya, N. (2007). Helping clients feel welcome: Principles of adapting treatment cross-culturally. *Alcoholism Treatment Quarterly, 25*, 11–30.

Venner, K. L., Feldstein, S. W., & Tafoya, N. (2008). Helping clients feel welcome: Principles of adapting treatment cross-culturally. *Alcoholism Treatment Quarterly, 25*(4), 11–30.

Venner, K. L., Greenfield, B. L., Hagler, K. J., Simmons, J., Shesche, J., Lupee, D., et al. (2016). Pilot outcome results of culturally tailored evidence-based substance use disorder treatment with a Southwest tribe. *Addictive Behavior Reports, 3*, 21–27.

Venner, K. L., Tonigan, J. S., Simmons, J., Greenfield, B. L., Hagler, K., Cloud, V., et al. (2016). *RCT outcomes from culturally tailored evidence-based treatments with a Southwestern tribe*. Paper presented at the Collaborative Perspective on Addiction, San Diego, CA.

Wallace, J. M., Jr., Bachman, J. G., O'Malley, P. M., Johnston, L. D., Schulenberg, J. E., & Cooper, S. M. (2002). Tobacco, alcohol, and illicit drug use: Racial and ethnic differences among U.S. high school seniors, 1976–2000. *Public Health Reports, 117*(Suppl. 1), S67–S75.

Walsh, M. L., & Baldwin, J. A. (2015). American Indian substance abuse prevention efforts: A review of programs, 2003–2013. *American Indian and Alaska Native Mental Health Research, 22*(2), 41–68.

Wang, B., Deveaux, L., Li, X., Marshall, S., Chen, X., & Stanton, B. (2014). The impact of youth, family, peer and neighborhood risk factors on developmental trajectories of risk involvement from early through middle adolescence. *Social Science and Medicine, 106,* 43–52.

Wei, M., Alvarez, A. N., Ku, T. Y., Russell, D. W., & Bonett, D. G. (2010). Development and validation of a Coping with Discrimination Scale: Factor structure, reliability, and validity. *Journal of Counseling Psychology, 57*(3), 328–344.

Whaley, A. L., & Davis, K. E. (2007). Cultural competence and evidence-based practice in mental health services: A complementary perspective. *The American Psychologist, 62*(6), 563–574.

Whitbeck, L. B., Chen, X., Hoyt, D. R., & Adams, G. W. (2004). Discrimination, historical loss and enculturation: Culturally specific risk and resiliency factors for alcohol abuse among American Indians. *Journal of Studies on Alcohol and Drugs,* 65(4), 409–418.

Whitbeck, L. B., Sittner Hartshorn, K. J., Crawford, D. M., Walls, M. L., Gentzler, K. C., & Hoyt, D. R. (2014). Mental and substance use disorders from early adolescence to young adulthood among indigenous young people: Final diagnostic results from an 8-year panel study. *Social Psychiatry and Psychiatric Epidemiology,* 49(6), 961–973.

Whitbeck, L. B., Sittner Hartshorn, K. J., & Walls, M. L. (2014). *Indigenous adolescent development.* New York: Routledge.

Yoder, K. A., Whitbeck, L. B., Hoyt, D. R., & LaFromboise, T. (2006). Suicidal ideation among American Indian youths. *Archives of Suicide Research, 10*(2), 177–190.

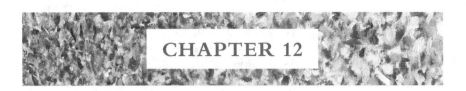

CHAPTER 12

Understanding and Addressing Alcohol and Substance Use in Sexual and Gender Minority Youth

Ethan H. Mereish, Kristi E. Gamarel, and Don Operario

Sexual and gender minority (SGM) communities in the United States have experienced a rise in visibility and social–political attention during the past decade. From popular culture to academic literature, awareness of SGM-related issues and experiences has provided unique opportunities to consider the psychological health and well-being of these communities. The 2011 report by the Institute of Medicine on the health of lesbian, gay, bisexual, transgender, and queer (LGBTQ) people articulated a groundbreaking research agenda and call for action to improve the health of SGM communities. It highlighted the relative lack of studies on SGM youth, especially SGM youth of color, and expressed concern about the behavioral health problems documented in research with these communities. Indeed, despite social media efforts to promote self-esteem and reduce SGM youth bullying, evidence of risk for alcohol and other substance use and co-occurring psychological problems in these populations demands research and intervention.

The aim of this chapter is threefold. First, we review literature on prevalence and etiology of substance use and misuse in SGM youth. Second, we describe strategies for reducing alcohol and other substance use in SGM youth, including relevant individual, family, and structural approaches. Finally, we provide recommendations for culturally competent counseling and services. The inclusive acronym SGM refers to two groups of youth: youth who experience same-sex attractions or same-sex behaviors (i.e., sexual minority [SM]), and/or youth whose gender identity or gender expression do not align with their sex assigned at birth (i.e., gender minority [GM]). Concepts or literature reviewed might be relevant for SGM youth as a collective group, or might be uniquely relevant to either SM or GM youth. Indeed, because of the paucity of literature on GM youth and the important distinctions between GM and SM youth, findings from studies of SM youth might not be generalizable to GM youth.

PREVALENCE OF SUBSTANCE USE
AND MISUSE AMONG SGM YOUTH

Studies show that SGM youth are at higher risk than heterosexual and non-transgender youth for substance use as well as many other poor mental health conditions (e.g., depression, anxiety, suicidality) and risky health behaviors (Corliss et al., 2014; Coulter et al., 2015; Goldbach, Mereish, & Burgess, 2017; Marshal et al., 2011; Reisner, Greytak, Parsons, & Ybarra, 2015; Rosario et al., 2013). For example, SM youth are more likely to use tobacco, marijuana, alcohol, and illicit drugs, as well as misuse prescription drugs than their heterosexual counterparts (Corliss et al., 2010, 2014; Goldbach et al., 2017; Rosario et al., 2013). In fact, results of a meta-analysis found that SM youth had 190% higher odds of any substance use than heterosexual youth (Marshal et al., 2008). This study also found that these risks are especially high within some SM youth subpopulations. Specifically, bisexual youth had 340% higher odds and SM females had 400% higher odds of substance use compared with heterosexual youth. Substance use is also prevalent among GM youth (Rowe, Santos, McFarland, & Wilson, 2015). Transgender youth are at greater risk for substance use, including alcohol, marijuana, and illicit drugs, and are more likely to have alcohol-related problems compared with nontransgender youth (Coulter et al., 2015; Reisner, Greytak, et al., 2015). Moreover, SM youth are twice as likely to be under the influence of substance use while having sex, putting them at greater risk for other adverse health outcomes such as sexually transmitted infections and HIV (Herrick, Marshal, Smith, Sucato, & Stall, 2011). With few exceptions (Corliss et al., 2014), a major limitation of this research is the lack of focus on SM youth of color and data identifying disparities among diverse GM youth.

ETIOLOGY OF SGM YOUTHS'
SUBSTANCE USE AND MISUSE

Several factors can inform the etiology of substance use and misuse among SGM youth. It is important to first note that SGM youth may use substances for similar reasons as their heterosexual and/or nontransgender counterparts (e.g., experimentation, peer pressure, to relieve tension or self-medicate, family history). However, there are unique factors that may explain elevated risk among SGM youth (Center for Substance Abuse Treatment, 2001; Green & Feinstein, 2012). For instance, the process of sexual or gender identity development might be especially stressful or challenging for SGM youth (Saewyc, 2011; Savin-Williams & Cohen, 2015), and substances may be used in an attempt to help ease this process.

SGM youth experience a range of adverse stressors as well as stigma-specific stressors. Meta-analyses show that SM youth are more likely than heterosexuals to have higher rates of traumatic stressors, such as childhood sexual abuse, parental physical abuse, assault at school, and verbal and physical victimization, and findings suggest these stressors are commonly associated with substance use (Friedman et al., 2011; Katz-Wise & Hyde, 2012). In addition, SM youth are more likely than heterosexual youth to experience interpersonal violence (i.e., physical, psychological, sexual, and cyber dating violence; Dank, Lachman, Zweig, & Yahner, 2014). Furthermore, GM youth experience higher rates of verbal and physical abuse by parents and peers (Grossman, D'Augelli, & Frank, 2011), and they experience higher rates of victimization (i.e., bullying and harassment) than nontransgender peers (Reisner, Greytak, et al., 2015). SGM youth are also disproportionately more likely to experience homelessness during adolescence (Corliss, Goodenow, Nichols, & Austin, 2011; Durso & Gates, 2012; Keuroghlian, Shtasel, & Bassuk, 2014).

In addition to the aforementioned adverse stressors, SGM youth experience unique and chronic stigma stressors (i.e., minority stressors) that are related to their stigmatized sexual or GM identities (Meyer, 2003), which also contribute to their risk for substance use (Collier, van Beusekom, Bos, & Sandfort, 2013; Goldbach, Fisher, & Dunlap, 2015; Goldbach, Tanner-Smith, Bagwell, & Dunlap, 2014; Rowe et al., 2015). According to the minority stress model, minority stressors range from direct experiences of stigma and discrimination (e.g., homophobic bullying, rejecting reactions from parents, victimization, or harassment) to the internalization of stigma (i.e., internalized heterosexism or transphobia), the development of expectations of stigma, and the concealment of one's SGM identity (Meyer, 2003). In one study, 81.9% of SM youth were verbally harassed, 38.3% were physically harassed, 18.3% were physically assaulted, and 55.2% were electronically harassed in the past year because of their sexual orientation (Kosciw, Greytak, Bartkiewicz, Boesen, & Palmer, 2012). Similarly, GM youth experience significant minority stressors and pervasive harassment and negative school climates (McGuire, Anderson, Toomey, & Russell, 2010).

A recent review of the literature found that the strongest risk factors for problematic substance use among SM youth were the combination of chronic adverse stressors, minority stressors, co-occurring internalizing and externalizing problem behaviors, homelessness, and a lack of supportive school and family environments (Goldbach et al., 2014). SGM youth may be using substances as a coping mechanism to deal with these chronic and adverse experiences (Bux, 1996). These stressors also "get under the skin" because they may cause emotional dysregulation, social and interpersonal problems, and maladaptive cognitive processes, which consequently put SGM youth at risk for problematic substance use and other poor health outcomes (Hatzenbuehler, 2009).

Etiological factors contributing to substance use among SGM youth also reside in the social environment. Due to a long history of limited access to affirming and safe social settings, SGM adults utilized bars as their main social outlets, and persistent bar patronage and bar-based communities may put them at greater risk for alcohol and other substance use (Green & Feinstein, 2012). In addition, there is evidence to show that companies (e.g., tobacco and alcohol industries) use targeted marketing of the LGBTQ community, even to SGM youth, and that SGM individuals are more likely to be exposed to substance use marketing than heterosexuals (Dilley, Spigner, Boysun, Dent, & Pizacani, 2008; Goebel, 1994; Washington, 2002). As a consequence of these environmental factors, substance use has become a part of the cultural norms of SGMs, affecting social norms and network dynamics related to substance use risk behaviors among SGM youth (Hatzenbuehler, Corbin, & Fromme, 2008; Hatzenbuehler, McLaughlin, & Xuan, 2015; Litt, Lewis, Rhew, Hodge, & Kaysen, 2015; Mereish, Goldbach, Burgess, & DiBello, 2017). For example, research shows that social networks of SM youth are more likely than heterosexual youth to comprise individuals who use alcohol and tobacco (Hatzenbuehler, McLaughlin, et al., 2015), and permissive social norms may help explain sexual orientation disparities in substance use (Mereish et al., 2017) .

EXISTING INTERVENTIONS TARGETING SUBSTANCE MISUSE

To prevent the onset and progression of substance use disorders (SUDs) among SGM youth, providers and programs must address the specific factors that cause SUDs in order to intervene directly to help young people. To date, few interventions have been developed and tested to intervene directly on substance use behaviors among SGM youth. Individual-level interventions with this population have been developed specifically to reduce HIV risk and co-occurring drug use among young adult SM men. Additional empirical evidence provides support for focusing beyond the individual, with family- and structural-level interventions designed to promote acceptance and changes in norms and social policies demonstrating strong potential for improving the health of SGM youth.

Individual Intervention Approaches

To our knowledge, there are no inperson individual-level intervention approaches developed and tested to specifically target SUDs among SGM youth. Given the increasing incidence of HIV among gay and bisexual male adolescents and young adults (Centers for Disease Control and Prevention, 2011, 2013), research has focused primarily on the development, implementation, and evaluation of HIV prevention programs that simultaneously target substance use (Harper, 2007). Reviews of HIV behavioral interventions highlight the paucity of empirically supported, youth-specific HIV prevention interventions, and particularly those that also target alcohol and other drug use (Harper & Riplinger, 2012; Mustanski, Newcomb, Du Bois, Garcia, & Grov, 2011).

Interventions for non-treatment-seeking SM populations need to be delivered in a nonjudgmental and nonthreatening manner in order to reach those who are ambivalent about changing their behavior (Parsons, Vial, Starks, & Golub, 2012). Thus, intervention approaches such as brief motivational interviewing (MI)—characterized by a collaborative, client-centered approach to enhancing motivation to change—have been commonly utilized to reduce HIV risk and co-occurring substance use behaviors (Parsons, Lelutiu-Weinberger, Botsko, & Golub, 2014). Despite the efficacy of MI in reducing substance use in adolescents (Barnett, Sussman, Smith, Rohrbach, & Spruijt-Metz, 2012), youth living with HIV (Murphy, Chen, Naar-King, & Parsons, 2011), and gay and bisexual adult males (Berg, Ross, & Tikkanen, 2011; Morgenstern et al., 2009), to our knowledge, only one study has tested the efficacy of a brief MI in reducing drug use and condomless anal sex among young HIV-negative gay and bisexual males ages 18–29 (Parsons et al., 2014). This specific MI consisted of four sessions, designed to provide information on club drugs and the risk of condomless sex with casual male partners, in order to enhance motivation and personal responsibility as well as establish goals for reducing both health behaviors. Participants who received MI showed reductions in club drug use and condomless sex over a 12-month period compared with those in a psychoeducation control condition, which included information only on club drug use and HIV risk (Parsons et al., 2014).

In the first session, the therapist provided an overview of the MI approach, as well as a "values card sort" exercise to identify values that were personally valued (Miller, C'de Baca, Matthews, & Wilbourne, 2001). Young men were asked which of two behaviors they wanted to focus on first (condomless sex or substance use), and the therapist elicited participants' views about the target behavior using MI techniques. Session 2 followed a similar format, with focus on the other target behavior, which was then followed by delivering personalized feedback about both target behaviors assessed during the baseline visit. Session 3 focused on facilitating participants' progress toward readiness to change, addressed motivations, and affirmed any commitments to change. The two target behaviors were discussed and participants were asked to reexamine their readiness to change and goals for both behaviors. The final session focused on termination and included a review and revisions of goals and the change plan. In this final session, participants were also provided with resources and services, as well as an emphasis on relapse prevention if any change had occurred.

Cognitive-behavioral therapy (CBT) approaches have also demonstrated promise in improving cognitive, affective, and behavioral minority stress processes and substance use behaviors in adult populations (Balsam, Martell, & Safren, 2006; Pachankis, 2015; Pachankis, Hatzenbuehler, Rendina, Safren, & Parsons, 2015; Safren, Hollander, Hart, & Heimberg, 2001). While there have been a number of case studies of LGB-affirmative CBT approaches applied to SM individuals' mental health (Kaysen, Lostutter, & Goines, 2005; Safren, 2005; Walsh & Hope, 2010), only one known study of this approach has been tested and demonstrated preliminary efficacy among young adult SM men ages 18–35 (Pachankis et al., 2015). CBT approaches place maladaptive behaviors in the context of their developmental function and environmental context, such as viewing substance use as a learned response for coping with minority stress, and can empower clients to cope with adversity such as minority stress (Pachankis, 2015; Pachankis et al., 2015). This intervention, Effective Skills to Empower Effective Men (ESTEEM), consisted of 10 inperson sessions based on *Unified Protocol for the Transdiagnostic Treatment of Emotion Disorders* (Barlow et al., 2010), which involves individually delivered CBT for reducing stress-sensitive mental disorders (e.g., anxiety and depression) by enhancing emotion regulation abilities; reducing maladaptive cognitive, affective, and behavioral patterns; and improving motivation and self-efficacy for enacting the desired behavior (Pachankis et al., 2015). The protocol was adapted to enhance young SM males' stigma coping by reducing minority stress (Pachankis et al., 2015). The program involved discussions of the impact of minority stress on health, strategies for mindful and present-focused reactions to minority stress, and a range of cognitive and emotional strategies for coping with minority stress (see Pachankis, 2015; Pachankis et al., 2015, for details). Findings illustrated that participation in ESTEEM reduced depressive symptoms, alcohol use problems, sexual compulsivity, and condomless anal sex with casual partners, and improved condom use self-efficacy compared to a wait-list comparison (Pachankis et al., 2015).

Like other adolescents and young adults, SGM youth often seek out health information online (Pingel, Bauermeister, Johns, Eisenberg, & Leslie-Santana, 2013; Pingel, Thomas, Harmell, & Bauermeister, 2013). As a result, e-Health interventions have garnered increasing attention as a potential model of substance use prevention, given their appeal to young people. In addition, in-office interventions may not sufficiently target those most at risk who are often not linked to services (Carballo-Diéguez, Miner, Dolezal, Rosser, & Jacoby, 2006; Hooper, Rosser, Horvath, Oakes, & Danilenko, 2008). Evidence indicates that SM young people are significantly more likely to delay or avoid seeking services compared with their heterosexual counterparts due to perceived provider bias and a relative lack of visibility of competent services and treatment providers (Krehely, 2009). We identified only one tailored, web-based intervention designed to prevent drug use among young SM males and females (Schwinn, Thom, Schinke, & Hopkins, 2015). This consisted of a three-session intervention in which animated narrators led youth through tailored content and practice scenarios that included interactive games, role-playing, and writing activities for identifying and managing stress, making decisions, and providing feedback on drug use prevalence information and refusal rates. The intervention arm demonstrated reductions in stress, peer drug use, and past-30-day illicit drug use, but no differences in alcohol, cigarette, and marijuana use were found at 3 months.

Given the impact of substance use on HIV risk behaviors, several e-health interventions have been designed for SM males. A systematic review identified nine published e-health interventions designed to address HIV and substance use (Young, Swendeman, Holloway, Reback, & Kao, 2015)—however, only one focused on young SM males. These nine studies used text messaging, interactive voice response, social media chats, smartphone apps, and websites to implement some or all intervention activities. These interventions used technology for self-monitoring, reminders, feedback, automated and tailored messaging, live chats on social media or text messaging, and social support. While these interventions hold promise in reducing substance use and HIV risk, only one study specifically focused on young SM males. Specifically, Motivational Interviewing Communication about Health, Attitudes, and Thoughts (MiChat) tested the feasibility, acceptability, and promise of a social media intervention designed to reduce substance use and condomless anal sex among young HIV-negative SM men ages 18–29 (Lelutiu-Weinberger et al., 2014). Guided by MI and CBT principles, MiChat consisted of eight sessions that delivered through the Facebook chat function with a live counselor. Guided by the inperson MI intervention (Parsons et al., 2014), MiChat used MI techniques to elicit change in both drug use and condomless sex. The first three sessions focused on building rapport, understanding participants' views of each of the target behaviors, and discussing their pros and cons. In Session 3, the therapist also explored sex and drug use through having participants complete a writing exercise in which they were asked to reflect on their sexual and substance use behaviors. Session 4 explored the influences on their sexual behaviors and drug use, and Session 5 reviewed progress and focused on identifying harm reduction skills. Sessions 6–7 reviewed progress, assessed barriers, and continued to discuss additional harm reduction skills. Results showed decreases in HIV risk as well as trends for alcohol and drug use over the 8-week intervention (Lelutiu-Weinberger et al., 2014).

While individual-level interventions hold promise in reducing substance use, research has yet to develop and test interventions for diverse SGM groups, such as young SM female adolescents, transgender individuals, and SGM youth under the age of 18. There is a real need to develop and test substance use prevention interventions outside of the context of HIV. This is particularly important as young SM females, and particularly bisexual females, demonstrate significant disparities in a range of substance use behaviors, such as tobacco, marijuana, and alcohol use (Marshal et al., 2008). While these individual-level intervention approaches show promise, substance use is initiated and sustained within a larger social context, including families, neighborhoods, peer groups, and schools (Stockdale et al., 2007).

Family Intervention Approaches

Given evidence illustrating strong associations between discrimination, victimization, and family rejection and substance use behaviors, interventions aimed at addressing family and social systems have also been developed for SGM youth. Evidence from the Family Acceptance Project® (FAP) illustrates that family rejection severely impacts the health of SGM youth, contributing to suicide attempts, depression, drug use, and condomless sex (Ryan, Huebner, Diaz, & Sanchez, 2009). Based on extensive research with LGB youth, young adults, and families (*http://familyproject.sfsu.edu*), FAP has developed family-focused intervention strategies, resources, and tools that can be used by health, social service, and school-based providers in different systems of care. FAP encourages providers to use their assessment tools so that at-risk SGM youth can be identified and families can receive help in increasing support, decreasing risk, reducing conflict, retaining youth in the home, and reconnecting families. Despite the promise of FAP, its efficacy has not been empirically tested.

Structural Intervention Approaches

Changes in norms, policies, and systems in order to reduce stigma and provide an affirming space for SGM youth have the potential to improve SUDs for these young people. Among adolescents and young adults, schools are a critical social context that contributes to the development of positive health. Over the last decade there has been a movement to be more inclusive of SGM youth in schools. Thousands of high schools across the United States have supported gay–straight alliance (GSA) organizations within school settings. A GSA is a school-based club that works to create a supportive school environment for all students, regardless of sexual orientation and/or gender identity and expression. A burgeoning body of literature suggests that attending a high school with a GSA can reduce the burden of minority stressors (Goodenow, Szalacha, & Westheimer, 2006; Heck et al., 2014; Poteat, Sinclair, DiGiovanni, Koenig, & Russell, 2013). Specifically, SGM youth attending schools with GSAs report experiencing less school-based victimization, a greater sense of school belonging, and less concealment of their SM statuses (Goodenow et al., 2006; Heck, Flentje, & Cochran, 2011). Importantly, GSAs have been shown to be associated with a reduced risk for suicide in adolescents (Goodenow et al., 2006), which extends into young adulthood (Toomey, Ryan, Diaz, & Russell, 2011). Furthermore, attending a school with a GSA has been linked to lower substance use behaviors among SGM youth and young adults (Heck et al., 2014; Poteat et al., 2013).

Notably, social policies addressing SGM persons have emerged over the last decade. For example, the U.S. Supreme Court's reversal of the Defense of Marriage Act (DOMA) in 2013 and the 2015 *Obergefell v. Hodges* decision that legally recognized same-sex marriage represent recent victories. While gay marriage has received the most attention, other policies have also been prominent in public discourse, including hate crime protections, employment discrimination, military service, gay adoption, migration equality, and the invalidation of state sodomy laws. In 2009, the U.S. Congress passed the Matthew Shepard Hate Crimes Prevention Act, which is a comprehensive hate crimes bill specifically protecting LGB people. Evidence indicates that LGB youth are at a lower risk of psychiatric disorders if they live in counties where a greater proportion of school districts have antibullying policies that include sexual orientation (Hatzenbuehler, Birkett, Van Wagenen, & Meyer, 2013; Hatzenbuehler & Keyes, 2013). Further evidence indicates that young SM males who live in states with fewer legal protections and more negative attitudes toward SMs have greater risk of substance use behaviors (Pachankis, Hatzenbuehler, & Starks, 2014). Such state-level policies that differentially exclude SGM people—such as the lack of employment nondiscrimination policies and negative attitudes toward SGM people—represent "structural stigma" (Hatzenbuehler & Link, 2014). In fact, one study found that SM adolescents are more likely to be at risk for marijuana and illicit drug use when living in states that have high structural stigma (i.e., fewer same-sex partner households, GSAs, and state-level policies related to the protection of SM people, as well as negative public opinion toward SMs) compared with adolescents who resided in states that had lower structural stigma (Hatzenbuehler, Jun, Corliss, & Bryn Austin, 2015).

To our knowledge, no studies have examined the impact of structural stigma on substance use among transgender and gender nonconforming youth. Recent years have witnessed a movement to be more inclusive of transgender people in nondiscrimination policies. For example, numerous states have passed laws to provide transgender people with equal protections in employment, housing, and education (Transgender Law and Policy Institute, 2012). While empirical work has yet to test the effects of these protective policies on the health of transgender people, one study of transgender adults in Massachusetts found that experiences of discrimination in health care settings were independently associated with adverse mental and physical symptoms, as well as with an increased risk of postponing needed care when sick or injured (Reisner, Hughto, et al., 2015). Additionally, access to gender transition-related care represents an important structural factor that can have a positive impact on the health of transgender people. In 2010, the Affordable Care Act (ACA) made it illegal for insurance companies to deny individuals on the basis of preexisting conditions and gender identity. The ACA provided low-income people with access to gender-affirmation therapies through Medicaid (Patient Protection and Affordable Care Act, 2010). Such structural-level interventions can promote immediate health benefits for transgender youth through increased access to care, as well as create a shift in societal attitudes by increasing public awareness of transgender issues (White Hughto, Reisner, & Pachankis, 2015).

RECOMMENDATIONS FOR SGM YOUTH-AFFIRMING AND CULTURALLY COMPETENT CLINICAL CARE

There are many important therapeutic considerations that clinicians should take into account when working with SGM youth. Here we review the literature related to LGBTQ-competent clinical care. It is important to note that some of this literature is specific to adult clients, and providers need to be sensitive to the developmental needs of their adolescents. Nonetheless, existing efficacious empirically supported treatments (e.g., MI; Barnett et al., 2012) that have been tested with the general adolescent population should also be considered with SGM youth. However, it is essential to culturally adapt these interventions to incorporate some of the aforementioned sociocultural etiological factors into treatment and continuously evaluate their efficacy, as well as practice from a culturally competent and LGBTQ-affirming approach (Center for Substance Abuse Treatment, 2001; Lee, 2015). Clinicians must be cognizant that SGM youths' treatment is complex and multifaceted, considering the developmental and sociocultural demands and stressors SGM youth face (Keuroghlian, Reisner, White, & Weiss, 2015; Saewyc, 2011). In fact, SGM adult clients seeking substance abuse treatment often have more severe substance abuse problems and psychiatric conditions compared with their heterosexual counterparts (Cochran & Cauce, 2006). The following two case vignettes are used to help illustrate our clinical recommendations.

Case Example 1

Max is a 13-year-old biracial young male. His parents recently divorced and he lives with his mother who struggles with alcoholism. Max is performing poorly academically, often refuses to go to school, and sometimes skips school altogether. He is involved with his local LGBTQ youth organization. At his intake, Max reports heavy drinking and marijuana use, much conflict with his mother, and relationship issues with his boyfriend, whom Max's mother is not aware that Max is dating.

Case Example 2

Kim is a 17-year-old white young transgender woman who is a patient at a substance use residential facility. Kim presents with a severe alcohol use disorder and a tobacco use disorder. At the intake session, the therapist asked Kim for her gender pronouns, as he asks of all his clients, and Kim identified her pronouns as she/her/hers and is also comfortable with they/them/their pronouns. Kim's gender expression is gender neutral. The therapist noticed that Kim's parents as well as other patients and some staff at the clinical facility have incorrectly used male pronouns when referring to Kim, such as he/him/his. At school, Kim does not have gender-neutral facilities and is forced to use men's bathrooms. She experiences a lot of transphobic bullying and family conflict related to coming out as transgender.

Similar to all adolescents, SGM youth value clinical providers who are respectful, honest, professional, nonjudgmental, and who will maintain confidentiality (Ginsburg et al., 2002; Hoffman, Freeman, & Swann, 2009). SGM youth also report that the provider's gender or sexual orientation has little importance to them (Hoffman et al., 2009). At the same time, SGM youth also value validating, affirming, and culturally competent clinicians who have knowledge in the unique issues experienced by SGM youth (Ginsburg et al., 2002; Hoffman et al., 2009). Being culturally competent involves reflecting on, acknowledging, and addressing one's own biases, stereotypes, privileges, and implicit and explicit prejudiced attitudes toward SGM youth and other oppressed groups. This is especially important because many treatment counselors, especially heterosexual providers, report negative or ambivalent attitudes toward LGBTQ clients (Cochran, Peavy, & Cauce, 2007; Eliason & Hughes, 2004). Clinical staff must also recognize SGM youth clients' other intersecting identities (e.g., race/ethnicity) and how they might be related to other forms of oppression and obstacles to treatment. Additionally, research shows that treatment counselors lack basic knowledge about the experiences of LGBTQ individuals (e.g., experiences of homophobia, coming out) and have little formal education regarding the needs of LGBTQ clients (Eliason & Hughes, 2004). Thus, there is a great need for ongoing training and education to help providers learn more about SGM youth clients' health needs, community, and culture, as well as effective and competent clinical care (Center for Substance Abuse Treatment, 2001). The National LGBT Health Education Center (*www. lgbthealtheducation.org*) offers LGBTQ trainings to providers, including online videos, learning modules, and webinars.

With the intention to be culturally competent, the therapist in Max's case spent a lot of time inquiring about Max being gay and conceptualized his presenting concerns to be related to his sexual orientation. However, this well-meaning therapist incorrectly assumed that Max's sexual orientation is primarily related to his presenting concerns, when in fact the etiology of his substance use is related to his preexisting family history of alcoholism, including his mother's heavy drinking, his parents' divorce, and school difficulties. The therapist also missed the opportunity to identify one of Max's strengths— his involvement in the LGBTQ organization. Finally, the therapist's sole focus on Max's sexual orientation prevented her from learning about the frequent racist microaggressive experiences he endures. Clearly, Max's therapist would benefit from further continuing education regarding LGBTQ care.

Safe and Affirming Therapeutic Milieus

Research points to the need for a safe and affirming therapeutic milieu for SGM youth clients (Hicks, 2000; Lombardi & van Servellen, 2000; Lyons et al., 2015; Rowan, Jenkins, & Parks, 2013; Senreich, 2011) and for affirmative practice that promotes self-acceptance (Center for Substance Abuse Treatment, 2001). It is the clinical staff's responsibility to maintain and protect the safety of all clients, especially SGM youth. Clinical staff can create safety for SGM youth by adopting and publicly posting nondiscrimination policies that explicitly include sexual orientation and gender identity, and by providing ongoing professional trainings for staff (Center for Substance Abuse Treatment, 2001). In Kim's case, the therapist must intervene with the other staff and patients to ensure that they are aware of Kim's correct pronouns and the importance of addressing all patients with appropriate pronouns. The staff would also benefit from cultural competency training in transgender and other GM health care.

In addition to program policies, clinicians might consider making the physical space of their facility a safe and welcoming space by displaying rainbow flags or stickers and putting LGBTQ-affirming magazines or posters in waiting rooms. SGM youth value when providers do not make assumptions about their sexual orientation or gender identity or about the cause of their substance use, and when providers do not pathologize their sexuality and gender expression (Ginsburg et al., 2002; Hoffman et al., 2009). Clinicians should not label clients' identities and allow clients' to describe themselves in terms of gender and sexual identity. In Max's case, the therapist had several LGBTQ-related materials publicly displayed in her office, which allowed Max to feel comfortable disclosing that he had a boyfriend. However, the therapist considered Max as gay because he has a boyfriend. Due to the therapist's lack of knowledge and awareness of bisexuality, she mistook Max as gay, when in fact he identifies as bisexual. She allowed her assumptions to influence her assessment of Max's sexual orientation without providing him the opportunity to inform her of his sexual orientation. Max's therapist would benefit from incorporating sexual orientation assessments in her intake forms.

Treatment Considerations

The Center for Substance Abuse Treatment (CSAT) of the Substance Abuse and Mental Health Services Administration (SAMHSA) published comprehensive guidelines and information for working with SGM youth clients (Center for Substance Abuse Treatment, 2001). CSAT recommends that substance abuse treatment staff evaluate their assessment practices, consider appropriate modalities, and develop effective discharge and aftercare plans for SGM youth. As with any substance abuse treatment, a comprehensive assessment is essential. Thus, staff should review their intake and assessment forms and protocols to be culturally sensitive, and include assessment questions regarding sexual orientation and gender identity as well as experiences of minority stressors and identity disclosure and transition. For example, clinicians are encouraged to assess three dimensions of sexual orientation: (1) sexual orientation self-identification such as lesbian, gay, bisexual, queer, and heterosexual; (2) sexual attractions; and (3) sexual behaviors. Based on much research, the Fenway Institute's suggestions on how to assess sexual orientation identity are illustrated in Figure 12.1 (Bradford, Cahill, Grasso, & Makadon, 2012). An "other" fill-in response option can also be added to allow youth to identify their sexual orientation in ways not provided (e.g., pansexual). Moreover, the Williams Institute has published a detailed report on how to assess other sexual orientation dimensions (Sexual Minority Assessment Research Team, 2009). In addition to sexual orientation, clinicians are encouraged to assess for gender identity using the two-step method of assessing current gender identity and assigned sex at birth (Cahill & Makadon, 2013). Figure 12.2 illustrates this method. An "other" fill-in response option for gender identity can also be added to allow youth to identify their gender identity in ways not listed (e.g., nonbinary, gender fluid). Both assessments can also be added to patients' medical records. Clinicians should emphasize building an affirming therapeutic relationship and provide comprehensive case management. An essential part of therapeutic relationships with adolescents is confidentiality, which at times might be complicated for SGM youth. Thus, clinicians must be transparent with clients about the terms of confidentiality and ways they will navigate their clients' privacy, especially related to their sexual orientation or gender identity. For Max, the therapist must discuss with him whether, and if necessary, how they should address him having a boyfriend with his mother, given her lack of awareness of his relationship and potentially his sexual orientation.

In considering therapeutic modalities, staff members must create a safe clinical context in group counseling and directly address any homophobia or transphobia that might come up. Family counseling is also another challenging but yet essential clinical factor to consider. Given that parents or other

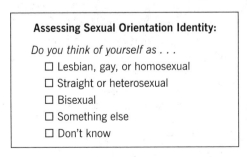

FIGURE 12.1. Suggested method to assess sexual orientation identity.

Assessing Gender Identity:

1. *What sex were you assigned at birth?*
   ☐ Male
   ☐ Female
   ☐ Decline to state

2. *What is your current gender identity?*
   ☐ Male
   ☐ Female
   ☐ Transgender boy/man/transboy/transman
   ☐ Transgender girl/woman/transgirl/transwoman
   ☐ Genderqueer
   ☐ Decline to state

FIGURE 12.2. Suggested two-step method to assess gender identity.

family members are crucial for SGM youths' resilience (Bouris et al., 2010), it is important that clinicians understand their client's comfort with discussing their SGM identities with their families and work to educate and support families. Other helpful family intervention tools may be adapted from the aforementioned FAP intervention.

In Kim's case, the therapist noticed her parents use the wrong pronouns. Therefore, with permission from Kim, the therapist must address these issues with her family. Moreover, given that Kim experiences much conflict with her family related to them misunderstanding her transgender identity, the therapist must advocate for Kim and provide her family with psychoeducation and resources regarding GM youth.

Finally, discharge and aftercare planning includes making appropriate referrals to SGM- affirming clinical providers, SGM-specific 12-step meetings, or community-based (e.g., Parents, Families and Friends of Lesbians and Gays [PFLAG]) or school-based organizations (e.g., GSAs) or other support services (e.g., legal supports from organizations such as GLBTQ Legal Advocates & Defenders). Given the high prevalence and negative effects of homophobic and transphobic bullying on youths' health and academic functioning (Poteat, Mereish, DiGiovanni, & Koenig, 2011), staff should help SGM youth who experience bullying and their families secure safe and supportive school services. In Kim's case, there are several aftercare planning steps that are needed for a successful discharge. Example aftercare planning includes connecting Kim with appropriate and culturally affirmative transgender medical and mental health care providers. In addition, given her bullying experiences and lack of access to gender-neutral facilities at school, discharge planning should include educating Kim and her family about her rights at school regarding bullying and access to facilities as well as advocating for Kim by contacting the school to set appropriate and affirmative services at school.

Conceptualizing and Contextualizing SGM Clients' Substance Misuse

Providers should, when appropriate, conceptualize their SGM clients' substance abuse concerns in the context of societal stigma, prejudice, and/or oppression. For example, in Kim's case, much of her addiction is related to the constant transphobic bullying and discrimination she experiences at home and school. Thus, she turned to alcohol and cigarettes as a way to numb and manage the negative emotions she experiences as a result of oppression. Young SGM clients may carry shame associated with their stigmatized identities and experiences of minority stress (Mereish & Poteat, 2015)—thus, clinicians should help them normalize their experiences and affirm their identities and experiences. Specifically, in order to work through recovery while addressing minority stressors, and guided by the *Unified Protocol for the Transdiagnostic Treatment of Emotion Disorders* (Barlow et al., 2010), the aforementioned ESTEEM treatment protocol might be a promising evidence-based treatment that providers may integrate into their existing clinical practices (Pachankis, 2015; Pachankis et al., 2015).

Additional Considerations for Young SM Clients

When working with SM youth, clinicians should be respectful of their clients' coming out process and validate their positioning in that process (Center for Substance Abuse Treatment, 2001). Although coming out is a source of resilience for SM youth, clinicians must not attempt to pressure clients to come out, especially since outness can be associated with higher rates of victimization (Kosciw, Palmer, & Kull, 2014). Moreover, it is important to recognize that adolescence is a developmental period for sexual orientation, sexuality, and identity exploration and development—thus, youth may be questioning of their identities and/or change how they identify during this process (Saewyc, 2011; Savin-Williams & Cohen, 2015). Additionally, as demonstrated with Max, clinicians must acknowledge the fluidity of sexual orientation as well as the validity and distinction of bisexuality or pansexuality from heterosexuality and homosexuality.

Additional Considerations for Young GM Clients

GM clients face unique challenges and obstacles with substance abuse treatment. Research shows that GM clients experience less access to treatment due to discrimination, less therapeutic support from clinicians, lower satisfaction with treatment, and poorer treatment outcomes than heterosexual and SM clients (Lombardi & van Servellen, 2000; Lyons et al., 2015; Senreich, 2011).

For example, consistent with Kim's experience, a recent study of transgender individuals who have been in residential addiction treatment found that many experienced social rejection, violence, and transphobia, which forced them to prematurely end treatment. Given these obstacles, it is crucial that clinicians receive formal training focused on GM health and ongoing clinical supervision and consultation when working with GM youth. In fact, transgender individuals who attended programs that are inclusive and respectful have positive treatment experiences (Lyons et al., 2015).

In addition to receiving further professional training, SAMHSA's CSAT has some specific clinical recommendations when working with GMs (Center for Substance Abuse Treatment, 2001). Clinical staff must allow GM youth to use appropriate facilities (e.g., restrooms, showers, bedrooms, or housing) that are congruent with the client's gender identity or create gender-neutral facilities (e.g., gender-neutral restrooms). In Kim's case, the therapist worked with the clinical staff to initially find a temporary room to house her until they arranged a roommate situation that was supportive of Kim. Moreover, the clinical staff turned a single- occupancy bathroom into a gender-neutral bathroom by posting a gender-neutral sign and informing patients in the residential facility about the gender-neutral bathroom. This allowed Kim to have safe access to a bathroom during her stay.

Clinicians should ask all clients for their pronouns and should treat all clients with respect by using the pronouns that the client identifies when talking to or about clients. In Kim's case, during the unit's community group meeting, the therapist asked all patients to introduce themselves and identify their pronouns, which is part of his customary group routine. This normalized pronoun disclosure helped Kim feel comfortable disclosing her gender pronouns, and educated all other patients about all patients' correct pronouns.

It is crucial that clinicians discuss with their transgender clients whether they are using hormones, such as testosterone or estrogen, and how they obtain them. Given that many transgender youth experience obstacles in receiving medical care, they often obtain hormones through underground or illicit methods, which also puts them at greater risk for substance use and HIV risk behaviors (Lombardi & van Servellen, 2000). Therefore, to further help with relapse prevention, clinicians should help transgender clients get connected to affirming medical care where they can obtain prescribed hormones (Center for Substance Abuse Treatment, 2001; Lombardi & van Servellen, 2000). As such, in Kim's case, the therapist inquired about Kim's hormone use and helped her become connected to a local doctor who prescribed hormones.

FUTURE DIRECTIONS

There is a growing need for specialized SGM-tailored substance abuse treatment programs and/or separate units or facilities (Bux, 1996; Cochran, Peavy,

& Robohm, 2007; Hicks, 2000; Rowan et al., 2013). Although specialized programs currently exist for SGM clients, a review of these treatment programs found that 71% of them provided services that are comparable to general programs and only a small percentage offered tailored services that meet the needs of LGBT clients (Cochran, Peavy, & Robohm, 2007). Thus, more tailored and specialized substance treatment programs are needed for SGM youth.

Research on SGM youth has focused on white and middle-class SM youth. There is much less research on GM youth, racially diverse SGM youth, bisexual and pansexual youth, and youth from socioeconomically disadvantaged backgrounds. Despite SM girls and bisexual youth being at greatest risk for substance abuse (Marshal et al., 2008), there is limited attention to their experiences in treatment. Research is needed to better understand these youths' substance use, other health needs, and treatment outcomes. Moreover, there is a need to utilize longitudinal studies to examine etiological factors associated with and trajectories of SGM youths' substance use from and throughout adolescence and into adulthood. Finally, considering the dearth of empirically based treatments for SGM youths' substance use, more research is needed to examine effective and affirming interventions for SGM youth.

REFERENCES

Balsam, K. F., Martell, C. R., & Safren, S. A. (2006). Affirmative cognitive-behavioral therapy with lesbian, gay, and bisexual people. In P. A. Hays & G. Y. Iwamasa (Eds.), *Culturally responsive cognitive-behavioral therapy: Assessment, practice, and supervision* (pp. 223–243). Washington, DC: American Psychological Association.

Barlow, D. H., Farchione, T. J., Fairholme, C. P., Ellard, K. K., Boisseau, C. L., Allen, L. B., et al. (2010). *Unified protocol for transdiagnostic treatment of emotional disorders: Therapist guide.* New York: Oxford University Press.

Barnett, E., Sussman, S., Smith, C., Rohrbach, L. A., & Spruijt-Metz, D. (2012). Motivational interviewing for adolescent substance use: A review of the literature. *Addictive Behaviors, 37*(12), 1325–1334.

Berg, R. C., Ross, M. W., & Tikkanen, R. (2011). The effectiveness of MI4MSM: How useful is motivational interviewing as an HIV risk prevention program for men who have sex with men?: A systematic review. *AIDS Education and Prevention, 23*(6), 533–549.

Bouris, A., Guilamo-Ramos, V., Pickard, A., Shiu, C., Loosier, P. S., Dittus, P., et al. (2010). A systematic review of parental influences on the health and well-being of lesbian, gay, and bisexual youth: Time for a new public health research and practice agenda. *Journal of Primary Prevention, 31*(5), 273–309.

Bradford, J., Cahill, S., Grasso, C., & Makadon, H. (2012). *How to ask about sexual orientation and gender identity in clinical settings.* Boston: Fenway Institute.

Bux, D. A. (1996). The epidemiology of problem drinking in gay men and lesbians: A critical review. *Clinical Psychology Review, 16*(4), 277–298.

Cahill, S., & Makadon, H. (2013). Sexual orientation and gender identity data collection in clinical settings and in electronic health records: A key to ending LGBT health disparities. *LGBT Health, 1*(1), 34–41.

Carballo-Diéguez, A., Miner, M., Dolezal, C., Rosser, B. R. S., & Jacoby, S. (2006). Sexual negotiation, HIV-status disclosure, and sexual risk behavior among Latino men who use the internet to seek sex with other men. *Archives of Sexual Behavior, 35*(4), 473–481.

Center for Substance Abuse Treatment. (2001). *A provider's introduction to substance abuse treatment for lesbian, gay, bisexual, and transgender individuals.* Washington, DC: U.S. Department of Health and Human Services, Substance Abuse and Mental Health Services Administration, Center for Substance Abuse Treatment.

Centers for Disease Control and Prevention. (2011). Diagnoses of HIV infection in the United States and dependent areas. *HIV Surveillance Report, 23.*

Centers for Disease Control and Prevention. (2013). HIV testing and risk behaviors among gay, bisexual, and other men who have sex with men—United States. *Morbidity and Mortality Weekly Report, 62*(47), 958–962.

Cochran, B. N., & Cauce, A. M. (2006). Characteristics of lesbian, gay, bisexual, and transgender individuals entering substance abuse treatment. *Journal of Substance Abuse Treatment, 30*(2), 135–146.

Cochran, B. N., Peavy, K. M., & Cauce, A. M. (2007). Substance abuse treatment providers' explicit and implicit attitudes regarding sexual minorities. *Journal of Homosexuality, 53*(3), 181–207.

Cochran, B. N., Peavy, K. M., & Robohm, J. S. (2007). Do specialized services exist for LGBT individuals seeking treatment for substance misuse?: A study of available treatment programs. *Substance Use and Misuse, 42*(1), 161–176.

Collier, K. L., van Beusekom, G., Bos, H. M. W., & Sandfort, T. G. M. (2013). Sexual orientation and gender identity/expression related peer victimization in adolescence: A systematic review of associated psychosocial and health outcomes. *Journal of Sex Research, 50*(3–4), 299–317.

Corliss, H. L., Goodenow, C. S., Nichols, L., & Austin, S. B. (2011). High burden of homelessness among sexual-minority adolescents: Findings from a representative Massachusetts high school sample. *American Journal of Public Health, 101*(9), 1683–1689.

Corliss, H. L., Rosario, M., Birkett, M. A., Newcomb, M. E., Buchting, F. O., & Matthews, A. K. (2014). Sexual orientation disparities in adolescent cigarette smoking: Intersections with race/ethnicity, gender, and age. *American Journal of Public Health, 104*(6), 1137–1147.

Corliss, H. L., Rosario, M., Wypij, D., Wylie, S. A., Frazier, A. L., & Austin, S. B. (2010). Sexual orientation and drug use in a longitudinal cohort study of U.S. adolescents. *Addictive Behaviors, 35*(5), 517–521.

Coulter, R. W. S., Blosnich, J. R., Bukowski, L. A., Herrick, A. L., Siconolfi, D. E., & Stall, R. D. (2015). Differences in alcohol use and alcohol-related problems between transgender- and nontransgender-identified young adults. *Drug and Alcohol Dependence, 154,* 251–259.

Dank, M., Lachman, P., Zweig, J., & Yahner, J. (2014). Dating violence experiences of lesbian, gay, bisexual, and transgender youth. *Journal of Youth and Adolescence, 43*(5), 846–857.

Dilley, J. A., Spigner, C., Boysun, M. J., Dent, C. W., & Pizacani, B. A. (2008). Does tobacco industry marketing excessively impact lesbian, gay and bisexual communities? *Tobacco Control, 17*(6), 385–390.

Durso, L. E., & Gates, G. J. (2012). *Serving our youth: Findings from a national survey of services providers working with lesbian, gay, bisexual and transgender youth who are homeless or at risk of becoming homeless.* Los Angeles: University of California, Los Angeles, Williams Institute.

Eliason, M. J., & Hughes, T. (2004). Treatment counselors' attitudes about lesbian, gay, bisexual, and transgendered clients: Urban vs. rural settings. *Substance Use and Misuse, 39*(4), 625–644.

Friedman, M. S., Marshal, M. P., Guadamuz, T. E., Wei, C., Wong, C. F., Saewyc, E. M., et al. (2011). A meta-analysis of disparities in childhood sexual abuse, parental physical abuse, and peer victimization among sexual minority and sexual nonminority individuals. *American Journal of Public Health, 101*(8), 1481–1494.

Ginsburg, K. R., Winn, R. J., Rudy, B. J., Crawford, J., Zhao, H., & Schwarz, D. F. (2002). How to reach sexual minority youth in the health care setting: The teens offer guidance. *Journal of Adolescent Health, 31*(5), 407–416.

Goebel, K. (1994). Lesbian and gays face tobacco targeting. *Tobacco Control, 3*(1), 65.

Goldbach, J. T., Fisher, B. W., & Dunlap, S. (2015). Traumatic experiences and drug use by LGB adolescents: A critical review of minority stress. *Journal of Social Work Practice in the Addictions, 15*(1), 90–113.

Goldbach, J. T., Mereish, E. H., & Burgess, C. (2017). Sexual orientation disparities in the use of emerging drugs. *Substance Use and Misuse, 52*(2), 265–271.

Goldbach, J. T., Tanner-Smith, E., Bagwell, M., & Dunlap, S. (2014). Minority stress and substance use in sexual minority adolescents: A meta-analysis. *Prevention Science, 15*(3), 350–363.

Goodenow, C., Szalacha, L., & Westheimer, K. (2006). School support groups, other school factors, and the safety of sexual minority adolescents. *Psychology in the Schools, 43*(5), 573–589.

Green, K. E., & Feinstein, B. A. (2012). Substance use in lesbian, gay, and bisexual populations: An update on empirical research and implications for treatment. *Psychology of Addictive Behaviors, 26*(2), 265–278.

Grossman, A. H., D'Augelli, A. R., & Frank, J. A. (2011). Aspects of psychological resilience among transgender youth. *Journal of LGBT Youth, 8*(2), 103–115.

Harper, G. W. (2007). Sex isn't that simple: Culture and context in HIV prevention interventions for gay and bisexual male adolescents. *American Psychologist, 62*(8), 806–819.

Harper, G. W., & Riplinger, A. J. (2012). HIV prevention interventions for adolescents and young adults: What about the needs of gay and bisexual males? *AIDS and Behavior, 17*(3), 1082–1095.

Hatzenbuehler, M. L. (2009). How does sexual minority stigma "get under the skin"?: A psychological mediation framework. *Psychological Bulletin, 135*(5), 707–730.

Hatzenbuehler, M. L., Birkett, M., Van Wagenen, A., & Meyer, I. H. (2013). Protective school climates and reduced risk for suicide ideation in sexual minority youths. *American Journal of Public Health, 104*(2), 279–286.

Hatzenbuehler, M. L., Corbin, W. R., & Fromme, K. (2008). Trajectories and determinants of alcohol use among LGB young adults and their heterosexual peers: Results from a prospective study. *Developmental Psychology, 44*(1), 81–90.

Hatzenbuehler, M. L., Jun, H.-J., Corliss, H. L., & Bryn Austin, S. (2015). Structural stigma and sexual orientation disparities in adolescent drug use. *Addictive Behaviors, 46*, 14–18.

Hatzenbuehler, M. L., & Keyes, K. M. (2013). Inclusive anti-bullying policies and reduced risk of suicide attempts in lesbian and gay youth. *Journal of Adolescent Health, 53*(Suppl. 1), S21–S26.

Hatzenbuehler, M. L., & Link, B. G. (2014). Introduction to the special issue on structural stigma and health. *Social Science and Medicine, 103*, 1–6.

Hatzenbuehler, M. L., McLaughlin, K. A., & Xuan, Z. (2015). Social networks and sexual orientation disparities in tobacco and alcohol use. *Journal of Studies on Alcohol and Drugs, 76*(1), 117–126.

Heck, N. C., Flentje, A., & Cochran, B. N. (2011). Offsetting risks: High school gay–straight alliances and lesbian, gay, bisexual, and transgender (LGBT) youth. *School Psychology Quarterly, 26*(2), 161–174.

Heck, N. C., Livingston, N. A., Flentje, A., Oost, K., Stewart, B. T., & Cochran, B. N. (2014). Reducing risk for illicit drug use and prescription drug misuse: High school gay–straight alliances and lesbian, gay, bisexual, and transgender youth. *Addictive Behaviors, 39*(4), 824–828.

Herrick, A. L., Marshal, M. P., Smith, H. A., Sucato, G., & Stall, R. D. (2011). Sex while intoxicated: A meta-analysis comparing heterosexual and sexual minority youth. *Journal of Adolescent Health, 48*(3), 306–309.

Hicks, D. (2000). The importance of specialized treatment programs for lesbian and gay patients. *Journal of Gay and Lesbian Psychotherapy, 3*(3–4), 81–94.

Hoffman, N. D., Freeman, K., & Swann, S. (2009). Healthcare preferences of lesbian, gay, bisexual, transgender and questioning youth. *Journal of Adolescent Health, 45*(3), 222–229.

Hooper, S., Rosser, B. R. S., Horvath, K. J., Oakes, J. M., & Danilenko, G. (2008). An online needs assessment of a virtual community: What men who use the internet to seek sex with men want in internet-based HIV prevention. *AIDS and Behavior, 12*(6), 867–875.

Katz-Wise, S. L., & Hyde, J. S. (2012). Victimization experiences of lesbian, gay, and bisexual individuals: A meta-analysis. *Journal of Sex Research, 49*(2–3), 142–167.

Kaysen, D., Lostutter, T. W., & Goines, M. A. (2005). Cognitive processing therapy for acute stress disorder resulting from an anti-gay assault. *Cognitive and Behavioral Practice, 12*(3), 278–289.

Keuroghlian, A. S., Reisner, S. L., White, J. M., & Weiss, D. (2015). Substance use and treatment of substance use disorders in a community sample of transgender adults. *Drug and Alcohol Dependence, 152*, 139–146.

Keuroghlian, A. S., Shtasel, D., & Bassuk, E. L. (2014). Out on the street: A public health and policy agenda for lesbian, gay, bisexual, and transgender youth who are homeless. *American Journal of Orthopsychiatry, 84*(1), 66–72.

Kosciw, J. G., Greytak, E. A., Bartkiewicz, M. J., Boesen, M. J., & Palmer, N. A. (2012). *The 2011 National School Climate Survey: The Experiences of Lesbian, Gay, Bisexual and Transgender Youth in Our Nation's Schools* (ERIC). New York: Gay, Lesbian and Straight Education Network.

Kosciw, J. G., Palmer, N. A., & Kull, R. M. (2014). Reflecting resiliency: Openness about sexual orientation and/or gender identity and its relationship to well-being and educational outcomes for LGBT students. *American Journal of Community Psychology, 55*(1), 167–178.

Krehely, J. (2009). How to close the LGBT health disparities gap. *Center for American Progress*, 1–9.

Lee, S. J. (2015). Addiction and lesbian, gay, bisexual and transgender (LGBT) issues. In N. el-Guebaly, G. Carrà, & M. Galanter (Eds.), *Textbook of addiction treatment: International perspectives* (pp. 2139–2164). Milan, Italy: Springer Milan.

Lelutiu-Weinberger, C., Pachankis, J. E., Gamarel, K. E., Surace, A., Golub, S. A., & Parsons, J. T. (2014). Feasibility, acceptability, and preliminary efficacy of a live-chat social media intervention to reduce HIV risk among young men who have sex with men. *AIDS and Behavior, 19*(7), 1214–1227.

Litt, D. M., Lewis, A., Rhew, I. C., Hodge, K. A., & Kaysen, D. L. (2015). Reciprocal relationships over time between descriptive norms and alcohol use in young adult sexual minority women. *Psychology of Addictive Behaviors, 29*(4), 885–893.

Lombardi, E. L., & van Servellen, G. (2000). Building culturally sensitive substance use prevention and treatment programs for transgendered populations. *Journal of Substance Abuse Treatment, 19*(3), 291–296.

Lyons, T., Shannon, K., Pierre, L., Small, W., Krüsi, A., & Kerr, T. (2015). A qualitative study of transgender individuals' experiences in residential addiction treatment settings: Stigma and inclusivity. *Substance Abuse Treatment, Prevention, and Policy, 10*(1), 1–6.

Marshal, M. P., Dietz, L. J., Friedman, M. S., Stall, R., Smith, H. A., McGinley, J., et al. (2011). Suicidality and depression disparities between sexual minority and heterosexual youth: A meta-analytic review. *Journal of Adolescent Health, 49*(2), 115–123.

Marshal, M. P., Friedman, M. S., Stall, R., King, K. M., Miles, J., Gold, M. A., et al. (2008). Sexual orientation and adolescent substance use: A meta-analysis and methodological review. *Addiction, 103*(4), 546–556.

McGuire, J. K., Anderson, C. R., Toomey, R. B., & Russell, S. T. (2010). School climate for transgender youth: A mixed method investigation of student experiences and school responses. *Journal of Youth and Adolescence, 39*(10), 1175–1188.

Mereish, E. H., Goldbach, J., Burgess, C., & DiBello, A. (2017). Sexual orientation, minority stress, social norms, and substance use among racially diverse adolescents. *Drug and Alcohol Dependence, 178*, 49–56.

Mereish, E. H., & Poteat, V. P. (2015). A relational model of sexual minority mental and physical health: The negative effects of shame on relationships, loneliness, and health. *Journal of Counseling Psychology, 62*(3), 425–437.

Meyer, I. H. (2003). Prejudice, social stress, and mental health in lesbian, gay, and bisexual populations: Conceptual issues and research evidence. *Psychological Bulletin, 129*(5), 674–697.

Miller, W., C'de Baca, J., Matthews, D., & Wilbourne, P. (2001). *Personal values card sort*. Albuquerque: University of New Mexico.

Morgenstern, J., Bux, D. A., Jr., Parsons, J., Hagman, B. T., Wainberg, M., & Irwin, T. (2009). Randomized trial to reduce club drug use and HIV risk behaviors among men who have sex with men. *Journal of Consulting and Clinical Psychology, 77*(4), 645–656.

Murphy, D. A., Chen, X., Naar-King, S., & Parsons, J. T. (2011). Alcohol and marijuana use outcomes in the healthy choices motivational interviewing intervention for HIV-positive youth. *AIDS Patient Care and STDs, 26*(2), 95–100.

Mustanski, B. S., Newcomb, M. E., Du Bois, S. N., Garcia, S. C., & Grov, C. (2011).

HIV in young men who have sex with men: A review of epidemiology, risk and protective factors, and interventions. *Journal of Sex Research, 48*(2–3), 218–253.

Pachankis, J. E. (2015). A transdiagnostic minority stress treatment approach for gay and bisexual men's syndemic health conditions. *Archives of Sexual Behavior, 44*(7), 1843–1860.

Pachankis, J. E., Hatzenbuehler, M. L., Rendina, H. J., Safren, S. A., & Parsons, J. T. (2015). LGB-affirmative cognitive-behavioral therapy for young adult gay and bisexual men: A randomized controlled trial of a transdiagnostic minority stress approach. *Journal of Consulting and Clinical Psychology, 83*(5), 875–889.

Pachankis, J. E., Hatzenbuehler, M. L., & Starks, T. J. (2014). The influence of structural stigma and rejection sensitivity on young sexual minority men's daily tobacco and alcohol use. *Social Science and Medicine, 103*, 67–75.

Parsons, J. T., Lelutiu-Weinberger, C., Botsko, M., & Golub, S. A. (2014). A randomized controlled trial utilizing motivational interviewing to reduce HIV risk and drug use in young gay and bisexual men. *Journal of Consulting and Clinical Psychology, 82*(1), 9–18.

Parsons, J. T., Vial, A. C., Starks, T. J., & Golub, S. A. (2012). Recruiting drug using men who have sex with men in behavioral intervention trials: A comparison of internet and field-based strategies. *AIDS and Behavior, 17*(2), 688–699.

Patient Protection and Affordable Care Act. (2010). Patient protection and Affordable Care Act. *Public Law, 111*–148.

Pingel, E. S., Bauermeister, J. A., Johns, M. M., Eisenberg, A., & Leslie-Santana, M. (2013). "A safe way to explore": Reframing risk on the internet amidst young gay men's search for identity. *Journal of Adolescent Research, 28*(4), 453–478.

Pingel, E. S., Thomas, L., Harmell, C., & Bauermeister, J. A. (2013). Creating comprehensive, youth centered, culturally appropriate sex education: What do young gay, bisexual, and questioning men want? *Sexuality Research and Social Policy, 10*(4), 293–301.

Poteat, V. P., Mereish, E. H., DiGiovanni, C. D., & Koenig, B. W. (2011). The effects of general and homophobic victimization on adolescents' psychosocial and educational concerns: The importance of intersecting identities and parent support. *Journal of Counseling Psychology, 58*(4), 597–609.

Poteat, V. P., Sinclair, K. O., DiGiovanni, C. D., Koenig, B. W., & Russell, S. T. (2013). Gay–straight alliances are associated with student health: A multischool comparison of LGBTQ and heterosexual youth. *Journal of Research on Adolescence, 23*(2), 319–330.

Reisner, S. L., Greytak, E. A., Parsons, J. T., & Ybarra, M. L. (2015). Gender minority social stress in adolescence: Disparities in adolescent bullying and substance use by gender identity. *Journal of Sex Research, 52*(3), 243–256.

Reisner, S. L., Hughto, J. M. W., Dunham, E. E., Heflin, K. J., Begenyi, J. B. G., Coffey-Esquivel, J., et al. (2015). Legal protections in public accommodations settings: A critical public health issue for transgender and gender-nonconforming people. *Milbank Quarterly, 93*(3), 484–515.

Rosario, M., Corliss, H. L., Everett, B. G., Reisner, S. L., Austin, S. B., Buchting, F. O., et al. (2013). Sexual orientation disparities in cancer-related risk behaviors of tobacco, alcohol, sexual behaviors, and diet and physical activity: Pooled youth risk behavior surveys. *American Journal of Public Health, 104*(2), 245–254.

Rowan, N. L., Jenkins, D. A., & Parks, A. (2013). What is valued in gay and lesbian specific alcohol and other drug treatment? *Journal of Gay and Lesbian Social Services, 25*(1), 56–76.

Rowe, C., Santos, G.-M., McFarland, W., & Wilson, E. C. (2015). Prevalence and correlates of substance use among trans*female youth ages 16–24 years in the San Francisco Bay area. *Drug and Alcohol Dependence, 147,* 160–166.

Ryan, C., Huebner, D., Diaz, R. M., & Sanchez, J. (2009). Family rejection as a predictor of negative health outcomes in white and Latino lesbian, gay, and bisexual young adults. *Pediatrics, 123,* 346–352.

Saewyc, E. M. (2011). Research on adolescent sexual orientation: Development, health disparities, stigma, and resilience. *Journal of Research on Adolescence, 21*(1), 256–272.

Safren, S. A. (2005). Affirmative, evidence-based, and ethically sound psychotherapy with lesbian, gay, and bisexual clients. *Clinical Psychology: Science and Practice, 12*(1), 29–32.

Safren, S. A., Hollander, G., Hart, T. A., & Heimberg, R. G. (2001). Cognitive-behavioral therapy with lesbian, gay, and bisexual youth. *Cognitive and Behavioral Practice, 8*(3), 215–223.

Savin-Williams, R. C., & Cohen, K. M. (2015). Developmental trajectories and milestones of lesbian, gay, and bisexual young people. *International Review of Psychiatry, 27*(5), 357–366.

Schwinn, T. M., Thom, B., Schinke, S. P., & Hopkins, J. (2015). Preventing drug use among sexual-minority youths: Findings from a tailored, web-based intervention. *Journal of Adolescent Health, 56*(5), 571–573.

Senreich, E. (2011). The substance abuse treatment experiences of a small sample of transgender clients. *Journal of Social Work Practice in the Addictions, 11*(3), 295–299.

Sexual Minority Assessment Research Team. (2009). *Best practices for asking questions about sexual orientation on surveys.* Los Angeles: Williams Institute.

Stockdale, S. E., Wells, K. B., Tang, L., Belin, T. R., Zhang, L., & Sherbourne, C. D. (2007). The importance of social context: Neighborhood stressors, stress-buffering mechanisms, and alcohol, drug, and mental health disorders. *Social Science and Medicine, 65*(9), 1867–1881.

Toomey, R. B., Ryan, C., Diaz, R. M., & Russell, S. T. (2011). High school gay–straight alliances (GSAs) and young adult well-being: An examination of GSA presence, participation, and perceived effectiveness. *Applied Developmental Science, 15*(4), 175–185.

Transgender Law and Policy Institute. (2012). *U.S. jurisdictions with laws prohibiting discrimination on the basis of gender identity or expression.* Brooklyn, NY: Author.

Walsh, K., & Hope, D. A. (2010). LGB-affirmative cognitive behavioral treatment for social anxiety: A case study applying evidence-based practice principles. *Cognitive and Behavioral Practice, 17*(1), 56–65.

Washington, H. A. (2002). Burning love: Big tobacco takes aim at LGBT youths. *American Journal of Public Health, 92*(7), 1086–1095.

White Hughto, J. M., Reisner, S. L., & Pachankis, J. E. (2015). Transgender stigma and health: A critical review of stigma determinants, mechanisms, and interventions. *Social Science and Medicine, 147,* 222–231.

Young, S. D., Swendeman, D., Holloway, I. W., Reback, C. J., & Kao, U. (2015). Use of technology to address substance use in the context of HIV: A systematic review. *Current HIV/AIDS Reports, 12*(4), 462–471.

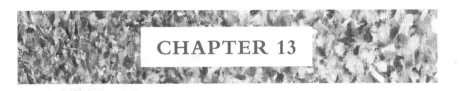

CHAPTER 13

Pharmacotherapy for Adolescent Substance Misuse

Robert Miranda Jr. and Hayley Treloar

Adolescence is a critical period for the early identification and treatment of substance misuse. Substance use disorders (SUDs) are developmentally linked phenomena that reach peak prevalence during late adolescence, and early substance use confers heightened risk for a multitude of psychosocial difficulties across the lifespan, including persistent problems with addiction (Johnston, O'Malley, Miech, Bachman, & Schulenberg, 2015; Lubman, Yucel, & Hall, 2007; Swendsen et al., 2012). This heightened vulnerability coincides with nearly 400 youth, ages 12–17 years, admitted to publicly funded substance abuse treatment facilities in the United States each day (National Institute on Drug Abuse, 2014). Despite recognition of the critical need for effective treatment options, the best available interventions have limitations. Several psychosocial interventions demonstrate efficacy with youth, including family-focused or systemic approaches, contingency management, cognitive-behavioral therapy (CBT), and motivational enhancement techniques (Bender, Tripodi, Sarteschi, & Vaughn, 2011; Winters, Tanner-Smith, Bresani, & Meyers, 2014). Yet, despite the modest effectiveness of these interventions, their beneficial effects often fade over time, and many youth do not respond to these treatments (Belendiuk & Riggs, 2014; Bender et al., 2011).

Pharmacotherapy is a key component of best-practice treatment guidelines for myriad psychiatric conditions in adolescents. Indeed, the number of adolescents prescribed psychotropic medication for many psychiatric conditions increased markedly over the past two decades, with nearly 7% of adolescents ages 12–19 years taking psychotropic medication (National Center for Health

Statistics, 2014). This reliance on medications to help treat adolescent psychopathology is driven, in part, by increased recognition of the mental health needs among youth and by considerable advances in medication development research with adolescents. Unlike the vast amount of pharmacotherapy research on adults with SUDs, however, there are very few well-controlled and adequately powered medication studies on adolescents with SUDs. Thus, it remains unclear how relevant pharmacotherapies are to the development of more effective, comprehensive care for adolescent substance misuse (Belendiuk & Riggs, 2014; Clark, 2012; Courtney & Milin, 2015; Waxmonsky & Wilens, 2005).

The U.S. Food and Drug Administration (FDA) has approved medications for treating adults with alcohol, opioid, and nicotine dependence. Although these efforts have advanced available treatment options for adults, no medication is indicated for adolescent substance use. This gap raises key questions about whether and how medications could benefit youth. Optimizing treatment options will require closing this important gap in medication development research. Research from several branches of medicine has demonstrated that the safety and efficacy of medication use with adolescents cannot be inferred from adult data (Bridge et al., 2007; Mayes et al., 2007; Safer, 2004). This concern may be especially important in the substance use field (Simkin & Grenoble, 2010). Adolescents differ considerably from adults in terms of their symptom presentation, course, and associated features of SUDs, and substantial neuronal remodeling that occurs during adolescence may account, in part, for these differences (Brown et al., 2008; Spear, 2014; Winters et al., 2014). Moreover, adolescents experience alcohol and possibly other drugs differently from adults, and these differences appear to heighten their vulnerability to heavy drinking and other drug use, and possibly impact how they respond to medications (Spear, 2014).

Since the publication of Monti, Colby, and O'Leary (2001), the number of pharmacotherapy studies with youth has markedly increased. Recent reviews have detailed this growing, yet still nascent, literature (Bailey et al., 2014; Belendiuk & Riggs, 2014; Courtney & Milin, 2015; Kim et al., 2011; Simkin & Grenoble, 2010). In this chapter, we begin by reviewing the best available scientific evidence regarding pharmacotherapy for adolescent SUDs. We focus on randomized clinical trials and then discuss how researchers and clinicians can leverage brief psychosocial interventions to help allay some of the barriers to successful pharmacotherapy. We believe that medications can dovetail well with psychosocial interventions in ways that can maximize both. Within this context, we review the details of the multimodal treatment approach we have employed for a number of years that combines pharmacotherapy with a psychosocial intervention. At the conclusion of this chapter, we discuss future directions. In doing so, our objective is to facilitate useful dialogue about how pharmacotherapies can be leveraged with the best available psychosocial interventions to enhance treatment options.

CURRENT STATUS OF THE FIELD

Randomized controlled trials (RCTs) are the gold standard for evaluating the safety and efficacy of psychosocial and pharmacological interventions. Most published reports on medications for adolescent SUDs, however, are limited to case reports and open-label studies in which patients and researchers know the treatment given. In the sections that follow, we provide an overview of the published RTCs that targeted adolescent substance misuse with pharmacological treatment. We then review medication trials that examined substance use secondary to a co-occurring psychiatric diagnosis, such as depression or attention-deficit/hyperactivity disorder (ADHD). Our review narrative is organized by substance type, and Tables 13.1 and 13.2 detail each study with special emphasis on whether and how medications were paired with psychosocial interventions. Tables 13.1 and 13.2 also describe potential issues associated with pharmacotherapy, such as medication adherence and treatment retention, as they pertain to each study. We include clinical trials that targeted youth ages 25 years and younger for two primary reasons. First, the FDA regards pediatric patients as individuals younger than age 22 years and defines adolescence as spanning ages 12–21 years (21 CFR 814.3; 79 FR 1740, January 10, 2014). Second, there is strong neurodevelopmental evidence that adolescence extends into the mid-20s (Brown et al., 2008; Giedd, 2004; Lisdahl, Shollenbarger, Sagar, & Gruber, Chapter 2, this volume; Windle et al., 2009).

Alcohol

Naltrexone is an opioid antagonist approved by the FDA for treatment of alcohol use disorder in adults (Miranda et al., 2014). We recently completed a preliminary within-subjects crossover study of naltrexone with adolescents ages 15–19 years. Results showed naltrexone reduced craving, blunted the pleasurable and enhanced sedating effects of drinking, and reduced likelihood of drinking and heavy drinking. Similar effects on drinking and craving were reported in an early open-label trial (Deas, May, Randall, Johnson, & Anton, 2005). In addition, Table 13.1 details a recent, well-executed RCT (and follow-ups) of heavy drinkers ages 18–25 years that paired naltrexone treatment, which was taken daily and when youth anticipated drinking (i.e., targeted), with an eclectic brief intervention that included a manualized Brief Alcohol Screening and Intervention for College Students (BASICS), medication management counseling, and personalized normative feedback about how their alcohol use patterns and consequences compared with peers of a similar age (O'Malley et al., 2015). Naltrexone treatment, particularly when targeted, was hypothesized to be well suited for use in this younger age group—they are generally more open to reducing drinking rather than abstaining and prefer taking medication as needed versus daily doses (Epler, Sher, Loomis, & O'Malley, 2009). Naltrexone decreases the reinforcing effects of alcohol and thus may

TABLE 13.1. Description of Randomized, Placebo-Controlled Trials of Adjunctive Pharmacotherapy for Adolescent Substance Use Treatment

Reference	Participants	Treatment		Duration and follow-up	Retention rates	Adherence monitoring
		Psychosocial	Pharmacological			
			Alcohol			
O'Malley et al. (2015)	140 heavy drinkers (≥4 binge-drinking days in past month); ages 18–25; recruited from community via Facebook ads and fliers	Brief, manualized BASICS counseling and medication management; 15–20 minutes every other week; personalized normative feedback; 1.5 hours at baseline	Naltrexone, 25 mg daily + 25 mg targeted (up to once daily)	8 weeks	*Medication group:* 7 discontinued tx (5 lost interest, 1 family emergency, 1 medical contraindication) *Placebo group:* 5 discontinued tx (4 lost interest, 1 medical contraindication)	Pill counts and daily diary reports; o medication adherence or counseling session differences
DeMartini et al. (2014)	118 completing follow-ups from O'Malley et al. (2015)	Follow-ups 3, 6, and 12 months post-tx	Differential loss to follow-up not reported			
			Cannabis			
Gray, Carpenter, Baker, et al. (2012)	116 treatment-seeking, cannabis-dependent youth; ages 15–21; clinical referrals and local media	CM and brief cessation counseling; <10 minutes weekly	N-acetylcysteine, 1,200 mg twice daily	8 weeks Follow-up 4 weeks post-tx	*Medication group:* 21 discontinued tx[a]; 8 more lost to follow-up[a] *Placebo group:* 25 discontinued tx[a]; 12 more lost to follow-up[a]	Pill counts and medication diaries; no medication adherence differences or differences in CM earnings for adherence

(continued)

TABLE 13.1. (continued)

| Reference | Participants | Treatment | | Duration and follow-up | Retention rates | Adherence monitoring |
		Psychosocial	Pharmacological			
Miranda et al. (2017)	66 heavy cannabis users; ages 15–24; recruited from community, primarily via posting ads and fliers	MET including personalized feedback; 50-minute sessions every other week	Topiramate; titrated to 200 mg daily target dose stabilized for final 2 weeks of trial	6 weeks	*Medication group:* 21 discontinued tx[b] (8 lost interest, 14 side effects, 1 new contraindicated med, 1 relocation) *Placebo group:* 6 discontinued tx (6 lost interest, 1 side effects)	Urinalysis weekly; no medication adherence differences; medication group received fewer MET sessions due to higher attrition
			Nicotine			
Hanson, Allen, Jensen, & Hatsukami (2003)	100 smokers (≥ 10 cigarettes/ day) interested in quitting; ages 13–19; recruited from schools, clinics, and larger community	CM and individual CBT; 10–15 minutes, once in first week, twice in second week, weekly for the next 6 weeks, and biweekly for last 4 weeks	Nicotine patch; stepped tx from 21 or 14 mg depending on level of prequit smoking frequency	10 weeks Follow-ups 1 and 6 months post-tx	*Medication group:* 25 discontinued tx[a] *Placebo group:* 22 discontinued tx[a] Follow-up rates among those who completed treatment were 49% at 14 weeks and 38% at 36 weeks	Self-reported nicotine patch use compliance; no patch adherence differences
Killen et al. (2001)	211 smokers (≥ 10 cigarettes/day) with 1+ failed quit attempts; ages 15–18; recruited from high schools	Group-based skills training; 45 minutes weekly	Bupropion SR + nicotine patch or placebo + patch; 150 mg daily bupropion SR for 1 week prior to quit day and 8 weeks after	9 weeks bupropion; 8 weeks patch Follow-up 1 and 16 weeks post-tx	*Medication group:* 20 discontinued tx[a]; 19 more lost to follow-up[a] *Placebo group:* 14 discontinued tx[a]; 24 more lost to follow-up[a]	Urinalysis and self-reported compliance; 38% positive urine week 5; 44% reported adhering to medication and 41% adhering to patch on ≤ 2 tx weeks; 80% attended 8+ tx sessions

332

Moolchan et al. (2005)	120 smokers (≥ 10 cigarettes/ day) desiring to quit; ages 13–17; recruited from community	Group CBT; 45 minutes weekly; individual counseling to address side effects and adherence; 3–4 minutes weekly	Nicotine patch, 21 mg; nicotine gum 2 or 4 mg as needed	12 weeks Follow-up 3 months post-tx	*Patch group:* 16 discontinued tx[a] *Gum group:* 27 discontinued tx[a] *Placebo group:* 24 discontinued tx[a] Follow-up rates not reported	Collected used and unused patches, self-report; 78.4% patch adherence, no group differences in proportion of patches used; 38.5% gum adherence, slightly less in active gum versus placebo
Roddy, Romilly, Challenger, Lewis, & Britton (2006)	98 smokers (≥ 1 cigarette/day or < 1 cigarette/day with withdrawal); ages 11–21; recruited from after-school program	Individual or small-group behavioral counseling; 10–15 minutes weekly	Nicotine patch; stepped tx from 15 mg	6 weeks Follow-up 5 weeks post-tx	Only 8 participants (3 active tx, 5 placebo) completed trial (of 90 who discontinued tx, 27 provided reasons for attrition: 2 side effects, 2 quit smoking, 1 perceived patches as ineffective, 22 changed mind about quitting)	Not reported
Muramoto, Leischow, Sherrill, Matthews, & Strayer (2007)	312 smokers (≥ 6 cigarettes/day) with 2+ failed quit attempts and motivated to quit smoking; ages 14–17; recruited from metropolitan community	Individual counseling to prepare for quitting smoking; 1 prequit session Medication adherence; on quit date, weekly, and 1 week post-tx	Bupropion SR, randomized to 150 mg daily or 300 mg daily	6 weeks Follow-up 20 weeks post-tx	*Bupropion SR 150 mg:* 18 discontinued tx (6 withdrew, 2 postrandomization exclusion, 10 lost to follow-up); 19 discontinued follow-up (1 protocol deviation, 1 withdrew, 17 lost) *Bupropion SR 300 mg:* 19 discontinued tx (3 adverse events, 1 protocol deviation, 11 withdrew, 4 lost to follow-up); 19 discontinued follow-up (1 protocol deviation, 2 withdrew, 16 lost)	Breath CO and urinalysis for smoking; medication adherence outcomes not reported

(continued)

TABLE 13.1. (continued)

Reference	Participants	Treatment		Duration and follow-up	Retention rates	Adherence monitoring
		Psychosocial	Pharmacological			
					Placebo group: 13 discontinued tx (2 protocol deviation, 6 withdrew, 1 postrandomization exclusion, 4 lost); 31 discontinued follow-up (2 protocol deviation, 6 withdrew, 23 lost)	
Gray et al. (2011)	134 smokers (≥ 5 cigarettes/day) interested in quitting; ages 12–21; recruited from schools and community	CM[c]; eligible for payment first week and twice weekly thereafter (11 total payments)	Bupropion SR[c] 150 mg twice daily	6 weeks Follow-up 6 weeks post-tx	*Medication + CM:* 8 discontinued tx (all due to schedule changes); 12 more lost to follow-up *Medication only:* 5 discontinued tx (4 schedule, 1 pregnancy); 13 more lost to follow-up *Placebo + CM:* 4 discontinued tx (all due to schedule changes); 14 more lost to follow-up *Placebo only:* 4 discontinued tx (3 schedule, 1 to take medication outside of study); 10 more lost to follow-up	Weekly pill counts and self-report diaries; no medication adherence differences; session attendance higher in medication groups

(continued)

Study	Sample	Counseling	Medication	Duration	Attrition	Compliance
Gray, Carpenter, Baker, et al. (2012)	29 smokers (≥ 5 cigarettes/day) interested in quitting including 1+ quit attempt; ages 15–20; recruited from community ads	Brief individual cessation counseling (≤ 10 minutes weekly)	Varenicline, titrated to 0.5 or 1 mg twice daily based on weight; bupropion XL, titrated from 150 mg first week to 300 mg daily target dose	8 weeks Follow-up 1 month post-tx	*Varenicline:* None discontinued medication, but 6 dropped out by week 8[a]; 11 lost to follow-up[a]. *Bupropion XL:* 2 discontinued tx due to side effects (1 anxiety, 1 feeling "too focused"); 7 dropped out by week 8[a]; 11 lost to follow-up[a]	Weekly pill counts and self-report diaries; 80% adherence to varenicline; 79% adherence to bupropion XL
Scherphof, van den Eijnden, Engels, & Vollebergh (2014)	257 smokers (≥ 7 cigarettes/day) motivated to quit; ages 12–18; recruited from 33 schools	None	Nicotine patch; stepped tx from 21 or 14 mg depending on level of prequit smoking frequency	15 days 1 day post-tx	*Patch group:* 5 lost at follow-up[a]. *Placebo group:* 11 lost at follow-up[a]; attrition more likely in placebo condition	Compliance with online surveys did not differ between groups
Rubinstein, Benowitz, Auerback, & Moscicki (2008)	40 smokers (≥ 7 cigarettes/day) with desire to quit; ages 15–18; recruited from area high schools	Group smoking cessation counseling; 8 sessions, 45–60 minutes, nearly weekly, 6–12 participants per group	Nicotine nasal spray as needed, ≤ 40 doses daily; 1 dose is 2 sprays ≈ 1 mg nicotine	12 weeks	*Medication group:* 4 discontinued tx (1 prior to tx, 3 left school before study end). *Counseling-only group:* 2 discontinued tx (2 left school before study end, 2 withdrew)	Self-report of number of sprays each day; 13 in tx group stopped spray after 1 week; no differences in tx completers

TABLE 13.1. (continued)

Reference	Participants	Treatment		Duration and follow-up	Retention rates	Adherence monitoring
		Psychosocial	Pharmacological			
			Opiates			
Marsch et al. (2005)	36 opioid-dependent youth; ages 13–18; self-referred	Individual behavioral counseling; 3 times weekly; CM; payments for negative urinalysis and session attendance	Buprenorphine hydrochloride, 6 or 8 mg sublingual dose (based on weight and pretrial opiate use); clonidine hydrochloride, titrated to 0.2 mg dose days 7–14, stepped down starting day 14	28 days	*Buprenorphine:* 5 discontinued tx[a] *Clonidine:* 11 discontinued tx[a]	Urinalysis; greater adherence in the buprenorphine group
Woody et al. (2008)	152 youth with physiological opioid dependence seeking tx; ages 15–21; self-referred	Drug counseling; 1 individual and 1 group session weekly or more frequently as needed	Buprenorphine–naloxone, randomized to ≤ 24 mg daily, taper in weeks 9–12 or ≤ 14 mg daily with taper ending day 14	12 weeks or 14-day detoxification	*12-week group:* 22 discontinued tx (16 nonadherent, 4 enrolled in other treatment, 1 voluntarily withdrew, 1 deceased) *14-day group:* 62 discontinued tx (32 nonadherent, 23 enrolled in other treatment, 2 voluntarily withdrew, 5 incarcerated)	Urinalysis; main reason for noncompletion was missing 2 counseling sessions; 12-week group attended more counseling sessions than detoxification group (average of 12 vs. 5, respectively)

Note. BASICS, brief alcohol screening and intervention for college students; CM, contingency management; tx, treatment; MET, motivational enhancement therapy; CBT, cognitive-behavioral therapy; CO, carbon monoxide.

[a]Specific reasons for loss not reported.

[b]Participants could withdraw for more than one reason, which explains why the sum of reasons for discontinuation exceeds the total number of participants who withdrew.

[c]Crossed treatment; buproprion with or without CM and placebo with or without CM.

TABLE 13.2. Description of Randomized, Placebo-Controlled Trials for Combined Treatment of Adolescent Substance Use and Other Psychiatric Comorbidity

		Treatment				
Reference	Participants	Psychosocial	Pharmacological	Duration[a]	Retention rates	Adherence monitoring
Riggs, Mikulich-Gilbertson, & Davies (2007)	126 youth with current MDD, lifetime CD, and 1+ current SUD; ages 13–19; recruited from community	Individual, manualized CBT for SUD; 1 hour weekly + up to 2 family sessions; medication monitoring	Fluoxetine hydrochloride, 20 mg daily	16 weeks	*Medication group:* 11 discontinued tx (4 incarcerated, 3 residential tx, 3 lost to follow-up, 1 relocated) *Placebo group:* 9 discontinued tx (1 incarcerated, 3 lost to follow-up, 3 relocated, 2 withdrew consent)	Pill counts, self-report, and medication events monitoring system; no differences in treatment completers or mean CBT session attendance
Cornelius et al. (2010)	70 youth with current MDD and CUD; ages 14–25; referrals from tx programs, community	Individual, manualized CBT for MDD/CUD and MET for CUD; baseline, weekly 4 weeks, then biweekly 4 weeks	Fluoxetine; 10 mg daily for 2 weeks, then 20 mg daily target dose	12 weeks	*Medication group:* 3 discontinued tx[b] *Placebo group:* 3 discontinued tx[b]	Urinalysis for cannabis; medication adherence outcomes not reported; none withdrew due to side effects
Cornelius et al. (2009)	50 youth with current MDD and AUD; ages 15–20; referrals from tx programs, community	Individual, manualized CBT for MDD/AUD and MET for AUD; baseline, weekly 4 weeks, then biweekly 4 weeks	Fluoxetine; 10 mg daily for 2 weeks, then 20 mg daily target dose	12 weeks	*Medication group:* 0 discontinued tx *Placebo group:* 3 discontinued tx (at suggestion of treatment team because of severe depressive symptoms)	Medication adherence outcomes not reported; none withdrew due to side effects

(continued)

TABLE 13.2. (continued)

| Reference | Participants | Treatment | | Duration[a] | Retention rates | Adherence monitoring |
		Psychosocial	Pharmacological			
Riggs, Hall, Mikulich-Gilbertson, Lohman, & Kayser (2004)	69 youth with current ADHD, lifetime CD, SUD; ages 13–19; recruited from community or former substance tx program	No formal treatment reported; 4 meetings with study physician and 8 with study coordinator	Pemoline, 1 (36.5 mg) capsule daily for 1 week, increased to 2 capsules week 2, and 3 capsules week 3 (target 112.5 mg)	12 weeks	*Medication group:* 2 discontinued before receiving tx; 14 discontinued tx (9 lost to follow-up, 2 adverse effects, 2 non-study-related illnesses) *Placebo group:* 1 discontinued before receiving tx; 16 discontinued tx (8 lost to follow-up, 3 adverse effects, 6 non-study-related illnesses)	Pill counts and self-report; medication adherence outcomes not reported, but no differences in treatment completers; 3 adverse events more likely in medication group (stomachaches, insomnia, skin "picking")
Thurstone, Riggs, Salomonsen-Sautel, & Mikulich-Gilbertson (2010)	70 youth with ADHD 1+ current non-tobacco SUD; ages 13–19; referral source not reported	Individual MI/CBT for SUD; 1 hour, weekly	Atomoxetine, < 70 kg at 0.5 mg/kg or 0.75 mg/kg daily increased by 25 mg/week to target 1.1 mg/kg–1.5 mg/kg; > 70 kg at 50 mg daily increased to 75–100 mg target	12 weeks	*Medication group:* 3 discontinued tx (all lost to follow-up) *Placebo group:* 2 discontinued tx (all lost to follow-up)	Pill counts and self-report; medication adherence did not differ between groups; both groups averaged 8 MI/CBT sessions

| Riggs et al. (2011) | 303 youth with ADHD and SUD; ages 13–18; recruited from range of community sources (clinics, schools, juvenile justice system, SUD tx programs) | Individual, manualized CBT + MET components for SUD | Osmotic-release methylphenidate; 18 mg daily titrated to 72 mg daily | 16 weeks | *Medication group:* 33 discontinued tx (11 withdrew, 3 relocated, 4 incarcerated, 9 lost to follow-up, 6 other)

 Placebo group: 43 discontinued tx (11 withdrew, 1 relocated, 5 incarcerated, 17 lost, 1 felt tx not working, 8 other) | Pill counts and self-report; no differences between groups in study completion, compliance with weekly sessions, CBT session attendance, or medication compliance |

Note. MDD, major depressive disorder; CD, conduct disorder; SUD, substance use disorder; CBT, cognitive-behavioral therapy; tx, treatment; CUD, cannabis use disorder; AUD, alcohol use disorder; MET, motivational enhancement therapy; MI, motivational interviewing. Underlined text denotes the primary psychosocial treatment target.

[a]No long-term follow-up.

[b]Specific reasons for loss not reported.

be especially effective for reducing use rather than maintaining abstinence. Adjunctive pharmacotherapy with naltrexone reduced the number of drinks per drinking day at completion of the 8-week trial (O'Malley et al., 2015), but gains were not maintained at 1-year follow-up (DeMartini et al., 2014). As shown in Table 13.1, loss of interest in the study was the most common barrier to retention, which ostensibly could have been addressed by including a focused, motivational component in the psychosocial intervention.

Cannabis

Two RCTs evaluated the potential for pharmacotherapies to reduce cannabis (marijuana) misuse among youth (see Table 13.1). The first tested the effects of N-acetylsysteine (NAC; 1,200 mg or placebo twice daily), an over-the-counter amino acid supplement, combined with brief cessation counseling and contingency management (CM) that targeted retention and cannabis abstinence for 8 weeks among cannabis-dependent youth ages 15–21 years who were interested in stopping use (Gray, Carpenter, Baker, et al., 2012). NAC appeared efficacious to promote abstinence in the short term, but effects were not maintained at 1 month. Adherence to NAC did not seem to be an issue, with no significant treatment group differences in medication adherence or CM earnings for adherence. Retention was low in both treatment groups, however, with a third of youth (36.2%) in the NAC group and nearly half (43%) of the placebo group dropping out prematurely. Attrition attributable to medication side effects was limited to one participant; other reasons for dropping out were not provided.

The second trial is our own recently completed RCT that tested topiramate versus placebo among youth ages 15–24 years. Topiramate is an antiepileptic medication shown to reduce alcohol, cocaine, and nicotine use in clinical trials with adults (Johnson et al., 2013; Kranzler et al., 2014; Miranda et al., 2008, 2016; Oncken et al., 2014). All participants also received a brief, four-session motivational enhancement therapy (MET) targeting cannabis use (Miranda et al., 2017). Topiramate reduced quantity of cannabis use, measured in grams, but did not influence overall frequency of use, which could support the use of topiramate for youth who would like to reduce use, but not necessarily for those with a cessation goal. However, across both groups, the percentage of days smoking cannabis per week decreased significantly and percentage of negative urinalysis increased over the trial. If our psychosocial intervention was responsible for reduced frequency of youth cannabis use, this may have set a high bar for topiramate to exceed. A larger trial comparing topiramate to placebo with and without MET could answer this question. Another trial with a longer follow-up is also needed to establish maintenance of effects. As for barriers to treatment, retention was poor, with only 48% of those receiving topiramate completing the trial, compared with 77% in the placebo group. Further, those dropping out received fewer MET sessions and thus missed the therapeutic benefits of this intervention. Adverse side effects were the most common reason youth in the topiramate condition discontinued treatment.

Nicotine

Considerably more research has been devoted to evaluating the efficacy of pharmacological aids for smoking cessation than to other substances. A recent review cited 13 studies, including one laboratory study of nicotine deprivation in teenagers 13–18 years of age (Killen et al., 2001), four open-label trials, two small RCTs, and six larger RCTs (Bailey et al., 2012). The larger RCTs are reviewed in Table 13.1 along with two additional recent RCTs (Gray, Carpenter, Lewis, Klintworth, & Upadhyaya, 2012; Scherphof, van den Eijnden, Engels, & Vollebergh, 2014). Most trials lasted at least 6 weeks and included at least one follow-up. Of note, studies to reduce tobacco use tended to have less intensive adjunctive psychosocial treatment relative to other substances. Although the FDA has approved several nicotine replacement therapies (NRTs; gum, inhaler, lozenge, nasal spray, patch) and two non-nicotinic pharmacotherapies (i.e., varenicline tartrate [Chantix], bupropion hydrochloride [Wellbutin/ Zyban]) for adults, none are approved for pediatric use.

In terms of treatment outcomes, a review of the literature concluded that the nicotine patch and buproprion produced beneficial effects immediately posttreatment (Bailey et al., 2012). Yet, these effects were transient, and no medication showed long-term effects on cessation. Further, a second review by Kim and colleagues (2011) involved a meta-analysis of the six RCTs also described by Bailey et al. (2012) and found no short- or midterm benefit of pharmacological treatment for adolescents. Since these reviews, three additional RCTs were published. Gray and colleagues (2011) tested the efficacy of bupropion, with and without CM, and found that the combination of bupropion and CM was superior to placebo plus CM in terms of abstinence rates. In a second study, Gray, Carpenter, Lewis, et al. (2012) showed improved smoking outcomes over time among adolescent smokers treated with varenicline or bupropion, but no differences were observed between the medication conditions. Most recently, Scherphof and colleagues (2014) examined the efficacy of the nicotine patch on smoking outcomes among 12- to 18-year-old youth. The patch, as compared to placebo, increased the odds of quitting smoking after 2 weeks of treatment.

Opiates

Two RCTs of pharmacological treatment for opiate dependence are published. One included 36 adolescents, ages 13–18 years, who self-referred to outpatient treatment (Marsch et al., 2005). Sublingual buprenorphine hydrochloride (Subutex) + placebo clonidine hypochloride patch was compared to clonidine hypochloride patch + placebo sublingual buprenorphine hypochloride. Both groups received thrice weekly behavioral counseling and CM. Buprenorphine was superior to clonidine both in terms of retention/adherence and urinalysis-verified abstinence at the end of the 28-day trial. There was no follow-up, however, and it remains unknown whether treatment gains would last. A larger

RCT of 152 youth ages 15–21 years with physiological opioid dependence who sought treatment compared extended and short-term buprenorphine-naloxone (Suboxone) treatment (12 weeks vs. 14 days; Woody et al., 2008). Longer-term treatment was more effective to prevent treatment dropout and promote abstinence relative to short-term detoxification. Those in the 12-week group also attended more counseling sessions, an important difference given that the most common reason for noncompletion was missed sessions.

Methamphetamines

Only one small, 8-week pilot RCT of 19 adolescents ages 14–21 years examined treatment of methamphetamine use disorder (Heinzerling et al., 2013). Participants were randomized in a 2:1 ratio to bupropion SR (150 mg twice daily) or placebo, and both were combined with twice weekly counseling. Abstinence was verified with urinalysis and adherence was evaluated based on session attendance and weekly pill counts. Results showed placebo was superior to bupropion in promoting abstinence and retention (trend of 33.3 days retained in bupropion treatment vs. 49.3 days for placebo). Given the small sample size, however, results should be interpreted with caution. Side effects were generally minor and included flu-like symptoms and abdominal pain. However, one participant receiving bupropion required hospitalization for suicidal ideation during a relapse.

Psychiatric Comorbidity

Substance misuse often co-occurs with other psychiatric disorders, and the presence of comorbid psychopathology may exacerbate misuse, impede treatment response, and increase risk of relapse. Given this overlap, it is not surprising that researchers have examined effects of pharmacotherapy for co-occurring psychiatric conditions, such as depression and ADHD, among adolescents with an SUD and examined its effects on outcome. An important consideration is to determine the treatment target. Is the pharmacological and, in many cases, the adjunctive psychosocial intervention meant to treat the comorbid psychiatric condition, substance misuse, or both? Of the six studies reviewed in Table 13.2, five included psychosocial interventions that targeted substance misuse, and of these, only two included manualized CBT to treat the comorbid condition (Cornelius et al., 2009, 2010). One study did not report any formal treatment outside of meetings with a study physician and study coordinator (Riggs et al., 2004).

Half of the RCTs evaluated the effects of the antidepressant fluoxetine, and half evaluated medications commonly used to treat ADHD (see Table 13.2)—only one study found a treatment effect (Riggs et al., 2011). Riggs and colleagues (2011) paired individual, manualized CBT with MET components with either osmotic-release methylphenidate (OROS-MPH) or placebo among youth with co-occurring ADHD and at least one nontobacco SUD. Although primary outcomes of self-reported substance use were not affected, the OROS-MPH group showed greater improvement in problem-solving and coping skills and had more negative urinalysis results at the end of the 16-week trial than placebo.

In summary, medication development research for adolescent substance misuse has shown limited effects of pharmacotherapies on substance use outcomes. Research in this area is scarce, however, and null findings may be attributed to inadequate sample sizes that might have rendered most studies underpowered. Moreover, the safety and tolerability of pharmacotherapy for adolescent SUDs remain largely unstudied. Information regarding the most efficacious medication dose, duration of treatment to maximize maintenance of beneficial effects, and strategies for integrating medications with psychosocial interventions is unknown. Although treatment differences were not found in many studies, substance use often decreased overall across medication and placebo conditions. This overall decrease in use may be attributable to the efficacy of the adjunctive psychosocial interventions. This possibility coincides with the fact that one of the two psychiatric comorbidity studies that did not show overall reductions in use did not include a psychosocial intervention (Riggs et al., 2004). Additional research is needed, however, to more fully understand how best to integrate psychosocial and pharmacological interventions in the treatment of adolescents.

FACILITATING PHARMACOTHERAPY
WITH BRIEF INTERVENTIONS

Brief psychosocial interventions encompass a variety of approaches that can be tailored to targeted patient populations by varying their intensity (i.e., number of sessions—typically six or fewer) and the types of strategies employed (Pettinati et al., 2005). Given their flexibility and brevity, they are often integrated in medication trials as a minimal behavioral treatment platform delivered across medication conditions to ensure all receive some form of active treatment (Miller, Locastro, Longabaugh, O'Malley, & Zweben, 2005). Within this context, however, researchers typically give little or no attention to the effects of the behavioral intervention because of primary focus on pharmacotherapy outcomes. Indeed, there may be concerns that a robust behavioral treatment might obscure medication effects.

An alternative and growing perspective is that pharmacological and psychosocial interventions offer unique benefits and may yield the best results when combined (Miller et al., 2005). Pharmacotherapies are thought to exert beneficial effects by easing withdrawal, blunting craving, or altering sensitivity to alcohol and other drugs (see Table 13.3). By contrast, the best available psychosocial interventions focus on enhancing motivation to reduce alcohol and other drug use and teaching skills and coping mechanisms to improve one's ability to adaptively regulate affect and behavior. Conceptually, developing and sharpening these skills can help patients initiate initial changes in their use and sustain beneficial treatment effects beyond the active phase of treatment (Miller et al., 2005).

Brief interventions can also help address common barriers to pharmacotherapy and enhance medication effects by boosting acceptance of medication as a viable component of treatment, facilitating compliance with prescribed medication regimens, and maximizing retention. Although nearly 7% of adolescents ages 12–19 years are prescribed psychiatric medication in the United States, most refuse or desist their medication regimen before it is even recommended (Jonas, Qiuping, & Albertorio-Diaz, 2013). Nonadherence is associated with poorer clinical outcomes across many medical conditions, including SUDs in adults (Swift, Oslin, Alexander, & Forman, 2011) and adolescents (Bentzley, Tomko, & Gray, 2015). Moreover, the accuracy of adolescents' insight into the severity of their difficulties as well as the benefits of treatment, their motivation to change, and concurrent engagement in behavioral treatment are key predictors of adherence to medication (Charach & Fernandez, 2013; Stein, Klein, Greenhouse, & Kogan, 2012). Thus, integrated treatment that combines pharmacological and psychosocial interventions may afford important opportunities to increase medication utilization and maximize treatment outcome by addressing complementary treatment targets (Sibley, Kuriyan, Evans, Waxmonsky, & Smith, 2014).

Despite potential advantages of a multimodal treatment approach, our knowledge regarding whether and how combining pharmacotherapy with a behavioral intervention affects treatment outcomes is limited. Few studies have systematically examined the value of using a multimodal approach that combines psychotherapy with medication to treat addiction (Anton et al., 2006; De Wildt et al., 2002; Donovan et al., 2008), and no studies have evaluated its utility with adolescents with SUD. Research on other disorders, however, has shown benefits of combining interventions for adolescents and adults (Karyotaki et al., 2016; Sibley et al., 2014). For example, studies have shown that combined interventions for depression produce better short- and long-term outcomes when compared with pharmacotherapy alone (Karyotaki et al., 2016; Pampallona, Bollini, Tibaldi, Kupelnick, & Munizza, 2004).

The Combined Pharmacotherapies and Behavioral Interventions (COMBINE) study is the largest and most comprehensive evaluation of whether combining behavioral and pharmacological therapies for alcoholism enhances outcome (Anton et al., 2006). Primary findings indicated that, in the 16-week active treatment period, adult patients who received (1) medical management plus naltrexone, (2) a behavioral treatment, or (3) both had better drinking outcomes than patients who received only medication management (Anton et al., 2006). The combination of naltrexone and behavioral therapy, however, had no incremental benefit over either alone. Effects were generally upheld during the year following active treatment with an emergence of a small but significant advantage of the behavioral intervention (Donovan et al., 2008).

TABLE 13.3. Purported Mechanisms of Action of Medications (Trade Names) for Treating Substance Misuse

Substance	FDA-approved medications[a]	Non-FDA-approved medications	Purported mechanisms of action to reduce substance use
Alcohol	Disulfiram (Antabuse)		Causes an aversive reaction to alcohol
	Naltrexone (ReVia, Vivitrol[b])		Blocks rewarding effects of alcohol; reduces craving
	Acamprosate (Campral)		Suppresses long-lasting withdrawal
		Topiramate (Topamax)	Reduces craving when using alcohol
Cannabis		Topiramate (Topamax)	Reduces craving when using cannabis
		N-acetylcysteine	Reduces craving
Nicotine	Nicotine (Nicorette, Nicoderm, others)		Substitution
	Bupropion[c] (Zyban, Wellbutrin)		Reduces craving
	Varenicline (Chantix)		Reduces craving
Opiates	Methadone (Dolophine)		Substitution for prolonged maintenance; detoxification or relief of withdrawal
	Buprenorphine (Subutex, Suboxone[d])		Substitution for prolonged maintenance; detoxification or relief of withdrawal
	Naltrexone		Blocks rewarding effects of opiates; reduces craving
Stimulants		Bupropion (Zyban, Wellbutrin)	Alleviates withdrawal symptoms; treatment of comorbid disorders

Note. FDA = U.S. Food and Drug Administration.
[a]The FDA has not approved any medication for treating substance use disorders in pediatric populations.
[b]Vivitrol is a long-acting form of naltrexone administered monthly by injection.
[c]The generic medication bupropion hydrocholoride is marketed as Zyban for smoking cessation and as Wellbutrin for depression.
[d]The Suboxone formulation includes naloxone in addition to buprenorphine.

Although the initial findings do not support the clinical utility of a multimodal approach for treating alcoholism, it is noteworthy that patients randomized to active medication or placebo received a robust nine-session medical management protocol that focused on patient education regarding alcohol misuse that included individualized information on how alcohol affects his or her medical status, the importance of adherence and strategies to facilitate compliance with the prescribed medication regimen, and support and optimism for recovery (Pettinati et al., 2005). The inclusion of medication management, which itself can be considered a psychosocial intervention, may have hampered the ability to detect any added benefit of combining medication with psychotherapy over either alone. Moreover, the emergence of a significant advantage of the behavioral intervention following the active treatment phase is consistent with the notion that skills learned during psychosocial treatment can help sustain beneficial effects beyond active treatment (Miller et al., 2005).

CLINICAL APPLICATION:
AN ILLUSTRATIVE CASE

The model we developed for our research over the past decade involves testing effects of medications as adjunctive treatments to brief interventions for adolescent alcohol and cannabis misuse. Major objectives of the psychosocial treatment component are twofold: (1) enhance motivation for behavior change and treatment engagement, and (2) teach skills to help facilitate and sustain reductions in drinking and other drug use. We chose this multimodal approach for several scientific and clinical reasons. First, and perhaps most importantly, we hold an ethical responsibility to provide active intervention to all participating in our clinical trials. Adolescence is a key period of vulnerability for developing pathological alcohol and other drug use, and there is strong evidence that early effective intervention yields long-term benefits. By providing all with an active behavioral intervention, we ensure that those randomized to placebo medication still receive some treatment. Second, we aim to test the efficacy of medications in professional and clinical contexts similar to actual clinical practice in order to maximize how well our findings generalize to real-world settings. Third, we believe it is important to test whether experimental medications produce any benefit beyond the effects of established psychosocial interventions. As compared to psychosocial interventions, medications can produce a host of adverse side effects. Medications that do not yield benefits beyond those produced by available interventions may carry limited clinical utility.

The psychosocial platform used in our pharmacotherapy trials consists of biweekly individually administered sessions, modeled after work by Monti, Colby, and Tevyaw (the editors of this volume). We selected this treatment frequency, which translates into three or four sessions depending on the trial, based on the dose–response relationship between the amount of person-to-person contact time and successful outcomes. The MET component incorporates the central principles described by Miller and Rollnick (2012).

The first of the first two sessions, both of which lasts approximately 60 minutes, focuses on enhancing motivation to cut down and quit alcohol or other drug use, using four primary components: establishing rapport, assessing motivation for change, enhancing motivation, and establishing goals for change. After providing an overview and establishing rapport, counselors, who are blind to the adolescent's medication condition, initiate a discussion about the adolescent's perceived pros and cons of drinking or other substance use. This facilitates a mutual understanding about the adolescent's decisional balance to use based on his or her perceived positive and negative consequences of alcohol or other drug use. Based on this information, the counselor individualizes the brief intervention to each youth in order to maximize ambivalence about his or her alcohol or other drug use and to enhance readiness for pharmacotherapy and behavior change. We use this approach given that adolescents are often very early in their readiness to change and commonly self-initiate few reasons for change (Miller & Rollnick, 2009).

During Session 2, youth receive a personalized feedback packet regarding their use, which is reviewed in the context of a motivational interviewing-style discussion about the content. Counselors review computer-generated, personalized feedback from youths' assessment data collected at the start of the clinical trial, including normative data on drinking or drug use, degree of physical dependence on alcohol or other substance use, and current consequences related to use. All youth receive a copy of the feedback forms, information about alcohol or drug use, and strategies for cutting down or quitting. Counselors then ask youth to imagine what would happen if their alcohol or other drug use stayed the same or if they decided to quit. Barriers to change are discussed and problems solved. Counselors and youth then develop an action plan for behavior change and, if appropriate, explore how medication may assist with this plan. Counselors provide youth with a menu of suggested goals and strategies, and develop short- and long-term goals for cutting down or quitting. Finally, counselors focus on enhancing self-efficacy by eliciting discussion about youths' past personal successes with behavior change and inquiring about their personal characteristics that demonstrate ability to change.

Sessions 3 and 4 (each approximately 30 minutes) follow a common format, using MET principles, focusing on progress made toward changing drinking or drug use behaviors and planning for the future. First, counselors review the prior session(s) and address questions. Then counselors and youth discuss progress toward the goals set in the prior session and any barriers encountered, and problem-solve and set new goals. Finally, counselors and youth identify triggers for drinking or drug use and review coping skills to handle high-risk situations. The same counselor conducts all sessions of the brief intervention, whenever possible, to enhance rapport, provide continuity of care, and minimize attrition.

We believe incorporation of adjunctive psychosocial treatment in medication trials with adolescents is imperative for advancing pharmacotherapy for youth. Inasmuch as our goal is to maximize the likelihood that youth will make lasting changes in their alcohol and other drug use, we must teach adolescents cognitive and behavioral skills to help them sustain, and possibly even enhance, initial medication-driven reductions. Behavioral strategies can also help enhance adherence. Adolescents must believe not only that pharmacotherapy can help them achieve their desired goals for behavior change but also understand how to implement new skills to augment treatment effectiveness.

CONCLUSIONS AND FUTURE DIRECTIONS

The treatment of adolescent substance misuse remains a challenge to clinicians and researchers alike, especially when alcohol and other drug use are resistant to the best available psychosocial interventions. Moreover, youth often present with multiple comorbid disorders, numerous psychosocial and academic problems, and engage in various other health-risk behaviors. As such, these youth may require integrated treatments that include both pharmacological agents and psychotherapy (Boylan, Romero, & Birmaher, 2007). Indeed, pharmacotherapy is a key component of evidence-based care of adults with certain addictions—namely, alcohol, nicotine, and opiates—and has been shown to be cost-effective (Gastfriend, 2014). With few exceptions, however, randomized pharmacotherapy trials with adolescents have inadequate sample sizes and only short-term or no follow-ups. This lack of research is particularly problematic when considering that adolescent substance misuse differs from adult use in myriad ways that could impact whether and how medications affect it. Our knowledge about how medications may help reduce substance use among youth (i.e., putative mechanisms of action) is limited and, at present, pharmacological intervention approaches with adolescents are based almost entirely on treatment targets identified in adult studies, such as the attenuation of craving. Thus, additional information is needed regarding the most salient treatment targets during adolescence in order to tailor interventions and maximize effects. Further adequately powered clinical trials with long-term follow-up assessments are needed to test the efficacy and safety of medications for adolescents. In addition, safety concerns and limited knowledge about the impact of medication on brain development, especially for long-term exposure, necessitate continued research.

In summary, over the past 20 years the scientific literature on pharmacotherapy for treating addiction in youth has expanded manifold. Despite this progress, our understanding of the role of medications in the clinical management of adolescent substance misuse remains inadequate, and recommendations regarding their use cannot be drawn from the literature. Although effective pharmacological treatments exist for adults, there are still few studies that examine the safety and efficacy of these medications with youth, and no medication is FDA approved for substance abuse treatment for adolescents. Further controlled clinical trials assessing efficacy of medications for treating adolescent substance misuse are necessary, with careful attention paid to the most effective ways to integrate pharmacotherapy within a broader scope of established behavioral and family interventions.

REFERENCES

Anton, R. F., O'Malley, S. S., Ciraulo, D. A., Cisler, R. A., Couper, D., Donovan, D. M., et al. (2006). Combined pharmacotherapies and behavioral interventions for alcohol dependence: The COMBINE study: A randomized controlled trial. JAMA, 295(17), 2003–2017.

Bailey, J. A., Samek, D. R., Keyes, M. A., Hill, K. G., Hicks, B. M., McGue, M., et al. (2014). General and substance-specific predictors of young adult nicotine dependence, alcohol use disorder, and problem behavior: Replication in two samples. Drug and Alcohol Dependence, 138, 161–168.

Bailey, S. R., Crew, E. E., Riske, E. C., Ammerman, S., Robinson, T. N., & Killen, J. D. (2012). Efficacy and tolerability of pharmacotherapies to aid smoking cessation in adolescents. Pediatric Drugs, 14(2), 91–108.

Belendiuk, K. A., & Riggs, P. (2014). Treatment of adolescent substance use disorders. Current Treatment Options in Psychiatry, 1(2), 175–188.

Bender, K., Tripodi, S. J., Sarteschi, C., & Vaughn, M. G. (2011). A meta-analysis of interventions to reduce adolescent cannabis use. Research on Social Work Practice, 21, 153–164.

Bentzley, J. P., Tomko, R. L., & Gray, K. M. (2015). Low pretreatment impulsivity and high medication adherence increase the odds of abstinence in a trial of N-acetylcysteine in adolescents with cannabis use disorder. Journal of Substance Abuse Treatment, 63, 72–77.

Boylan, K., Romero, S., & Birmaher, B. (2007). Psychopharmacologic treatment of pediatric major depressive disorder. Psychopharmacology, 191, 27–38.

Bridge, J. A., Iyengar, S., Salary, C. B., Barbe, R. P., Birmaher, B., Pincus, H. A., et al. (2007). Clinical response and risk for reported suicidal ideation and suicide attempts in pediatric antidepressant treatment: A meta-analysis of randomized controlled trials. JAMA, 297(15), 1683–1696.

Brown, S. A., McGue, M., Maggs, J., Schulenberg, J., Hingson, R., Swartzwelder, S., et al. (2008). A developmental perspective on alcohol and youths 16 to 20 years of age. Pediatrics, 121(Suppl. 4), S290–S310.

Charach, A., & Fernandez, R. (2013). Enhancing ADHD medication adherence: Challenges and opportunities. Current Psychiatry Reports, 15(7), 371.

Clark, D. B. (2012). Pharmacotherapy for adolescent alcohol use disorder. CNS Drugs, 26(7), 559–569.

Cornelius, J. R., Bukstein, O. G., Douaihy, A. B., Clark, D. B., Chung, T. A., Daley, D. C., et al. (2010). Double-blind fluoxetine trial in comorbid MDD-CUD youth and young adults. Drug and Alcohol Dependence, 112(1–2), 39–45.

Cornelius, J. R., Bukstein, O. G., Wood, D. S., Kirisci, L., Douaihy, A., & Clark, D.

B. (2009). Double-blind placebo-controlled trial of fluoxetine in adolescents with comorbid major depression and an alcohol use disorder. *Addictive Behaviors, 34*(10), 905–909.

Courtney, D. B., & Milin, R. (2015). Pharmacotherapy for adolescents with substance use disorders. *Current Treatment Options in Psychiatry, 2*(3), 312–325.

De Wildt, W. A., Schippers, G. M., Van Den Brink, W., Potgieter, A. S., Deckers, F., & Bets, D. (2002). Does psychosocial treatment enhance the efficacy of acamprosate in patients with alcohol problems? *Alcohol and Alcoholism, 37*(4), 375–382.

Deas, D., May, M. P., Randall, C., Johnson, N., & Anton, R. (2005). Naltrexone treatment of adolescent alcoholics: An open-label pilot study. *Journal of Child and Adolescent Psychopharmacology, 15*(5), 723–728.

DeMartini, K. S., Gueorguiva, R., Leeman, R. F., Corbin, W. R., Fucito, L. M., Kranzler, H. R., et al. (2014). Naltrexone for non-treatment seeking young adult drinkers: One-year outcomes. *Alcoholism: Clinical and Experimental Research, 38*(Suppl. 1), 212A.

Donovan, D. M., Anton, R. F., Miller, W. R., Longabaugh, R., Hosking, J. D., Youngblood, M., et al. (2008). Combined pharmacotherapies and behavioral interventions for alcohol dependence (the COMBINE study): Examination of posttreatment drinking outcomes. *Journal of Studies on Alcohol and Drugs, 69*(1), 5–13.

Epler, A. J., Sher, K. J., Loomis, T. B., & O'Malley, S. S. (2009). College student receptiveness to various alcohol treatment options. *Journal of American College Health, 58*(1), 26–32.

Gastfriend, D. R. (2014). A pharmaceutical industry perspective on the economics of treatments for alcohol and opioid use disorders. *Annals of the New York Academy of Sciences, 1327*(1), 112–130.

Giedd, J. N. (2004). Structural magnetic resonance imaging of the adolescent brain. *Annals of the New York Academy of Sciences, 1021*, 77–85.

Gray, K. M., Carpenter, M. J., Baker, N. L., DeSantis, S. M., Kryway, E., Hartwell, K. J., et al. (2012). A double-blind randomized controlled trial of N-acetylcysteine in cannabis-dependent adolescents. *American Journal of Psychiatry, 169*(8), 805–812.

Gray, K. M., Carpenter, M. J., Baker, N. L., Hartwell, K. J., Lewis, A. L., Hiott, D. W., et al. (2011). Bupropion SR and contingency management for adolescent smoking cessation. *Journal of Substance Abuse Treatment, 40*(1), 77–86.

Gray, K. M., Carpenter, M. J., Lewis, A. L., Klintworth, E. M., & Upadhyaya, H. P. (2012). Varenicline versus bupropion XL for smoking cessation in older adolescents: A randomized, double-blind pilot trial. *Nicotine and Tobacco Research, 14*(2), 234–239.

Hanson, K., Allen, S., Jensen, S., & Hatsukami, D. (2003). Treatment of adolescent smokers with the nicotine patch. *Nicotine and Tobacco Research, 5*(4), 515–526.

Heinzerling, K. G., Gadzhyan, J., van Oudheusden, H., Rodriguez, F., McCracken, J., & Shoptaw, S. (2013). Pilot randomized trial of bupropion for adolescent methamphetamine abuse/dependence. *Journal of Adolescent Health, 52*(4), 502–505.

Johnson, B. A., Ait-Daoud, N., Wang, X. Q., Penberthy, J. K., Javors, M. A., Seneviratne, C., et al. (2013). Topiramate for the treatment of cocaine addiction: A randomized clinical trial. *JAMA Psychiatry, 70*(12), 1338–1346.

Johnston, L. D., O'Malley, P. M., Miech, R. A., Bachman, J. G., & Schulenberg, J. E. (2015). *Monitoring the Future national results on adolescent drug use: Overview of key findings, 2014.* Ann Arbor: Institute for Social Research, University of Michigan.

Jonas, B. S., Qiuping, G., & Albertorio-Diaz, M. A. (2013). *Psychotropic medication use among adolescents: United States, 2005–2010* (NCHS Data Brief No. 135). Hyattsville, MD: National Center for Health Statistics

Karyotaki, E., Smit, Y., Holdt Henningsen, K., Huibers, M. J., Robays, J., de Beurs, D., et al. (2016). Combining pharmacotherapy and psychotherapy or monotherapy for major depression?: A meta-analysis on the long-term effects. *Journal of Affective Disorders, 194,* 144–152.

Killen, J. D., Ammerman, S., Rojas, N., Varady, J., Haydel, F., & Robinson, T. N. (2001). Do adolescent smokers experience withdrawal effects when deprived of nicotine? *Experimental and Clinical Psychopharmacology, 9*(2), 176–182.

Kim, Y., Myung, S. K., Jeon, Y. J., Lee, E. H., Park, C. H., Seo, H. G., et al. (2011). Effectiveness of pharmacologic therapy for smoking cessation in adolescent smokers: Meta-analysis of randomized controlled trials. *American Journal of Health-System Pharmacy, 68*(3), 219–226.

Kranzler, H. R., Covault, J., Feinn, R., Armeli, S., Tennen, H., Arias, A. J., et al. (2014). Topiramate treatment for heavy drinkers: Moderation by a GRIK1 polymorphism. *American Journal of Psychiatry, 171*(4), 445–452.

Lubman, D. I., Yucel, M., & Hall, W. D. (2007). Substance use and the adolescent brain: A toxic combination? *Journal of Psychopharmacology, 21*(8), 792–794.

Marsch, L. A., Bickel, W. K., Badger, G. J., Stothart, M. E., Quesnel, K. J., Stanger, C., et al. (2005). Comparison of pharmacological treatments for opioid-dependent adolescents: A randomized controlled trial. *Archives of General Psychiatry, 62*(10), 1157–1164.

Mayes, T. L., Tao, R., Rintelmann, J. W., Carmody, T., Hughes, C. W., Kennard, B. D., et al. (2007). Do children and adolescents have differential response rates in placebo-controlled trials of fluoxetine? *CNS Spectrums, 12*(2), 147–154.

Miller, W. R., Locastro, J. S., Longabaugh, R., O'Malley, S., & Zweben, A. (2005). When worlds collide: Blending the divergent traditions of pharmacotherapy and psychotherapy outcome research. *Journal of Studies on Alcohol Supplement, 15,* 17–23, discussion 6–7.

Miller, W. R., & Rollnick, S. (2009). Ten things that motivational interviewing is not. *Behavioural and Cognitive Psychotherapy, 37*(2), 129–140.

Miller, W. R., & Rollnick, S. (2012). *Motivational interviewing: Helping people change* (3rd ed.). New York: Guilford Press.

Miranda, R., Jr., MacKillop, J., Monti, P. M., Rohsenow, D. J., Tidey, J., Gwaltney, C., et al. (2008). Effects of topiramate on urge to drink and the subjective effects of alcohol: A preliminary laboratory study. *Alcoholism: Clinical and Experimental Research, 32*(3), 489–497.

Miranda, R., Jr., MacKillop, J., Treloar, H., Blanchard, A., Tidey, J. W., Swift, R. M., et al. (2016). Biobehavioral mechanisms of topiramate's effects on alcohol use: An investigation pairing laboratory and ecological momentary assessments. *Addiction Biology, 21*(1), 171–182.

Miranda, R., Jr., Ray, L., Blanchard, A., Reynolds, E. K., Monti, P. M., Chun, T., et al. (2014). Effects of naltrexone on adolescent alcohol cue reactivity and sensitivity: An initial randomized trial. *Addiction Biology, 19*(5), 941–954.

Miranda, R., Jr., Treloar, H., Blanchard, A., Justus, A., Monti, P. M., Chun, T., et al. (2017). Topiramate and motivational enhancement therapy for cannabis use among youth: A randomized placebo-controlled pilot study. *Addiction Biology, 22*(3), 779–790.

Monti, P. M., Colby, S. M., & O'Leary, T. A. (Eds.). (2001). *Adolescents, alcohol, and substance abuse: Reaching teens through brief interventions.* New York: Guilford Press.

Moolchan, E. T., Robinson, M. L., Ernst, M., Cadet, J. L., Pickworth, W. B., Heishman, S. J., & Schroeder, J. R. (2005). Safety and efficacy of the nicotine patch and gum for the treatment of adolescent tobacco addiction. *Pediatrics, 115*(4), 407–414.

Muramoto, M. L., Leischow, S. J., Sherrill, D., Matthews, E., & Strayer, L. J. (2007). Randomized, double-blind, placebo-controlled trial of 2 dosages of sustained-release bupropion for adolescent smoking cessation. *Archives of Pediatrics and Adolescent Medicine, 161*(11), 1068–1074.

National Center for Health Statistics. (2014). *Health, United States, 2013: With special reature on prescription drugs.* Hyattsville, MD: Centers for Disease Control and Prevention.

National Institute on Drug Abuse. (2014). Principles of adolescent substance use disorder treatment: A research-based guide (14-7953). Retrieved from *https://d14rmg-trwzf5a.cloudfront.net/sites/default/files/podata_1_17_14.pdf.*

O'Malley, S. S., Corbin, W. R., Leeman, R. F., DeMartini, K. S., Fucito, L. M., Ikomi, J., et al. (2015). Reduction of alcohol drinking in young adults by naltrexone: A double-blind, placebo-controlled, randomized clinical trial of efficacy and safety. *Journal of Clinical Psychiatry, 76*(2), e207–e213.

Oncken, C., Arias, A. J., Feinn, R., Litt, M., Covault, J., Sofuoglu, M., et al. (2014). Topiramate for smoking cessation: A randomized, placebo-controlled pilot study. *Nicotine and Tobacco Research, 16*(3), 288–296.

Pampallona, S., Bollini, P., Tibaldi, G., Kupelnick, B., & Munizza, C. (2004). Combined pharmacotherapy and psychological treatment for depression. *Archives of General Psychiatry, 61,* 714–719.

Pettinati, H. M., Weiss, R. D., Dundon, W., Miller, W. R., Donovan, D., Ernst, D. B., et al. (2005). A structured approach to medical management: A psychosocial intervention to support pharmacotherapy in the treatment of alcohol dependence. *Journal of Studies on Alcohol, 15*(Suppl.), 170–178, discussion 168–169.

Riggs, P. D., Hall, S. K., Mikulich-Gilbertson, S. K., Lohman, M., & Kayser, A. (2004). A randomized controlled trial of pemoline for attention-deficit/hyperactivity disorder in substance-abusing adolescents. *Journal of the American Academy of Child and Adolescent Psychiatry, 43*(4), 420–429.

Riggs, P. D., Mikulich-Gilbertson, S. K., & Davies, R. D. (2007). A randomized controlled trial of fluoxetine and cognitive behavioral therapy in adolescents with major depression, behavior problems, and substance use disorders. *Archives of Pediatrics and Adolescent Medicine, 161*(11), 1026–1034.

Riggs, P. D., Winhusen, T., Davies, R. D., Leimberger, J. D., Mikulich-Gilbertson, S., Klein, C., et al. (2011). Randomized controlled trial of osmotic-release methylphenidate with cognitive-behavioral therapy in adolescents with attention-deficit/ hyperactivity disorder and substance use disorders. *Journal of the American Academy of Child and Adolescent Psychiatry, 50*(9), 903–914.

Roddy, E., Romilly, N., Challenger, A., Lewis, S., & Britton, J. (2006). Use of nicotine replacement therapy in socioeconomically deprived young smokers: A community-based pilot randomised controlled trial. *Tobacco Control, 15*(5), 373–376.

Rubinstein, M. L., Benowitz, N. L., Auerback, G. M., & Moscicki, A. B. (2008) A randomized trial of nicotine nasal spray in adolescent smokers. *Pediatrics, 122*(3), 595–600.

Safer, D. J. (2004). A comparison of risperidone-induced weight gain across the age span. *Journal of Clinical Psychopharmacology, 24*(4), 429–436.

Scherphof, C. S., van den Eijnden, R. J., Engels, R. C., & Vollebergh, W. A. (2014). Short-term efficacy of nicotine replacement therapy for smoking cessation in adolescents: A randomized controlled trial. *Journal of Substance Abuse Treatment, 46*(2), 120–127.

Sibley, M. H., Kuriyan, A. B., Evans, S. W., Waxmonsky, J. G., & Smith, B. H. (2014). Pharmacological and psychosocial treatments for adolescents with ADHD: An updated systematic review of the literature. *Clinical Psychology Review, 34*(3), 218–232.

Simkin, D. R., & Grenoble, S. (2010). Pharmacotherapies for adolescent substance use disorders. *Child and Adolescent Psychiatric Clinics of North America, 19*(3), 591–608.

Spear, L. P. (2014). Adolescents and alcohol: Acute sensitivities, enhanced intake, and later consequences. *Neurotoxicology and Teratology, 41*, 51–59.

Stein, B. D., Klein, G. R., Greenhouse, J. B., & Kogan, J. N. (2012). Treatment of attention-deficit hyperactivity disorder: Patterns of evolving care during the first treatment episode. *Psychiatric Services, 63*(2), 122–129.

Swendsen, J., Burstein, M., Case, B., Conway, K. P., Dierker, L., He, J., et al. (2012). Use and abuse of alcohol and illicit drugs in US adolescents: Results of the National Comorbidity Survey—Adolescent Supplement. *Archives of General Psychiatry, 69*(4), 390–398.

Swift, R., Oslin, D. W., Alexander, M., & Forman, R. (2011). Adherence monitoring in naltrexone pharmacotherapy trials: A systematic review. *Journal of Studies on Alcohol and Drugs, 72*(6), 1012–1018.

Thurstone, C., Riggs, P. D., Salomonsen-Sautel, S., & Mikulich-Gilbertson, S. K. (2010). Randomized, controlled trial of atomoxetine for ADHD in adolescents with substance use disorder. *Journal of the American Academy of Child and Adolescent Psychiatry, 49*(6), 573–582.

Waxmonsky, J. G., & Wilens, T. E. (2005). Pharmacotherapy of adolescent substance use disorders: A review of the literature. *Journal of Child and Adolescent Psychopharmacology, 15*(5), 810–825.

Windle, M., Spear, L. P., Fuligni, A. J., Angold, A., Brown, J. D., Pine, D., et al. (2009). Transitions into underage and problem drinking: Summary of developmental processes and mechanisms: Ages 10–15. *Alcohol Research and Health, 32*(1), 30–40.

Winters, K. C., Tanner-Smith, E. E., Bresani, E., & Meyers, K. (2014). Current advances in the treatment of adolescent drug use. *Adolescent Health, Medicine and Therapeutics, 5*, 199–210.

Woody, G. E., Poole, S. A., Subramaniam, G., Dugosh, K., Bogenschutz, M., Abbott, P., et al. (2008). Extended vs short-term buprenorphine-naloxone for treatment of opioid-addicted youth: A randomized trial. *JAMA, 300*(17), 2003–2011.

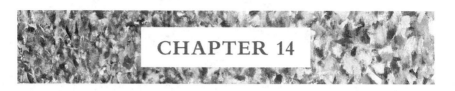

CHAPTER 14

Group–Based Interventions for Youth

Elizabeth J. D'Amico and Sarah W. Feldstein Ewing

*E*xploration and development of identity, autonomy, sexuality, academic functioning, and peer relationships are important age-appropriate tasks of adolescence (Ingersoll & Feldstein Ewing, 2011). Some of this exploration and experimentation may include alcohol and other drug (AOD) use and related risk behavior, including normative and nonpathological experimentation with alcohol and marijuana (e.g., Tucker, Ellickson, Collins, & Klein, 2006). Often, the AOD use and related risk behavior of some adolescents interferes with their health and development (Schulenberg & Maggs, 2002). Adolescent group work can help teens think about their lifestyle choices, such as unhealthy drinking patterns and AOD use, and reroute adolescents toward healthy life choices and skills through listening to both the group facilitator and their peers (D'Amico et al., 2015; D'Amico, Houck, et al., 2013; Kaminer, 2005; Vaughn & Howard, 2004).

EMPIRICAL DATA IN SUPPORT OF
ADOLESCENT GROUP INTERVENTIONS

In most adolescent AOD treatment settings, the group format is used to help teens examine and discuss their AOD use (Kaminer, 2005; Vaughn & Howard, 2004). Group work is typically conducted because it is economical (French, Zavala, McCollister, Waldron, & Ozechowski, 2008; Sobell, Sobell, & Agrawal, 2009) and enables practitioners to reach a larger number of youth in a shorter amount of time. There are several efficacious group interventions for youth. Because a comprehensive review of all such interventions is beyond the scope of this chapter, we focus on cognitive-behavioral therapy (CBT) and motivational interviewing (MI) group interventions. We also discuss the group process.

CBT approaches purport that AOD use is a learned behavior that is often initiated and maintained due to environmental context (Kaminer, Spirito, & Lewander, 2011). Therapy involves identifying certain triggers, such as settings, situations, or feelings that may lead to AOD use (Marlatt & Gordon, 1985). There is a great deal of work examining effects of individual CBT on an adolescent's AOD use in randomized controlled trials (RCTs), with most studies finding positive effects of CBT (see Waldron & Turner, 2008, for a review). Studies that have conducted RCTs of group CBT for adolescents have also found that CBT is effective in reducing AOD use, and this may be due in part to increased self-efficacy and better coping (e.g., (Battjes et al., 2004; Kaminer, Blitz, Burleson, Sussman, & Rounsaville, 1998; Kaminer, Burleson, Burke, & Litt, 2014; Kaminer, Burleson, & Goldberger, 2002; Ramo, Myers, & Brown, 2010; Waldron & Kaminer, 2004; Waldron, Slesnick, Brody, & Peterson, 2001).

CBT may also be combined with other treatments. One of the larger RCTs to date, the Cannabis Youth Treatment (CYT) study (Dennis et al., 2004) compared several different types of treatments, including CBT, among a sample of 600 adolescents. Youth were randomized across four treatment sites and there were two trials that compared different treatments, including motivational enhancement therapy (MET) MET-CBT 5 sessions (MET-CBT 5), MET-CBT 12 sessions (MET-CBT 12); family support network (FSN); adolescent community reinforcement approach (ACRA); or multidimensional family therapy (MDFT). MET is an adaptation of MI that includes one or more sessions in which normative feedback is presented to the client and discussed in an explicitly nonconfrontational manner (Miller, 2000). MET-CBT 5 consisted of two individual MET sessions and three group CBT sessions, MET-CBT 12 included an additional seven CBT sessions. FSN added six parent education group meetings focused on improving parent knowledge and skills relevant to adolescent problems and family functioning, four therapeutic home visits, referral to self-help support groups, and case management to the MET-CBT 12. ACRA consisted of 10 individual sessions with the youth, four sessions with caregivers (two of which are with the whole family), and limited case management provided by the therapist over a period of 12–14 weeks. MDFT included 12–15 sessions (typically six with the adolescent, three with parents, and six with the whole family) and case management provided over a period of 12–14 weeks.

Adolescents in both trials completed a baseline and 3-, 6-, 9-, and 12-month follow-up assessments. The two clinical outcomes assessed were days of abstinence between the randomization date and the 12-month follow-up interview and whether the adolescent was in recovery at the end of the study. Being in recovery at the end of the study was defined as living in the community (vs. incarceration, inpatient treatment, or other controlled environment) and reporting no past-month substance use, abuse, or dependence problems at the 12-month interview. Overall, there were significant reductions in cannabis use and negative consequences of use for all treatment conditions from pretreatment to the 3-month follow-up, and these reductions were sustained at 12 months. They also found that youth in the MET-CBT 5 had the highest percentage in recovery. When they examined cost-effectiveness for the different treatments, they found that MET-CBT 5 and MET-CBT 12 were more cost-effective than FSN, ACRA was more cost-effective than MET-CBT 5 and MDFT, and MET-CBT 5 was more cost effective than MDFT (Dennis et al., 2004).

A 2011 evaluation of the CYT study compared adolescents in the CYT trial who received the MET-CBT 5 with youth who received outpatient treatment from one of three community-based programs selected for evidence of efficacy (Ramchand, Griffin, Suttorp, Harris, & Morral, 2011). The authors of this study used data from youth in the CYT study who received MET-CBT 5, and then identified a new population of adolescents who received community-based outpatient treatment whose pretreatment characteristics were closely matched with the youth who received MET-CBT 5 in the original trial. They examined six outcome domains at 12 months: substance use problems, substance use frequency, emotional problems, illegal activities, recovery, and institutionalization. They found that youth who received MET-CBT 5 had significantly better outcomes for substance use frequency, substance use problems, and criminal activity than those who received care in the three outpatient settings. They did not find differences with regard to emotional problems or institutionalization rates. The authors suggest that the relatively low cost of MET-CBT 5 makes it a promising option for treating adolescents with cannabis-related disorders compared with more intensive, longer-term approaches (Ramchand et al., 2011).

In sum, research supports the effectiveness of CBT in treating youth who use AOD. The focus on modeling, behavioral rehearsal, and coping skills can help youth learn how to better self-regulate their behavior and develop problem-solving skills (Kaminer et al., 2011; Winters, Botzet, & Fahnhorst, 2011), which may lead to greater self-efficacy and better coping and thus decreased AOD use.

STEP-BY-STEP CLINICAL GUIDELINES FOR DELIVERING BRIEF INTERVENTIONS

Conducting group interventions with young people is an interactive and invigorating process. In contrast to individual interventions, *the group is the client*, which makes it especially important for the facilitator to be in tune with the group process. With their new skills in hypothesis generation and evaluation, adolescents are adept at examining situations from different angles. In addition, they are keenly aware of the behaviors of those around them, and how those behaviors compare with their own (e.g., Ingersoll & Feldstein Ewing, 2011). These two areas of heightened attention make group approaches especially salient for this developmental age group. Below, we give an example of a 1- to 2-hour adolescent MI group focused on reducing health risk behaviors. We provide specific suggestions for different types of strategies (e.g., providing normative feedback, discussing pros and cons of use) that we have used in our sessions to increase engagement in the group (see *www.groupmiforteens.org* for an introduction to using MI in groups and curricula for prevention and intervention for youth).

It is fairly common for adolescents and young adults to overestimate the amount of substances consumed by their peers, which may contribute to later AOD use (e.g., Pedersen et al., 2013). Exploring the validity of estimations of peer risk behavior can be an important starting point for group approaches including MI. Moreover, having group members shout out their guesses regarding their friends' and peers' risk behavior has the wonderful effect of generating group dialogue in a nonthreatening and nonconfrontational manner. Youth tend to be quite playful when discussing how much risk behavior occurs among their peers (particularly if they are from different social groups), and it sets an excellent foundation for talking about adolescents' own behavior. The target here is to allow exploration of topics not typically discussed regarding AOD use, but with an eye toward identifying and pulling for client language in favor of change. We explore steps to manage negative cross-talk, for example, when youth may begin to discuss how fun it is to party or use substances, in the section on "Issues Regarding Treatment Engagement" below.

Opening the Group

Depending on the reason for holding the group, the opening will vary. As a group leader, it is important to clearly and openly lay out the context and the parameters of the group (i.e., Will the group be confidential? When would confidentiality have to be violated? How long will the group run? How many times?). Transparency from the leaders facilitates a safe, genuine, and comfortable atmosphere. After laying out the parameters, it is important to have group members generate rules for the session. With adolescents, this approach has two positive effects. First, it gets them talking, which warms them up for more sensitive topics. Second, it gives them a sense of ownership and control over the group. To validate their thoughts and contributions, we write, display, and occasionally reference the rules that they generated. This strategy also helps manage negative behaviors within the group, as members tend to be sensitive to violations of rules that they generated.

> "Thank you for coming today. I know that you have lots of things that you could be doing, and I appreciate that you came here. For the next hour, we will be talking together about different risk-taking behaviors like drinking, drug use, and sexual risk behaviors. This is a confidential group, which means

that we won't tell your parents, teachers, or anyone else what you say, unless you mention that you are being hurt (by yourself or anybody else), or that you are hurting someone else. If that comes up, we have to tell someone to make sure that you and those around you are safe. By confidential, we also mean that we don't want you to discuss anything that anyone says in here with anyone else. It's OK to talk about today's topics with other people once you leave, because these topics are important and we want you to be thinking about them, but it is not OK to say who said what. What do you think about that? Can we agree to that? Also, for the group to be a safe, respectful, purposeful place, we need some rules. What rules do you think would be important to have today?"

The rules that a leader would want established are generally generated by the group. Those rules include "No name calling," "No interrupting," "Respect each person's opinion," and "Make sure everybody has a chance to talk." If the leader finds that he or she would like to include a rule that has not been suggested by the group, the leader can check in with the group to see whether it would be OK to include it.

"You have come up with some great rules for today. I'm impressed. There is one other rule that we would like to see. That rule is to make sure that we don't judge anyone else's experiences. Would it be OK with the group if we add it to the rule list?"

Once rules have been established, it is also important to get to know the members of the group. This is particularly important if participants in the group are unfamiliar with one another. One way to begin is by asking members to introduce themselves, say something that they like about themselves, and mention at least one of their future goals. This information helps establish a positive group dynamic focused on self-efficacy, with a foundation for developing healthy prosocial behaviors. It's easiest to model this by having one of the group leaders start:

"Hi, my name is Sarah. I work at [insert place] with teens. One thing that I like about myself is that I always say what I'm thinking. For the future, my goal is to create programs that help teens stay healthy. Angie, you're next."

If adolescents mention that they don't have anything that they like about themselves, a group leader can reflect:

"You can't come up with something right now. At the same time, you're here and willing to participate in the group, which is pretty cool. Let's start with that for now."

If they can't generate a future goal, the leader can reflect:

"It's hard to know where you're heading. We'll keep talking about what you might like to do in the future. OK, Paco. You're up. Tell us about you."

One activity that is often part of adolescent group work for AOD use is to compare members' ideas about the prevalence of risk behaviors. The key is to do this without raising resistance, and in a nonconfrontational, genuinely curious manner. With health risk behaviors, you can start very broadly, openly exploring the local states' rates of alcohol, marijuana, and tobacco use, and sexual risk behaviors. It is critical to provide information about demographically matched comparison groups when possible. In the United States, the Centers for Disease Control and Prevention (CDC) website (*www.cdc.gov*) is a great resource for finding age- and demographically matched health risk information. With adolescents in the United States, the CDC's Youth Risk Behavior Surveillance System (*www.cdc.gov/HealthyYouth/yrbs/index.htm*) is one resource for comparison data. For youth of other nations, the World Health Organization offers a database for finding drinking data by age group and geographic region (*www.who.int/globalatlas/DataQuery/default.asp*).

We begin to discuss comparison data by exploring members' guesses about how many people may be engaged in the target behavior. We might say:

"We are curious about how what you've seen and experienced compares with what's happening with other teens in [insert place]. So, from what you've seen, how many 16-year-old teens do you think drank alcohol during the past month?"

After posing the question, we wait for responses. If no responses are generated, we reflect:

"You aren't sure how many teens your age are drinking."

With their evaluative skills, adolescents might need time to determine the worth of participating in the group (e.g., Will my friends still like me if I participate?). To join with the group, it is important to give them time to explore the leaders and their fellow peers, without pushing against their lack of participation. It may take time for them to warm up. If after reflecting, they still don't respond, it is OK to move along to the next behavior.

"OK. How many teens do you think smoked marijuana in the past month? How about smoked cigarettes? How many teens your age have had sexual intercourse?"

Encourage their guesses and reflect back their hypotheses.

"It seems like almost everybody is using marijuana, every day. Who else would like to guess?"

After exploring adolescents' current perspectives on risk-taking behavior, we turn our focus toward broadening those perspectives and eliciting motivation to change. We focus our efforts on three elements: (1) raising doubt, (2) exploring reasons and need to change, and (3) increasing self-efficacy to change. Within the group environment, this shift is subtle and we do not draw attention to it to prevent unnecessarily eliciting resistance and sustain talk (e.g., where youth may argue that they don't want to change and instead focus on the benefits of using substances). Specifically, once we've generated lots of guesses about peer behavior patterns, we present a poster or individual handouts (that we generated previously) that have comparative rates of behavior for AOD use and risky sexual behaviors. We wonder with the group about how rates on the board compare with their guesses.

Many will have questions about the data or reply that the data are wrong. This is normal and should be expected. First, we use the opportunity to reflect the discrepancy.

> "This doesn't fit with your experience. The people on this chart aren't like the people you know."

It is also appropriate to mention some characteristics of the survey (e.g., size, year conducted, referent group). However, leaders should be careful to avoid arguing with the group about the data. We also use this opportunity to encourage responses from members who may have seen less risk behavior.

> "We know that people have different experiences. What do the rest of you think of this?"

It is important to maintain that the group is your client—for example, where exploring ambivalence from within the same person works for individual brief interventions, leaders should not be pulled toward one person in group approaches. It is also important to ensure that most members are participating. If a few are doing most of the talking, encourage others by looking at them when you ask questions or asking them directly:

> "Josie, tell us what you make of all this."

Of course, the goal is not to convince young people that their perceptions are wrong or that they should give up all risk behaviors. This approach is designed to raise doubts for them about assumptions of what others do, about what is normal, and about choices that they may want to make in the future. Also following the guiding approach of brief MI interventions in which there is a strong emphasis on reflections and working collaboratively, it is important to summarize the ideas that have been discussed before moving on to the next activity so youth know that they have been heard. A summary could sound like:

"OK, about half of you know teens who drink every day, and the rest of you don't know anybody who drinks. And we've found that the information for teens in [insert place] is somewhere in the middle. In terms of marijuana— about half know teens who smoke marijuana pretty often and the rest of you don't have friends who are smoking. Again, the information from [insert place] says that about 30% of teens (three out of 10) are smoking weed, so it makes sense that it's more than some of you have seen, but less than others of you have seen. Across the board, it looks like almost all of you have friends who smoke cigarettes. That is a lot more than most teens your age in [insert place]. The alcohol and marijuana experiences of your friends are right on target with the state information for [insert place], and the cigarette use of your friends is much higher. What else?"

We also use comparison data to explore ambivalence and discrepancies from within the group. After summarizing their peers' experiences, we wonder about how the behavior of their peers might compare with their own behavior.

"So we noticed that the people you know use more tobacco than similar teens in [insert place]. How does the tobacco use of your friends compare with your own experiences?"

Some members may be reluctant to respond, particularly if the group is being conducted in any type of juvenile or criminal justice context. To alleviate concerns, we remind participants that the group is confidential and their responses are private and contained to the group. Many adolescents may respond in a polarized way, stating that their friends drink more than they do, or that they are drinking at high levels and have never had any problems.

Once group responses are on the table, the leaders can explore them.

"You have a wide range of experiences. It looks like some of you feel like your friends are drinking a lot more than you, and some of you feel like you're drinking and not experiencing any problems and are not quite sure what the big deal is."

For adolescents whose friends are engaged in greater levels of risk behavior compared with their own, it is worthwhile to explore peer norms, behaviors, beliefs, and comparisons. For example:

"Your friends are drinking every weekend. And, that's kind of what people do in your school. What would you say that your friends expect of you? What happens to teens in your friend group who don't drink? What would happen to you if you didn't drink?"

Genuinely and empathically, we explore all of the angles of this behavior and are curious about the ramifications of the behavior with the group. Again, here is an area where you can encourage the group to generate ideas among themselves.

> "Paco, what thoughts do you have about Mary's friends' expectations for her to drink?"

If the group becomes encouraging of negative behaviors, then the group leaders can step in and intervene and move on to the next topic.

> "OK, so lots of your friends drink, and yet many of you have said that people don't drink or that you choose not to drink. How do you make that happen?"

With their relatively brief risk histories, it is not unusual for adolescents to have experienced only positive effects of risk behavior. We operate under the idea that people use substances and engage in risk behavior for valid reasons. These behaviors might help them develop friendships (it's easier to meet and talk to people in the small social groups of smokers), navigate social settings (it's easier to interact at a party if you're intoxicated), or move through the fears that may accompany new relationships (it might be easier to just have sex than to talk about feelings, needs, or desires). Therefore, joining with this other side of the group's ambivalence is important.

> "Let's switch gears for a moment. Some of you mentioned that you have been drinking without experiencing any problems. How would you know when problems started happening? What would that look like?"

If the group is unable to generate ideas, the leaders can move on to reflecting potential negative consequences, with openness and genuineness.

> "So you haven't had anything bad happen when you've had unprotected sex. It's hard to imagine anything scary happening to you or anyone you know because of sex."

The messages that they get from adults in their lives can also be helpful in this activity.

> "Tell us what your parents, teachers, and/or doctors said about having sex. What are they worried about?"

Once some negative consequences are generated, the leaders can explore how those negative consequences might fit with future goals. Pulling from what the participants' said at the introduction of the group, a leader could say;

> "OK, so you haven't had anything bad happen to you or anybody you know after having sex. Your mom mentioned that teens can sometimes get sexually

transmitted infections and diseases. How does getting HIV from unprotected sex fit with going to college or being a soccer star?"

Summaries that collect each contribution from the group members are critical. We want to reflect, in a clear manner, the group's reasons for risk behavior and end with the group's ideas about the negative consequences of risk behavior, checking in to see whether we missed any contributions. It is always important to acknowledge both sides, and using double-sided reflections is one way to encourage change talk (D'Amico et al., 2015)—for example:

"Many of you said that it's really fun to smoke marijuana, and yet, you also said that it's gotten you into trouble with your parents and at school."

We then let the group know that we will come back to this discussion, but that we would like to do something else for a moment.

Before moving into the next phase of this brief group, it is important to bolster youths' sense of self-efficacy. We do this because we are asking youth to make active decisions to (1) not engage in a behavior, (2) engage in a lower level of a behavior, and/or (3) engage in a different behavior. Each is difficult and likely discrepant from the prevalent behaviors of their peer groups. Before asking them to take on these behavioral changes, we want to increase their belief in their *ability* to enact these changes. We have found that three approaches work particularly well in adolescent groups. The first approach is the "characteristics of successful adolescents' sheet." This activity can be introduced in the following manner:

"We are going to hand out a sheet of paper. This paper contains a list of adjectives that describes adolescents like you. These adolescents face all of the pressures of high school and still decide to make healthy choices. We'd like for each of you to take a moment and circle all of the adjectives on this sheet that describe you."

Once the pencils have stopped moving, we encourage adolescents to go around the room and pick their favorite five adjectives to share. As they are speaking, it can be very powerful to write these adjectives on a sheet of paper for the whole group to see. Once all have shared their adjectives, we can reflect the strength of the room.

"You're a pretty incredible group. You're 'alive,' and 'honest,' and 'smart' . . . With this kind of strength and ability, you could do anything that you put your mind to."

Adolescents rarely get to say what they think is wonderful and powerful about themselves—it is even rarer to hear about their positive attributes from their peers. Therefore, the second approach, exploring strengths of fellow group members, encourages adolescents to highlight the positive attributes about their fellow group members. This activity can be introduced by saying:

> "Well, at the start of today, we each said something that we liked about ourselves. Now, I'd like each of you to mention a strength you noticed of one of your fellow group members. I'll begin by saying that at the start of group today, Paco said that he's honest. And, I think that's pretty cool. I have also noticed that Paco really thinks hard about tough topics—he is also very smart. Josie, do you remember what Mary said at the start of group?"

The third approach, change success stories, can also be very powerful in a group context. In this MI approach, youth are encouraged to state a time that they were able to do something that they thought they could not do. This tends to be very powerful for the speaker. It also generates a feeling of self-efficacy throughout the group. We introduce this activity by saying:

> "Now, I'd like for us to think about a time when we were able to do something that we had originally thought that we could not do. I'll give us a minute to think about it. We'll have Eric start, and then go around the room sharing our stories."

If a member is not able to generate a success story, the leader might lower the bar.

> "Mary—no worries. This doesn't have to be a change-the-world kind of event, it might just be a time that you didn't think that you could get up that morning and face the world, but you did anyway. Why don't we move on to Jason and come back to you in a minute?"

As with individual brief interventions, some members of a group may not be ready to make formal change plans, and it is important not to push beyond the group's readiness. However, it is helpful to have the group generate ideas of what a person could do *if* he or she wanted to make any behavior changes. We introduce this approach by revisiting the cons of the behavior (through our summary from the negative consequences section), bolstering members' self-efficacy (by summarizing the strengths of the group and their expertise in their own lives), and exploring potential options.

> "Earlier today, when we talked about drinking, we noticed that half of you have a lot of friends who drink frequently. You also mentioned that while you know that drinking can lead to accidents, like falling off of the roof at a party or getting in a car accident, if you were to stop drinking, you're not sure that your friends would still be your friends. We also know that you guys are smart, alive, and creative. And, you're the experts on how these things go at your school. You're the ones who know these situations best. So, let's have you

all put your heads together and think about ways to manage drinking situations so that you don't lose your friends *and also* so that you don't get hurt because of drinking. If you're at a party, and you don't want to drink, but all your friends are expecting you to drink—and will give you a hard time if you don't—what could you do?"

By this time, group members are likely to generate great ideas. We like to encourage silly ideas or ideas of what they should *not* do, to get the group laughing and talking. It is helpful for the leaders to have some ideas as well, in the event that the group struggles with generating possibilities. If they do encounter problems in brainstorming ideas, the leaders can go through the steps of elicit–provide–elicit—a standard approach in MI-based interventions (Miller & Rollnick, 2012) focused on eliciting information from the group, providing information as needed, and continuing to elicit information from the group (Feldstein Ewing, Walters, & Baer, 2012). When working with adolescents toward harm reduction, the three strategies that we keep in our back pocket are (1) how to be at a party without drinking heavily—*glasses half-full (of soda)*, (2) how to get home from a party safely—*designated drivers and planned (safe) sleepovers,* and (3) how to reduce sexual risk taking—*having friend chaperones at parties (particularly for girls).*

> "So there are lots of situations when we might need to take steps to be safe, and it's hard to figure out what those steps might be. Eric and I have some ideas. Would it be OK if we share them with the group?"

If the group does not consent to hearing leaders' ideas, you can close this activity by reflecting in a genuine manner.

> "You have a pretty good handle on these situations and don't need to hear any other ideas about what might work."

If the group consents, it is possible to go on.

> "So, you want to go to this party because the boy you like is going to be there, but you don't want to have sex yet. It can be hard when you feel like his group of friends are all sexually active, and they might pressure you to go further than you want to. One of the things that you could do is have an assigned friend know where you are and check up on you. How might this approach work for you?"

It is appropriate for youth to still be developing their problem-solving skills. So, working through problem-solving strategies together is worthwhile. The steps for problem solving include (1) identifying the problem, (2) generating several (five or so) possible solutions, (3) identifying the top three possibilities, (4) going through each possibility systematically to determine possible

obstacles, (6) generating solutions to possible obstacles, (7) updating each possibility with the new information, and (8) firming up the final strategies. This
can be augmented by adding role plays to try out the strategies, to determine
the possible obstacles and final strategies. This activity might sound like:

> "So the group came up with three ways of getting home from a party when
> intoxicated. You could call your parents or your older sibling, or walk home.
> Part of figuring out how these strategies might work is really thinking through
> what it might look like to do that. Let's do that together. Paco, you came up
> with the call-your-older-sibling strategy. Let's have Mary pretend to be you
> and you can be your older brother. Let's see how that goes.
>
> " . . . So, lots of times your older brother is busy with his girlfriend and
> won't come to get you. And, Josie, you mentioned that you don't have an older
> sibling to call, so this strategy might be tougher for you. At the same time,
> calling someone to pick you up is a great idea. What could we do to make this
> strategy work better?"

At the end of this activity, we write their ideas on a board or poster board,
and verbally review the strategies. Overall, we find that these different activities make for an engaging group discussion that generates lots of dialogue about
different risk behaviors and how to make changes if youth are willing and ready.

Issues Regarding Treatment Engagement/Establishing a Working Alliance

We recommend keeping groups small, capping them at six to eight participants. Having two leaders can also help with attending to the needs of the
group—however, many groups are conducted with just one facilitator, and this
is fine. We also like to keep the groups brief; some of this may depend upon
the setting. To encourage positive interactions, leaders may have to be vocal
in fostering and maintaining a positive and judgment-free climate. Finally, as
with individual brief interventions, most of the content should be generated by
the group.

As participants arrive with a wide range of needs, it is important to
have an established reason for holding the group (and maintaining that focus
throughout the group). To manage potentially less productive behaviors, such
as discussion of the latest party, or funny stories about what happens when
people use, we have found it worthwhile to be deliberate in assembling the
group composition. Groups that consist primarily of high-risk individuals (e.g.,
youth who have a first-time alcohol or drug offense, youth who are mandated
to come to group because of an infraction) may be more difficult to conduct,
as leaders will likely need to be vigilant about managing (and intervening)
with divisive and/or negative cross-talk. This is critical for preventing potentially iatrogenic effects (see below for further discussion on group process). For

high-risk adolescents who engage in lots of negative talk and are not amenable to decreasing that type of commentary, individual MI sessions may be more appropriate. In addition, many group exercises are aimed at developing discrepancies between current behaviors and goals. These work well, provided that leaders are aware that discussing certain beliefs—for example, that drinking is cool, or that everyone smokes pot—may elicit resistance. When youth feel challenged, they may argue against change (either out loud or silently) to preserve their beliefs. Part of the art of group interventions is to gently explore participants' beliefs without increasing resistance. This can often be done by using MI-consistent behaviors, such as asking open-ended questions and giving reflections (D'Amico et al., 2015). We raise these points because arguments against change may be vocalized and supported by other group members. Leaders need to encourage participation and open exchanges with the awareness that group exchanges can elicit arguments against change. This might take the form of members talking proudly about their wild nights, chuckling about someone else's drinking behavior, or arguing with the leaders or fellow members. Therefore, leaders need to listen for arguments both for and against change in all exchanges, and selectively reinforce the former and respectfully minimize the latter.

The Importance of Ensuring Developmental and Cultural Relevance

Given that many groups will include youth of different ages, it's important to consider each adolescent's developmental status along with relevant sociocultural factors (Burrow-Sánchez, Minami, & Hops, 2015; Wagner, 2009; Winters et al., 2011). For example, we have found that the needs of middle and high school youth are different, and the activities and discussion should be developmentally relevant. Specifically, younger adolescents tend to enjoy doing role plays to act out potential high-risk situations, whereas older youth prefer to just discuss these situations and how they would respond (D'Amico et al., 2005). Furthermore, prevention and intervention programming aimed at non-treatment-seeking youth must engage high-risk and high-need youth who would otherwise not receive services. For example, youth from lower-income families and from ethnic-minority backgrounds tend to participate less in structured after-school activities compared with higher-income and white youth (Harvard Family Research Project, 2007). At-risk youth, such as those who have already initiated AOD use, may also be less likely to access services (Sterling, Weisner, Hinman, & Parthasarathy, 2010; Wu, Hoven, Tiet, Kovalenko, & Wicks, 2002). Thus, innovative and creative approaches are needed to reach these high-need and underserved youth (D'Amico, Green, et al., 2012).

MI is one evidence-based approach that tends to resonate with minority youth (Becker et al., 2012; Dickerson, Brown, Johnson, Schweigman, & D'Amico, 2015)—however, there are also aspects of MI, such as the focus on the individual, rather than the community, that may make it potentially less efficacious, particularly for youth in collectivistic cultures. Research is needed to determine how to evaluate and improve the efficacy of interventions like MI with minority youth (Feldstein Ewing, Wray, Mead, & Adams, 2012). The most recent meta-analysis of MI interventions targeting AOD use among adolescents was conducted in 2011. As of this date, there were 21 MI outcome trials, and only five of these studies included samples with more than 50% nonwhite youth (Jensen et al., 2011). Few of these trials explicitly evaluated the role of race, ethnicity, or culture in prevention and intervention outcomes. Preliminary evidence suggests that cultural factors (e.g., level of ethnic mistrust, cultural orientation, ethnic pride) may influence adolescents' response to MI-based interventions (Gil, Wagner, & Tubman, 2004).

In addition, recent work by one of us (S. W. F. E.) has indicated that providers may not conduct MI in the same way with minority versus non-minority youth (Feldstein Ewing, Gaume, Ernst, Rivera, & Houck, 2015). In one study, we found that providers exhibited significantly fewer MI-consistent behaviors and statements (i.e., lower scores on MI spirit, support of autonomy, complex reflections, and evocation) with Hispanic versus non-Hispanic youth, which in turn predicted poorer outcomes, specifically in experiencing alcohol-related problems. However, despite the lower levels of MI-consistent practitioner behaviors, equivalent treatment outcomes were observed for Hispanic and white youth for the other key 3-month outcomes, including alcohol use, cannabis use, and cannabis-related problems (Feldstein Ewing, Gaume, et al., 2015). One possibility is that Hispanic youth bring something to the treatment equation that evokes fewer MI-consistent efforts from their therapists. To this end, our findings may reflect the operation of different cultural scripts for Hispanic youth (defined as patterns of social interactions that are predominant within different cultural groups; Triandis, Marin, Lisansky, & Betancourt, 1984). For example, Hispanic youth may desire a power distance with their health providers (Gallo, Penedo, Espinosa de los Monteros, & Arguelles, 2009). Thus, given what is known about cultural scripts, theory and anecdote indicate that Hispanic youth may work to develop and protect a clinical distance between their provider and themselves (e.g., Lopez-Viets, 2007). These youth behaviors may, in turn, elicit a different set of therapist responses (Barnett, Spruijt-Metz, et al., 2014). Future work would benefit from examining cultural scripts to see how these factors influence therapeutic interactions in group settings.

Furthermore, empirical research has shown that, although the instruments that exist to assess metrics of adolescent treatment response in MI and other group interventions is parallel between minority and nonminority youth (Feldstein Ewing, Montanaro, Gaume, Caetano, & Bryan, 2015), we still do not have a good understanding of the cultural mechanisms that might underlie adolescents' successful treatment response (Salvador, DeVargas, & Feldstein Ewing, 2015; Salvador, Goodkind, & Feldstein Ewing, 2016). Overall, recent work in this area emphasizes that gaining a stronger understanding of the role of key, but often underexamined, variables in the therapeutic process, such as cultural scripts noted above, may be important to include in the adaptation of MI for minority youth (Feldstein Ewing, Wray, et al., 2012).

MI IN GROUP FORMATS

In the last decade, research on MI (Miller & Rollnick, 2012) with adolescents has grown (Jensen et al., 2011; Lundahl & Burke, 2009), especially with non-white youth (Becker et al., 2012; Clair et al., 2013; Dickerson et al., 2015; Feldstein Ewing, Gaume, et al., 2015; Feldstein Ewing, Wray, et al., 2012; Gilder et al., 2011). The brevity and transportability of this intervention has made it ideal in reaching youth across a variety of settings, including juvenile justice, medical clinics, homeless shelters, and schools (Cushing, Jensen, Miller, & Leffingwell, 2014; Jensen et al., 2011; Lundahl, Kunz, Brownell, Tollefson, & Burke, 2010). Not only is this brief, empathic, and strength-based intervention highly transportable, it is also highly effective across a number of substance use and health risk behaviors (Hettema, Steele, & Miller, 2005; Jofre-Bonet & Sindelar, 2001; Lundahl et al., 2010).

MI is typically used in one-on-one situations—however, in the last several years, MI has been utilized more frequently in group settings with youth (D'Amico, Feldstein Ewing, et al., 2010; D'Amico, Osilla, et al., 2012; Wagner & Ingersoll, 2012). To date, there are two published RCTs that have examined MI in a group setting with at-risk youth. One study included a single session of group MET to enhance an intervention targeting risky sexual behavior among youth ($n = 484$) in detention centers (Schmiege et al., 2009). Youth randomized to the augmented intervention received an additional component addressing risky alcohol use and its relation to sexual risk-taking behavior. They were provided with feedback regarding their alcohol use and a discussion followed using MET procedures. Outcomes at 3 months showed that youth who received the additional MET session reduced their sexual risk behavior compared with youth who only received the sexual risk reduction intervention (Schmiege et al., 2009), suggesting the efficacy of group MI to reduce risk behaviors.

We conducted the second study of group MI intervention, called Free Talk (D'Amico, Osilla, & Hunter, 2010), with ethnically diverse youth with a first-time AOD offense. The study goals were to (1) understand youth acceptance of Free Talk, (2) determine the feasibility of training facilitators to deliver MI in a group setting by examining treatment integrity and adherence, and (3) conduct a preliminary evaluation of Free Talk's efficacy (D'Amico, Hunter, Miles, Ewing, & Osilla, 2013). First, youth felt that the quality of the MI group was superior compared with usual care groups. Fidelity to MI was also high, as facilitators were able to use reflections and open-ended questions and were not confrontational when teens discussed their AOD use. Evaluation results showed that both the control and MI groups reduced their AOD use. We only had a short-term follow-up of 3 months and recognize having this kind of "teachable moment" (e.g., intervening in close proximity to teens getting into trouble with the police, going to teen court, being sentenced by peers, participating in 6 weeks of classes, and getting drug tested) is likely a very powerful experience for both teens and parents. Thus, this type of experience may be enough in the short term to create some positive change, perhaps because parents increase their monitoring and/or teens cut back on their AOD use because of these intense consequences. We did find, however, that recidivism was slightly lower in the Free Talk group 12 months later compared with usual care, suggesting that the youth who received MI may be doing better in the long term (D'Amico, Hunter, et al., 2013).

In sum, preliminary work examining the effects of group MI on adolescent risk behaviors appears promising. Further work is needed with larger samples and longer-term follow-up periods to provide a better indication of the effectiveness of group MI with this age group.

EMPIRICAL DATA ANALYZING
THE ADOLESCENT GROUP PROCESS

Given the plethora of adolescent group intervention work, it is interesting to note that very little is known about what may distinguish effective and ineffective group interventions (Engle & Macgowan, 2009). Some research has suggested that group work for youth may have iatrogenic effects—that it can increase risk behaviors, due to negative peer behavior that may occur in a group session (Arnold & Hughes, 1999; Dishion, McCord, & Poulin, 1999; Dodge, Dishion, & Lansford, 2006). This may be due to youth responding positively in the group setting to bravado about use, such as "I'll never quit" or "Smoking pot is a good way to relax" (Engle, Macgowan, Wagner, & Amrhein, 2010), and in part, to how the facilitator may respond to these types of situations (described below). It is important to note that the majority of studies have shown that working with at-risk youth in a group setting is safe, effective, and comparable to working with youth individually (Burleson, Kaminer, & Dennis, 2006; D'Amico, Hunter, et al., 2013; Kaminer, 2005; Lee & Thompson, 2009; Schmiege et al., 2009; Waldron & Turner, 2008).

Equivocal findings for adolescent group interventions may be due, in part, to what actually happens during the group—that is, the "group process." However, adolescent group process has rarely been studied. In a review of the relevant literature, Engle and Macgowan (2009) found that only one out of 13 RCTs of adolescent group work administered any kind of group process measure. Thus, there is a paucity of research on process, group structures, and facilitator behavior for adolescent group treatment in general and for adolescent AOD use in particular. It is important to understand the group process so that clinicians and researchers can optimize outcomes with youth in the group setting.

Recent work has begun to examine the group process for youth who receive group MI interventions. Specifically, research has examined youth change talk (CT) and sustain talk (ST) in the group setting, and how CT (e.g., "I am thinking that I might need to cut back on my drinking") and ST (e.g., "Smoking pot is fun and it hasn't affected my school work at all") may affect an adolescent's subsequent AOD use. Engle and colleagues (2010) examined positive commitment language (e.g., "I'm quitting for the summer") and negative commitment language (e.g., "I'll never quit") and peer reinforcement of this language (e.g., "That's great") in 19 adolescent group sessions. Their sample comprised 108 youth ages 10–19 receiving AOD treatment (Engle et al., 2010). Correlational data indicated that when youth expressed positive commitment language *and* peer response was also positive (e.g., "That's cool"), teens reported reduced marijuana use—the more positive and less negative the peer responses, the greater the reduction in marijuana use. Group facilitator empathy (measured globally on a scale from 1 to 7 using the Motivational Interviewing Treatment Integrity [MITI; version 2.0] scale) was also correlated with more positive commitment language and peer responses to commitment language (Engle et al., 2010). This study was an important first step in trying to understand the adolescent group process when using MI—however, it was exploratory and had some limitations. For example, they were able to examine outcomes only at the group level—thus, their total sample size for analysis was 19 (for the number of groups), which limited their power and their ability to find significant associations.

Our group is one of the few teams to take an in-depth look at group process, and we have published several papers describing adolescent group dynamics in MI and the effects of those dynamics on AOD use outcomes (D'Amico, Houck, et al., 2013; Houck et al., 2015; Osilla et al., 2015). In these studies, we accounted for group membership to increase statistical power and also analyzed individual AOD use outcomes. This work is important for both research and clinical practice as it provides a better understanding of what makes adolescent groups "work" and informs practitioners how to modify their behaviors to improve AOD group treatment for youth.

In a seminal study, we examined how facilitator and peer behavior affected CT in a group setting for at-risk adolescents, and how CT during group affected an adolescent's individual AOD use outcomes (D'Amico et al., 2015). It was the first study to use sequential coding to assess adolescent group dynamics by evaluating the specific transitions that occurred during the group—for example, what happened in the group right after the facilitator reflected ST, CT, or asked a closed-ended question. We coded 129 group sessions attended by 110 individuals using the Motivational Interviewing Skill Code (MISC 2.5; Houck, Moyers, Miller, Glynn, & Hallgren, 2010) and CASAA Application for Coding Treatment Interactions (CACTI; Glynn, Hallgren, Houck, & Moyers, 2012) and examined outcomes 3 months later. Overall, we found that CT (e.g., "Drinking alcohol is affecting my schoolwork, so I don't think I want to drink during the week anymore") was associated with significant decreases in past 30-day alcohol use, heavy drinking in the past 30 days, and in intentions to use alcohol 3 months later. There was also a trend whereby greater CT was associated with lower positive expectancies for alcohol. ST (e.g., "I haven't had any problems because of using") in the group setting was associated with reductions in motivation to change, increases in intentions to use marijuana, and positive expectancies for alcohol and marijuana at 3-month follow-up. There was also a trend whereby greater ST was associated with increased marijuana use in the past 30 days at follow-up. We believe that the group facilitator's reflections that increased CT *were specific to CT*—that is, the reflections focused on the adolescent's desire to change (e.g., "You have thought a lot about cutting back on smoking pot"). Thus, our data emphasize that how the facilitator responds to adolescents' ambivalence surrounding their AOD use is crucial in determining the subsequent group response.

In a second study, we examined whether session content, such as discussion of normative feedback, decisional balance, or education on how AOD use affects the brain, was associated with CT/ST and whether different subtypes of CT/ST were associated with subsequent AOD use outcomes 3 months later. Subtypes of CT include statements indicating desire (e.g., "I want to quit doing drugs"), ability (e.g., "I can do it . . . . this is doable"), reasons (e.g., "I hate the way cigarettes smell"), need ("I need to stop"), commitment (e.g., "I stopped seeing him so I wouldn't smoke"), and taking steps ("This week, I won't go to any parties"). Each of these subtypes can also be a subtype of ST if it is expressed in opposition of change. For example, desire ST would indicate not wanting to change (e.g., "I do not want to quit") and reason ST would offer reasons why one continues to use (e.g., "I like smoking because it relaxes me").

Overall, we found that session content was not associated with CT—however, some session content was associated with higher percentages of ST (e.g., normative feedback). This is important as many youth may express disbelief regarding feedback on their AOD use as they are typically surrounded by other youth who "use just as much." We noted this earlier in our discussion of presenting this information. Thus, the facilitator must skillfully handle this ST by reflecting his or her surprise and trying to determine whether or not the adolescent is willing to make a change in his or her AOD use based on this feedback. We also found that particular subtypes of CT such as commitment (e.g., "I stopped seeing him so I wouldn't drink") and reason (e.g., "Marijuana affects my ability to focus") were associated with improved AOD use outcomes. In contrast, ability subtype remarks (e.g., "I can change") were related to increased marijuana use, intentions, and consequences. Previous research examining subtypes of CT found that ability CT may function differently from the other subtypes of CT (Gaume, Gmel, Faouzi, & Daeppen, 2009; Martin, Christopher, Houck, & Moyers, 2011), and may be interpreted as client confidence versus motivation to change (Barnett, Moyers, et al., 2014). For example, some youth who reported using marijuana would often state in group that although changing their marijuana use was not important to them at this time, they were very confident that they *could* stop smoking marijuana if they needed to stop (D'Amico et al., 2015). Ability language may therefore require differential response and further research is needed to understand its influence on the association between self-efficacy and AOD use outcomes (Barnett, Moyers, et al., 2014).

Finally, in terms of understanding the adolescent group process, Houck et al. (2015) examined temporal variation in facilitator and client behavior— that is, does the facilitator's speech in group affect adolescent speech differentially during different parts of the group session (e.g., beginning, middle, end)? Results indicated effects of facilitator speech on client speech only at the beginning and end of the group sessions, when open-ended questions respectively suppressed and enhanced adolescents' expressions of CT. Findings, therefore, emphasize that group MI sessions clinicians cannot "coast" on the strength of an initial positive exchange that may include many adolescent expressions of CT and facilitator reflections of CT. Instead, they must remain attentive throughout the session, continually focusing on reinforcing adolescent CT, and using open-ended questions to elicit CT if the adolescent does not offer it spontaneously, particularly near the end of the session.

In sum, the recent work in this area emphasizes the importance of the adolescent group process and the critical role of the clinician in helping adolescents think about whether they are ready to change their AOD use behavior. Findings highlight the significance of reflecting adolescents' CT during the group, helping adolescents come up with reasons for change and how they might commit to that change, and the importance of remaining attentive throughout the session and reinforcing CT.

IMPLICATIONS FOR TREATMENT OF ADOLESCENT SUBSTANCE ABUSE

The group process is particularly important in understanding whether youth may be willing and ready to make changes in their AOD use. This is especially relevant for youth who are in treatment for abuse or dependence. Work in this area has generally shown that group work is an effective modality for youth with substance use disorders (Burleson et al., 2006; Weiss et al., 2005). One thing to consider when conducting treatment groups is the comorbidity of other disorders as this could affect the group process. For example, one analysis of CYT study data (Dennis et al., 2004) found that there was a slight advantage for youth with high levels of conduct disorder (CD) to be included in groups with youth with lower levels of CD (Burleson et al., 2006). Having youth with more problems in the group did *not* create an iatrogenic effect for youth with fewer problems, and may have been beneficial for those youth with greater problems. Other work has also shown that having mixed groups (e.g., groups with low and high risk) are not harmful to the low-risk youth and actually benefit the high-risk youth (Ang & Hughes, 2001). This is consistent with the recent group process work indicating that positive peer interactions in the group can increase CT (D'Amico et al., 2015; Engle et al., 2010).

FUTURE DIRECTIONS

Group approaches are a promising avenue for work with adolescents and emerging adults. However, work has only begun in this area. Future research on group intervention outcomes, particularly by group composition, type of content, and delivery, will ultimately help determine what types of group approaches are most effective, for which behaviors, and for whom. In addition, future work on mechanisms of change (including youth CT, therapist language) in group interventions will likely follow the recent work on mechanisms of change in individual brief intervention outcomes. For instance, future studies might examine group activities such as raising ambivalence, normative comparisons, and skill building that are almost always used together in a group format. Research might also compare different group sizes, participant composition, race/ethnic matching between group facilitators and youth, and group leadership strategies. Past group research has demonstrated that certain MI-consistent counselor behaviors, including levels of empathy and questions-to-reflections ratios, can predict subsequent client change (D'Amico et al., 2015; Engle et al., 2010). Furthermore, client language about change has also been associated with better outcomes in studies of adolescents and adults in both individual and group interventions (e.g., Apodaca & Longabaugh, 2009; D'Amico et al., 2015; Moyers, Martin, Houck, Christopher, & Tonigan, 2009; Walker et al., 2011). Further research is needed to understand the adolescent- and group facilitator-level processes during group sessions. There are many challenges in examining the group process—however, a greater understanding of this process is an important step in bridging the gap between research and clinical practice and in providing crucial information on how groups function to help youth work toward positive change.

REFERENCES

Ang, R. P., & Hughes, J. N. (2001). Differential benefits of skills training with antisocial youth based on group composition: A meta-analytic investigation. *School Psychology Review, 31*, 164–185.

Apodaca, T. R., & Longabaugh, R. (2009). Mechanisms of change in motivational interviewing: A review and preliminary evaluation of the evidence. *Addiction, 104*(5), 705–715.

Arnold, M. E., & Hughes, J. N. (1999). First do no harm: Adverse effects of grouping deviant youth for skills training. *Journal of School Psychology, 37*, 99–115.

Barnett, E., Moyers, T. B., Sussman, S., Smith, C., Rohrbach, L. A., Sun, P., et al. (2014). From counselor skill to decreased marijuana use: Does change talk matter? *Journal of Substance Abuse Treatment, 46*(4), 498–505.

Barnett, E., Spruijt-Metz, D., Moyers, T. B., Smith, C., Rohrbach, L. A., Sun, P., et al. (2014). Bidirectional relationships between client and counselor speech: The importance of reframing. *Psychology of Addictive Behaviors, 28*(4), 1212–1219.

Battjes, R. J., Gordon, M. S., O'Grady, K. E., Kinlock, T. W., Katz, E. C., & Sears, E. A. (2004). Evaluation of a group-based substance abuse treatment program for adolescents. *Journal of Substance Abuse Treatment, 27*, 123–134.

Becker, S., Spirito, A., Hernandez, L., Barnett, N., Eaton, C., Lewander, W., et al. (2012). Trajectories of adolescent alcohol use after brief treatment in an emergency department. *Drug and Alcohol Dependence, 125*, 103–109.

Burleson, J. A., Kaminer, Y., & Dennis, M. L. (2006). Absence of iatrogenic or contagion effects in adolescent group therapy: Findings from the Cannabis Youth Treatment (CYT) study. *American Journal on Addictions, 15*, 4–15.

Burrow-Sánchez, J. J., Minami, T., & Hops, H. (2015). Cultural accommodation of group substance abuse treatment for Latino adolescents: Results of an RCT. *Cultural Diversity and Ethnic Minority Psychololgy, 21*(4), 571–583.

Clair, M., Stein, L. A., Soenksen, S., Martin, R. A., Lebeau, R., & Golembeske, C. (2013). Ethnicity as a moderator of motivational interviewing for incarcerated adolescents after release. *Journal of Substance Abuse Treatment, 45*(4), 370–375.

Cushing, C. C., Jensen, C. D., Miller, M. B., & Leffingwell, T. R. (2014). Meta-analysis of motivational interviewing for adolescent health behavior: Efficacy beyond substance use. *Journal of Consulting and Clinical Psychology, 82*(6), 1212–1218.

D'Amico, E. J., Ellickson, P. L., Wagner, E. F., Turrisi, R., Fromme, K., Ghosh-Dastidar, B., et al. (2005). Developmental considerations for substance use interventions from middle school through college. *Alcoholism: Clinical and Experimental Research, 29*, 474–483.

D'Amico, E. J., Feldstein Ewing, S. W., Engle, B., Hunter, S., Osilla, K. C., & Bryan, A. D. (2010). Group alcohol and drug treatment. In S. Naar-King & M. Suarez (Eds.), *Motivational interviewing with adolescents and young adults* (pp. 151–157). New York: Guilford Press.

D'Amico, E. J., Green, H. D. J., Miles, J. N. V., Zhou, A. J., Tucker, J. A., & Shih, R. A. (2012). Voluntary after school alcohol and drug programs: If you build it right, they will come. *Journal of Research on Adolescence, 22*(3), 571–582.

D'Amico, E. J., Houck, J. M., Hunter, S. B., Miles, J. N. V., Osilla, K. C., & Ewing, B. A. (2015). Group motivational interviewing for adolescents: Change talk and alcohol and marijuana outcomes. *Journal of Consulting and Clinical Psychology, 83*(1), 68–80.

D'Amico, E. J., Houck, J. M., Miles, J. N. V., Hunter, S. B., Osilla, K. C., & Ewing, B. A. (2013). What happens during group and does it matter?: An analysis of change talk of at-risk adolescents in a teen court setting. *Alcoholism: Clinical and Experimental Research, 37*(Suppl. 2), 276a.

D'Amico, E. J., Hunter, S. B., Miles, J. N. V., Ewing, B. A., & Osilla, K. C. (2013). A randomized controlled trial of a group motivational interviewing intervention for adolescents with a first time alcohol or drug offense. *Journal of Substance Abuse Treatment, 45*(5), 400–408.

D'Amico, E. J., Osilla, K. C., & Hunter, S. B. (2010). Developing a group motivational interviewing intervention for adolescents at-risk for developing an alcohol or drug use disorder. *Alcoholism Treatment Quarterly, 28,* 417–436.

D'Amico, E. J., Osilla, K. C., Miles, J. N. V., Ewing, B., Sullivan, K., Katz, K., et al. (2012). Assessing motivational interviewing integrity for group interventions with at-risk adolescents. *Psychology of Addictive Behaviors, 26*(4), 994–1000.

Dennis, M., Godley, S. H., Diamond, G., Tims, F. M., Babor, T., Donaldson, J., et al. (2004). The Cannabis Youth Treatment (CYT) study: Main findings from two randomized trials. *Journal of Substance Abuse Treatment, 27,* 197–213.

Dickerson, D. L., Brown, R. A., Johnson, C. L., Schweigman, K., & D'Amico, E. J. (2015). Integrating motivational interviewing and traditional practices to address alcohol and drug use among urban American Indian/Alaska Native youth. *Journal of Substance Abuse Treatment, 65,* 26–35.

Dishion, T. J., McCord, J., & Poulin, F. (1999). When interventions harm: Peer groups and problem behavior. *American Psychologist, 54,* 755–764.

Dodge, K. A., Dishion, T. J., & Lansford, J. E. (2006). *Deviant peer influences in programs for youth.* New York: Guilford Press.

Engle, B., & Macgowan, M. J. (2009). A critical review of adolescent substance abuse group treatments. *Journal of Evidence-Based Social Work, 6*(3), 217–243.

Engle, B., Macgowan, M. J., Wagner, E. F., & Amrhein, P. (2010). Markers of marijuana use outcomes within adolescent substance abuse group treatment. *Research on Social Work Practice, 20,* 271–282.

Feldstein Ewing, S. W., Gaume, J., Ernst, E. B., Rivera, L., & Houck, J. M. (2015). Do therapist behaviors differ with Hispanic youth?: A brief look at within-session therapist behaviors and youth treatment response. *Psychology of Addictive Behaviors, 29*(3), 779–786.

Feldstein Ewing, S. W., Montanaro, E. A., Gaume, J., Caetano, R., & Bryan, A. D. (2015). Measurement invariance of alcohol use instruments with Hispanic youth. *Addictive Behaviors, 46,* 113–120.

Feldstein Ewing, S. W., Walters, S. T., & Baer, J. S. (2012). Motivational interviewing groups for adolescents and emerging adults. In C. C. Wagner & K. S. Ingersoll (Eds.), *Motivational interviewing in groups* (pp. 387–406). New York: Guilford Press.

Feldstein Ewing, S. W., Wray, A. M., Mead, H. K., & Adams, S. K. (2012). Two approaches to tailoring treatment for cultural minority adolescents. *Journal of Substance Abuse Treatment, 43,* 190–213.

French, M. T., Zavala, S. K., McCollister, K. E., Waldron, H. B., & Ozechowski, T. J. (2008). Cost-effectiveness analysis of four interventions for adolescents with a substance use disorder. *Journal of Substance Abuse Treatment, 34,* 272–281.

Gallo, L. C., Penedo, F. J., Espinosa de los Monteros, K., & Arguelles, W. (2009). Resiliency in the face of disadvantage: Do Hispanic cultural characteristics protect health outcomes? *Journal of Personality, 77*(6), 1707–1746.

Gaume, J., Gmel, G., Faouzi, M., & Daeppen, J.-B. (2009). Counselor skill influences outcomes of brief motivational interventions. *Journal of Substance Abuse Treatment, 37,* 151–159.

Gil, A. G., Wagner, E. F., & Tubman, J. G. (2004). Culturally sensitive substance abuse intervention for Hispanic and African American adolescents: Empirical examples from the Alcohol Treatment Targeting Adolescents in Need (ATTAIN) project. *Addiction, 99*(Suppl. 2), 140–150.

Gilder, D. A., Luna, J. A., Calac, D., Moore, R. S., Monti, P. M., & Ehlers, C. L. (2011). Acceptability of the use of motivational interviewing to reduce underage drinking in a Native American community. *Substance Use and Misuse, 46*(6), 836–842.

Glynn, L. H., Hallgren, K. A., Houck, J. M., & Moyers, T. B. (2012). CACTI: Free, open-source software for the sequential coding of behavioral interactions. *PLOS ONE, 7*(7), e39740.

Harvard Family Research Project. (2007). *Findings from HFRP's study of predictors of participation in out-of-school time activities: Fact sheet.* Cambridge, MA: Harvard Graduate School of Education.

Hettema, J., Steele, J., & Miller, W. R. (2005). Motivational interviewing. *Annual Review of Clinical Psychology, 1*(1), 91–111.

Houck, J. M., Hunter, S. B., Benson, J. G., Cochrum, L. L., Rowell, L. N., & D'Amico, E. J. (2015). Temporal variation in facilitator and client behavior during group motivational interviewing sessions. *Psychology of Addictive Behaviors, 29*(4), 941–949.

Houck, J. M., Moyers, T. B., Miller, W. R., Glynn, L. H., & Hallgren, K. A. (2010). Motivational Interviewing Skill Code (MISC) version 2.5. Retrieved from *http://casaa.unm.edu/download/misc25.pdf.*

Ingersoll, K. S., & Feldstein Ewing, S. W. (2011). Vulnerability to addictive disorders and substance abuse in adolescence and emerging adulthood. In B. A. Johnson (Ed.), *Addiction medicine* (pp. 1329–1344). New York: Springer Science + Business Media.

Jensen, C. D., Cushing, C. C., Aylward, B. S., Craig, J. T., Sorell, D. M., & Steele, R. G. (2011). Effectiveness of motivational interviewing interventions for adolescent substance use behavior change: A meta-analytic review. *Journal of Consulting and Clinical Psychology, 79*(4), 433–440.

Jofre-Bonet, M., & Sindelar, J. L. (2001). Drug treatment as a crime fighting tool. *Journal of Mental Health Policy and Economics, 4,* 175–188.

Kaminer, Y. (2005). Challenges and opportunities of group therapy for adolescent substance abuse: A critical review. *Addictive Behaviors, 30*(9), 1765–1774.

Kaminer, Y., Blitz, C., Burleson, J., Sussman, J., & Rounsaville, B. J. (1998). Psychotherapies for adolescent substance abusers: Treatment outcome. *Journal of Nervous and Mental Disease, 186,* 684–690.

Kaminer, Y., Burleson, J. A., Burke, R., & Litt, M. D. (2014). The efficacy of contingency management for adolescent cannabis use disorder: A controlled study. *Substance Abuse, 35*(4), 391–398.

Kaminer, Y., Burleson, J., & Goldberger, R. (2002). Psychotherapies for adolescent substance abusers: Short- and long-term outcomes. *Journal of Nervous and Mental Disease, 190,* 737–745.

Kaminer, Y., Spirito, A., & Lewander, W. (2011). Brief motivational interventions, cognitive-behavioral therapy, and contingency management for youth substance use disorders. In Y. Kaminer & K. C. Winters (Eds.), *Clinical manual of adolescent substance abuse treatment* (pp. 213–237). Arlington, VA: American Psychiatric Publishing.

Lee, B. R., & Thompson, R. (2009). Examining externalizing behavior trajectories of youth in group homes: Is there evidence for peer contagion? *Journal of Abnormal Child Psychology, 37*(1), 31–44.

Lopez-Viets, V. (2007). CRAFT: Helping Latino families concerned about a loved one. *Alcoholism Treatment Quarterly, 25*(4), 111–123.

Lundahl, B., & Burke, B. L. (2009). The effectiveness and applicability of motivational interviewing: A practice-friendly review of four meta-analyses. *Journal of Clinical Psychology, 65*(11), 1232–1245.

Lundahl, B. W., Kunz, C., Brownell, C., Tollefson, D., & Burke, B. L. (2010). A meta-analysis of motivational interviewing: Twenty-five years of empirical studies. *Research on Social Work Practice, 20*(2), 137–160.

Marlatt, G. A., & Gordon, J. R. (Eds.). (1985). *Relapse prevention: Maintenance strategies in the treatment of addictive behaviors.* New York: Guilford Press.

Martin, T., Christopher, P. J., Houck, J. M., & Moyers, T. B. (2011). The structure of client language and drinking outcomes in project match. *Psychology of Addictive Behaviors, 25*(3), 439–445.

Miller, W. R. (2000). Motivational enhancement therapy: Description of a counseling approach. In J. J. Boren, L. S. Onken, & K. M. Caroll (Eds.), *Approaches to drug abuse counseling* (pp. 89–93). Bethesda, MD: National Institute on Drug Abuse.

Miller, W. R., & Rollnick, S. (2012). *Motivational interviewing: Helping people change* (3rd ed.). New York: Guilford Press.

Moyers, T. B., Martin, T., Houck, J. M., Christopher, P. J., & Tonigan, J. S. (2009). From in-session behaviors to drinking outcomes: A causal chain for motivational interviewing. *Journal of Consulting and Clinical Psychology, 77,* 1113–1124.

Osilla, K. C., Ortiz, J. A., Miles, J. N. V., Pedersen, E. R., Houck, J., & D'Amico, E. J. (2015). How group factors affect adolescent change talk and substance use outcomes: Implications for motivational interviewing training. *Journal of Counseling Psychology, 62*(1), 79–86.

Pedersen, E. R., Miles, J. N. V., Ewing, B. A., Tucker, J. S., Shih, R. A., & D'Amico, E. J. (2013). A longitudinal examination of alcohol, marijuana, and cigarette perceived norms among middle school adolescents. *Drug and Alcohol Dependence, 133*(2), 647–653.

Ramchand, R., Griffin, B. A., Suttorp, M., Harris, K. M., & Morral, A. (2011). Using a cross-study design to assess the efficacy of motivational enhancement therapy–cognitive behavioral therapy 5 (MET/CBT 5) in treating adolescents with cannabis-related disorders. *Journal of Studies on Alcohol and Drugs, 72*(3), 380–389.

Ramo, D. E., Myers, M. G., & Brown, S. A. (2010). Self-efficacy mediates the relationship between depression and length of abstinence after treatment among youth but not among adults. *Substance Use and Misuse, 45*(13), 2301–2322.

Salvador, J. G., DeVargas, E. C., & Feldstein Ewing, S. W. (2015). Who are Hispanic youth?: Considerations for adolescent addiction clinical research and treatment. *Alcoholism Treatment Quarterly, 33,* 348–362.

Salvador, J. G., Goodkind, J., & Feldstein Ewing, S. W. (2016). Perceptions and use of community- and school-based behavioral health services among urban American Indian/Alaska Native youth and families. *American Indian and Alaska Native Mental Health Research, 23*(3), 221–247.

Schmiege, S. J., Broaddus, M. R., Levin, M., Taylor, S. C., Seals, K. M., & Bryan, A. (2009). Sexual and alcohol risk reduction among incarcerated adolescents: Mechanisms underlying the effectiveness of a brief group-level motivational interviewing-based intervention. *Journal of Consulting and Clinical Psychology, 77,* 38–50.

Schulenberg, J., & Maggs, J. L. (2002). A developmental perspective on alcohol use and heavy drinking during adolescence and the transition to young adulthood. *Journal of Studies on Alcohol, 14*(Suppl.), 54–70.

Sobell, L. C., Sobell, M. B., & Agrawal, S. (2009). Randomized controlled trial of a cognitive-behavioral motivational intervention in a group versus individual format for substance use disorders. *Psychology of Addictive Behaviors, 23,* 672–683.

Sterling, S., Weisner, C., Hinman, A., & Parthasarathy, S. (2010). Access to treatment for adolescents with substance use and co-occurring disorders: Challenges and opportunities. *Journal of the American Academy of Child and Adolescent Psychiatry, 49,* 637–646.

Triandis, H. C., Marin, G., Lisansky, J., & Betancourt, H. (1984). Simpatia as a cultural script of Hispanics. *Journal of Personality and Social Psychology, 47*(6), 1363–1375.

Tucker, J. S., Ellickson, P. L., Collins, R. L., & Klein, D. J. (2006). Are drug experimenters better adjusted than abstainers and users?: A longitudinal study of adolescent marijuana use. *Journal of Adolescent Health, 39,* 488–494.

Vaughn, M. G., & Howard, M. O. (2004). Adolescent substance abuse treatment: A synthesis of controlled evaluations. *Research on Social Work Practice, 14*(5), 325–335.

Wagner, C. C., & Ingersoll, K. S. (2012). *Motivational interviewing in groups.* New York: Guilford Press.

Wagner, E. F. (2009). Improving treatment through research: Directing attention to the role of development in adolescent treatment success. *Alcohol and Research Health, 32*(1), 67–75.

Waldron, H. B., & Kaminer, Y. (2004). On the learning curve: The emerging evidence supporting cognitive-behavioral therapies for adolescent substance abuse. *Addiction, 99,* 93–105.

Waldron, H. B., Slesnick, N., Brody, J. L., & Peterson, T. R. (2001). Treatment outcomes for adolescent substance abuse 4- and 7-month assessments. *Journal of Consulting and Clinical Psychology, 69,* 802–813.

Waldron, H. B., & Turner, C. W. (2008). Evidence-based psychosocial treatments for adolescent substance abuse. *Journal of Clinical Child and Adolescent Psychology, 37*(1), 238–261.

Walker, D. D., Stephens, R., Roffman, R., DeMarce, J., Lozano, B., Towe, S., et al. (2011). Randomized controlled trial of motivational enhancement therapy with nontreatment-seeking adolescent cannabis users: A further test of the teen marijuana check-up. *Psychology of Addictive Behaviors, 25*(3), 474–484.

Weiss, B., Caron, A., Ball, S., Tapp, J., Johnson, M., & Weisz, J. R. (2005). Iatrogenic effects of group treatment for antisocial youth. *Journal of Consulting and Clinical Psychology, 73,* 1036–1044.

Winters, K. C., Botzet, A. M., & Fahnhorst, T. (2011). Advances in adolescent substance abuse treatment. *Current Psychiatry Reports, 13*(5), 416–421.

Wu, P., Hoven, C. W., Tiet, Q., Kovalenko, P., & Wicks, J. (2002). Factors associated with adolescent utilization of alcohol treatment services. *American Journal of Drug and Alcohol Abuse, 28,* 353–369.

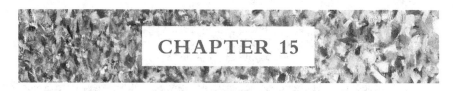

CHAPTER 15

Integrated 12-Step Facilitation to Promote Adolescent Mutual-Help Involvement

John F. Kelly, Julie Cristello, and Brandon Bergman

*D*rug and alcohol misuse and related use disorders are the top cause of premature mortality and morbidity among young people in high-income countries globally (Gore et al., 2011). Providing effective intervention for youth with substance use disorders (SUDs) has become a top public health priority, yet engaging young people in treatment has proven challenging (Kaminer & Gordon, 2014; Physician Leadership on National Drug Policy, 2002; Smith, Godley, Godley, & Dennis, 2011; Tanner-Smith, Wilson, & Lipsey, 2013). Once engaged, professional treatment does often produce modest initial salutary changes in adolescents' substance use (Dennis et al., 2004; Miller & Wilbourne, 2002; Tanner-Smith et al., 2013), but the short-term nature of most SUD treatment along with the prodigious and chronic burden of disease attributable to alcohol and other drugs mean that, by itself, professionally delivered interventions often lack the ability to sustain long-term behavioral change (Humphreys & Tucker, 2002; Kelly & White, 2011). As a result, briefer professional interventions often attempt to stimulate patients' engagement with ongoing community-based supports that can help sustain long-term SUD remission (Roman & Blum, 1999).

Peer-based 12-step mutual-help organizations (MHOs), such as Alcoholics Anonymous (AA), Narcotics Anonymous (NA), and Marijuana Anonymous (MA), have emerged and proliferated during the past 80 years in the United States and in approximately 150 countries worldwide (Humphreys, 2004; Kelly & Yeterian, 2013). Non-12-step MHOs, such as SMART Recovery, LifeRing, and Women for Sobriety, have also emerged and grown globally. These MHOs provide a ubiquitous, free, community-based recovery resource that can aid recovery and help enhance and extend professional treatment effects (Fiorentine & Hillhouse, 2000; Humphreys, 2004; Kelly & Myers, 2007). AA and other MHOs are the oldest and largest and have been subjected to the most scientific scrutiny. AA initially attracted and catered to severe and chronic, middle-age, alcohol-dependent individuals (Alcoholics Anonymous, 2001). However, with cultural changes since the 1960s in many Western societies in the acceptance of, and access to, alcohol and other drugs among youth, as well as greater knowledge and acceptance of alcohol addiction as a disease, AA and other MHOs increasingly began to receive younger referrals and to engage young people, often before the onset of severe health problems and associated disabilities (Alcoholics Anonymous, 1981).

Several prospective studies, including work from our group, suggest that 12-step MHO attendance is safe and beneficial for young people, with significant, modest correlations between greater attendance and better outcomes (Alford, Koehler, & Leonard, 1991; Chi, Kaskutas, Sterling, Campbell, & Weisner, 2009; Dow & Kelly, 2013; Hsieh, Hoffmann, & Hollister, 1998; Kelly, Dow, Yeterian, & Myers, 2011; Kelly & Myers, 2007; Kelly & Urbanoski, 2012; Kennedy & Minami, 1993; Mundt, Parthasarathy, Chi, Sterling, & Campbell, 2012). In one 8-year prospective study on adolescent inpatients, for example, we found that adolescents gained an average of 2 days of abstinence for each AA or NA meeting attended, over and above all other factors associated with better outcomes (Kelly, Brown, Abrantes, Kahler, & Myers, 2008). Our study also found that an average "dose" of two to three meetings per week was associated with complete abstinence across the 8-year follow-up.

Another important aspect of MHO referral and participation for patients with SUDs is that they can simultaneously reduce health care use and related costs in adults (Humphreys & Moos, 2001, 2007) and adolescents (Mundt et al., 2012). A 7-year prospective study with adolescents found that those who participated in 12-step MHOs following treatment had significantly better substance use outcomes. For every MHO meeting attended, a saving of approximately $145 in health care costs was observed (Mundt et al., 2012).

To varying degrees, most residential SUD treatment for adolescents in the United States also incorporates the 12-step philosophy and practices of AA and NA and helps prepare young people for engagement with groups like AA and NA following discharge (Jaffe & Kelly, 2010; Knudsen, Ducharme, Roman, & Johnson, 2008; White, 2014). These programs are often referred to as "Minnesota Model" programs, reflecting where the model originated (McElrath, 1997). To help illustrate how 12-step-based treatment might fit within a contemporary clinical approach, Table 15.1 lists the 12-step process, followed by interpretations of the broader themes on which each step is based and a more simplified, youth-focused translation of each step. The final column lists the potential therapeutic outcomes that may result from successfully completing each step.

Given the old-fashioned and ostensibly religious language used in the 12 steps, we want to translate the concepts involved and use more mundane terms for easier understanding.

While popular, data on the relative effectiveness of this model of treatment is limited, especially for adolescents. One of the earliest studies of 12-step-based treatment for adolescents found greater 6-month rates of abstinence (males = 71%, females = 79%) for treatment "completers," with abstinence rates still high but declining at 1-year (48%) and 2-year (40%) follow-ups (Alford et al., 1991). Other studies of inpatient/residential 12-step treatments found similar 1-year abstinence rates, ranging from 47 to 53% (Hsieh et al., 1998; Kennedy & Minami, 1993; Winters, Stinchfield, Latimer, & Lee, 2007). Due to the absence of a comparison condition in these studies, however, it is not possible to determine whether these 12-step treatments were superior to other treatments or no treatment. In an attempt to partially redress these prior limitations, Winters and colleagues (Winters et al., 2007; Winters, Stinchfield, Opland, Weller, & Latimer, 2000) assessed adolescents who received either a 12-step-based treatment or a separate "wait-list" group that was assessed but received no treatment during the study. At the 1-year follow-up, 53% of treatment patients were abstinent or had experienced only a minor lapse, compared with 28% of wait-list adolescents (Winters et al., 2000). Also, these differences were substantially greater at a 5-year, 5-month follow-up, when improvements on substance use were sustained by approximately one-third of the treatment sample (35%) but almost none of the wait-list sample (5%; Winters et al., 2007). While the lack of randomization still limits conclusions from this quasi-experimental study, the groups were not statistically different at intake on any variables examined, including socioeconomic status. This lends support to the interpretation that attending treatment (vs. not attending treatment) *caused* the observed differences in abstinence rates. In the absence of more rigorous randomized controlled trials, the results from these studies provide some preliminary evidence for the effectiveness of 12-step-based residential treatment and suggest that about half of adolescent patients who complete such a program remain abstinent up to 1 year following treatment.

Consistent with their treatment orientation and goals, 12-step-based residential programs appear to be effective in linking patients with community-based MHOs, with generally declining attendance rates as patients are further removed in time from treatment. In our work, we found that 72% of adolescent inpatients ($N = 74$) attended at least one MHO meeting during the first 3 months after discharge, with an average attendance rate of two times per week. During the next 3 months (i.e., 4- to 6-months postdischarge), the attendance rate dropped to 54%, with average attendance around once per week (Kelly, Myers, & Brown, 2002). In our 8-year prospective study mentioned above with adolescent inpatients ($N = 166$), rates of MHO meeting attendance were very high in the first 6-months posttreatment (91% attended at least once, 83% at least monthly, 65% at least weekly), but rates dropped off in the next 6-month

TABLE 15.1. Interpretation and Potential Therapeutic Outcome of the 12-Step Process

Step	Theme	Youth-focused interpretation	Therapeutic outcome
1. We admitted we were powerless over our addiction—that our lives had become unmanageable.	Honesty	I've got an alcohol/drug problem	Liberation/ relief
2. Came to believe that a Power greater than ourselves could restore us to sanity	Open-mindedness	Help is available; change is possible	Instillation of hope
3. Made a decision to turn our will and our lives over to the care of God, *as we understood Him.*	Willingness	Decide to get help	Self-efficacy
4. Made a searching and fearless moral inventory of ourselves.	Self-assessment and appraisal	Take a look at what's bothering you and why	Insight and discovery
5. Admitted to God, to ourselves, and to another human being the exact nature of our wrongs.	Self-forgiveness	Talk about what's bothering you and why with someone you trust and who can help you	Reduced shame and guilt
6. Were entirely ready to have God remove all these defects of character.	Readiness to change	Start to make the necessary changes	Greater consistency between values and behaviors
7. Humbly asked Him to remove our shortcomings.	Making changes	Continue to make the necessary changes	Greater consistency between values and behaviors
8. Made a list of all persons we had harmed and became willing to make amends to them all.	Taking responsibility and forgiveness of others	Attempt to rectify sources of guilt/shame	Peace of mind; reduced guilt
9. Made direct amends to such people whenever possible except when to do so would injure them or others.	Restitution to others	Talk to those concerned and make amends where necessary	Peace of mind; diminution of guilt and self-esteem
10. Continued to take personal inventory and when we were wrong promptly admitted it.	Emotional balance	Keep on taking a look at yourself and correct mistakes as you go	Self-monitoring; affect regulation; self-efficacy
11. Sought through prayer and meditation to improve our conscious contact with God, *as we understood Him,* praying only for knowledge of his will for us and the power to carry that out.	Connectedness and emotional balance	Stay connected; stay mindful	Awareness; psychological well-being
12. Having had a spiritual awakening as the result of these steps, we tried to carry this message to alcoholics and to practice these principles in all our affairs.	Helping others achieve recovery	Continue to access help, work on yourself, and try to help others	Self-esteem; confidence and mastery

period (i.e., 6- to 12-months posttreatment; 59% attended at least once, 48% at least monthly, 33% at least weekly) and continued to decline steadily across the 8-year follow-up period. By 6–8 years after treatment, only 31% attended at least once, 19% at least monthly, and 6% at least weekly (Kelly, Brown, et al., 2008).

During the past 20 years there has been a major shift from residential to outpatient treatment for adults and adolescents. In 2012, for example, approximately 83% of all adolescent SUD treatment admissions were in outpatient settings (Substance Abuse and Mental Health Services Administration, 2014). Many of these outpatient programs are theoretically and technically eclectic—they use various elements from cognitive-behavioral therapy (CBT), motivational interviewing, and family therapy, in addition to 12-step-based approaches. Regardless of theoretical orientation, however, linkage to MHOs by outpatient treatment providers remains a popular clinical practice. Among adolescent SUD programs nationally, while only a small percentage base their treatment solely on 12-step philosophy and practices (9%), nearly half (47%) require participation in community-based MHOs during treatment, and 85% link adolescents with AA or NA groups as a continuing care resource (Drug Strategies, 2003; Kelly, Yeterian, & Myers, 2008; Knudsen et al., 2008). Thus, most outpatient professional treatment agencies appear to view nonprofessional community MHOs as important continuing care resources and encourage patients' participation in these groups.

Adolescent patients treated in outpatient programs, however, do not appear to engage as much with MHOs as those coming from 12-step-based residential programs. This could reflect differences in (1) the degree of clinical emphasis placed on MHO participation across these different levels of care; (2) differences in patients' addiction severity and complexity, as a major predictor of continuing participation in MHOs among adolescents and adults is greater addiction severity; or (3) some combination (Kelly, Brown, et al., 2008; Kelly & Myers, 2007). A 3-year follow-up of 357 adolescents in intensive outpatient treatment found that at 1-year postintake, only 29% reported having attended 10 or more MHO meetings in the past 6 months. At 3-years postintake, this number dropped to 14% (Chi et al., 2009). In a 6-month follow-up of 127 adolescents in low-intensity outpatient SUD treatment, just over one-quarter of patients (28%) attended at least one MHO meeting during the 3 months postintake, whereas from 4- to 6-months postintake, that figure dropped to 24%. At intake, we found that fewer than half (43%) of participants had ever been to an MHO meeting (Kelly, Dow, Yeterian, & Kahler, 2010). Also, in contrast with the roughly 50% of adolescents who are abstinent about 1 year after 12-step residential treatment, only approximately 25% of adolescents in outpatient treatment for cannabis use disorder were abstinent in the past 30 days at 1-year follow-up (Dennis et al., 2004). Thus, while clinical linkage to enhance engagement with MHOs is common in adolescent outpatient treatment, more systematic and developmentally sensitive approaches may be needed to engage adolescent outpatients with these freely available recovery support resources.

THE DEVELOPMENT OF BRIEF INTERVENTIONS
TO ENGAGE INDIVIDUALS WITH MHOS

Findings on MHOs for adults, including relapse prevention and recovery support potential and cost-effectiveness (Humphreys & Moos, 2001, 2007; Kelly & Yeterian, 2012, 2013), has led to the development and testing of clinical strategies to maximize the chances of patients' engagement with them. These clinical strategies collectively have become known as "Twelve-Step Facilitation" (TSF) interventions, and several of these have been tested and validated among adult outpatients suffering from SUDs (e.g., Kahler et al., 2004; Kaskutas, Subbaraman, Withrodt, & Zemore, 2009; Litt, Kadden, Kabela-Cormier, & Petry, 2009; Manning et al., 2012; Project MATCH Research Group, 1997; Timko, Debenedetti, & Billow, 2006; Walitzer, Dermen, & Barrick, 2009). These TSF interventions can be short, single-session format, consisting of brief advice or a brief motivation-enhancing discussion along with linkage with existing 12-step members (e.g., Kahler et al., 2004; Timko et al., 2006) or multisession treatments that attempt to engage, monitor, and manage continued MHO engagement in weekly sessions over a period of 2–3 months (e.g., Project MATCH Research Group, 1997; Walitzer et al., 2009).

Given the lack of knowledge on TSF for adolescents, including a paucity of well-established guidelines for its implementation, below we describe some formative clinical guidelines and pilot outcomes based on our preliminary work developing and testing the first integrated TSF for young people. First, however, we outline some important life-stage developmental factors that were considered in developing this youth-focused TSF treatment.

STATUS OF THE FIELD
AND DEVELOPMENTAL CONSIDERATIONS

From a clinical and public health standpoint, MHO participation and clinical practices designed to stimulate engagement with MHOs makes a lot of sense. Despite this, there are a number of life-stage developmental factors that should be considered when tailoring adult-based TSF interventions to engage youth in these mostly adult-oriented entities.

Heterogeneity in Addiction Severity and the Problem of "Powerlessness"

Compared with adults, adolescents typically have shorter, less severe, and less complex clinical histories. They also tend to have less intrinsic motivation to be in treatment, engage in continuing care, or change alcohol/drug use (Dennis et al., 2004). Many adolescents also do not have as much difficulty controlling substance use when they want to. In addition, adolescent treatment programs cater to a broad and wide-ranging clientele, from younger adolescents

(14–15 years old)—who, while meeting criteria for (mild) SUDs, have relatively low levels of substance involvement and impairment—up to older teens and young adults (e.g., 19- to 20-year-olds), who have clinically severe problems and experience significant withdrawal symptoms. Adolescents with less severe problems or who have not yet experienced severe medical or psychological consequences of substance use may be less likely to identify with the 12-step ideas of "powerlessness" over a substance and the need for abstinence. Adolescents who engage with MHOs tend to have more severe substance use histories and are more likely to have an abstinence goal and recognize and admit having a substance problem (Kelly, Brown, et al., 2008). In addition, having received treatment for either substance use or mental health issues in the past also predicts 12-step meeting attendance (Grella, Joshi, & Hser, 2004; Kelly, Brown, et al., 2008). From a theoretical standpoint, this fits well with the health beliefs model construct of "perceived severity," whereby the more severe someone perceives him- or herself to be, the more likely he or she is to seek help (Finney & Moos, 1995). The clinical implication of these differences means that the notion of powerlessness over the ability to maintain abstinence from a substance may be true only for a subset of adolescents in treatment. For this subset, MHOs may be a more natural and better fit, but for those less impaired, the emphasis may need to be placed more on the "unmanageability" aspect of this first step ("We admitted we were powerless over our addiction—that our lives had become *unmanageable*") that focuses on the consequences of substance use. In other words, while some teens may still be able to control their impulses to use drugs, and are therefore not technically "powerless," their use of substances, nevertheless, has caused significant problems in their lives resulting in "unmanageability" and SUD treatment admission.

Polysubstance versus Single-Substance Focus

Compared with adults, adolescents are more likely to use multiple substances simultaneously and often present with several co-occurring SUD diagnoses. In one study of adolescents presenting for inpatient treatment, rates of alcohol and marijuana dependence were 72 and 86%, respectively (Winters et al., 2007). In a separate study, 54% of adolescents attending intensive outpatient treatment were using both alcohol and other drugs at intake, and more than half were using multiple drugs (Campbell, Chi, Sterling, Kohn, & Weisner, 2009). Since many 12-step meetings are structured around the discussion of one particular substance (e.g., alcohol in AA, marijuana in MA, cocaine in Cocaine Anonymous [CA]), polysubstance-using adolescents may find these substance-specific meetings to be less tailored to their needs. On the other hand, NA addresses use of all substances (including alcohol) as it focuses on "addiction" rather than any particular substance, and thus may be a more fitting referral for young people. Also, despite cannabis being a prominently used drug among adolescents, there are as yet few MA meetings in most communities.

Spirituality/Religiosity

Another developmental factor to consider is that while religiosity has been found to be a protective factor against the onset of an SUD (Miller, Davies, & Greenwald, 2000; Ouimette et al., 2001; Vaughan, de Dios, Steinfeldt, & Kratz, 2011) and is predictive of a better treatment response among adolescents treated for an SUD (Kelly, Pagano, Stout, & Johnson, 2011), the quasi-religious language inherent in 12-step fellowships may not appeal to some adolescents treated for an SUD (Kelly & Myers, 2007). This may constitute a further barrier for young people who may be more preoccupied and interested with more mundane pursuits and social factors. Because MHOs are not religious, but spiritual, encouraging a personally defined spirituality to aid recovery and talking to youth about myths relating to NA or AA being "religious" organizations can help remove this barrier. This has been done in TSF interventions with adults by discussing the broad meaning of spirituality and how MHOs allow for an entirely personal construction of its definition and place in recovery (e.g., Kaskutas, Ye, Greenfield, Witbrodt, & Bond, 2008).

Logistical Barriers

Most adolescents do not have independent transportation or the freedom to attend 12-step meetings at will, even if they wanted to. Thus, parents and guardians need to be onboard with the notion that providing their teens transportation to and from 12-step meetings is a worthwhile investment. For youth under age 18 years old, this means obtaining buy in from parents about the value and safety of MHO participation as part of the intervention. Some clinicians and parents might be concerned about potential predatory behavior at AA or NA meetings, but MHO participation among young people has been found to be safe and valuable. Teens attending AA and NA meetings report some instances where they have been harassed but it is rare (Kelly, Brown, et al., 2008; Kelly, Dow, et al., 2011).

Older Age Composition of Most 12-Step Meetings and Challenges with Identification

Adolescents also face barriers in becoming engaged with 12-step MHOs because the majority of members are significantly older. The average AA and NA member is 47 and 43 years old, respectively, with only 2% of members under 21 (Alcoholics Anonymous World Services, 2014; Narcotics Anonymous World Services, 2013). Given that adults face different life-stage challenges than adolescents (e.g., work, children, marriage, housing problems) and typically have longer and more severe addiction histories and different life contexts and preferences, looking at a sea of older adult faces at a meeting may present a formidable barrier to feeling comfortable and identifying with other members, even if teens are motivated to attend (Kelly, Myers, & Brown, 2005; Labbe, Slaymaker, & Kelly, 2014). In one study , teens who attended AA and NA meetings consisting of a substantial proportion of teenagers had significantly better attendance rates and better substance use outcomes 3-months posttreatment than those who attended predominantly adult meetings (Kelly et al., 2005). Similarity in age and life stage may increase identification and a sense of belonging and instill hope that change is both positive and acceptable for young people. Another larger study with more than 300 young adults observed a similar relationship (Labbe, Greene, Bergman, Hoeppner, & Kelly, 2013). This suggests that clinically making efforts to locate and link young people with young persons' MHO meetings initially is likely to yield higher rates of engagement and better substance use outcomes. Listings of young persons' meetings can be obtained online through the local/regional central offices of AA and NA or other 12-step MHOs. If no young persons' meetings are available, keeping lists of former young patients who are AA/NA members who might serve as contacts can be helpful in getting youth engaged in meetings. There are online recovery meetings, too, such as *www.intherooms.org*, which has about 350,000 online members about one-third of whom are under age 30 years old.

Challenges in Finding Recovering or Low-Risk Social Network Members Even within MHOs

Social contexts are particularly influential in helping to establish and maintain the heavy and frequent patterns of substance use that can result in the development of an SUD. Conversely, youths' social contexts also play a pivotal role in the successful recovery from SUDs. Whereas in adults, the precursors to relapse typically involve negative affect (e.g., depression, anger) and interpersonal conflict (e.g., disagreements or quarrels with a partner), the vast majority of relapse for adolescents occurs in social contexts where alcohol and other drugs are present (Brown, 1993). Hence, recovery-specific social resources, such as NA, may provide a rare and concentrated group of supportive peers with whom young people can socialize and thus lower the influence of this potent relapse risk (Kelly, Brown, et al., 2008). In fact, mobilizing changes in social network ties and social activities appears to be one of the major mechanisms through which AA conveys its beneficial effects on sustaining remission and recovery among adults with SUDs (Kelly, Magill, & Stout, 2009; Litt et al., 2009). Yet, while 12-step MHO participation appears to confer recovery benefits (Kelly, Stout, & Slaymaker, 2012), and may reduce negative high-risk social network members (Kelly, Stout, Greene, & Slaymaker, 2014), MHOs may be unable to provide new social network member friends in recovery because there are fewer young people attending 12-step MHOs (Hoeppner, Hoeppner, & Kelly, 2014; Kelly et al., 2014). Consequently, while some young people will meet new friends in recovery at 12-step meetings, it may still be important nonetheless to emphasize finding additional low-risk peers to socialize with even though those individuals may not be in recovery. Clinically this might be done by brainstorming about identifying stable, higher-functioning young people from school, community, or college who might make suitable low-risk supportive acquaintances. These might be new friends, or old friends who were once not considered by the adolescent because they were not using substances. It could also involve encouraging participation in sports and recreational activities with other young people, all while helping the young person stay mindful about maintaining remission and staying in recovery.

Differences in the Types of Addiction Recovery Needs and Derived Therapeutic 12-Step Benefits

There are a number of addiction- and life-stage-specific differences between adolescents and adults. There also appear to be differences in the ways that adolescents may benefit from MHOs. In analyses of 12-step participation with adolescents, the effects of meeting attendance on future substance use were found to be explained by maintaining and boosting motivation for abstinence over time, but not by boosting adolescents' abstinence-focused coping or self-efficacy during the follow-up period (Kelly, Myers, & Brown, 2000). This is in contrast to adult studies that find that AA recovery benefits are explained by boosting coping, abstinence self-efficacy, and recovery motivation (e.g., Morgenstern, Labouvie, McCrady, Kahler, & Frey, 1997). In another study, motivation for abstinence also helped explain the effects of *active* 12-step involvement (e.g., having a sponsor, reading literature, working the 12 steps) on posttreatment substance use (Kelly et al., 2002), suggesting that both continued attendance as well as active involvement helps adolescents reduce substance use by maintaining their motivation for abstinence over time. A separate study also found evidence for recovery-specific social support as an important factor in explaining the effects of greater 12-step attendance and activities on better 3-year alcohol and drug use outcomes (Chi et al., 2009). While there are many potential factors that may explain the effects of participating in AA or NA at different levels (e.g., social, psychological, neurobiological), it appears that both intrinsic (e.g., motivation) and extrinsic (e.g., social network) factors can at least partially explain the relationship between MHO attendance and improved substance use outcomes among young people, but MHOs may operate more centrally for young people by sustaining abstinence motivation over time. Motivation for recovery is a key variable for treatment and continuing care engagement and is generally very low among youth. Consequently, this is valuable knowledge and can be helpful particularly in informing parents more concretely about how AA or NA participation might benefit their son or daughter and lead to better outcomes. For example, clinically encouraging parents to assist their son or daughter to participate in MHOs and offer to give them a ride to meetings could help young people participate. Parents and young people might also be told that going to meetings enhances the chances of remission and better functioning and less trouble and that it tends to work by helping young people to stay motivated over time.

These life-stage differences between adolescents and adults indicate that a developmentally tailored intervention that considers these factors could help young people become more involved in MHOs. Next, we describe how this knowledge has been used clinically to inform interventions and develop best-practice guidelines for engaging young people with MHOs.

CLINICAL APPLICATIONS

Due to the existing acceptance of MHO philosophy among the majority of youth treatment programs in the United States, and the common practice of referring patients to MHOs even among eclectic or non-12-step programs, a manualized TSF intervention shown to be efficacious could be readily disseminated, adopted, and implemented by adolescent SUD providers (Glasgow, Lichtenstein, & Marcus, 2003). Given the limited amount of formal research regarding TSF specifically for adolescents, below we provide clinical guidelines based in part on the results of the development of the first youth-focused motivational/cognitive-behavioral integrated TSF (iTSF) treatment conducted by one of us (J. F. K.). This intervention was developed in an iterative manner over the course of six group cycles run over 17 months. Prior to the first cycle, a preliminary iTSF manual was created that incorporated elements from evidence-based treatments (TSF, motivational enhancement therapy [MET], CBT; e.g., Kaskutas et al., 2008; Walitzer et al., 2009) as well as clinical experience and research focused specifically on youth and 12-step programs (e.g., Kelly & Myers, 2007). A brief outpatient intervention that integrates TSF with MET-CBT was deemed optimal given the broad heterogeneity in the degrees of substance involvement and impairment among outpatient youth, and many younger adolescents with less severe problems were deemed unlikely to want or need MHOs but may still need other skills and support provided by MET-CBT, an intervention shown to be efficacious for adolescents with cannabis use disorders (Dennis et al., 2004). This preliminary iTSF manual was then modified over time based on participant feedback and therapist impressions following each group, resulting in a 12-week protocol, consisting of 10 group therapy sessions and two individual therapy sessions (Kelly, Yeterian, et al., 2016).

GUIDELINES FOR DELIVERING TSF INTERVENTIONS FOR ADOLESCENTS

Provide Information about 12–Step Meetings

In contrast to adults, adolescents typically enter treatment with little or no prior exposure to or knowledge of 12-step meetings, particularly in outpatient settings. Consequently, providing information about what the organizations are, who they are for, and where to find them is important. Therapists should inquire about adolescents' knowledge of or prior experience with meetings, and provide a brief overview of meetings and a recommendation to attend during treatment. Over time, patients can be encouraged to include attending 12-step meetings as a written "step to take" toward their treatment goal, so as to elicit a verbal and written commitment to attend during treatment.

Providing information regarding what to expect at the first meeting—including discussing types of meetings, typical meeting format, and 12-step culture—is advisable. When adolescent group members attend 12-step meetings, it is useful to have them describe their experience during the next session, in order to provide a firsthand account to other group members. Introducing 12-step concepts in relation to group topics is helpful in assisting participants to understand things they might hear at meetings. These can include common slogans such as "One day at a time" and "This too shall pass," as well as sayings such as "If you sit in a barbershop long enough, you'll end up getting a haircut," and discussion of the Serenity Prayer and the different meanings of "God" and "Higher Power" in 12-step programs.

Provide a Rationale for Attending 12-Step Meetings during and after Treatment

It is useful to elicit the rationale for 12-step attendance from the adolescents themselves. This can be done by asking, "Why do we talk about attending 12-step meetings in treatment?" and allow members to generate answers. The rationale that treatment is short term and sustained recovery-specific social support is needed to maintain sobriety over time can be stated if youth themselves do not generate it. Say something like "This treatment is really short and will be over before you know it; so what do you do then?" Discussing ways in which attending 12-step meetings can help with each group topic covered (i.e., effective communication, social support, coping with urges and cravings, coping with feelings, coping with the challenges of sobriety) is recommended to help participants draw connections and understand what they could gain by attending. For example, when discussing avoiding risky people, places, and things in recovery, discuss how attending 12-step meetings can provide access to new sober supports and help avoid high-risk social situations or times of the week (e.g., attending a meeting on a Friday night, socializing with sober young people after the meetings).

Facilitate In-House Presentations by Young Existing Members of 12-Step Organizations

It is strongly advisable to invite members of 12-step organizations into treatment to share their stories of recovery with adolescents in treatment. This provides exposure to young recovering role models and can go a long way in effectively addressing myths and misconceptions of recovery or MHO stereotypes.

We recommend inviting speakers who are young to increase the chances that group members can relate to them and allow them to provide targeted information on being a young person in an MHO program (e.g., how to find good young persons' meetings). Such speakers can be invited through the local central office for NA, MA, AA, and others. It is also advisable to invite speakers who are a good match for the types of drug-using experiences represented by the majority of your adolescent patients. For example, if most use cannabis as their primary substance, invite speakers from MA and NA to facilitate greater identification.

Incorporate Elements of MHO Meetings into Treatment Wherever Possible

Several strategies can be implemented in treatment groups that mirror 12-step meetings and participants can be informed of these similarities. For example, having and reading aloud a specific group "preamble" and "closing statement" outlining the rationale and goals of the group at the start and end of each group, mirroring the preamble and closing with the Twelve Promises read at actual 12-step community meetings can help prepare youth for what to expect (see Figures 15.1 and 15.2).

"Chips" or tokens for meeting attendance can also be given out, similar to the way chips are given at 12-step meetings for sobriety milestones. Also, members who are new to the treatment group can be asked to briefly share their personal story for 10 minutes during check-in. This type of story sharing again

---

Group Preamble

The goal of this group is to help us with the problems that brought us into this program. This group is designed to give us support and information to help us with drinking- and drug-related problems.

Each one of us is the expert on our own life and we each have something important to contribute to the group.

In order for everyone in this group to feel comfortable and respected, we will:
- Come to group on time and sober.
- Turn off our cell phones, and place them in the basket until the end of group in order to remain focused on the group.
- Listen to one another. Only one person speaks at a time.
- Respect one another. Do not threaten or harass other group members.
- Not glorify our drug and alcohol use. We will be straightforward about it.
- Maintain one another's confidentiality. What is said in group stays in group.

FIGURE 15.1. Example of group preamble.

Group Closing Statement

Recovery from the disease of drug and alcohol addiction is challenging, and it is very possible, especially when we take it 1 week, 1 day, and when necessary, even 1 hour at a time. The "HOW" of recovery is Honesty, Open-mindedness, and Willingness: Honesty with ourselves and others, Openness to accept and try new things, and Willingness to do whatever it takes. A life free of drug and alcohol problems is achievable. The rewards are great. Those who succeed are those who never stop trying. Keep trying—keep coming back!

FIGURE 15.2. Example of group closing statement.

is typical of what they might hear at a meeting, and also a way for members to get to know other members, including their history and why they are attending treatment. Finally, many elements of the in-house presentations by young 12-step MHO members noted above are similar to the meeting format, such as the story sharing, opportunities to express "identification" with the story, and the "no cross-talk" rule while the speaker is talking.

Have Adolescents Set Weekly Sober Activity Goals and Strongly Encourage MHO Attendance

At the end of each group, it is advisable to have youth set a goal to complete at least one sober activity in the following week. Writing this on a worksheet and stating his or her goal aloud to the group also solidifies this practice, because making a public commitment to change can increase the likelihood of making that change. During check-in each week, it is a good idea to ask group members to reread their prior week's goal and state whether they met it. These sober activity goals can include participating in fun activities with a sober friend or attending a 12-step meeting. The intent here is to have youth engage in a safe and sober activity and participate in other recovery activities in addition to 12-step meetings. Giving adolescents the choice to attend meetings is typically appreciated. Using a flexible sober activity plan also allows participants not yet ready to attend a 12-step meeting to use group time productively to think through what they want to accomplish in the week ahead.

Have a Structured Check-In That Mimics 12-Step Meetings

Having a structured check-in mimics 12-step meetings. For example, the leader can ask a volunteer to read the group preamble and then have group members read aloud their past week's treatment goal from their worksheet and state whether or not they have met their goal—briefly reflecting on obstacles or things that were helpful is useful. This practice of reading goals (treatment goals and sober activity goals) aloud during check-in encourages participants to be accountable to the group and to decrease vague and unhelpful descriptions about the past week (e.g., "It was fine").

Incorporate a Behavior Chain of Substance Use and Relate It to 12-Step Philosophy and Practices

CBT often includes a behavior chain model of substance use (i.e., "triggers—thoughts—feelings—behaviors—positive consequences—negative consequences") to help participants understand the function of their substance use (the "behavior" in the behavior chain). In this model, substance use is understood by contextualizing it within a chronological sequence of events, including the triggers, thoughts, and feelings that precede substance use and the positive and negative results that occur after substance use. Adolescents readily grasp this model. It is useful as an overarching model to anchor any group topic to a specific link in the behavior chain. This can be done by asking participants "Where does [group topic] fit on the behavior chain?" For example, when the topic is coping with urges and cravings, participants can identify that urges and cravings can take the form of thoughts and feelings that precede substance use and are influenced by triggers. As noted above, it is also a good idea to link how MHOs can help youth cope with these risk factors (e.g., call a sponsor or other trusted member when feeling an urge to smoke marijuana).

ISSUES REGARDING TREATMENT ENGAGEMENT AND ESTABLISHING A WORKING THERAPEUTIC ALLIANCE

As noted previously, most adolescents do not feel positively about being in SUD treatment, and it can be very challenging to engage them in the therapeutic process. There are a number of strategies that are useful to help foster engagement and enhance the therapeutic working alliance.

Use a Socratic Therapeutic Intervention Style

In some cases, therapists provide a great deal of information to participants in lecture style in order to teach skills. Adolescents can quickly lose interest when therapists speak for long periods (i.e., more than a few sentences), so using a consistent Socratic dialogue (i.e., posing questions to patients) rather than lecturing is more fruitful at keeping young people's attention. For example, instead of therapists stating the reasons for discussing 12-step meetings during a particular treatment session, these questions are pitched to the adolescent participants: "Why do treatment programs discuss the importance of attending

12-step meetings during treatment?" or "Why would people view addiction as a disease?" When given the opportunity, participants are almost always able to generate the information that the therapist provides. Using this style also helps participants to stay much more engaged in the group process, as they take an active role in generating the content throughout the group. This may help members also feel more empowered by making valid contributions to group content and process.

Enlist Parental Support for 12–Step Meeting Attendance

In order to facilitate adolescents' attendance at 12-step meetings during and after treatment, parents/guardians of minor participants should be invited into at least a portion of individual treatment sessions (e.g., the last 15 minutes). It is ideal to have both the parents and their child in the room at the same time so that both the adolescent and their parents are all privy to any information and recommendations communicated by therapists. This helps avoid any perceptions that the adolescent may have of "secret communication" between his or her therapist and the parents and helps maintain and strengthen the therapeutic alliance. During this conjoint session time, therapists can provide information about 12-step meetings, including research results, ideally graphically presented, showing that adolescents who attend tend to have better treatment outcomes, and problem solving around any barriers to parents driving or arranging transportation for their teens to 12-step meetings during treatment. The aim here is to help parents understand the potential therapeutic value of their child's attendance at meetings and to enlist their support for providing transportation to meetings.

Allow for Flexible Timing of Individual TSF Sessions

To minimize dropout from treatment, the timing of any individual sessions can be altered, such that participants complete just one individual session prior to entering group and complete a second or more individual session at the midway point of treatment. Doing this also allows goal setting to occur in the first session and for the second (or more) individual session to be used as a time to check in about whether the participant is making progress toward his or her treatment goal and touch base about other progress, barriers, or concerns. At the first iTSF individual session, youth are asked about any prior experiences with 12-step MHOs and their thoughts about them. Information is also presented about what they are and youth are asked why these are often recommended and why they might be helpful: "Why do we talk about groups like AA and NA in treatment? How might they help someone with an alcohol or drug problem?" If the young person is unable to generate answers, the clinician can provide the rationale, but in our experience this is seldom necessary. Also, aspects of 12-step MHOs are discussed such as what is a sponsor, the "12-steps," the different types of meetings, how long they last, and so on. Also, it is stated clearly by the clinician: "I'd like you to attend some of these (AA/NA/MA, etc.) meetings while you are here in treatment." The second session can be used to check in on progress on attending MHO meetings and discussion of experiences.

EMPIRICAL DATA
IN SUPPORT OF INTERVENTIONS

As noted in the introduction to this chapter, there have been several studies suggesting adolescents can benefit from both 12-step-based residential treatment and community-based MHO participation. Yet, none of these studies were based on replicable, manualized treatments or used randomized controlled trials to test the efficacy of TSF interventions for young people. Consequently, below we describe some of the results from our study of iTSF for youth ages 14–21, which compared this novel TSF approach with MET-CBT—an existing evidence-based treatment for adolescents (Dennis et al. 2004). First, we describe some of the results from the phase I treatment development study. This is followed by some preliminary results from the randomized controlled clinical trial where we compared the integrated iTSF treatment (which included elements of MET, CBT, and TSF) with a combination of MET and CBT (without TSF).

12-Step Attendance and Abstinence

The first phase of developing the iTSF treatment involved recruiting adolescents to receive SUD treatment. Ads were placed on radio, in newspapers, and on buses, and local residential adolescent SUD treatment agencies were notified, as were drug courts and criminal justice settings. The treatment was developed over several group cycles with about 40 youth who all received different variations of the iTSF treatment as it was being developed and improved. Among the adolescents at entry into this initial phase of the study, 24% of participants had previously attended a 12-step meeting, with 10% attending within the past 3 months. When excluding meetings that were attended as part of an inpatient/residential treatment program, these percentages dropped to 19 and 5%, respectively. During treatment, 40% of participants attended a 12-step meeting, with 33% attending outside of an inpatient/residential setting. Adolescents attended AA (22%), NA (19%), and MA (15%) meetings. Adolescents' abstinent days increased significantly from an average of about 25 out of 90 days at baseline to an average of about 40 out of 90 days at 3-month follow-up. There was a significant positive correlation between greater MHO attendance during treatment and greater abstinence at 3-month follow-up, when considering both total meetings and noninpatient meetings only.

Participants' Reactions to 12-Step Inservices

Using a 1–5 scale, participants rated the MA ($M = 3.96$, $SD = 0.78$) and NA ($M = 4.04$, $SD = 0.70$) inservices as most helpful, and rated the AA inservices as less helpful ($M = 2.75$, $SD = 0.71$). Of the 20 participants exposed to an MA inservice, 18 found it to be the most helpful part of the session. One participant wrote that it was helpful "Hearing from someone with similar problems as mine. Hearing that MA is more mellow than AA." Another stated, "MA people . . . knew what they were talking about. [I] connected with them. They were really chill." Participants' views on NA were more mixed, with 67% viewing it as the most helpful part of the session. Participants tended to view the AA inservice as unhelpful (80%). It is unclear whether this could be due to aspects related to the specific speakers themselves, since the younger AA speaker on several occasions was accompanied by a much older member.

Clinical Trial Results

Preliminary results showed that, compared with participants randomized to MET-CBT ($n = 30$), those randomized to iTSF ($n = 29$) had similar improvements on percentage of days abstinent across the 9-month follow-up, but significantly greater improvement on substance use consequences and marginally better rates of continuous abstinence. Also, consistent with the purported mechanisms of action in a TSF approach, iTSF participants were more likely to attend an MHO meeting during treatment, although this effect decayed posttreatment (Kelly, Kaminer, et al., 2016). Because a considerable number of patients in the MET/CBT condition also attended community 12-step meetings—despite not being specifically linked to such groups—we analyzed the effect of 12-step meting participation irrespective of treatment condition and found a positive benefit with significantly increased days abstinent with greater attendance.

IMPLICATIONS FOR TREATMENT
OF ADOLESCENT SUBSTANCE USE

We have found that the use of MET and CBT concepts and practices in the same context with TSF can work well for adolescent outpatients with SUDs. Outpatient adolescents have wide-ranging clinical histories and presentations. The integration of practices from evidence-based interventions mean that there is a variety of therapeutic tools that clinicians can use to help adolescents address substance use at specific stages of recovery (e.g., precontemplation, contemplation, preparation, or action; Prochaska, DiClemente, & Norcross, 1992).

In keeping with treatment process evaluations (Finney, 1995; Suchman, 1967), the broad underlying theory of iTSF is that the intervention will increase community MHO participation and, in turn, this will lead to better substance use outcomes. A key immediate outcome of iTSF, therefore, is patients' participation in MHOs, which should be associated with improved substance use outcomes. As anticipated, 30% more patients attended MHO meetings in the iTSF compared to the MET-CBT condition (Kelly, Kaminer, et al., 2016). Furthermore, MHO participation was associated with better substance use outcomes during and following treatment. This suggests that the theory of this iTSF treatment was supported even among these clinically less severe outpatient adolescents with generally low motivation for treatment engagement or abstinence. Thus, iTSF, a developmentally tailored and integrative approach, may be an effective clinical strategy to enhance adolescent outpatients' MHO participation and clinical outcomes.

OTHER INNOVATIVE STRATEGIES TO FACILITATE ADOLESCENTS' MHO PARTICIPATION: MOBILE AND INTERNET-BASED TECHNOLOGIES

In addition to this face-to-face treatment innovation to enhance adolescents' MHO participation, recent studies have shown that sociodigital technologies, which are very popular strategies that adolescents use to connect socially with one another (Lenhart, 2015), might also be leveraged to promote MHO and other recovery-support activity participation. For example, in a 6-week pilot study of the continuing care smartphone application Addiction–Comprehensive Health Enhancement Support System (A-CHESS), among adolescents (14–18 years old) discharged from residential SUD treatment ($N = 29$), Dennis, Scott, Funk, and Nicholson (2015) showed that patients participated in six brief recovery support activities (e.g., discussion groups, reaching out to others, and locating mutual-help meetings) per day on average, and at least 80% rated each activity as useful or very useful. Those who participated in two or more activities within an hour of an automatic prompt assessing relapse risk factors (e.g., craving) were about *half as likely* to use alcohol or other drugs during the following week. Although this study did not measure MHO participation specifically, it suggests technology-based interventions can help link adolescents to online, recovery-enhancing, peer-supportive resources like MHOs.

Also, Gonzales, Ang, Murphy, Glik, and Anglin (2014) recently tested a text-message-based continuing care intervention called Educating and Supporting Inquisitive Youth in Recovery (Project ESQYIR), which assesses relapse risk factors and automatically provides recovery coping tips as needed, compared with continuing care as usual in a 12-week randomized trial among adolescents and young adult SUD inpatients and outpatients ($N = 81$). On average, those randomized to receive ESQYIR were *half as likely* to use their primary drug and had lower levels of substance use severity while receiving the intervention and through 90-day follow-up. Importantly, the intervention group also had significantly more days attending mutual-help meetings (9 days in the intervention group vs. 3 days in the comparison group), but this effect decreased to nonsignificance by 90-day follow-up *when the texting intervention was no longer being delivered* (7 vs. 5 days, respectively). This suggests ongoing strategies to facilitate adolescents' MHO participation may be needed. It is possible that the text-message application enhanced outcomes, in part, through its ability to facilitate MHO participation, though this has not yet been tested. Overall, these two recent studies of technology-based interventions for adolescents highlight the potential reach and impact of text-message and smartphone applications as tools that may help engage youth with recovery support services and MHO meetings—more specifically, improving their likelihood of recovery and remission in a cost-efficient framework. In addition to these interventions, there are several emerging platforms for online MHOs, including those with video format and within the structure of a social network site similar to Facebook but catering to individuals with SUDs (e.g., *www.intherooms.org*). However, these are designed largely for adults (i.e., ages 18+), and tests of their effectiveness have not been conducted.

FUTURE DIRECTIONS

In reviewing the range of evidence for 12-step-based residential treatment, outpatient treatment, and during- and posttreatment MHO participation, it appears that clinically facilitating linkage to groups like MA, NA, and AA during treatment is likely to result in higher rates of MHO participation and better substance use outcomes following discharge. Also, from a health care system perspective, this practice is likely to be cost-effective. For the first time, there is now a brief, manualized replicable treatment that incorporates MET-CBT with TSF to cater to the broad range of clinical severity in presentation among adolescents with SUDs that simultaneously capitalizes on the widespread recovery support available through MHOs such as MA, NA, and AA. Given the compatibility with current SUD treatment practices among youth treatment providers (Kelly, Yeterian, et al., 2008; Knudsen et al., 2008), iTSF treatment could be relatively easily adopted, implemented, and sustained, providing an evidence-based option that would support current practice.

REFERENCES

Alcoholics Anonymous. (1981). *Twelve steps and twelve traditions.* New York: Alcoholics Anonymous World Services.

Alcoholics Anonymous. (2001). *Alcoholics Anonymous: The story of how many thousands of men and women have recovered from alcoholism* (4th ed.). New York: Alcoholics Anonymous World Services.

Alcoholics Anonymous World Services. (2014). 2014 membership survey. Retrieved September 25, 2015, from *www.aa.org/assets/en_US/p-48_membershipsurvey.pdf.*

Alford, G. S., Koehler, R. A., & Leonard, J. (1991). Alcoholics Anonymous–Narcotics Anonymous model inpatient treatment of chemically dependent adolescents: A 2-year outcome study. *Journal of Studies on Alcohol and Drugs, 52*(2), 118–126.

Brown, S. A. (1993). Recovery patterns in adolescent substance abuse. In G. A. Marlatt & J. S. Baer (Eds.), *Addictive behaviors across the life span: Prevention, treatment, and policy issues* (pp. 161–183). Newbury Park, CA: SAGE.

Campbell, C. I., Chi, F., Sterling, S., Kohn, C., & Weisner, C. (2009). Self-initiated tobacco cessation and substance use outcomes among adolescents entering substance use treatment in a managed care organization. *Addictive Behaviors, 34*(2), 171–179.

Chi, F. W., Kaskutas, L. A., Sterling, S., Campbell, C. I., & Weisner, C. (2009). Twelve-step affiliation and 3-year substance use outcomes among adolescents: Social support and religious service attendance as potential mediators. *Addiction, 104*(6), 927–939.

Dennis, M., Godley, S. H., Diamond, G., Tims, F. M., Babor, T., Donaldson, J., et al. (2004). The Cannabis Youth Treatment (CYT) study: Main findings from two randomized trials. *Journal of Substance Abuse Treatment, 27*(3), 197–213.

Dennis, M., Scott, C. K., Funk, R. R., & Nicholson, L. (2015). A pilot study to examine the feasibility and potential effectiveness of using smartphones to provide recovery support for adolescents. *Substance Abuse, 36,* 486–492.

Dow, S. J., & Kelly, J. F. (2013). Listening to youth: Adolescents' reasons for substance use as a unique predictor of treatment response and outcome. *Psychology of Addictive Behaviors, 27*(4), 1122–1131.

Drug Strategies. (2003). *Treating teens: A guide to adolescent programs.* Washington, DC: Author.

Finney, J. W. (1995). Enhancing substance abuse treatment evaluations: Examining mediators and moderators of treatment effects. *Journal of Substance Abuse, 7*(1), 135–150.

Finney, J. W., & Moos, R. H. (1995). Entering treatment for alcohol abuse: A stress and coping model. *Addiction, 90*(9), 1223–1240.

Fiorentine, R., & Hillhouse, M. P. (2000). Drug treatment and 12-step program participation: The additive effects of integrated recovery activities. *Journal of Substance Abuse Treatment, 18*(1), 65–74.

Glasgow, R. E., Lichtenstein, E., & Marcus, A. C. (2003). Why don't we see more translation of health promotion research to practice?: Rethinking the efficacy-to-effectiveness transition. *American Journal of Public Health, 93*(8), 1261–1267.

Gonzales, R., Ang, A., Murphy, D. A., Glik, D. C., & Anglin, M. D. (2014). Substance use recovery outcomes among a cohort of youth participating in a mobile-based texting aftercare pilot program. *Journal of Substance Abuse Treatment, 47,* 20–26.

Gore, F. M., Bloem, P. J. N., Patton, G. C., Ferguson, J., Joseph, V., Coffey, C., et al. (2011). Global burden of disease in young people aged 10–24 years: A systematic analysis. *The Lancet, 377*(9783), 2093–2102.

Grella, C. E., Joshi, V., & Hser, Y. (2004). Effects of comorbidity on treatment processes and outcomes among adolescents in drug treatment programs. *Journal of Child and Adolescent Substance Abuse, 13*(4), 13–32.

Hoeppner, B. B., Hoeppner, S. S., & Kelly, J. F. (2014). Do young people benefit from AA as much, and in the same ways, as adults aged 30+?: A moderated multiple mediation analysis. *Drug and Alcohol Dependence, 143,* 181–188.

Hsieh, S., Hoffmann, N. G., & Hollister, C. D. (1998). The relationship between pre-, during-, post-treatment factors, and adolescent substance abuse behaviors. *Addictive Behaviors, 23*(4), 477–488.

Humphreys, K. (2004). *Circles of recovery: Self-help organizations for addictions.* Cambridge, UK: Cambridge University Press.

Humphreys, K., & Moos, R. H. (2001). Can encouraging substance abuse patients to participate in self-help groups reduce demand for health care?: A quasi-experimental study. *Alcoholism: Clinical and Experimental Research, 25*(5), 711–716.

Humphreys, K., & Moos, R. H. (2007). Encouraging posttreatment self-help group involvement to reduce demand for continuing care services: Two-year clinical and utilization outcomes. *Alcoholism: Clinical and Experimental Research, 31*(1), 64–68.

Humphreys, K., & Tucker, J. A. (2002). Toward more responsive and effective intervention systems for alcohol-related problems. *Addiction, 97*(2), 126–132.

Jaffe, S., & Kelly, J. F. (2010). Twelve-step mutual help programs for adolescents: A guide for clinicians. In Y. Kaminer & K. Winters (Eds.), *Handbook of clinical interventions for adolescents.* Washington, DC: American Psychiatric Association Press.

Kahler, C. W., Read, J. P., Ramsey, S. E., Stuart, G. L., McCrady, B. S., & Brown, R. A. (2004). Motivational enhancement for 12-step involvement among patients undergoing alcohol detoxification. *Journal of Consulting and Clinical Psychology, 72*(4), 736–741.

Kaminer, Y., & Gordon, A. J. (2014). It is getting late here early: Youth substance abuse theory and practice. *Substance Abuse, 35*(4), 329–330.

Kaskutas, L. A., Subbaraman, M. S., Withrodt, J., & Zemore, S. E. (2009). Effectiveness of making Alcoholics Anonymous easier: A group format 12-step facilitation approach. *Journal of Substance Abuse Treatment, 37,* 228–239.

Kaskutas, L. A., Ye, Y., Greenfield, T. K., Witbrodt, J., & Bond, J. (2008). Epidemiology of Alcoholics Anonymous participation. In M. Galanter & L. A. Kaskutas (Eds.), *Research on Alcoholics Anonymous and spirituality in addiction recovery: Recent developments in alcoholism* (pp. 261–282). New York: Springer Science + Business Media.

Kelly, J. F., Brown, S. A., Abrantes, A., Kahler, C. W., & Myers, M. (2008). Social recovery model: An 8-year investigation of adolescent 12-step group involvement following inpatient treatment. *Alcoholism: Clinical and Experimental Research, 32*(8), 1468–1478.

Kelly, J. F., Dow, S. J., Yeterian, J. D., & Kahler, C. W. (2010). Can 12-step group participation strengthen and extend the benefits of adolescent addiction treatment?: A prospective analysis. *Drug and Alcohol Dependence, 110,* 117–125.

Kelly, J. F., Dow, S. J., Yeterian, J. D., & Myers, M. (2011). How safe are adolescents at Alcoholics Anonymous and Narcotics Anonymous meetings?: A prospective investigation with outpatient youth. *Journal of Substance Abuse Treatment, 40*(4), 419–425.

Kelly, J. F., Kaminer, Y., Kahler, C. W., Hoeppner, B., Yeterian, J., Cristello, J. V., et al. (2017). A pilot randomized clinical trial testing integrated 12-step facilitation (iTSF) treatment for adolescent substance use disorder. *Addiction, 112,* 2155–2166.

Kelly, J. F., Magill, M., & Stout, R. L. (2009). How do people recover from alcohol dependence?: A systematic review of the research on mechanisms of behavior change in Alcoholics Anonymous. *Addiction Research and Theory 17*(3), 236–259.

Kelly, J. F., & Myers, M. G. (2007). Adolescents' participation in Alcoholics Anonymous and Narcotics Anonymous: Review, implications and future directions. *Journal of Psychoactive Drugs, 39*(3), 259–269.

Kelly, J. F., Myers, M. G., & Brown, S. A. (2000). A multivariate process model of adolescent 12-step attendance and substance use outcome following inpatient treatment. *Psychology of Addictive Behaviors, 14*(4), 376–389.

Kelly, J. F., Myers, M. G., & Brown, S. A. (2002). Do adolescents affiliate with 12-step groups?: A multivariate process model of effects. *Journal of Studies on Alcohol, 63*(3), 293–304.

Kelly, J. F., Myers, M. G., & Brown, S. A. (2005). The effects of age composition of 12-step groups on adolescent 12-step participation and substance use outcome. *Journal of Child and Adolescent Substance Abuse, 15*(1), 63–72.

Kelly, J. F., Pagano, M. E., Stout, R. L., & Johnson, S. M. (2011). Influence of religiosity on 12-step participation and treatment response among substance-dependent adolescents. *Journal of Studies on Alcohol and Drugs, 72*(6), 1000–1011.

Kelly, J. F., Stout, R. L., Greene, M. C., & Slaymaker, V. (2014). Young adults, social networks, and addiction recovery: Post treatment changes in social ties and their role as a mediator of 12-step participation. *PLOS ONE, 9*(6), e100121.

Kelly, J. F., Stout, R. L., & Slaymaker, V. (2012). Emerging adults' treatment outcomes in relation to 12-step mutual-help attendance and active involvement. *Drug and Alcohol Dependence, 129*(1–2), 151–157.

Kelly, J. F., & Urbanoski, K. (2012). Youth recovery contexts: The incremental effects of 12-step attendance and involvement on adolescent outpatient outcomes. *Alcoholism: Clinical and Experimental Research, 36*(7), 1219–1229.

Kelly, J. F., & White, W. L. (Eds.). (2011). *Addiction recovery management: Theory, research, and practice.* New York: Spring Science + Business Media.

Kelly, J. F., & Yeterian, J. D. (2012). Empirical awakening: The new science on mutual help and implications for cost containment under health care reform. *Journal of Substance Abuse, 33*(2), 85–91.

Kelly, J. F., & Yeterian, J. D. (2013). Mutual-help groups for alcohol and other substance use disorders. In B. S. McCrady & E. E. Epstein (Eds.), *Addictions: A comprehensive guidebook* (2nd ed.). New York: Oxford University Press.

Kelly, J. F., Yeterian, J. D., Cristello, J. V., Kaminer, Y., Kahler, C. W., & Timko, C. (2016, June). *Developing and testing twelve-step facilitation for adolescents with substance use disorder: Manual development and preliminary outcomes.* Presentation at the Research Society of Alcoholism Conference, New Orleans, LA.

Kelly, J. F., Yeterian, J. D., & Myers, M. G. (2008). Treatment staff referrals, participation expectations, and perceived benefits and barriers to adolescent involvement in twelve-step groups. *Alcoholism Treatment Quarterly, 26*(4), 427–449.

Kennedy, B. P., & Minami, M. (1993). The Beech Hill Hospital/Outward Bound Adolescent Chemical Dependency Treatment Program. *Journal of Substance Abuse Treatment, 10*(4), 395–406.

Knudsen, H. K., Ducharme, L. J., Roman, P. M., & Johnson, J. A. (2008). *Service delivery and use of evidence-based treatment practices in adolescent substance abuse treatment settings.* Project report: Robert Wood Johnson Foundation's Substance Abuse Policy Research Program (Grant No. 53130).

Labbe, A. K., Greene, C., Bergman, B. G., Hoeppner, B., & Kelly, J. F. (2013). The importance of age composition of 12-step meetings as a moderating factor in the relation between young adults' 12-step participation and abstinence. *Drug and Alcohol Dependence, 133*(2), 541–547.

Labbe, A. K., Slaymaker, V., & Kelly, J. F. (2014). Toward enhancing 12-step facilitation among young people: A systematic qualitative investigation of young adults' 12-step experiences. *Substance Abuse, 35*(4), 399–407.

Lenhart, A. (2015). *Teens, social media & technology overview 2015* (pp. 1–47). Washington, DC: Pew Research Center.

Litt, M. D., Kadden, R. M., Kabela-Cormier, E., & Petry, N. M. (2009). Changing network support for drinking: Network support project 2-year follow-up. *Journal of Consulting and Clinical Psychology, 77*(2), 229–242.

Manning, V., Best, D., Faulkner, N., Titherington, E., Morinan, A., Keaney, F., et al. (2012). Does active referral by a doctor or 12-step peer improve 12-step meeting attendance?: Results from a pilot randomised control trial. *Drug and Alcohol Dependence, 126*(1–2), 131–137.

McElrath, D. (1997). The Minnesota model. *Journal of Psychoactive Drugs, 29*(2), 141–144.

Miller, L., Davies, M., & Greenwald, S. (2000). Religiosity and substance use and abuse among adolescents in the National Comorbidity Survey. *Journal of the American Academy of Child and Adolescent Psychiatry, 39*(9), 1190–1197.

Miller, W. R., & Wilbourne, P. L. (2002). Mesa Grande: A methodological analysis of clinical trials of treatments for alcohol use disorders. *Addiction, 97*(3), 265–277.

Morgenstern, J., Labouvie, E., McCrady, B. S., Kahler, C. W., & Frey, R. M. (1997). Affiliation with Alcoholics Anonymous after treatment: A study of its therapeutic effects and mechanisms of action. *Journal of Consulting and Clinical Psychology, 65*(5), 768–777.

Mundt, M. P., Parthasarathy, S., Chi, F. W., Sterling, S., & Campbell, C. I. (2012). 12-step participation reduces medical use costs among adolescents with a history of alcohol and other drug treatment. *Drug and Alcohol Dependence, 126*(1–2), 124–130.

Narcotics Anonymous World Services. (2013). Narcotics Anonymous 2013 Membership Survey. Retrieved September 25, 2015, from *www.na.org/admin/include/spaw2/uploads/pdf/PR/NA_Membership_Survey.pdf*.

Ouimette, P., Humphreys, K., Moos, R. H., Finney, J. W., Cronkite, R., & Federman, B. (2001). Self-help group participation among substance use disorder patients with posttraumatic stress disorder. *Journal of Substance Abuse Treatment, 20*, 25–32.

Physician Leadership on National Drug Policy. (2002). *Adolescent substance abuse: A public health priority*. Providence, RI: PLNDP Project Office, Brown University, Center for Alcohol and Addiction Studies.

Prochaska, J. O., DiClemente, C. C., & Norcross, J. C. (1992). In search of how people change: Applications to addictive behaviors. *American Psychologist, 47*(9), 1102–1114.

Project MATCH Research Group. (1997). Matching alcoholism treatments to client heterogeneity: Project MATCH posttreatment drinking outcomes. *Journal of Studies on Alcohol, 58*(1), 7–29.

Roman, P. M., & Blum, T. C. (1999). *National Treatment Center Study* (Summary 3). Athens: University of Georgia.

Smith, D. C., Godley, S. H., Godley, M. D., & Dennis, M. L. (2011). Adolescent community reinforcement approach outcomes differ among emerging adults and adolescents. *Journal of Substance Abuse Treatment, 41*(4), 422–430.

Substance Abuse and Mental Health Services Administration. (2014). *Treatment Episode Data Set (TEDS) 2002–2012: National admissions to substance abuse treatment services* (BHSIS Series: S-71, HHS Publication No. [SMA] 14-4850). Rockville, MD: Author.

Suchman, E. A. (1967). *Evaluative research: Principles and practice in public service and social action programs.* New York: Russell Sage Foundation.

Tanner-Smith, E. E., Wilson, S. J., & Lipsey, M. W. (2013). The comparative effectiveness of outpatient treatment for adolescent substance abuse: A meta-analysis. *Journal of Substance Abuse Treatment, 44*(2), 145–158.

Timko, C., Debenedetti, A., & Billow, R. (2006). Intensive referral to 12-step self-help groups and 6-month substance use disorder outcomes. *Addiction, 101*(5), 678–688.

Vaughan, E. L., de Dios, M. A., Steinfeldt, J. A., & Kratz, L. M. (2011). Religiosity, alcohol use attitudes, and alcohol use in a national sample of adolescents. *Psychology of Addictive Behaviors, 25*(3), 547–553.

Walitzer, K. S., Dermen, K. H., & Barrick, C. (2009). Facilitating involvement in Alcoholics Anonymous during out-patient treatment: A randomized clinical trial. *Addiction, 104*(3), 391–401.

White, W. L. (2014). *Slaying the dragon: The history of addiction treatment and recovery in America* (2nd ed.). Bloomington, IL: Chestnut Health Systems/Lighthouse Institute.

Winters, K. C., Stinchfield, R., Latimer, W. W., & Lee, S. (2007). Long-term outcome of substance-dependent youth following 12-step treatment. *Journal of Substance Abuse Treatment, 33*(1), 61–69.

Winters, K. C., Stinchfield, R. D., Opland, E., Weller, C., & Latimer, W. W. (2000). The effectiveness of the Minnesota model approach in the treatment of adolescent drug abusers. *Addiction, 95*(4), 601–612.

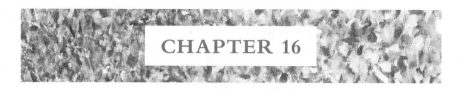

CHAPTER 16

Brief Interventions to Reduce College Student Drinking

Nadine R. Mastroleo

As individuals enter and attend college, a variety of concerns surface regarding alcohol use and associated harms. The stage of late adolescence, or emerging adulthood (Arnett, 2000), encompasses most first-year and early-stage college students and is marked by a variety of developmental tasks such as identity formation and forming more mature interpersonal relationships (Arnett, 2000; Schulenberg & Maggs, 2002). In addition, the transition from high school to college presents a new environment in which students explore their independence, adjust to a new living arrangement, and establish new friends and social networks (Cantor, Norem, Niedenthal, Langston, & Brower, 1987; Pascarella & Terenzini, 1991). The new influences offer opportunities for, as well as, expectations of alcohol use. As such, alcohol is routinely cited as the most pervasively misused substance in colleges.

Work spanning decades has focused on the role of risky alcohol use among college students (Kilmer, Cronce, & Larimer, 2014; Perkins, 2002). National studies consistently document significant prevalence rates of past-month alcohol consumption (68% consumed alcohol) and alcohol misuse (40% report having "been drunk"; Johnston, O'Malley, Bachman, & Schulenberg, 2013). More concerning are the rates of extremely heavy drinking within the past 2 weeks: 37% of students had five or more drinks in a row, 13% had 10 or more, and 5% had 15 or more (Johnston et al., 2013). When comparing emerging adults who are in college with those who are not, college students exhibit higher rates of drinking (68% vs. 54%) and heavy episodic drinking (4 drinks for women, 5 drinks for men over 2 hours; 37% vs. 29%, respectively; Johnston et al., 2013). Along with the high consumption rates for college students there are also high rates of alcohol-related harm and negative consequences, which are due, in part, to college students' engagement in heavy episodic drinking.

ALCOHOL-RELATED HARM

There is a well-established association between heavy drinking in college and alcohol use disorders later in life (e.g., National Center on Addiction and Substance Abuse, 2007; Jennison, 2004). However, colleges tend to focus on the immediate need to reduce alcohol-related harm to individual students who consume alcohol, as well as the larger university community that is also impacted by college student drinking. There are a range of consequences related to alcohol use among college students, including sexual aggression and assault, impaired academic performance, vandalism, physical assaults and injuries, motor vehicle crashes and fatalities, and transmission of sexual diseases (Hingson, Heeren, Winter, & Wechsler, 2005; Hingson, Zha, & Weitzman, 2009). Although not all alcohol-related problems are brought to the attention of the university administration, a large number of students are cited for violating alcohol policies following arrests, medical transports (being taken to a hospital emergency room by ambulance due to intoxication), and/or campus citations from residence hall staff and other members of the campus life administration (Hoover, 2003; Nicklin, 2000). As the majority of students consume alcohol (American College Health Association, 2013), research efforts have continued to evaluate prevention and intervention approaches to reduce consumption and related harms in the college environment. While effective strategies have been identified (Cronce & Larimer, 2011; Larimer & Cronce, 2002, 2007), challenges exist in implementing and maintaining such approaches. This chapter identifies and discusses specific groups at particularly high risk for heavy drinking and alcohol-related harm, presents the research evidence behind various levels of campus responses, provides guidelines for delivering interventions, and suggests future directions.

First-Year College Students and Alcohol

One specific group at high risk for engaging in heavy drinking behaviors and high rates of alcohol-related negative consequences are first-year college students. As matriculation to college is associated with increases in alcohol use over a very short period of time (first few weeks of college; Beets et al., 2009; National Institute on Alcohol Abuse and Alcoholism, 2002), first-year students are at high risk for accidental injury, poor academic performance, sexual violence, and crime (Hingson et al., 2009). This time period has the potential to influence two groups of first-year students: those who begin college with already established heavy drinking patterns and students who were either light or nondrinkers in high school. Patterns of previous heavy-drinking high school students may be maintained or increased during this time (White et al., 2006), while light/nondrinking high school students may begin to engage in heavy drinking (Weitzman, Nelson, & Wechsler, 2003). There are a number of reasons for the increased risk of alcohol use and negative consequences among first-year students as this group of emerging adults is meeting new people, joining new social groups, and attending social events where alcohol may be available. Further, research has shown that first-year college students—while increasing alcohol use—also decrease use of protective behavioral strategies (strategies used to reduce harm associated with alcohol use) during the same time period (Nguyen, Walters, Wyatt, & DeJong, 2011). When considering the increase in drinking, the access to alcohol, and a decrease in protective behavioral strategies by first-year college students, support for targeted intervention approaches is necessary to reduce the harm associated with this high-risk population of college students.

College Student Athletes and Alcohol

Collegiate student athletes (defined as students who are participating members of a varsity and university-supported athletic team) are at an even greater risk for heavy drinking and alcohol-related harms than the typical college student (Grossbard et al., 2009; Meilman, Leichliter, & Presley, 1999; Turrisi et al., 2009; Wechsler, Davenport, Dowdall, Grossman, & Zanakos, 1997). Participation in athletics at the collegiate level has been associated with elevated risk for consuming higher levels of alcohol, and, in turn, experiencing more negative alcohol consequences than nonathletes (Leichliter, Meilman, Presley, & Cashin, 1998; Meilman et al., 1999; Nattiv & Puffer, 1991; Wechsler et al., 1997; Yusko, Buckman, White, & Pandina, 2008). Specifically, compared with drinking among student nonathletes, the patterns of student-athlete drinking show higher rates of 2-week, heavy episodic drinking (college athletes: 53–57%, nonathletes: 36–43%), average drinks per week (college athletes: 7.6 drinks, nonathletes: 4.1 drinks), and higher rates of alcohol-related negative consequences (Leichliter et al., 1998; Nelson & Wechsler, 2001; Wechsler et al., 1997). These high drinking rates have been found across sport types (e.g., football, ice hockey, volleyball, basketball) and National Collegiate Athletic Association (NCAA; 2014) level of participation (i.e., Division I, II, and III). So, despite the wide range of sports and institution member types, heavy drinking is a pervasive issue across the spectrum of college student athletes. However, there are individual subgroup differences within the broader athlete population. Athlete alcohol consumption differs by race/ethnicity (Brenner & Swanik, 2007; Overman & Terry, 1991) and by gender (Damm & Murray, 1996; Hoeppner et al., 2012; Leichliter et al., 1998; Milroy et al., 2014). Although scarce research on racial and ethnic differences exists among student athletes, research has previously shown white athletes consuming alcohol more frequently than black athletes (Overman & Terry, 1991). Specifically, white male student athletes are significantly more likely to engage in heavy episodic drinking than their nonwhite counterparts (Ford, 2007). The NCAA reported high levels of heavy episodic drinking by 44% of male student athletes, while 33% of female student athletes surveyed consumed four or more drinks on one occasion (Burnsed, 2014).

A recent study compared student athletes with nonathletes and found athletes had significantly higher rates of heavy episodic drinking, peak and average estimated blood alcohol concentration (eBAC), higher rates of negative consequences and sex consequences, and higher reported rates of pregaming (drinking alcohol prior to attending an event or social function; Logan, Mastroleo, & Barnett, 2015). Specifically, the intoxication level (eBAC) for student athletes was twice the legal limit, and almost one in five students reported having an alcohol-related sexual consequence (e.g., unprotected sex, gotten into sexual situations he or she later regretted) in the past 2 weeks. Examination of athlete and nonathlete weekly drinking identified that student athletes were more likely than nonathletes to consume alcohol on Saturdays, Sundays, and Wednesdays, whereas nonathletes were more likely to drink on Tuesdays and Fridays. There were no differences between drinking rates on Mondays or Thursdays. This may be due to the specific competition schedules of student athletes and may be related to team rules regarding alcohol use prior to a competition (Logan, Mastroleo, et al., 2015). Athletes in their competitive season are more similar to nonathletes in their drinking as they drink less frequently, consume fewer drinks per week, and have fewer problems compared with when they are out of season. However, when in-season athletes do drink, they get as intoxicated as when out of season. Reasons behind why athletes drink more than their nonathlete peers when out of season has been studied with no one clear explanation emerging. It is likely a result of a combination of risk characteristics such as elevated sensation seeking and risk taking (Mastroleo, Scaglione, Mallett, & Turrisi, 2013), athletic identity and competitiveness (Grossbard et al., 2009), higher enhancement and drinking-coping motives (Yusko et al., 2008), and sports-related achievement motivation (Weaver et al., 2013). More research is needed to understand the underlying mechanisms of alcohol use among college student athletes, as this information is important for the development and implementation of intervention.

Greek Social Organization Members

Another subsample of high-risk students are members of social fraternities and sororities (Baer, 2002; Cashin, Presley, & Meilman, 1998; McCabe et al., 2005). Members of Greek life organizations are more likely to engage in high-risk drinking and other substance use and experience-related problems (Turrisi et al., 2009). In particular, men living in social fraternity houses drink more alcohol and drink more often, and as a result experience more negative consequences than non-Greek life students (Borsari & Carey, 1999). McCabe and colleagues (2005) found that significantly more Greek life members (70% of men, 50% of women) engaged in heavy episodic drinking during the past 2 weeks compared with non-Greek life students (42% of men, 29% of women). In addition, Cashin et al. (1998) reported that the average number of drinks consumed per week was significantly higher for Greek life members (men: 12 drinks per week, women: six drinks per week) than non-Greek life members (men: six drinks, women: two drinks). Furthermore, Greek life men and women report experiencing alcohol-related negative consequences (e.g., hangovers, blackouts, academic problems) at a much higher rate than non-Greeks. While less research has focused on interventions aimed at reducing alcohol use among Greek life members, the rates of heavy drinking and negative consequences suggest work in this area is needed and may be useful for overall reductions of drinking on college campuses.

UNIVERSAL PREVENTION APPROACHES

At the most fundamental level, colleges are charged with educating students about campus rules and regulations and the effects of alcohol. As a primary method of preventing alcohol misuse on campus, colleges focus on educating students through the implementation of basic awareness and general education programs. Programs for underage and heavy drinking on college campuses are often delivered at orientation sessions for new students; alcohol awareness weeks and other special events; and, in some instances, instructors include alcohol-related facts and issues in regular academic courses (Dejong, Larimer, Wood, & Hartman, 2009). The benefit of this approach is the opportunity to reach a large number of students at a low cost. However, this category of prevention approaches has been found ineffective when conducted in isolation (Larimer & Cronce, 2002). There remains a need to investigate the way in which these programs can be used in conjunction with and contribute to the impact of more comprehensive programs.

More recently, research has explored the role of living communities (specialized housing areas focused on specific topics or values; e.g., substance-free housing) as a means of prevention for increased drinking during college. In one study, the effects of living in a residential learning community (RLC) was evaluated and found that students who opted to live in the RLC showed smaller increases in drinking over time and were less likely to fit into a group defined as demonstrating a trajectory of high-risk drinking. In contrast, non-RLC students reported continued increases in maximum drinks per occasion over four semesters of college attendance (Cranford et al., 2009). These findings should be viewed with caution because of a number of limitations, including a lack of randomization and the potential for self-selection bias (e.g., students who chose to live in the RLC were less likely to drink before college than non-RLC students). However, it is important to note that students interested in limiting their exposure to alcohol use may need opportunities to select a living community that supports substance-free housing to more closely match their goals and exposure to students who choose to consume alcohol.

INDIVIDUALIZED INTERVENTIONS

As noted, the majority of college students report drinking within the past semester (American College Health Association, 2013). Colleges typically focus on ways to impact current drinkers using harm reduction models of intervention. Most research has focused on in-person and counselor-delivered brief motivational interventions aimed at reducing harm associated with heavy alcohol use. Studies have shown these motivational interventions, delivered in either an individual or group format by professional or peer counselors, are effective at reducing drinking behavior among college students (e.g., Borsari & Carey, 2005; Fromme & Corbin, 2004; Larimer et al., 2001) with effects lasting up to 2-years postintervention (Marlatt et al., 1998). However, the implementation of such programs can be costly, and limits the number of students who may receive such intervention approaches. More recent work has aimed to identify effective, low-cost scalable intervention approaches in an effort to reach a larger number of students, while also taking into consideration the limited resources on college campus to address all student drinking concerns (e.g., Cunningham, Hendershot, Murphy, & Neighbors, 2012; Larimer et al., 2007; Neighbors et al., 2016).

Brief Alcohol Screening and Intervention for College Students

One successful program used to reduce alcohol use in college students is the Brief Alcohol Screening and Intervention for College Students (BASICS; Dimeff, Baer, Kivlahan, & Marlatt, 1999). The National Institute on Alcohol Abuse and Alcoholism (NIAAA) Call to Action (2002) report identified BASICS (Dimeff et al., 1999) as a Tier I intervention approach. This Substance Abuse and Mental Health Services Administration (SAMHSA) model program (SAMHSA Model Programs, 2005) is a manualized treatment protocol that has been successful in reducing drinking and negative consequences when delivered in a controlled research environment (Larimer et al., 2001; Marlatt et al., 1998). BASICS is based upon the concepts of motivational interviewing (MI; Miller & Rollnick, 1991, 2002) and was designed as a brief, professionally led, motivational enhancement intervention aimed at reducing drinking and alcohol-related harm among heavy- and hazardous-drinking college students. The original model consisted of two 50-minute individual counseling sessions and combined assessment of the student's drinking behaviors, related attitudes about alcohol, motivation to change drinking behavior, feedback about personal risk factors, and advice about ways to moderate drinking. A computer-generated, personalized graphic feedback form is created using the student's information from responses to a comprehensive assessment battery that summarizes drinking behaviors, comparisons to general college student drinking norms, risk factors (e.g., family history), cognitive factors (e.g., beliefs about drinking effects), and consequences associated with drinking. The feedback offers an outline and structure for client discussions about current and past drinking. More recently, BASICS has been modified to a briefer approach in which counselors meet individually for one 50-minute motivational feedback intervention with an aim of reducing current heavy-drinking practices and related negative outcomes.

Peer-Led BASICS

In order to make delivery of BASICS cost-effective and widely scalable, thus increasing its potential reach to the large number of heavy-drinking students on college campuses, peer-delivered and group-based BASICS have also been tested. In the first study to test a peer-delivered BASICS, Larimer and colleagues (2001) compared peer- (fellow undergraduates who are trained to deliver the intervention) and professionally led (master's or higher degree) BASICS with first-year members of Greek social organizations. Students were assigned to either a brief individualized feedback session with a peer or professional counselor, or an assessment-only control condition. Findings showed the fraternity members in the treatment group had a decrease in drinks per week (from 15.5 to 12) and peak eBAC (from .12 to .08%), whereas the control group had an increase in drinks per week (from 14.5 to 17) and no change in peak eBAC over time. Peer providers were at least as effective as professional providers in reducing average drinks consumed per week (Larimer et al., 2001). The findings in this study lend support for widespread dissemination of a lower-cost BASICS across U.S. college campuses through the use of peers as intervention providers. The Larimer et al. (2001) study implemented peer BASICS using rigorous training and supervision approaches that are typically not used on college campuses using peer-based interventions (Mastroleo, Mallett, Ray, & Turrisi, 2008), raising questions about how a "real-world" application of this research may impact college student drinking.

Following this work, Mastroleo, Turrisi, Carney, Ray, and Larimer (2010) tested the role of supervision and training on implementing peer-led BASICS, first with voluntary heavy-drinking first-year college students, and then with students mandated to intervention following a campus alcohol violation (Mastroleo, Magill, Barnett, & Borsari, 2014). In both studies, students who received the peer-led BASICS reduced alcohol consumption. Although no reductions in negative consequences were found, the short follow-up time (3 months) and the fact that many college students do not consider hangovers and other reported consequences as negative (Mallett, Bachrach, & Turrisi, 2008) may be associated with this result. This low-cost implementation with minimal training and campus resources offers support for the use of peer counselors to implement evidence-based treatment approaches for high-risk and heavy-drinking students (Mastroleo et al., 2010, 2014). Surprisingly, the supervision of peer counselors did not play a factor in the impact on drinking outcomes lending support for a low-resource implementation strategy in which minimal staff time in training and supervising peers may still result in drinking reductions.

Implementation Considerations

There are a range of considerations when making the decision to implement an individually based alcohol intervention. Although a number of evidence-based individual interventions have manuals to guide practitioners, they typically include only the necessary components for implementing the intervention without offering guidelines on training and continued counselor supervision. First, a decision regarding who will be conducting the intervention is necessary. As noted, both professionals (master's or higher degree) and peers (fellow undergraduate students) have successfully implemented MI aimed at reducing college student alcohol use. However, within the context of rigorous research trials, specific training and supervision protocols were implemented to ensure intervention fidelity (Mastroleo et al., 2008). For both peer and professionally delivered interventions, initial training included a minimum of 8–12 hours of didactic training over 2 days incorporating alcohol information, accurate normative information, drinking reduction techniques, and MI principles. Initial training was followed with one or two supervised interventions to practice delivering the intervention prior to meeting with any college students.

When considering the specific content of counselor training, it ideally should include training in the use of active listening, empathic responses, genuineness in sessions, positive regard for clients, relationship-building skills, nonverbal behavior training, role-playing, communication skills, job-specific training, and the integration of skills (Mastroleo & Eaton Short, 2012). Specific training for each element should be decided by program directors and trainers based on the individual needs for each program. The needs of individual counselors will vary. Undergraduate peer counselors will likely need more time and attention to help develop counseling skills, where, in contrast, professional counselors or advanced graduate students may need less time on counseling skills. All interventionists (peer, professional, student affairs staff) will likely need specific training on alcohol content and the specific components of the intervention. Once trained, research suggests all counselors meet a threshold of baseline competency requirements for intervention fidelity, often evaluated using the Motivational Interviewing Treatment Integrity scale (Moyers, Martin, Manuel, Hendrickson, & Miller, 2005). As counselors begin to work with students, offering ongoing supervision to support counselors' work has been widely supported. Supervision can be conducted in a group format or individual basis and should offer counselors feedback on their skills, discussion of challenging cases, and feedback on practical aspects of delivering MI on campus. However, as previously noted, research suggests supervision for peer counselors may not have an effect on student outcomes. There are additional benefits of supervision as it does offer support to peer counselors as they work with heavy-drinking undergraduates.

A second area of consideration when deciding to offer one-on-one intervention sessions for college students is the availability of resources on campus to support the programming. A critical requirement is a private room that will ensure privacy and confidentiality. Implementation also requires the ability to create personalized feedback for college students, which will include each student completing a survey prior to a scheduled meeting. A number of programs exist commercially that would allow colleges to integrate a survey that creates personalized feedback. A final decision is which population of students would the university want to receive the intervention? Traditionally, it is used with students mandated to an alcohol intervention, but some schools have successfully implemented it with first-year students (Turrisi et al., 2009) and Greek life members (Larimer et al., 2001). The resources and time commitment is high for this level of intervention, and voluntary students often do not attend meetings (Mastroleo et al., 2010). As such, student affairs administrators should decide upon a specific target population prior to beginning planning for implementation.

Case Example

Tony is a first-year college student and member of the university baseball team. During the fall semester (his nontraditional season), he and some friends went out to a house party on a Saturday night. Tony drank some alcohol in high school, but never with the goal of getting drunk. This first night out he and his friends decided to have a few drinks before heading to the party. Tony ended up having two beers and doing two shots of hard liquor. When he got to the party around 10 P.M., he continued to drink beer out of red "keg" cups and thinks he had somewhere between four and six drinks. He remembers having a great time, dancing, meeting a lot of new people, but doesn't remember heading home from the party. He does know he threw up a few times after making it home and eventually passed out in his bed. He woke up the next morning with a bad headache and feeling sick to his stomach, and didn't feel 100% again until 2 days later.

In working with Tony in a one-on-one intervention and following the principles of BASICS and MI, the first step would be letting Tony know you are there to listen and not judge him—your goal is not to tell him what to do. Instead, it is to simply have a conversation about his experience, and if at all during the conversation there are things he would like to change about his drinking going forward, you are there to help him with that and be a partner in the process. It is best to next let Tony tell you, in his own words, what he recalls about that Saturday night and the different feelings he may have about the overall experience and outcome. As the interventionist, the goal is to listen for opportunities to reflect (let Tony know what you hear him saying) and identify opportunities to point out comments he makes that might suggest areas in which he can adjust his behavior to avoid future negative experiences (e.g., "I hear you saying you don't ever want to wake up feeling that sick again"). Over the course of the conversation, it is also important to understand the things Tony "likes" and "doesn't like" so much about alcohol use. By exploring both sides you will have a clearer understanding of the role alcohol may play in his life.

Once the interventionist understands the context of Tony's drinking, it is important to ask questions about his goals, and how he sees alcohol playing a part in his life. These initial aspects are an important part of any interaction with a student, regardless of gender, age, race/ethnicity, or student status (athlete, Greek life, etc). As Tony is an athlete, there are specific topics that are also important to address, such as how this may impact his standing on his team, the way in which alcohol effects his body as an athlete, and how his coaches may react to the event. All of this information is discussed as a way to help Tony identify the way in which alcohol will play a role in meeting his goals academically, personally, and athletically. Finally, an important aspect of the conversation will include some psychoeducation, offered when appropriate and in a manner consistent with a collaborative relationship. Topics include normative-based information on campus, standard drink sizes, the way eBAC is impacted by his drinking (including the importance of knowing how many drinks over how much time), the expectancies he may have around alcohol, and identifying protective behaviors (e.g., counting drinks, eating before going out) and the role they can play in reducing harm and negative consequences.

As the session comes to a close, asking Tony about his experience in the meeting and helping him to identify concrete behavioral goals regarding his future alcohol use as he moves forward is important. It may also be appropriate to offer Tony some additional campus resources should he indicate a need for them in the future.

GROUP INTERVENTIONS

The Alcohol Skills Training Program (ASTP; Baer, Kivlahan, Blume, McKnight, & Marlatt, 2001) was the first group-based alcohol intervention designed and tested to reduce alcohol consumption in college students. Similar to BASICS, ASTP incorporates education on basic alcohol information relevant to a student's personal experience; builds motivation to change drinking; challenges expectancies about alcohol's effects; corrects misperceptions through normative feedback; provides cognitive-behavioral skills training, including how to monitor daily alcohol consumption and stress management; and develops a tailored plan for reducing alcohol use and/or harm. The overarching premise is a belief that college students can learn to moderate their drinking behavior and reduce harm associated with alcohol use, acknowledging that any step toward reducing risk is a step in the right direction. Within the eight-session curriculum, information and exercises focus on the topics of addiction, individual drinking cues, skills for resisting alcohol offers, and strategies for relaxation and stress management. To stimulate students' consideration of changing their drinking behavior, ASTP facilitators elicit students identifying personally relevant reasons for change. This is often done by considering the short-term unwanted consequences (e.g., hangovers, embarrassment), rather than the longer-term physiological or extreme effects, as emerging adults are often more influenced by proximal consequences than by consequences that are far in the future. Facilitators also include the discussion of protective behavioral strategies to mitigate potential harm from heavy drinking. Although the program was initially designed as eight 90-minute sessions, the schedule does allow flexibility to adjust to specific campus needs.

Multiple studies have tested the effects of ASTP in comparison to control and other active experimental conditions. Consistent reductions in use, eBAC, and negative consequences have been found to offer strong support for this harm reduction approach with high-risk college student drinkers (Baer et al., 1992; Fromme, Marlatt, Baer, & Kivlahan, 1994; Logan, Kilmer, King, & Larimer, 2015). Modifications have been made to reduce the curriculum from eight sessions to six (Fromme et al., 1994) to two sessions (Miller, 1999), with continued support for alcohol use reduction and efficacy of the brief intervention. As ASTP was the original model for group-based alcohol interventions for college students, a number of adaptations have been tested in the effort to reduce the time and effort needed to deliver it.

A recent study tested a one-session group intervention, modeled after BASICS, compared to a one-on-one BASICS session (Hustad et al., 2014) with mandated students. Participants in both conditions reported a lower peak eBAC and fewer alcohol-related consequences at 1-, 3-, and 6-months postintervention, while no change was observed for number of drinks per week. There were no differences between the individual and group interventions, an important finding regarding the potential for cost savings by implementing group-based interventions, where multiple students can be treated simultaneously. In another study, high-risk mandated students completed an individual BASICS session (I-BASICS; 5+ past-month alcohol problems and 2+ past-month heavy-drinking episodes), while low-risk mandated students were assigned to a group BASICS session (G-BASICS; all others; Bernstein et al., 2017). Results of the 1-month follow-up assessment found both high-risk (assigned to I-BASICS) and low-risk (assigned to G-BASICS) students reported substantially less alcohol involvement at follow-up when compared with baseline alcohol use reports.

Further, alcohol use reduction was strongest for high-risk students. This study supports the feasibility of implementation as it was conducted with minimal resources and within the context of typical practice in a university setting as counselors were psychology graduate students trained over one weekend. Although both I-BASICS and G-BASICS sessions are effective in reducing college student alcohol use, research suggests individual sessions are modestly better than group sessions (Carey, Scott-Sheldon, Carey, & DeMartini, 2007). As I-BASICS sessions require a great deal of resources that may limit the ability to implement this prevention and intervention approach, alternative approaches are needed to reduce the resource strain placed on university communities.

Implementation Considerations

Training counselors to implement a group intervention includes learning MI skills, alcohol content knowledge, specific campus normative information, and the specific intervention protocol. Once the counselor establishes the skill set necessary to implement the protocol, training is transitioned to using these skills within a group setting. Special attention is aimed at preparing counselors to effectively manage groups while adhering to the treatment protocol. Techniques include initiating group discussion with an open-ended question, actively listening to the group members' responses, and reflecting (when appropriate) to direct the discussion back to the group. In groups, counselors should be especially aware of avoiding an instructional, purely didactic psychoeducation model, as this approach is less successful in impacting behavior change than actively engaging group members in the discussion (Miller & Rollnick, 2002; Walters & Baer, 2005). The goal is for counselors to create individual interactions with group members and encourage members to share experiences while adding to the overall discussion. Counselors should be trained to use summary statements to synthesize and reflect the various contributions of group members (e.g., "Through our conversation I see many of you have identified specific protective behaviors you use when you drink alcohol to reduce problems—things like spacing out your drinks, keeping track of how many drinks you have, and making sure to go home with a friend"). To ensure intervention fidelity, counselors should conduct role plays until they are comfortable and proficient in the intervention delivery and engage in supervision to discuss clinical and procedural issues (e.g., see Miller, Kilmer, Kim, Weingardt, & Marlatt, 2001, for an ASTP implementation model).

COMPUTER-BASED
INDIVIDUAL INTERVENTIONS

Given the importance of reaching a large number of students while minimizing financial and clinical burdens within overextended departments, universities have implemented computer- and web-based intervention approaches aimed at reducing drinking among heavy-drinking students (Larimer & Cronce, 2007). Students receive personalized normative feedback (PNF) about their own drinking behaviors that then compares their drinking to normative drinking rates of students on campus. The computerized feedback also includes suggestions on ways to reduce consumption and minimize harm if the student chooses to make changes. Results indicate that students receiving the PNF report significantly fewer drinking days and significantly less heavy drinking compared with those who do not (see Cronce & Larimer, 2011; Larimer & Cronce, 2007). Initial studies mailed PNF reports to students' mailboxes (Larimer et al., 2007), while more recent versions have delivered PNF in "real time" immediately to students via computer or smartphone technology (Neighbors, Larimer, & Lewis, 2004; Patrick, Lee, & Neighbors, 2014; Rodriguez et al., 2015). Findings from these studies suggest web-based alcohol interventions with personalized feedback is an effective way to reach large populations of college and university students with minimal cost and personnel effort needed for implementation.

A range of studies have tested the use of PNF with a variety of student drinking populations and targeted high-risk-drinking time periods. Research emphasizes the importance of gender-specific normative interventions where women and men are offered specific feedback about college students of their same gender on campus (Lewis & Neighbors, 2007). A recent study also examined effects of athlete-specific normative information to reduce alcohol use among college student athletes (Martens, Kilmer, Beck, & Zamboanga, 2010). Martens and colleagues (2010) found student athletes who received a targeted PNF (normative information presented was athlete specific) reported lower peak eBAC at 6-month follow-up compared with individuals who received nontargeted PNF or education only. When looking specifically at heavy-drinking students in the targeted PNF condition, this group reported a lower peak eBAC than those in the other conditions at 1-month follow-up and a lower peak eBAC than those in the education-only condition at 6 months. To date, no specific PNF interventions focused on Greek life students have been published, but work with college student athletes offers support for testing this approach with other high-risk student groups.

Finally, work testing the effects of computerized PNF has also been explored for high-risk drinking events specific to heavy alcohol use by college students (Neighbors et al., 2007). Specific dates and time frames for college students add heightened risk for heavy episodic drinking and associated consequences. Spring break, 21st birthdays, and holidays such as July 4th and New Year's result in higher than typical drinking (Neighbors et al., 2011). Interventions targeting both 21st-birthday celebrations (Neighbors et al., 2012; Neighbors, Lee, Lewis, Fossos, & Walter, 2009) and spring break (Lee et al., 2014; Patrick et al., 2014) have been tested. There has been little support across a number of studies for PNF interventions focused on 21st-birthday celebrations to reduce quantities of alcohol consumed. These interventions were, however, associated with significant reductions in eBAC levels but with very small effects (Steinka-Fry, Tanner-Smith, & Grant, 2015). When considering the effects of PNF on spring break drinking for students who went on a spring break trip with friends and planned to drink at least 1 day, the spring break web BASICS (with and without friend participation) was not effective in reducing spring break drinking. There was some support for an in-person BASICS session focused on spring break drinking—however, web-based interventions were not associated with reduced drinking (Lee et al., 2014).

Implementation Considerations

Challenges to computer-delivered interventions are decisions about implementation methods and the potential for mandatory participation by various student subgroups (e.g., first-year students, athletes). With the range of commercialized, computer-delivered alcohol intervention approaches, the decision of which intervention to choose should be based upon the needs of each specific campus. Using interventions that offer specific campus normative information may enhance the effectiveness of the intervention. There is a wide range of costs associated with each program, which may also influence choices made by individual colleges.

FUTURE DIRECTIONS

The support for interventions aimed at reducing college student drinking is strong, and a wide variety of choices exist to best meet the needs of each university. One challenge, despite the large number of research studies testing various intervention approaches, is a lack of understanding regarding how the interventions designed and tested under research protocols may work when delivered in practice without the high level of resources typically associated with research studies. More research examining the impact of drinking interventions in daily practice are needed to expand our understanding of intervention implementation and effectiveness. In order to accomplish this, universities must collect data on pre- and postintervention drinking behaviors to test how specific interventions function within the context of a real-world setting. This is important to advance the knowledge of implementation practice to colleges, but also to test for negative or iatrogenic effects that may occur in the absence of testing. Support for evaluation may be offered from academic departments or offices of institutional research.

Given the large number of available interventions, a better understanding of how and for whom they work is a natural next step in unpacking their potential. Studies that explore the individual characteristics of college students who respond to individual, group, or computerized intervention are needed to help tailor interventions more specifically to the needs of particular students. Further, examining the interactions between counselors and college students within an intervention session may elucidate our understanding of how to better train counselors to deliver interventions that are more effective in reducing student drinking. As research has shown, the relationship between counselors and students, as well as the way in which alcohol use is discussed and challenged, may have important implications for developing and enhancing the future of brief alcohol interventions for college students.

REFERENCES

American College Health Association. (2013, Fall). American College Health Association National College Health Assessment (ACHA-NCHA) web summary. *http://www.acha-ncha.org/docs/ACHA-NCHA-II_ReferenceGroup_Executive Summary_Fall2013.pdf*

Arnett, J. J. (2000). Emerging adulthood: A theory of development from the late teens through the twenties. *The American Psychologist, 55*(5), 469–480. Retrieved from *www.ncbi.nlm.nih.gov/pubmed/10842426*.

Baer, J. S. (2002). Student factors: Understanding individual variation in college drinking. *Journal of Studies on Alcohol Supplement, 14*, 40–53. Retrieved from *www.ncbi.nlm.nih.gov/pubmed/12022729*.

Baer, J. S., Kivlahan, D. R., Blume, A. W., McKnight, P., & Marlatt, G. A. (2001). Brief intervention for heavy-drinking college students: 4-year follow-up and natural history. *American Journal of Public Health, 91*, 1310–1316.

Baer, J. S., Marlatt, G. A., Kivlahan, D. R., Fromme, K., Larimer, M. E., & Williams, E. (1992). An experimental test of three methods of alcohol risk reduction with young adults. *Journal of Consulting and Clinical Psychology, 60*, 974–979.

Beets, M. W., Flay, B. R., Vuchinich, S., Li, K. K., Acock, A., Snyder, F. J., et al. (2009). Longitudinal patterns of binge drinking among first year college students with a history of tobacco use. *Drug and Alcohol Dependence, 103*(1–2), 1–8.

Bernstein, M. H., Baird, G. L., Mastroleo, N. R., Yusufov, M., Carey, K. B., Graney, D. D., et al. (2017). A novel approach for streamlining delivery of brief motivational interventions to mandated college students: Using group and individual sessions matched to level of risk. *Substance Use and Misuse, 16*, 1–9.

Borsari, B. E., & Carey, K. B. (1999). Understanding fraternity drinking: Five recurring themes in the literature, 1980–1998. *Journal of American College Health, 48*(1), 30–37.

Borsari, B., & Carey, K. B. (2005). Two brief alcohol interventions for mandated college students. *Psychology of Addictive Behaviors, 19*(3), 296–302.

Brenner, J., & Swanik, K. (2007). High-risk drinking characteristics in collegiate athletes. *Journal of American College Health, 56*(3), 267–272.

Burnsed, B. (2014). Rates of excessive drinking among student-athletes falling. *Media Center.* Retrieved from *www.ncaa.org/about/resources/media-center/news/rates-excessive-drinking-among-student-athletes-falling*.

Cantor, N., Norem, J. K., Niedenthal, P. M., Langston, C. A., & Brower, A. M. (1987).

Life tasks, self-concept ideals, and cognitive strategies in a life transition. *Journal of Personality and Social Psychology, 53,* 1178–1191.

Carey, K. B., Scott-Sheldon, L. A., Carey, M. P., & DeMartini, K. S. (2007). Individual-level interventions to reduce college student drinking: A meta-analytic review. *Addictive Behaviors, 32*(11), 2469–2494.

Cashin, J. R., Presley, C. A., & Meilman, P. W. (1998). Alcohol use in the Greek system: Follow the leader? *Journal of Studies on Alcohol, 59*(1), 63–70. Retrieved from *www.ncbi.nlm.nih.gov/pubmed/9498317.*

Cranford, J. A., McCabe, S. E., Boyd, C. J., Lange, J. E., Reed, M. B., & Scott, M. S. (2009). Effects of residential learning communities on drinking trajectories during the first two years of college. *Journal of Studies on Alcohol and Drugs, 16*(Suppl.), 86–95.

Cronce, J. M., & Larimer, M. E. (2011). Individual-focused approaches to the prevention of college student drinking. *Alcohol Research and Health, 34*(2), 210–221.

Cunningham, J. A., Hendershot, C. S., Murphy, M., & Neighbors, C. (2012). Pragmatic randomized controlled trial of providing access to a brief personalized alcohol feedback intervention in university students. *Addiction Science and Clinical Practice, 7,* 21.

Damm, J., & Murray, P. (1996). Alcohol and other drug use among college student-athletes. In E. F. Etzel, A. P. Ferrante, & J. W. Pinkney (Eds.), *Counseling college student-athletes: Issues and interventions* (Vol. 1996, pp. 185–220). Morgantown, WV: Fitness Information Technology.

Dejong, W., Larimer, M. E., Wood, M. D., & Hartman, R. (2009). NIAAA's rapid response to college drinking problems initiative: Reinforcing the use of evidence-based approaches in college alcohol prevention. *Journal of Studies on Alcohol and Drugs, 16*(Suppl.), 5–11. Retrieved from *www.ncbi.nlm.nih.gov/pubmed/19538907.*

Dimeff, L. A., Baer, J. S., Kivlahan, D. R., & Marlatt, G. A. (1999). *Brief alcohol screening and intervention for college students: A harm reduction approach.* New York: Guilford Press.

Ford, J. A. (2007). Alcohol use among college students: A comparison of athletes and nonathletes. *Substance Use and Misuse, 42*(9), 1367–1377.

Fromme, K., & Corbin, W. (2004). Prevention of heavy drinking and associated negative consequences among mandated and voluntary college students. *Journal of Consulting and Clinical Psychology, 72*(6), 1038–1049.

Fromme, K., Marlatt, G. A., Baer, J. S., & Kivlahan, D. R. (1994). The Alcohol Skills Training Program: A group intervention for young adult drinkers. *Journal of Substance Abuse Treatment, 11*(2), 143–154. Retrieved from *www.ncbi.nlm.nih.gov/pubmed/8040918.*

Grossbard, J. R., Geisner, I. M., Mastroleo, N. R., Kilmer, J. R., Turrisi, R., & Larimer, M. E. (2009). Athletic identity, descriptive norms, and drinking among athletes transitioning to college. *Addictive Behaviors, 34*(4), 352–359.

Hingson, R., Heeren, T., Winter, M., & Wechsler, H. (2005). Magnitude of alcohol-related mortality and morbidity among U.S. college students ages 18–24: Changes from 1998 to 2001. *Annual Review of Public Health, 26,* 259–279.

Hingson, R. W., Zha, W., & Weitzman, E. R. (2009). Magnitude of and trends in alcohol-related mortality and morbidity among U.S. college students ages 18–24,

1998–2005. *Journal of Studies on Alcohol and Drugs Supplement, 16,* 12–20. Retrieved from *www.ncbi.nlm.nih.gov/pubmed/19538908.*

Hoeppner, B. B., Barnett, N. P., Jackson, K. M., Colby, S. M., Kahler, C. W., Monti, P. M., et al. (2012). Daily college student drinking patterns across the first year of college. *Journal of Studies on Alcohol and Drugs, 73*(4), 613–624. Retrieved from *www.ncbi.nlm.nih.gov/pmc/articles/PMC3364328.*

Hoover, E. (2003). Drug and alcohol arrests increased on campuses in 2001. *Chronicle of Higher Education, 49.*

Hustad, J. T., Mastroleo, N. R., Kong, L., Urwin, R., Zeman, S., Lasalle, L., et al. (2014). The comparative effectiveness of individual and group brief motivational interventions for mandated college students. *Psychology of Addictive Behaviors, 28*(1), 74–84.

Jennison, K. M. (2004). The short-term effects and unintended long-term consequences of binge drinking in college: A 10-year follow-up study. *American Journal of Drug and Alcohol Abuse, 30*(3), 659–684. Retrieved from *www.ncbi.nlm.nih.gov/entrez/query.fcgi?cmd=Retrieve&db=PubMed&dopt=Citation&list_uids=15540499.*

Johnston, L. D., O'Malley, P. M., Bachman, J. G., & Schulenberg, J. E. (2013). *Monitoring the Future national survey results on drug use, 1975–2012.* Ann Arbor: Institute for Social Research, University of Michigan.

Kilmer, J. R., Cronce, J. M., & Larimer, M. E. (2014). College student drinking research from the 1940s to the future: Where we have been and where we are going. *Journal of Studies on Alcohol and Drugs Supplement, 75*(Suppl. 17), 26–35. Retrieved from *www.ncbi.nlm.nih.gov/pubmed/24565309.*

Larimer, M. E., & Cronce, J. M. (2002). Identification, prevention and treatment: A review of individual-focused strategies to reduce problematic alcohol consumption by college students. *Journal of Studies on Alcohol, 14*(Suppl.), 148–163. Retrieved from *www.ncbi.nlm.nih.gov/pubmed/12022721.*

Larimer, M. E., & Cronce, J. M. (2007). Identification, prevention, and treatment revisited: Individual-focused college drinking prevention strategies 1999–2006. *Addictive Behaviors, 32*(11), 2439–2468.

Larimer, M. E., Lee, C. M., Kilmer, J. R., Fabiano, P. M., Stark, C. B., Geisner, I. M., et al. (2007). Personalized mailed feedback for college drinking prevention: A randomized clinical trial. *Journal of Consulting and Clinical Psychology, 75*(2), 285–293.

Larimer, M. E., Turner, A. P., Anderson, B. K., Fader, J. S., Kilmer, J. R., Palmer, R. S., et al. (2001). Evaluating a brief alcohol intervention with fraternities. *Journal of Studies on Alcohol, 62*(3), 370–380. Retrieved from *www.ncbi.nlm.nih.gov/pubmed/11414347.*

Lee, C. M., Neighbors, C., Lewis, M. A., Kaysen, D., Mittmann, A., Geisner, I. M., et al. (2014). Randomized controlled trial of a spring break intervention to reduce high-risk drinking. *Journal of Consulting and Clinical Psychology, 82*(2), 189–201.

Leichliter, J. W., Meilman, P. W., Presley, C. A., & Cashin, J. R. (1998). Alcohol use and related consequences among students with varying levels of involvement in college athletics. *Journal of American College Health, 46*(6), 257–262.

Lewis, M. A., & Neighbors, C. (2007). Optimizing personalized normative feedback: The use of gender-specific referents. *Journal of Studies on Alcohol and Drugs, 68*(2), 228–237. Retrieved from *www.ncbi.nlm.nih.gov/pubmed/17286341.*

Logan, D. E., Kilmer, J. R., King, K. M., & Larimer, M. E. (2015a). Alcohol interventions for mandated students: Behavioral outcomes from a randomized controlled pilot study. *Journal of Studies on Alcohol and Drugs, 76*(1), 31–37. Retrieved from *www.ncbi.nlm.nih.gov/pubmed/25486391*.

Logan, D. E., Mastroleo, N. R., & Barnett, N. P. (2015b). *Alcohol-related risks among college student-athletes: Demographic and seasonal influences.* Paper presented at the annual meeting of Collaborative Perspectives on Addiction, Baltimore, MD.

Mallett, K. A., Bachrach, R. L., & Turrisi, R. (2008). Are all negative consequences truly negative?: Assessing variations among college students' perceptions of alcohol related consequences. *Addictive Behaviors, 33*(10), 1375–1381.

Marlatt, G. A., Baer, J. S., Kivlahan, D. R., Dimeff, L. A., Larimer, M. E., Quigley, L. A., et al. (1998). Screening and brief intervention for high-risk college student drinkers: Results from a 2-year follow-up assessment. *Journal of Consulting and Clinical Psychology, 66*(4), 604–615. Retrieved from *www.ncbi.nlm.nih.gov/pubmed/9735576*.

Martens, M. P., Kilmer, J. R., Beck, N. C., & Zamboanga, B. L. (2010). The efficacy of a targeted personalized drinking feedback intervention among intercollegiate athletes: A randomized controlled trial. *Psychology of Addictive Behaviors, 24,* 660–669.

Mastroleo, N. R., & Eaton Short, E. (2012). The role of training and supervision in delivering empirically supported treatments for college student drinkers. In C. Correia, J. G. Murphy, & N. P. Barnett (Eds.), *College student alcohol abuse: A guide to assessment, intervention, and prevention.* Hoboken, NJ: Wiley.

Mastroleo, N. R., Magill, M., Barnett, N. P., & Borsari, B. (2014). A pilot study of two supervision approaches for peer-led alcohol interventions with mandated college students. *Journal of Studies on Alcohol and Drugs, 75*(3), 458–466. Retrieved from *www.ncbi.nlm.nih.gov/pubmed/24766758*.

Mastroleo, N. R., Mallett, K. A., Ray, A. E., & Turrisi, R. (2008). The process of delivering peer-based alcohol intervention programs in college settings. *Journal of College Student Development, 49*(3), 255–259.

Mastroleo, N. R., Scaglione, N., Mallett, K. A., & Turrisi, R. (2013). Can personality account for differences in drinking between college athletes and non-athletes?: Explaining the role of sensation seeking, risk-taking, and impulsivity. *Journal of Drug Education, 43*(1), 81–95. Retrieved from *www.ncbi.nlm.nih.gov/pubmed/24855885*.

Mastroleo, N. R., Turrisi, R., Carney, J. V., Ray, A. E., & Larimer, M. E. (2010). Examination of posttraining supervision of peer counselors in a motivational enhancement intervention to reduce drinking in a sample of heavy-drinking college students. *Journal of Substance Abuse Treatment, 39*(3), 289–297.

McCabe, S. E., Schulenberg, J. E., Johnston, L. D., O'Malley, P. M., Bachman, J. G., & Kloska, D. D. (2005). Selection and socialization effects of fraternities and sororities on US college student substance use: A multi-cohort national longitudinal study. *Addiction, 100*(4), 512–524.

Meilman, P. W., Leichliter, J. S., & Presley, C. A. (1999). Greeks and athletes: Who drinks more? *Journal of American College Health, 47,* 187–190.

Miller, E. T. (1999). *Preventing alcohol abuse and alcohol-related negative consequences among freshman college students: Using emerging computer technology to deliver and evaluate the effectiveness of brief intervention efforts.* Unpublished doctoral dissertation, University of Washington, Seattle, WA.

Miller, E. T., Kilmer, J. R., Kim, E. L., Weingardt, K. R., & Marlatt, G. A. (2001). Alcohol skills training for college students. In P. M. Monti, S. M. Colby, & T. O'Leary (Eds.), *Adolescents, alcohol, and substance abuse: Reaching teens through brief interventions* (pp. 183–215). New York: Guilford Press.

Miller, W. R., & Rollnick, S. (1991). *Motivational interviewing: Preparing people to change addictive behavior.* New York: Guilford Press.

Miller, W. R., & Rollnick, S. (2002). *Motivational interviewing: Preparing people to change addictive behavior* (2nd ed.). New York: Guilford Press.

Milroy, J. J., Orsini, M. M., Wyrick, D. L., Fearnow-Kenney, M., Kelly, S. E., & Burley, J. (2014). A national study of the reasons for use and non-use of alcohol among college student-athletes by sex, race, and NCAA division. *Journal of Alcohol and Drug Education, 58*(3), 67–87.

Moyers, T. B., Martin, T., Manuel, J. K., Hendrickson, S. M., & Miller, W. R. (2005). Assessing competence in the use of motivational interviewing. *Journal of Substance Abuse Treatment, 28*(1), 19–26.

National Center on Addiction and Substance Abuse. (2007). *Wasting the best and brightest: Substance abuse at America's colleges and universities.* New York: Author.

National Collegiate Athletic Association. (2014, June). NCAA study of substance use habits of college student athletes. Retrieved November 16, 2017, from *www.ncaa. org/sites/default/files/Substance%20Use%20Final%20Report_FINAL.pdf.*

National Institute on Alcohol Abuse and Alcoholism. (2002). *A call to action: Changing the culture of drinking at US colleges* (NIH Publication No. 02-5010). Rockville, MD: Author.

Nattiv, A., & Puffer, J. C. (1991). Lifestyles and health risk of collegiate athletes. *Journal of Family Practice, 33*(6), 585–590.

Neighbors, C., Atkins, D. C., Lewis, M. A., Lee, C. M., Kaysen, D., Mittmann, A., et al. (2011). Event-specific drinking among college students. *Psychology of Addictive Behaviors, 25*(4), 702–707.

Neighbors, C., Larimer, M. E., & Lewis, M. A. (2004). Targeting misperceptions of descriptive drinking norms: Efficacy of a computer-delivered personalized normative feedback intervention. *Journal of Consulting and Clinical Psychology, 72*(3), 434–447.

Neighbors, C., Lee, C. M., Atkins, D. C., Lewis, M. A., Kaysen, D., Mittmann, A., et al. (2012). A randomized controlled trial of event-specific prevention strategies for reducing problematic drinking associated with 21st birthday celebrations. *Journal of Consulting and Clinical Psychology, 80*(5), 850–862.

Neighbors, C., Lee, C. M., Lewis, M. A., Fossos, N., & Walter, T. (2009). Internet-based personalized feedback to reduce 21st-birthday drinking: A randomized controlled trial of an event-specific prevention intervention. *Journal of Consulting and Clinical Psychology, 77*(1), 51–63.

Neighbors, C., Lewis, M. A., LaBrie, J., DiBello, A. M., Young, C. M., Rinker, D. V., et al. (2016). A multisite randomized trial of normative feedback for heavy drinking: Social comparison versus social comparison plus correction of normative misperceptions. *Journal of Consulting and Clinical Psychology, 84*(3), 238–247.

Neighbors, C., Walters, S. T., Lee, C. M., Vader, A. M., Vehige, T., Szigethy, T., et al. (2007). Event-specific prevention: Addressing college student drinking during known windows of risk. *Addictive Behaviors, 32*(11), 2667–2680.

Nelson, T. F., & Wechsler, H. (2001). Alcohol and college athletes. *Medicine and Science in Sports and Exercise, 33*(1), 43–47. Retrieved from *www.ncbi.nlm.nih.gov/pubmed/11194110.*

Nguyen, N., Walters, S. T., Wyatt, T. M., & DeJong, W. (2011). Use and correlates of protective drinking behaviors during the transition to college: Analysis of a national sample. *Addictive Behaviors, 36*(10), 1008–1014.

Nicklin, J. L. (2000). Arrests at colleges surge for alcohol and drug violations. *Chronicle of Higher Education,* A48–A58.

Overman, S. J., & Terry, T. (1991). Alcohol use and attitudes: A comparison of college athletes and nonathletes. *Journal of Drug Education, 21*(2), 107–117. Retrieved from *http://proxy.binghamton.edu/login?url=http://search.ebscohost.com/login.aspx?direct=true&db=mnh&AN=1886047&site=ehost-live.*

Pascarella, E. T., & Terenzini, P. T. (1991). *How college affects students: Findings and insights from twenty years of research.* San Francisco: Jossey-Bass.

Patrick, M. E., Lee, C. M., & Neighbors, C. (2014). Web-based intervention to change perceived norms of college student alcohol use and sexual behavior on spring break. *Addictive Behaviors, 39*(3), 600–606.

Perkins, H. W. (2002). Surveying the damage: A review of research on consequences of alcohol misuse in college populations. *Journal of Studies on Alcohol, 14*(Suppl.), 91–100. Retrieved from *www.ncbi.nlm.nih.gov/pubmed/12022733.*

Rodriguez, L. M., Neighbors, C., Rinker, D. V., Lewis, M. A., Lazorwitz, B., Gonzales, R. G., et al. (2015). Remote versus in-lab computer-delivered personalized normative feedback interventions for college student drinking. *Journal of Consulting and Clinical Psychology, 83*(3), 455–463.

SAMHSA Model Programs. (2005, March 7). BASICS: Brief alcohol screening and intervention for college students. Retrieved from *www.modelprograms.samhsa.gov/template_cf.cfm?page=model&pkProgramID=89.*

Schulenberg, J. E., & Maggs, J. L. (2002). A developmental perspective on alcohol use and heavy drinking during adolescence and the transition to young adulthood. *Journal of Studies on Alcohol, 14*(Suppl.), 54–70. Retrieved from *www.ncbi.nlm.nih.gov/pubmed/12022730.*

Steinka-Fry, K. T., Tanner-Smith, E. E., & Grant, S. (2015). Effects of 21st birthday brief interventions on college student celebratory drinking: A systematic review and meta-analysis. *Addictive Behaviors, 50,* 13–21.

Turrisi, R., Larimer, M. E., Mallett, K. A., Kilmer, J. R., Ray, A. E., Mastroleo, N. R., et al. (2009). A randomized clinical trial evaluating a combined alcohol intervention for high-risk college students. *Journal of Studies on Alcohol and Drugs, 70*(4), 555–567. Retrieved from *www.ncbi.nlm.nih.gov/pubmed/19515296.*

Walters, S. T., & Baer, J. S. (2005). *Talking with college students about alcohol: Motivational strategies for reducing abuse.* New York: Guilford Press.

Weaver, C. C., Martens, M. P., Cadigan, J. M., Takamatsu, S. K., Treloar, H. R., & Pedersen, E. R. (2013). Sport-related achievement motivation and alcohol outcomes: An athlete-specific risk factor among intercollegiate athletes. *Addictive Behaviors, 38*(12), 2930–2936.

Wechsler, H., Davenport, A. E., Dowdall, G. W., Grossman, S. J., & Zanakos, S. I. (1997). Binge drinking, tobacco, and illicit drug use and involvement in college athletics: A survey of students at 140 American colleges. *Journal of American College Health, 45*(5), 195–200.

Weitzman, E. R., Nelson, T. F., & Wechsler, H. (2003). Taking up binge drinking in college: The influences of person, social group, and environment. *Journal of Adolescent Health, 32*(1), 26–35. Retrieved from *www.ncbi.nlm.nih.gov/pubmed/12507798*.

White, H. R., McMorris, B. J., Catalano, R. F., Fleming, C. B., Haggerty, K. P., & Abbott, R. D. (2006). Increases in alcohol and marijuana use during the transition out of high school into emerging adulthood: The effects of leaving home, going to college, and high school protective factors. *Journal of Studies on Alcohol, 67*(6), 810–822. Retrieved from *www.ncbi.nlm.nih.gov/pubmed/17060997*.

Yusko, D. A., Buckman, J. F., White, H. R., & Pandina, R. J. (2008). Risk for excessive alcohol use and drinking-related problems in college student athletes. *Addictive Behaviors, 33*(12), 1546–1556.

PART III

FUTURE DIRECTIONS

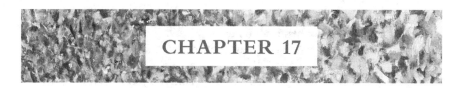

Future Research Opportunities for Screening and Brief Alcohol Interventions with Adolescents

Ralph Hingson and Aaron White

As the previous chapters indicate, in recent years research and practice of substance use screening and brief interventions (SBIs) has advanced to the point that population-level prevention using this approach has become a realistic objective. This chapter (1) highlights emerging evidence about the effectiveness of SBIs among youth, (2) notes gaps in SBI implementation, (3) identifies barriers that need to be overcome to increase implementation, and (4) points to research needs to improve effectiveness and expand the use of SBIs in various health care practice settings.

Considerable research indicates that alcohol SBIs can be effective, but research with adolescents needs further development. Established in 1984, the U.S. Preventive Services Task Force (USPSTF; 2012), an independent panel of nonfederal experts in prevention and evidence-based medicine, comprehensively addresses evidence and recommendations about the effectiveness of clinical preventive services, including screening tests; counseling about healthful behaviors; and preventive medications for children, adolescents, adults, older adults, and pregnant women.

The USPSTF (2012) recommends tobacco use counseling and intervention for adults and pregnant women with an A grade. The USPSTF also recommends alcohol misuse screening and behavioral counseling for adults and pregnant women with a B grade (Jonas et al., 2012). An A means there is a high certainty that the net benefit of the activity is substantial, while a B means there is a high certainty that the net benefit is moderate or there is a moderate certainty that the net benefit is moderate to substantial. Services receiving these recommendations are eligible (at the time of this writing) for Medicaid reimbursement under the Patient Protection and Affordable Care Act (ACA).

At the same time, the USPSTF (2012) concludes that the current evidence is insufficient to assess the balance of benefits and harms of the following services: alcohol misuse screening and behavioral counseling for adolescents in primary care; illicit drug use screening for adults, adolescents, and pregnant women; and prevention of motor vehicle occupant injuries through counseling in a primary care setting for driving under the influence of alcohol. Considerable evidence supports the recommendations for tobacco use counseling among adults and pregnant women (Land et al., 2012) and for alcohol misuse screening and behavioral counseling for adults and pregnant women (Jonas et al., 2012; O'Donnell et al., 2014).

Among adolescents, those ages 18–20 are most likely to meet alcohol-dependence criteria and hence be in need of treatment (U.S. Department of Health and Human Services, 2007). However, despite evidence linking SBIs to reductions in drinking and related problems, a recent meta-analysis of 13 studies found no evidence for increased use of substance use treatment services following an SBI (Glass et al., 2015). This may partially explain Saitz's (2010) finding of a lack of evidence that an SBI is effective for heavy users or alcohol-dependent drinkers. This suggests further SBI research should include receipt of treatment as an outcome if recommended.

NEW EVIDENCE FOR ALCOHOL SBIs FOR ADOLESCENTS

Evidence is expanding regarding the efficacy of alcohol SBIs for adolescents. Tripodi, Bender, Litschge, and Vaughn (2010) conducted a meta-analysis of 16 interventions targeting ages 16–19 published between 1994 and 2008. Outcomes included alcohol abstinence, frequency and quantity of drinking, and alcohol-related problems. The authors reported large benefits for brief interventions with adolescents and with adolescents and their parents. More recently, Tanner-Smith and Lipsey (2015) identified 185 experimental studies of brief interventions (universal, selective, or indicated) aimed at reducing alcohol use or alcohol-related problems among adolescents ages 11–18 and young adults ages 19–30. The authors reported that, overall, brief interventions were linked to significant reductions in alcohol consumption and alcohol-related problems. Effects persisted up to 1 year and did not vary across demographics. Adolescents already experiencing heavy or hazardous consumption experienced larger intervention effects. For adolescents, a motivational interviewing (MI)/ enhancement intervention in a high school setting in a single session for more than 15 minutes yielded the greatest reduction. Among adolescents, effects were larger when using the timeline follow-back (Tanner-Smith & Risser, 2016).

For young adults, a self-administered computerized expectancy challenge conducted on a university campus indicating blood alcohol concentration (BAC) information yielded the greatest reductions. Notably, reductions were greater in studies of adolescents than in studies of young adults.

As noted in the previous chapter on college students (Mastroleo, Chapter 16, this volume), literature reviews have found alcohol SBIs can reduce drinking and related problems among college students (e.g., Cronce & Larimer, 2011; National Institute on Alcohol Abuse and Alcoholism, 2015b). This has been observed both with students mandated for screening and counseling for alcohol or behavioral infractions and those screened voluntarily. Exceptions included efforts to reduce drinking and related problems in Greek organizations (Scott-Sheldon, Carey, Kaiser, Knight, & Carey, 2016) and 21st-birthday drinking reduction interventions (Steinka-Fry, Tanner-Smith, & Grant, 2015). In the most recent comprehensive review, Scott-Sheldon, Carey, Elliott, Garey, and Carey (2014) examined 41 studies with 62 individual or group interventions among first-year students. They reported that, compared with controls, recipients of interventions exhibited reductions in alcohol consumption and related problems up to 4-years postintervention on most outcomes. Individual and group interventions yielded comparable results. However, individual interventions reduced heavy drinking more than group interventions. The most effective intervention components were personalized drinking feedback, protective strategies to moderate drinking, setting alcohol-related goals, and challenging alcohol expectancies. The most effective interventions were those with the most components. The authors concluded that SBI approaches were so effective that they should be done with all incoming students. Because most students have at least one health service visit per year, if screening and brief interventions were routine in those settings, the potential for population-level effects would be great.

GAPS IN IMPLEMENTATION OF SBIs

Unfortunately, however, SBIs with adults, adolescents, or college students are not routine. A national survey of 18- to 39-year-olds (Hingson, Heeren, Edwards, & Saitz, 2012) found that two-thirds of respondents had seen a physician in the past year. Of those, only 14% were asked both about their drinking and given advice about what drinking patterns pose risk for health. Respondents ages 18–25 were less likely to have been asked about drinking (34% vs. 56%) than other age groups and especially those under age 21 (26%). But people ages 18–24 are most likely to exceed the National Institute on Alcohol Abuse and Alcoholism's (NIAAA; 2009) low-risk drinking guidelines compared with the general population (68% vs. 54%, respectively).

According to the 2012–2013 National Epidemiologic Survey on Alcohol and Related Conditions (Chen, Slater, Castle, & Grant, 2016), the group with the highest percentage meeting the fifth edition of the *Diagnostic and Statistical*

Manual of Mental Disorders's (DSM-5; American Psychiatric Association, 2013) alcohol use disorder (AUD) criteria is ages 18–24, with 35% meeting criteria versus 19% of all others over age 18. In fact, 10% of 18- to 24-year-olds met severe AUD criteria relative to 5% of all others.

According to the Centers for Disease Control and Prevention (CDC), the National Commission of Prevention Priorities lists SBIs for alcohol among the five most effective clinical services. Further, the ACA allows for health insurance coverage for alcohol SBIs. Nonetheless, according to the CDC Risk Factor Surveillance System in 2011 (N = 166,753, ages 18 and older), only 17% of U.S. adults reported discussing alcohol use with a physician in the past year, and only 25% of binge drinkers did so (McKnight-Eily et al., 2014).

The NEXT Generation Health Study, a national prospective study of 2,519 tenth graders, average age 16 at baseline, reported that 82% saw a physician in the previous year. At their last visit, over 50% were asked about drinking alcohol, smoking, and other drug use. Forty percent were advised about risks related to drinking alcohol, smoking, and drug use, but only 17% were advised to reduce or stop. Among those deemed as frequently (six or more times per month) getting drunk, smoking, or using drugs, only 24% were advised to reduce or stop alcohol use, 36% smoking, and 42% drug use (Hingson, Zha, Iannotti, & Simons-Morton, 2013).

A follow-up 1 year past high school indicated 71% had seen a physician in the past year and 77% of them were asked about drinking, 81% smoking, and 76% drug use. Forty-nine percent were advised about the risks of drinking, 50% smoking risks, and 48% drug use risks. Physicians advised only 20% to reduce or stop drinking, smoking, or drug use. Thirty-six percent of those who were frequently drunk (six or more times in the past month), 45% of frequent smokers, and 31% of frequent illicit drug users were asked to reduce or stop. Notably, comparing respondents in 4-year to those in 2-year colleges and those not in college, 4-year students were the least likely to be advised about risks of using those substances and least likely to be advised to reduce or stop using even though they reported the highest levels of drinking (Hingson, Zha, White, & Simons-Morton, 2015).

BARRIERS TO SUBSTANCE USE: SBI IMPLEMENTATION

Many barriers exist to implementation of SBIs for substance use. It takes time to ask screening questions and counsel patients about substance use. Some youth may fear loss of confidentiality of their responses, particularly if their substance use prompts referral to treatment, for which their parents may ultimately pay. The lack of physician training and reimbursement are also issues. The NIAAA has published guides on alcohol screening and counseling for adolescents and adults (National Institute on Alcohol Abuse and Alcoholism, 2011) and some reliable screening tools, such as the CRAFFT Substance Abuse Screening Test for both alcohol and drugs (Knight, Sherritt, Shrier, Harris, & Chang, 2002). Finally, while reimbursement issues could be addressed by the ACA, this may vary according to how each state implements it. Efforts are needed to remove these barriers to screening for all substances, particularly for alcohol misuse by youth, the leading contributor to injuries, which are the leading cause of death in that age group.

Clearly, research is needed to identify barriers to widespread adoption of SBIs for substance use in general medical practice. Trials are needed to test the efficacy of interventions to widen adoption of substance abuse SBIs. For example, the Veterans Administration has adopted electronic medical records with space devoted to questions about physician/provider discussion with patients about their use. Whether use of electronic medical records increases the proportions of patients receiving substance use, SBIs deserve systematic study.

DRUG USE SBI EFFICACY

Research on SBIs for drugs is much less developed than for alcohol, despite increases in drug deaths in recent years, mostly from painkillers (opiates) and sedatives. Preventing drug deaths has become an important prevention priority because deaths have totaled over 64,000 in 2016 (National Institute on Drug Abuse, 2017) (mostly overdoses) annually and have surpassed traffic deaths as the leading cause of injury death. It is well-known that heavy alcohol and drug use often occur simultaneously. A study of the Nationwide Inpatient Sample, a probability sample of U.S. community hospitals, identified 1.6 million hospitalizations for overdoses (180,000 among those ages 18–24) in 2008, with over half involving alcohol, usually in combination with other drugs (White, Hingson, Pan, & Yi, 2011). People with co-occurring alcohol and drug problems may have impaired judgment, prompting them to take higher, potentially more lethal doses. Further, alcohol can pharmacologically potentiate the effects of drugs, particularly sedatives and opiates. Also, one can overdose with lower BACs if he or she is taking other drugs.

Concerns have also increased about driving after drug use, particularly in combination with alcohol. The latest National Roadside Survey, conducted by the National Highway on Traffic Safety Administration, tested drivers for both alcohol and drugs. A higher percentage tested positive for drugs (22.5%) than for alcohol (8.3%). Driving after drug use had increased between the 2007 and 2013/2014 surveys, while percentage driving after drinking decreased.

Persons who drive after drug use are also much more likely to drive after drinking. Systematic reviews of experimental laboratory *studies of performing tasks* necessary to safely operate a motor vehicle found significant psychomotor impairment after use of benzodiazepines and cannabis with dose-dependent effects of cannabis on both experienced and novice drivers (Strand, Gjerde, & Mørland, 2016). The study also revealed that interactions of alcohol and tetrahydrocannabinol (THC) increased impairment, as did combined use of alcohol and methamphetamines. A review of 27 studies published since January 1960 examined randomized trials, cohort studies, case-control studies, and case-control-type studies to explore whether medications increase traffic crash risk. Of 53 medications investigated, the following 15 were associated with increased crash risk: buprenorphine, codeine, dihydrocodeine, methadone, tramadol, levocitirizine, diazepam, flunitrazepam, flurazepam, lorazepam, temazepam, triazolam, carisoprodol, zolpidem, and zopiclone (Rudisill, Zhu, Kelley, Pilkerton, & Rudisill, 2016).

A review of epidemiological studies by Gjerde, Strand, and Mørland (2015) found the following drugs increased traffic crash risk: benzodiazepines and z-hypnotics (in 25/28 studies), cannabis (in 23/36 studies), opioids (in 17/25 studies), amphetamines (in 8/10 studies), and simultaneous multiple drug use (in 12/12 studies). At the time of publication, nine states and the District of Columbia have legalized recreational marijuana use for adults (McCausland, 2018); which may further increase adolescent use. The authors concluded that, after alcohol, which poses the greatest traffic crash risk, amphetamines are the next single substance with highest risk. Combined use of drugs poses greater crash risk than any single drug, and the combined use of alcohol and a psychoactive drug poses the greatest risk (World Health Organization, 2016).

A much smaller number of studies have looked at SBIs for drugs other than alcohol, and results have been less consistent. A number have shown no benefit (e.g., Bogenschutz et al., 2014; Roy-Byrne et al., 2014; Saitz et al., 2014; White, Kraus, & Swartzwelder, 2006). The first three studies in JAMA were rigorously conducted. Each was done in a low-income, middle-age, inner-city population with large percentages unemployed, single, male, and having psychiatric comorbidities. In contrast, several studies of SBIs for drugs have shown some benefit (e.g., Bashir, King, & Ashworth, 1994; Gelberg et al., 2015; Winters, Lee, Botzet, Fahnhorst, & Nicholson, 2014). Of note, the Gelberg et al. (2015) study, like the three widely publicized studies in JAMA, was conducted in a low-income, inner-city population with similar characteristics as the JAMA studies.

Tanner-Smith, Steinka-Fry, Hennessy, Lipsey, and Winters (2015) recently published a meta-analysis of 30 studies focusing on adolescent and young adult populations. Seven of the studies focused on alcohol only, while 23 targeted both alcohol and drugs. The SBI studies targeting alcohol misuse yielded reductions only in drinking, with little variability across studies, but no carryover effects on drug use. Those that focused on both alcohol and drugs achieved alcohol reductions comparable to alcohol-only interventions. The alcohol and drug interventions also obtained reductions in marijuana and other drugs with the greatest reductions in other drugs. Clearly, this shows promise and remains a high-priority research area.

Steinka-Fry, Tanner-Smith, and Hennessy (2015) reviewed 12 experimental or quasi-experimental studies with 16 intervention groups ($N = 5,664$, mean age 17) to assess SBIs focused on reducing drinking and driving after drinking. The studies were published between 1991 and 2011. Compared with controls, participants in brief interventions experienced modest but significant reductions in drinking, driving after drinking, and related consequences.

We are unaware of any studies of SBIs that focus on reducing driving after drug use or driving after drugs in combination with alcohol. The research cited earlier by Strand et al. (2016), Rudisill et al. (2016), and Gjerde et al. (2015) indicates crash risk is linked to those behaviors, as does a recent review by the World Health Organization (2016). Research on SBIs for driving after substance use should also be a high research priority.

AREAS REQUIRING ADDITIONAL RESEARCH

The USPSTF (2012) identified these questions for future study in alcohol SBI research:

1. What are longer-term effects of SBI on morbidity, mortality, and quality of life?
2. Can those who screen gain positive benefit from behavioral counseling in primary care?
3. Which specific components of behavioral counseling are effective?
4. How should treatment decisions be individualized?

In a review by Foxcroft et al. (2016), priority questions for SBI research were as follows:

1. What is the optimal content of MI interventions and treatment exposure?
2. What is the optimal amount of MI that should be delivered?
3. Is MI, in conjunction with other prevention efforts, worthwhile?

Numerous suggestions for needed research were provided in several chapters of this volume. A common theme is that SBIs, and especially referral to treatment, can be enhanced by identifying treatments with proven efficacy. Examples of research needs from those chapters are listed below.

- "Despite widespread enthusiasm for SBIRT across service settings, questions persist regarding the model's effectiveness, feasibility, and developmental appropriateness for adolescents under age 18" (Becker, Ozechowski, & Hogue, Chapter 5, p. 134).
- "[B]rief interventions simultaneously targeting adolescent SUDs [substance use disorders] (alcohol; cannabis; other hard, illicit drugs) and comorbid conditions have not been tested" (Esposito-Smythers, Rallis, Machell, Williams, & Fischer, Chapter 7, p. 205).

- "Brief interventions for substance use treatment are largely untested with CINI youth, which is a significant gap given that 80% of all arrested youth never reach detention or incarceration and many CINI youth and families do not have the time or resources to participate in intensive, longer-term intervention" (Dauria, McWilliams & Tolou-Shams, Chapter 8, pp. 233–234).
- "[F]ew clinical trials have included sufficient numbers of ethnic/racial-minority children to permit generalization across cultures" (Hernandez & Moreno, Chapter 10, p. 267).

The most recent funding opportunity announcement (FOA) for SBI research from the NIAAA (2015c), lists the following series of unanswered questions:

1. What are the cost offsets? How much savings can be realized by SBI? European analysis identified savings (Angus, Thomas, Anderson, Meier, & Brennan, 2017) but U.S. studies are needed.
2. Can these effects be measured using typical administrative data?
3. How large does an effect size have to be to show a positive balance against the costs?
4. Can delivery be assisted by computerization?
5. How can uniformity of quality and fidelity to a protocol be best achieved when implementing SBI in a larger health care system?

The FOA also calls for the following types of studies:

1. Studies of the duration of effects and whether those effects can be enhanced by boosters. Will boosters or other changes lengthen duration?
2. Studies of the appropriate counseling that should be paired with screening and studies exploring how elements of this counseling might best be tailored to individuals.
3. Studies examining reasons for response and nonresponse to brief interventions (e.g., neurocognitive processes, parental involvement, or peer networks).
4. Studies of ways to combine alcohol screening with drug and smoking screening.
5. Studies adopting SBI for nonclinical settings, such as schools and the military.
6. Studies that examine implementation processes and contextual factors that hinder or facilitate adoption and sustainability.
7. Studies that evaluate the effectiveness of SBI in health disparities populations, which elements of the interventions increase effectiveness in those populations, and interventions *developed and tested explicitly for those populations.*

Other important questions or areas of inquiry not mentioned in the FOA include:

1. Who can most effectively offer the intervention? Do different types of interventions work better with certain subpopulations?
2. Including SBI research in other populations and venues, such as emergency departments, prenatal clinics, mental health clinics, the workplace, and foster care.
3. Is it effective to combine expansion of SBIs with more rigorous implementation of evidence-based environmental/policy interventions? Is there a relation between environmental alcohol and drug policies in place and effectiveness of substance use SBIs?
4. Do SBIs reduce alcohol consumption on heaviest drinking days at Levels 2–3 and three or more times the binge threshold (the equivalent of 8–11 and 12 or more drinks for women and 10–14 and 15 or more drinks for men over a 2-hour period)?

A few comments regarding the latter two suggestions are warranted. First, research is lacking regarding the effects of combining environmental policy interventions with expansion of SBIs. There is a sizable literature indicating a variety of policies aimed at reducing alcohol-impaired driving (e.g., the minimum legal drinking age of 21, lower legal BAC limits, zero-tolerance laws, and administrative license revocation), effectively reducing percentages engaging in risky drinking and related traffic crashes (see Goodwin et al., 2015). Also, reductions in risky drinking behaviors are achieved by policies that limit availability of alcohol, such as *raising* the legal drinking age to 21 (e.g., DeJong & Blanchette, 2014; Hingson & White, 2014; Wagenaar & Toomey, 2002), reducing alcohol outlet density (e.g., Campbell et al., 2009; Gruenewald, Ponicki, Holder, & Romelsjö, 2006; Zhang et al., 2015), and increasing alcohol taxes and price (e.g., Chaloupka, Grossman, & Saffer, 2002; Wagenaar, Salois, & Komro, 2009; World Health Organization, 2009).

As noted in this volume, great progress has been made in making SBIs for alcohol misuse more effective in reducing risky drinking and related problems, but studies are lacking that examine whether alcohol SBIs have larger or longer-term effects if done in jurisdictions with evidence-based alcohol policies and vigorous implementation. Komro's (2011–2016) project titled Cherokee Nation Prevention Trial: Interactive Effects of Environment and SBIRT explores this by conducting a multifactorial study to combine greater enforcement of minimum legal drinking age with annual school-based SBIs to reduce underage drinking.

Komro et al. (2017) randomly assigned six communities in eastern Oklahoma to a control, community-organized policy implementation, school-based universal SBI, and combined policy implementation and school-based intervention. A full-time social worker in each intervention community high school conducted a brief one-on-one health consultation with each student each semester based on the NIAAA's Alcohol Screening and Brief Intervention for Youth practitioner's guide (2015a).

The brief session used MI to encourage health behavior change related to alcohol consumption, including feedback on normative behavior and discussion of personal goals. Students reporting risky drinking attended a follow-up session approximately 2 weeks later, and students were referred to ongoing follow-up support or specialty treatment when appropriate. Postcards with behavioral tips were mailed three times per year to high school students' primary residences. Posters were placed throughout communities in commonly frequented venues, such as restaurants and places of worship. Based on quarterly surveys from 2012 to 2015, students in the community organization policy implementation showed a significant reduction in 30-day alcohol use (25%), heavy episodic drinking (24%), and alcohol-related consequences (8%). In the SBI groups, there was a reduction in past-30-day alcohol use (22%), heavy episodic drinking (19%), and alcohol-related consequences (4%). Overall reductions relative to the control community were 22–25% in the community-organized policy intervention group, 19–23% in the SBI group, and 12–15% in the combined group. This was the largest alcohol prevention intervention conducted to date with populations including high percentages of Native American youth, and notably achieved effects in target populations over 2.5 years. Effects were comparable in Native American and general population students.

Finally, a series of studies on high school seniors and college-age persons have recently been published indicating that a sizable minority drink at levels that substantially exceed the threshold for binge drinking (e.g., Dawson, Goldstein, Saha, & Grant, 2015; White, Morgan, et al., 2006). Dawson et al. (2015), in a national survey of adults ages 18 and older, reported that, from 2001/2002 to 2012/2013, percentages greatly exceeding the binge threshold increased in the United States. However, SBI studies have not looked at drinking at levels that substantially exceed the standard binge threshold as an outcome, and such research is warranted.

CONCLUSIONS

In summary, although the USPSTF says there is insufficient evidence that alcohol SBIs are effective with adolescents, a growing body of literature is emerging that indicates effectiveness in adolescent and college populations. However, more research with adolescents is needed. A new review by the USPSTF is planned.

While there is strong evidence regarding the effectiveness of SBIs to reduce alcohol misuse and related problems in *adult primary care* and growing evidence with adolescents, follow-up on referrals for specialty treatment has been lacking, which may also be an issue for adolescents. Consequently, more research is needed to overcome patient unwillingness to seek treatment and system barriers.

The USPSTF also indicates there is insufficient evidence that SBIs are effective for drugs for either adolescents or adults. This area has received much less attention than alcohol SBIs and results have not been consistently positive. More research on combining SBIs for alcohol and other drugs and smoking is warranted.

In all of the areas cited above, research is needed to identify brief interventions that achieve greater substance use and related harm reductions and that sustain the reductions over time. Cost-effectiveness studies are also lacking. Given that SBIs for substance misuse are not routinely conducted in adolescent or adult primary care, research is needed to identify and overcome barriers to their widespread use. Barriers to be addressed include time to screen and counsel, lack of provider training, patient confidentiality, availability of appropriate effective treatment/programs for referral, and reimbursement for brief interventions and referral.

The USPSTF has called for more research on the effects of SBIs for alcohol misuse on morbidity, mortality, quality of life, and further identification of the most effective, specific components of interventions and studies on treatment decisions.

Authors of several chapters in this volume and others have underscored the need for more SBI substance misuse screening and treatment referral in specific populations, such as adolescents, persons in the juvenile justice system, racial- and ethnic-minority groups, persons with conduct problems and comorbid mental health problems, persons at risk for HIV and sexually transmitted infections, persons in foster care, military personnel, sexual minority youth, school students, persons convicted of alcohol- or drug-impaired driving, persons attending emergency departments, visitors of prenatal and mental health clinics, workplace employees, and persons who greatly exceed the standard alcohol binge threshold. A common theme across several chapters is the need not only to improve brief interventions and identify which are most effective with specific populations, but also to improve behavioral and medication treatments to enhance patient willingness to follow up on referrals.

Finally, given the growing literature on both effective environmental policy interventions to reduce substance use and related problems and the progress being made with SBIs and referral for substance use, studies are needed to assess whether substance misuse SBIs will be even more effective when conducted in areas that have adopted and vigorously implemented evidence-based substance misuse prevention policies. Sufficient progress is being made on SBIs for substance misuse that it is a realistic future goal to explore how the best, most cost-effective interventions can be implemented on a wide-enough scope and with sufficient fidelity that they can achieve population-level substance abuse reduction and prevention effects.

REFERENCES

American Psychiatric Association. (2013). *Diagnostic and statistical manual of mental disorders* (5th ed.). Arlington, VA: Author.

Angus, C., Thomas, C., Anderson, P., Meier, P. S., & Brennan, A. (2017). Estimating the cost-effectiveness of brief interventions for heavy drinking in primary health care across Europe. *European Journal of Public Health, 27*(2), 345–351.

Bashir, K., King, M., & Ashworth, M. (1994). Controlled evaluation of brief intervention by general practitioners to reduce chronic use of benzodiazepines. *British Journal of General Practice, 44*(386), 408–412.

Bogenschutz, M. P., Donovan, D. M., Mandler, R. N., Perl, H. I., Forcehimes, A. A., Crandall, C., et al. (2014). Brief intervention for patients with problematic drug use presenting in emergency departments: A randomized clinical trial. *JAMA, 174*(11), 1736–1745.

Campbell, C. A., Hahn, R. A., Elder, R., Brewer, R., Chattopadhyay, S., Fielding, J., et al. (2009). The effectiveness of limiting alcohol outlet density as a means of reducing excessive alcohol consumption and alcohol-related harms. *American Journal of Preventive Medicine, 37*(6), 556–569.

Chaloupka, F. J., Grossman, M., & Saffer, H. (2002). The effects of price on alcohol consumption and alcohol-related problems. *Alcohol Research and Health, 26*(1), 22–34.

Chen, C. M., Slater, M. E., Castle, I.-J. P., & Grant, B. F. (2016). *Alcohol use and alcohol use disorders in the United States: Main findings from the 2012–2013 National Epidemiologic Survey on Alcohol and Related Conditions–III (NESARC-III)* (NIH Publication No. 16-AA-8020). Bethesda, MD: National Institute on Alcohol Abuse and Alcoholism.

Cronce, J. M., & Larimer, M. E. (2011). Individual-focused approaches to the prevention of college student drinking. *Alcohol Research and Health, 34*(2), 210–221.

Dawson, D. A., Goldstein, R. B., Saha, T. D., & Grant, B. F. (2015). Changes in alcohol consumption: United States, 2001–2002 to 2012–2013. *Drug and Alcohol Dependence, 148*, 56–61.

DeJong, W., & Blanchette, J. (2014). Case closed: Research evidence on the positive public health impact of the age 21 minimum legal drinking age in the United States. *Journal of Studies on Alcohol and Drugs Supplement, 75*(Suppl. 17), 108–115.

Foxcroft, D. R., Coombes, L., Wood, S., Allen, D., Almeida Santimano, N. M., & Moreira, M. T. (2016). Motivational interviewing for the prevention of alcohol misuse in young adults. *Cochrane Database of Systematic Reviews, 7*, CD007025.

Gelberg, L., Andersen, R. M., Afifi, A. A., Leake, B. D., Arangua, L., Vahidi, M., et al. (2015). Project QUIT (Quit Using Drugs Intervention Trial): A randomized controlled trial of a primary care-based multi-component brief intervention to reduce risky drug use. *Addiction, 110*(11), 1777–1790.

Gjerde, H., Strand, M. C., & Mørland, J. (2015). Driving under the influence of non-alcohol drugs—an update: Part I. Epidemiological studies. *Forensic Science Review, 27*(2), 89–113.

Glass, J. E., Hamilton, A. M., Powell, B. J., Perron, B. E., Brown, R. T., & Ilgen, M. A. (2015). Specialty substance use disorder services following brief alcohol intervention: A meta-analysis of randomized controlled trials. *Addiction, 110*(9), 1404–1415.

Goodwin, A., Thomas, L., Kirley, B., Hall, W., O'Brien, N., & Hill, K. (2015). *Counter-measures that work: A highway safety countermeasures guide for state highway safety offices* (8th ed.). Washington, DC: National Highway Traffic Safety Administration.

Gruenewald, P. J., Ponicki, W. R., Holder, H. D., & Romelsjö, A. (2006). Alcohol prices, beverage quality, and the demand for alcohol: Quality substitutions and price elasticities. *Alcoholism: Clinical and Experimental Research, 30*(1), 96–105.

Hingson, R. W., Heeren, T., Edwards, E. M., & Saitz, R. (2012). Young adults at risk for excess alcohol consumption are often not asked or counseled about drinking alcohol. *Journal of General Internal Medicine, 27*(2), 179–184.

Hingson, R., & White, A. (2014). New research findings since the 2007 surgeon general's call to action to prevent and reduce underage drinking: A review. *Journal of Studies on Alcohol and Drugs, 75*(1), 158–169.

Hingson, R. W., Zha, W., Iannotti, R. J., & Simons-Morton, B. (2013). Physician advice to adolescents about drinking and other health behaviors. *Pediatrics, 131*(2), 249–257.

Hingson, R., Zha, W., White, A., & Simons-Morton, B. (2015). Screening and brief alcohol counseling of college students and persons not in school. *JAMA Pediatrics, 169*(11), 1068–1070.

Jonas, D. E., Garbutt, J. C., Amick, H. R., Brown, J. M., Brownley, K. A., Council, C. L., et al. (2012). Behavioral counseling after screening for alcohol misuse in primary care: A systematic review and meta-analysis for the U.S. Preventive Services Task Force. *Annals of Internal Medicine, 157*(9), 645–654.

Knight, J. R., Sherritt, L., Shrier, L. A., Harris, S. K., & Chang, G. (2002). Validity of the CRAFFT Substance Abuse Screening Test among adolescent clinic patients. *Archives of Pediatrics and Adolescent Medicine, 156*(6), 607–614.

Komro, K. (2011–2016). Cherokee Nation Prevention Trial: Interactive effects of environment and SBIRT (NIH Project No. 5R01AA020695-04). Retrieved from *https://projectreporter.nih.gov/project_info_description.cfm?aid=8693880&icde=0.*

Komro, K. A., Livingston, M. D., Wagenaar, A. C., Kominsky, T. K., Pettigrew, D. W., Garrett, B. A., et al. (2017). Multilevel prevention trial of alcohol use among high school students in the Cherokee Nation. *American Journal of Public Health, 107*(3), 453–459.

Land, T. G., Rigotti, N. A., Levy, D. E., Schilling, T., Warner, D., & Li, W. (2012). The effect of systematic clinical interventions with cigarette smokers on quit status and the rates of smoking-related primary care office visits. *PLOS ONE, 7*(7), e41649.

McCausland, P. (2018, February 4). Stymied legalization process for marijuana opens door to gray market. NBC News. Retrieved from *https://www.nbcnews.com/news/us-news/stymied-legalization-process-marijuana-opens-door-gray-market-n844436.*

McKnight-Eily, L. R., Liu, Y., Brewer, R. D., Kanny, D., Lu, H., Denny, C. H., et al. (2014). Vital signs: Communication between health professionals and their patients about alcohol use—44 states and the District of Columbia, 2011. *Morbidity and Mortality Weekly Report, 63*(1), 16–22.

National Institute on Alcohol Abuse and Alcoholism. (2009). *Rethinking drinking: Alcohol and your health* (NIH Publication No. 15-3770). Bethesda, MD: U.S. Department of Health and Human Services.

National Institute on Alcohol Abuse and Alcoholism. (2011). *Alcohol screening and brief intervention for youth: A practitioner's guide* (NIH Publication No. 11-7805). Bethesda, MD: U.S. Department of Health and Human Services.

National Institute on Alcohol Abuse and Alcoholism. (2015a). *Alcohol screening and brief intervention for youth: A practitioner's guide* (NIH Publication No. 11-7805). Bethesda, MD: Author.

National Institute on Alcohol Abuse and Alcoholism. (2015b). *Planning alcohol interventions using NIAAA's CollegeAIM Alcohol Intervention Matrix* (NIH Publication No. 15-AA-8017). Bethesda, MD: National Institutes of Health.

National Institute on Alcohol Abuse and Alcoholism. (2015c). Screening and brief alcohol interventions in underage and young adult populations (R01, R03, R21). Retrieved from *http://grants.nih.gov/grants/guide/search_results.htm?scope=pa&year=active*.

National Institute on Drug Abuse. (2017). Overdose death rates. Retrieved from *www.drugabuse.gov/related-topics/trends-statistics/overdose-death-rates*.

O'Donnell, A., Anderson, P., Newbury-Birch, D., Schulte, B., Schmidt, C., Reimer, J., et al. (2014). The impact of brief alcohol interventions in primary healthcare: A systematic review of reviews. *Alcohol and Alcoholism, 49*(1), 66–78.

Roy-Byrne, P., Bumgardner, K., Krupski, A., Dunn, C., Ries, R., Donovan, D., et al. (2014). Brief intervention for problem drug use in safety-net primary care settings: A randomized clinical trial. *JAMA, 312*(5), 492–501.

Rudisill, T. M., Zhu, M., Kelley, G. A., Pilkerton, C., & Rudisill, B. R. (2016). Medication use and the risk of motor vehicle collisions among licensed drivers: A systematic review. *Accident Analysis and Prevention, 96*, 255–270.

Saitz, R. (2010). Alcohol screening and brief intervention in primary care: Absence of evidence for efficacy in people with dependence or very heavy drinking. *Drug and Alcohol Review, 29*(6), 631–640.

Saitz, R., Palfai, T. P., Cheng, D. M., Alford, D. P., Bernstein, J. A., Lloyd-Travaglini, C. A., et al. (2014). Screening and brief intervention for drug use in primary care: The ASPIRE randomized clinical trial. *JAMA, 312*(5), 502–513.

Scott-Sheldon, L. A., Carey, K. B., Elliott, J. C., Garey, L., & Carey, M. P. (2014). Efficacy of alcohol interventions for first-year college students: A meta-analytic review of randomized controlled trials. *Journal of Consulting and Clinical Psychology, 82*(2), 177–188.

Scott-Sheldon, L. A., Carey, K. B., Kaiser, T. S., Knight, J. M., & Carey, M. P. (2016). Alcohol interventions for Greek letter organizations: A systematic review and meta-analysis, 1987 to 2014. *Health Psychology, 35*(7), 670–684.

Steinka-Fry, K. T., Tanner-Smith, E. E., & Grant, S. (2015). Effects of 21st birthday brief interventions on college student celebratory drinking: A systematic review and meta-analysis. *Addictive Behaviors, 50*, 13–21.

Steinka-Fry, K. T., Tanner-Smith, E. E., & Hennessy, E. A. (2015). Effects of brief alcohol interventions on drinking and driving among youth: A systematic review and meta-analysis. *Journal of Addiction and Prevention, 3*(1), 11.

Strand, M. C., Gjerde, H., & Mørland, J. (2016). Driving under the influence of non-alcohol drugs—an update: Part II. Experimental studies. *Forensic Science Review, 28*(2), 79–101.

Tanner-Smith, E. E., & Lipsey, M. W. (2015). Brief alcohol interventions for adolescents and young adults: A systematic review and meta-analysis. *Journal of Substance Abuse Treatment, 51*, 1–18.

Tanner-Smith, E. E., & Risser, M. D. (2016). A meta-analysis of brief alcohol interventions for adolescents and young adults: Variability in effects across alcohol measures. *American Journal of Drug and Alcohol Abuse, 42*(2), 140–151.

Tanner-Smith, E. E., Steinka-Fry, K. T., Hennessy, E. A., Lipsey, M. W., & Winters, K. C. (2015). Can brief alcohol interventions for youth also address concurrent illicit drug use?: Results from a meta-analysis. *Journal of Youth and Adolescence, 44*(5), 1011–1023.

Tripodi, S. J., Bender, K., Litschge, C., & Vaughn, M. G. (2010). Interventions for reducing adolescent alcohol abuse: A meta-analytic review. *Archives of Pediatrics and Adolescent Medicine, 164*(1), 85–91.

U.S. Department of Health and Human Services. (2007). *The surgeon general's call to action to prevent and reduce underage drinking.* Rockville, MD: U.S. Department of Health and Human Services, Office of the Surgeon General.

U.S. Preventive Services Task Force. (2012). Second annual report to Congress on high-priority evidence gaps for clinical preventive services. Retrieved from *www.uspreventiveservicestaskforce.org/Page/Name/second-annual-report-to-congress-on-high-priority-evidence-gaps-for-clinical-preventive-services.*

Wagenaar, A. C., Salois, M. J., & Komro, K. A. (2009). Effects of beverage alcohol price and tax levels on drinking: A meta-analysis of 1003 estimates from 112 studies. *Addiction, 104*(2), 179–190.

Wagenaar, A. C., & Toomey, T. L. (2002). Effects of minimum drinking age laws: Review and analyses of the literature from 1960 to 2000. *Journal of Studies on Alcohol, 14*(Suppl.), 206–225.

White, A. M., Hingson, R. W., Pan, I. J., & Yi, H. Y. (2011). Hospitalizations for alcohol and drug overdoses in young adults ages 18–24 in the United States, 1999–2008: Results from the Nationwide Inpatient Sample. *Journal of Studies on Alcohol and Drugs, 72*(5), 774–786.

White, A. M., Kraus, C. L., & Swartzwelder, H. (2006). Many college freshmen drink at levels far beyond the binge threshold. *Alcoholism: Clinical and Experimental Research, 30*(6), 1006–1010.

White, H. R., Morgan, T. J., Pugh, L. A., Celinska, K., Labouvie, E. W., & Pandina, R. J. (2006). Evaluating two brief substance-use interventions for mandated college students. *Journal of Studies on Alcohol, 67*(2), 309–317.

Winters, K. C., Lee, S., Botzet, A., Fahnhorst, T., & Nicholson, A. (2014). One-year outcomes and mediators of a brief intervention for drug abusing adolescents. *Psychology of Addictive Behaviors, 28*(2), 464–474.

World Health Organization. (2009). *Evidence for the effectiveness and cost-effectiveness of interventions to reduce alcohol-related harm.* Geneva, Switzerland: Author.

World Health Organization. (2016). *Drug use and road safety.* Geneva, Switzerland: Author.

Zhang, X., Hatcher, B., Clarkson, L., Holt, J., Bagchi, S., Kanny, D., et al. (2015). Changes in density of on-premises alcohol outlets and impact on violent crime, Atlanta, Georgia, 1997–2007. *Preventing Chronic Disease, 12,* E84.

Index